FUNDING IN AGING

FUNDING IN AGING

A Guide to Giving by Foundations, Corporations, & Charitable Organizations

First Edition

Edited by Elizabeth H. Rich

Contributing Editors
Jeffrey A. Falkenstein, L. Victoria Hall,
Linda Tobiasen & Michael Tuller

40th Year
THE FOUNDATION CENTER

CONTRIBUTING STAFF

Vice President for Publications	Frederick Schoff
Director of Reference Book Publishing	Margaret Derrickson
Senior Database Editor	Margaret Feczko
Manager of Information Control	Annette Johnson
Project Coordinator	Jose Santiago
Editorial Associate	Louis Au
Database Operations Manager	Lin Lin
Database Operations Assistant	Veronique A. Topping

The editors gratefully acknowledge the many other Foundation Center staff who contributed support, encouragement, and information that was indispensable to the preparation of this volume. Special mention should be made of the staff members of the New York, Washington, D.C., Cleveland, San Francisco, and Atlanta libraries who assisted in tracking changes in foundation information. We would like to express our appreciation as well to the many foundations that cooperated fully in updating information prior to the compilation of this volume.

ISBN 0-87954-663-8
Printed and bound in the United States of America
Cover design by Apicella Design

CONTENTS

INTRODUCTION

The graying of America has become a well-documented and highly publicized phenomenon. The number of elderly persons has grown, and for the next forty years will continue to grow, more rapidly than the total population. It is estimated that the number of Americans over the age of 65 will grow to 31 million in the year 2000, and about 55 million by the year 2030. Similarly, the percentage of elderly persons in our society is expected to increase to 12.2 percent by the end of the century and to peak at about 18.8 percent by the year 2030.

These demographic shifts have serious political and sociological implications and are already placing growing demands on health, education, and human service providers. Meeting the needs of this growing elderly population will require planning and creativity that cut across professional domains and parochial interests. New solutions and stronger collaborative efforts are being sought by the agencies that serve older Americans and the public and private providers that grant essential funding for these services.

For more than 20 years, beginning with the publication of the *Grant Guide in Aging* (formerly *Comsearch*), the Foundation Center has displayed an ongoing commitment to serving the needs of the grantseeker in the field of aging. *Funding in Aging: A Guide to Giving by Foundations, Corporations, and Charitable Organizations,* the successor to the *National Guide to Funding in Aging,* is designed to provide essential information on public and private sources of support for programs and services for the older adult. Information has been compiled on corporate and foundation funding sources for nonprofit organizations concerned with the elderly and, to a lesser extent, funding assistance available for older individuals, as well as a listing of voluntary associations, religious groups, and academic and research centers concerned with aging.

Those who are familiar with the predecessor to *Funding in Aging: A Guide to Giving by Foundations, Corporations, and Charitable Organizations* will notice that information on federal programs for the elderly is not included in this publication. Because this information is so readily available through the *Catalog of Federal Domestic Assistance* both in print and now through electronic formats, it was decided to forego including redundant information on government funding for aging in this reference work. The field owes a debt of gratitude to the Nassau County Department of Senior Citizen Affairs for their initial ground-breaking work in collating the federal government information for the earlier volumes.

DESCRIPTIVE DIRECTORY OF GRANTMAKERS

The listings of private and community foundations with an interest in programs related to the elderly were compiled by the Foundation Center from its publications database. The *Guide* contains a total of 1,073 entries including 893 grantmaking foundations, 58 direct corporate giving programs and 122 public charities (including 107 community foundations) that have expressed an interest in the elderly as part of their stated purpose or through the actual grants they reported to the Center.

Entries include the foundation's name and address; most currently available fiscal information (assets, expenditures, total grants paid, etc.); purpose and activities; names and titles of officers and members of its governing body; application information; any state restrictions on the giving program; any publication(s) about its giving program distributed by the organization; and, where available, the number of staff employed. A listing of 1,332 grants awarded in the field of aging are included for 348 foundations that reported grants to the Foundation Center in 1994 or 1995. Grant listings include the size of the award, the name and location (if available) of the agency receiving the grant, the year the grant was awarded, and a brief description of the purpose of the grant (if provided).

In addition, the Foundation Center's Bibliographic Information Service has compiled a selected bibliography from its database. This bibliography includes books, journal articles, and research studies on funding in aging.

VOLUNTARY ORGANIZATIONS

Although very few private voluntary organizations provide direct financial support to the elderly, many do offer valuable technical assistance or information to older Americans and the agencies that serve them. We have included basic descriptions of 85 private organizations in Section II, arranged in four categories: Academic and Research Centers; Denominational Organizations; Gerontological Organizations; and Professional and Service Organizations. For this edition of *Funding in Aging: A Guide to Giving by Foundations, Corporations, and Charitable Organizations,* organizations were contacted and asked to provide current information.

STATE GOVERNMENT AGENCIES

The appendix is included as a resource for state government funding programs and services. The entries are arranged alphabetically by state or territory and include the name, address, and, where available, the contact and telephone number of the state agency or agencies that administer services and funds for the elderly. For this edition of *Funding in Aging: A Guide to Giving by Foundations, Corporations, and Charitable Organizations,* state agencies were contacted and asked to confirm or update information. In many cases, the only funding available for the elderly is through the Older Americans Act or other Federal allocation.

ACKNOWLEDGEMENTS

The editor gratefully acknowledges the cooperation and assistance of the staff members of the state government offices, foundations, corporations, and other voluntary organizations who provided current information for inclusion in this edition. Special thanks to the many other Foundation Center staff members who contributed support, encouragement, and information that was indispensable to the preparation of this volume.

FUNDING IN AGING BIBLIOGRAPHY

This selected bibliography is compiled from the Foundation Center's bibliographic database. Many of the items are available for free reference use in the Foundation Center's New York City, Washington, D.C., Cleveland, San Francisco, and Atlanta libraries as well as in many of its cooperating libraries throughout the United States. For further references, see *The Literature of the Nonprofit Sector: A Bibliography with Abstracts,* Vols. I–8. New York: The Foundation Center, 1989–1996.

Bramwell, R.D. "Seniors As Volunteers and Their Training." *Journal of Volunteer Administration* 12 (Fall-Winter 1993-1994): 47-57.

Catalog of Federal Domestic Assistance. Washington: Government Printing Office, 1996.

Chambre, Susan Maizel. "Older Volunteers: Trends." *Leadership* (October-December 1993): 16-8, 25.

Chambre, Susan Maizel. "Volunteerism by Elders: Past Trends and Future Prospects." *Gerontologist* 33 (1993): 221-8.

Chernesky, Roslyn H., and Irene A. Gutheil. "Foundation Grantmaking in the 1980s: How Three Human Service Fields Fared." *Journal of Sociology and Social Welfare* 21 (June 1994): 153-60.

Elling, Ronald, and Gerald L. Glandon. *Making Dollars & Sense Out of Fees for Service.* Chicago: Illinois Alliance for the Aging, 1991.

Ellis, Susan J. "Adapting to Older Volunteers." *Nonprofit Times* 7 (November 1993): 8, 10.

Espy, Siri N. "The Aging of America: Implications for Nonprofit Planning." *Nonprofit World* 10 (March-April 1992): 31-3.

Galvin, Dallas. "Jobs in Nonprofits." *New Choices for the Best Years* 31 (December-January 1992).

Gillen, Lynette. "Elder Abuse Peer Support Partners: A Family Violence Prevention Strategy Utilizing Volunteers." *Journal of Volunteer Administration* 13 (Winter 1995): 26-9.

"Grant Makers Create Alliances to Share Ideas and Collaborate on Programs." *Foundation Giving Watch* 11 (November 1991): 1-2.

Grants for the Aging. Grant Guide, no. 1. New York: Foundation Center, 1995.

Greene, Elizabeth. "For Elderly Women, a Chance to Talk." *Chronicle of Philanthropy* 4 (21 April 1992): 6-7, 10.

Greene, Elizabeth. "Quality of Health Care for the Elderly Found to Be a Top Concern of Foundations." *Chronicle of Philanthropy* 3 (24 September 1991): 22.

Huber, Ruth, F. Ellen Netting, and Ruth Nelson Paton. "In Search of the Impact of Staff Mix on Long-Term Care Ombudsman Programs." *Nonprofit and Voluntary Sector Quarterly* 22 (Spring 1993): 69-91.

Jenkins, Robert K., ed. *Grant Funding for Elderly Health Services.* Wall Township, NJ: Health Resources Publishing, 1993.

Knauft, E.B. Senior Citizens As Volunteers. Washington: *Independent Sector,* [1994].

Millar, Bruce. "Day Care for Children and the Elderly Gains in United Way Giving Priorities." *Chronicle of Philanthropy* 4 (3 December 1991): 14.

Morris, Robert. "Productive Retirement: Stimulating Greater Volunteer Efforts to Meet National Needs." *Grassroots Fundraising Journal* 14 (Winter 1996): 5-13.

Nelson, H. Wayne, Clara C. Pratt, Charles E. Carpenter, et al. "Factors Affecting Volunteer Long-Term Care Ombudsman Organizational Commitment and Burnout." *Nonprofit and Voluntary Sector Quarterly* 24 (Fall 1995): 213-234.

Prince, Russ Alan and Karen Maru File. *The Seven Faces of Philanthropy.* San Francisco: Jossey-Bass, 1994.

"Profile: Wealthy Donors to Organizations for the Elderly." *Chronicle of Philanthropy* 6 (19 April 1994): 10.

Stevens, Ellen S. "Older Women Who Volunteer: Tapping a Valuable Woman Resource." *Journal of Volunteer Administration* 11 (Summer 1993): 9-14.

Wilson, Laura B. "Using the Future Search Process for Senior Volunteer Services in Long-Term Care." *Journal of Volunteer Administration* 14 (Fall 1995): 33-8.

Zinn, Richard. "An Unwise Habit of Too Many Nonprofits." *Fund Raising Management* 23 (December 1992): 17-8.

PUBLICATIONS AND SERVICES OF THE FOUNDATION CENTER

The Foundation Center is a national service organization founded and supported by foundations to provide a single authoritative source of information on foundation and corporate giving. The Center's programs are designed to help grantseekers select those funders which may be most interested in their projects from the more than 40,000 active U.S. foundations. Among its primary activities toward this end are publishing reference books on foundation and corporate philanthropy and disseminating information on grantmaking through a nationwide public service program.

Publications of the Foundation Center are the primary working tools of every serious grantseeker. They are also used by grantmakers, scholars, journalists, and legislators—in short, by anyone seeking any type of factual information on philanthropy. All private foundations and a significant number of corporate grantmakers actively engaged in grantmaking, regardless of size or geographic location, are included in one or more of the Center's publications. The publications are of three kinds: directories that describe specific funders, characterizing their program interests and providing fiscal and personnel data; grants indexes that list and classify by subject recent foundation and corporate awards; and guides, monographs, and bibliographies that introduce the reader to funding research, elements of proposal writing, and nonprofit management issues.

Foundation Center publications may be ordered from the Foundation Center, 79 Fifth Avenue, New York, NY 10003-3076. For more information about any aspect of the Center's program or for the name of the Center's library collection nearest you, call 1-800-424-9836.

GENERAL RESEARCH DIRECTORIES

THE FOUNDATION DIRECTORY, 1996 Edition

The Foundation Directory has been widely known and respected in the field for more than 35 years. It includes the latest information on all foundations whose assets exceed $2 million or whose annual grants total $200,000 or more. The 1996 Edition includes over 7,500 of these foundations, over 700 of which are new to this edition. *Directory* foundations hold more than $178 billion in assets and award $10 billion in grants annually, accounting for 90 percent of all U.S. foundation dollars awarded in 1994.

Each *Directory* entry contains precise information on application procedures, giving limitations, types of support awarded, the publications of each foundation, and foundation staff. In addition, each entry features such vital data as the grantmaker's giving interests, financial data, grant amounts, address, and telephone number. This edition includes over 40,000 selected grants for over 55 percent of the entries. The Foundation Center works closely with foundations to ensure the accuracy and timeliness of the information provided.

The *Directory* includes indexes by foundation name; subject areas of interest; names of donors, officers, and trustees; geographic location; international interests; and types of support awarded. Also included are analyses of the foundation community by geography, asset and grant size, and the different foundation types.

March 1996
Softbound: ISBN 0-87954-670-0 / $185
Hardbound: ISBN 0-87954-654-9 / $210
Published annually

THE FOUNDATION DIRECTORY PART 2, 1996
5th Edition

Following in the tradition of *The Foundation Directory, The Foundation Directory Part 2* brings you the same thorough coverage for the next largest set of foundations, those with assets from $1 million and less than $2 million or grant programs from $50,000 and less than $200,000. It includes *Directory*-level information on mid-sized foundations, an important group of grantmakers responsible for millions of dollars in funding annually. Essential data on over 5,000 foundations is included along with more than 28,000 recently awarded foundation grants, providing an excellent overview of the foundations' giving interests. Quick access to foundation entries is facilitated by six indexes, including foundation name; subject areas of interest; names of donors, officers, and trustees; geographic location; international interests; and types of support awarded.

March 1996 / ISBN 0-87954-655-7 / $180
Published annually

THE FOUNDATION DIRECTORY SUPPLEMENT

The Foundation Directory Supplement provides the latest-breaking information on *Foundation Directory* and *Foundation Directory Part 2* grantmakers six months after those volumes are published. Each year, thousands of policy and staff changes occur at these foundations. Fundraisers need to know about these crucial changes as rapidly as possible, as they may affect the way fundraisers prepare their grant proposals. The *Supplement* ensures that users of the *Directory* and *Directory Part 2* always have the latest addresses, contact names, policy statements, application guidelines, and financial data for the foundations they're approaching for funding.

September 1996 / ISBN 0-87954-668-9 / $125
Published annually

GUIDE TO U.S. FOUNDATIONS, THEIR TRUSTEES, OFFICERS, AND DONORS, 1996 Edition

This powerful fundraising reference tool provides fundraisers with current, accurate information on over 38,800 private grantmaking foundations in the U.S. The two-volume set also includes a master list of the names of the people who establish, oversee, and manage those institutions. With access to this information, fundraisers can facilitate their funding research by discovering the philanthropic connections of current donors, board members, volunteers, and prominent families in their geographic area. Because it provides a comprehensive list of U.S. foundations and the people who govern them, the *Guide to U.S. Foundations* also helps fundraisers follow up on any giving leads they may uncover. Each entry includes asset and giving amounts as well as geographic limitations, allowing fundraisers to quickly determine whether or not to pursue a particular grant source.

The *Guide to U.S. Foundations* is the only source of published data on thousands of local foundations. (It includes more than 26,000 grantmakers not covered in other Foundation Center publications.) Each entry also tells you whether you can find more extensive information on the grantmaker in another Foundation Center reference work.

April 1996 / 0-87954-658-1 / $225
Published annually

THE FOUNDATION 1000

Nonprofit fundraisers and other researchers have access to annually published, comprehensive reports on the 1,000 largest foundations in the country. *The Foundation 1000* provides access to extensive and accurate information on this set of powerful funders, a group of grantmakers responsible for distributing more than 65 percent of all foundation grant dollars. *Foundation 1000* grantmakers hold over $139 billion in assets and each year award nearly $7 billion and more than 210,000 grants to nonprofit organizations nationwide.

The Foundation 1000 provides the most thorough analyses available of the 1,000 largest foundations and their extensive grant programs, including all the data fundraisers need most when applying for grants from these top-level foundations. Each multi-page foundation profile features a full foundation portrait, a detailed breakdown of the foundation's grant programs, and extensive lists of recently awarded foundation grants.

Five indexes give fundraisers the opportunity to target potential funders in a variety of ways: by subject field, type of support, geographic location, international giving, and the names of foundation officers, donors, and trustees.

October 1996 / ISBN 0-87954-665-4 / $295
Published annually

NATIONAL DIRECTORY OF CORPORATE GIVING, 4th Edition

Each year, corporations donate billions of dollars to nonprofit organizations. To help fundraisers tap into this vital source of funding, the 4th Edition of the *National Directory of Corporate Giving* offers authoritative information on more than 2,600 corporate foundations and direct-giving programs.

Fundraisers who want access to current, accurate fundraising facts on corporate philanthropies will benefit from the full range of data in this volume. The *National Directory of Corporate Giving* features detailed portraits of 1,972 corporate foundations plus an additional 670 direct-giving programs. Fundraisers will find essential information on these corporate grantmakers, including application information, key personnel, types of support generally awarded, giving limitations, financial data, and purpose and activities statements. Also included in the 4th Edition are more than 9,900 selected grants. These grants give you the best indication of a grantmaker's funding priorities by identifying nonprofits it has already funded. The volume also provides data on the corporations that sponsor foundations and direct-giving programs—essential background information for corporate grant searches. Each entry gives the company's name and address, a listing of its types of business, its financial data (complete with *Forbes* and *Fortune* ratings), a listing of its subsidiaries, divisions, plants, and offices and a charitable-giving statement.

The *National Directory of Corporate Giving* also features an extensive bibliography to guide you to further research on corporate funding. Six essential indexes help you target funding prospects by geographic region; types of support; subject area; officers, donors, and trustees; types of business; and the names of the corporation, its foundation, and its direct-giving program.

October 1995 / ISBN 0-87954-646-8 / $195
Published biennially

CORPORATE FOUNDATION PROFILES, 9th Edition

This biennially updated volume includes comprehensive information on 235 of the largest corporate foundations in the U.S., grantmakers who each give at least $1.25 million annually. Each profile includes foundation giving interests, application guidelines, recently awarded grants, information on the sponsoring company, and many other essential fundraising facts. A section on financial data provides a summary of the size and grantmaking capacity of each foundation and contains a list of assets, gifts or contributions, grants paid, operating programs, expenditures, scholarships, and loans. A quick-scan appendix lists core financial data on some 1,200 additional corporate foundations, all of which give at least $50,000 in grants every year. Three indexes help grantseekers search for prospective funders by subject area, geographic region, and types of support favored by the foundation.

February 1996 / ISBN 0-87954-653-0 / $155
Published biennially

NATIONAL DIRECTORY OF GRANTMAKING PUBLIC CHARITIES, 1st Edition

The first publication to cover this diverse segment of the philanthropic community, the 1st Edition of this volume features current information on over 800 public charities—grantmakers that, up to now, have been difficult to locate or have been simply overlooked. With the *National Directory of Grantmaking Public Charities*, grantseekers have easy reference to these potential sources of funding, a set that includes 450 community foundations, all of which offer some form of financial support to nonprofit organizations or individuals, whether it be grants, scholarships, fellowships, loans, or in-kind gifts. The *National Directory* includes descriptions of over 1,200 selected grants, which often provide the best indication of giving interests. Indexes help grantseekers target the most likely grant sources by subject interest, types of support, geographic preferences, and names of officers and trustees.

October 1995 / ISBN 0-87954-651-4 / $95

GUIDE TO GREATER WASHINGTON D.C. GRANTMAKERS, 2nd Edition

The *Guide to Greater Washington D.C. Grantmakers,* a comprehensive source of information on funding sources in the District and surrounding counties, provides current, accurate data on over 1000 grantmakers—foundations, corporate giving programs, and public charities. Each grantmaker portrait includes an application address, financial data, giving limit-ations, and the names of key officials. For larger foundations—those that give at least $50,000 in grants annually—application procedures and giving interest statements are also provided. In addition, over 1,800 descriptions of recently awarded grants, provide further insight into a grantmaker's funding priorities.

July 1996 / ISBN 0-87954-664-6 / $60

NEW YORK STATE FOUNDATIONS: A Comprehensive Directory, 4th Edition

New York State Foundations offers fundraisers complete coverage of over 5,300 independent, corporate, and community foundations throughout New York State in one comprehensive source. Every entry has been drawn from the most current sources of information available, including IRS 990-PF returns and, in many cases, the foundations themselves. Many entries also include descriptions of recently awarded grants, the best indication of a grantmaker's giving interests. A separate section covers hundreds of out-of-state grantmakers that fund nonprofits in New York State. Six time-saving indexes offer quick access to foundations according to their fields of interest; international interests; types of support awarded; city and county; names of donors, officers, and trustees; and foundation names.

May 1995 / ISBN 0-87954-609-3/ $175
Published biennially

DIRECTORY OF MISSOURI GRANTMAKERS, 1st Edition

The *Directory of Missouri Grantmakers* provides a comprehensive guide to grantmakers in the state—over 800 foundations, corporate giving programs, and public charities—from the largest grantmakers to local family foundations. The volume will facilitate your grantseeking with information-filled entries that list giving amounts, fields of interest, purpose statements, selected grants, and much more. Indexes help you target the most appropriate funders by subject interest, types of support, and names of key personnel. Missouri nonprofits simply cannot afford to conduct their grant-seeking without this valuable book!

June 1995 / ISBN 0-97954-612-3 / $75

FOUNDATION GRANTS TO INDIVIDUALS, 9th Edition

The only publication devoted entirely to foundation grant opportunities for qualified individual applicants, the 9th Edition of this volume features more than 2,600 entries, all of which profile foundation grants to individuals. Entries include foundation addresses and telephone numbers, financial data, giving limitations, and application guidelines. This edition—the largest ever published, with over 550 entirely new grantmakers featured—will save individual grantseekers countless hours of research.

May 1995 / ISBN 0-87954-604-2 / $65
Published biennially

SUBJECT DIRECTORIES

The Foundation Center's National Guide to Funding series is designed to facilitate grantseeking within specific fields of nonprofit activity. Each of the directories described below performs the crucial first step of fundraising research by identifying a set of grantmakers that have already stated or demonstrated an interest in a particular field. Fact-filled entries provide access to foundation addresses, financial data, giving priorities, application procedures, contact names, and key officials. Many entries also feature recently awarded grants, the best indication of a grantmaker's funding priorities. A variety of indexes help fundraisers target potential grant sources by subject area, geographic preferences, types of support, and the names of donors, officers, and trustees.

AIDS FUNDING: A Guide to Giving by Foundations and Charitable Organizations, 4th Edition

This volume covers more than 600 foundations, corporate giving programs, and public charities that support AIDS- and HIV-related nonprofit organizations involved in direct relief, medical research, legal aid, preventative education, and other programs to empower persons with AIDS and AIDS-related diseases. Grants lists showing the types of projects funded by grantmakers accompany 312 entries.

December 1995 / ISBN 0-87954-647-6 / $75

FUNDING IN AGING: A Guide to Giving by Foundations, Corporations, and Charitable Organizations

The all new *Funding in Aging* provides essential facts on more than 1,000 grantmakers with a specific interest in the field of aging. This funding tool includes up-to-date addresses, financial data, giving priorities statements, application procedures, contact names, and key officials. The volume also provides recent grants lists with descriptions of more than 900 grants for over 300 foundation entries. Section II of this volume includes basic descriptions and contact information for nearly 100 voluntary organizations which offer valuable technical assistance or information to older Americans and the agencies that serve them.

October 1996 / ISBN 0-87954-663-8 / $95

GUIDE TO FUNDING FOR INTERNATIONAL AND FOREIGN PROGRAMS, 3rd Edition

The 3rd Edition of the *Guide to Funding for International and Foreign Programs* covers over 700 foundations and corporate direct-giving programs interested in funding projects with an international focus, both within the U.S. and abroad. Program areas covered include international relief, disaster assistance, human rights, civil liberties, community development, education, and much more. The volume also includes descriptions of more than 6,000 recently awarded grants.

May 1996 / ISBN 0-87954-657-3 / $115

NATIONAL GUIDE TO FUNDING IN ARTS AND CULTURE, 4th Edition

The 4th Edition of this volume covers more than 4,000 grantmakers with an interest in funding art-colonies, dance companies, museums, theaters, and countless other types of arts and culture projects and institutions. The volume also includes more than 11,000 descriptions of recently awarded grants.

June 1996 / ISBN 0-87954-660-3 / $145

NATIONAL GUIDE TO FUNDING FOR CHILDREN, YOUTH AND FAMILIES, 3rd Edition

The *National Guide to Funding for Children, Youth and Families* provides access to essential facts on some 3,400 foundations and corporate direct-giving programs that together award millions of dollars each year to organizations committed to causes involving children, youth, and families. Each entry includes the grantmaker's address and contact person, purpose statement, and application guidelines. Grantseekers will also find useful descriptions of over 13,000 sample grants recently awarded by many of these foundations.

April 1995 / ISBN 0-87954-603-4 / $145

NATIONAL GUIDE TO FUNDING FOR COMMUNITY DEVELOPMENT, 1st Edition

The new *National Guide to Funding for Community Development* contains essential facts on over 2,500 foundations and corporate direct-giving progams. Entries feature crucial information: address and contact names, giving interest statements, current financial data, key personnel, application guidelines, and, in many cases, examples of recently awarded grants—8,000+ descriptions of recently awarded grants provide unique insight into foundation funding priorities. Indexes help you find the most appropriate funders by subject field, geographic area, and type of support.

May 1996 / ISBN 0-87954-659-X / $95

NATIONAL GUIDE TO FUNDING FOR THE ECONOMICALLY DISADVANTAGED

The *National Guide to Funding for the Economically Disadvantaged* provides essential facts on more than 1,400 foundations and corporate direct-giving programs, each with a history of awarding grant dollars to programs for the economically disadvantaged, employment programs, homeless shelters, hunger relief, welfare initiatives, and dozens of other subject categories. The volume also includes more than 2,000 recently awarded grants.

May 1993 / ISBN 0-87954-494-5 / $85

NATIONAL GUIDE TO FUNDING FOR ELEMENTARY AND SECONDARY EDUCATION, 3rd Edition

With the publication of the 3rd Edition of this volume, fundraisers for elementary and secondary education have access to information on more than 2,000 foundations and corporate giving programs that support nursery schools, bilingual education initiatives, remedial reading/math programs, drop-out prevention services, educational testing programs, and many other nonprofit organizations and initiatives. The volume also includes descriptions of nearly 6,400 recently awarded grants, the best indication of a grantmaker's funding interests.

May 1995 / ISBN 0-87954-607-7 / $135

NATIONAL GUIDE TO FUNDING FOR THE ENVIRONMENT AND ANIMAL WELFARE, 3rd Edition

The 3rd Edition of this guide covers over 1,700 foundations and corporate direct-giving programs that fund nonprofits involved in international conservation, ecological research, waste reduction, animal welfare, and much more. The volume includes descriptions of over 4,000 recently awarded grants.

May 1996 / ISBN 0-87954-662-X / $95

NATIONAL GUIDE TO FUNDING IN HEALTH, 4th Edition

The 4th Edition of the *National Guide to Funding in Health* contains essential facts on more than 3,400 foundations and corporate direct-giving programs interested in funding hospitals, universities, research institutes, community-based agencies, national health associations, and a broad range of other health-related programs and services. The volume also includes descriptions of more than 13,800 recently awarded grants.

March 1995 / ISBN 0-87954-600-X / $145

NATIONAL GUIDE TO FUNDING IN HIGHER EDUCATION, 4th Edition

The 4th Edition of the *National Guide to Funding in Higher Education* includes information on over 4,500 grantmakers with an interest in funding colleges, universities, graduate programs, and research institutes, as well as descriptions of more than 15,000 recently awarded grants.

June 1996 / ISBN 0-87954-661-1 / $145

NATIONAL GUIDE TO FUNDING FOR LIBRARIES AND INFORMATION SERVICES, 3rd Edition

Fundraisers for libraries and information services will benefit from the 3rd Edition of this volume, which provides essential data on over 600 foundations and corporate direct-giving programs that support a wide range of organizations and initiatives, from the smallest public libraries to major research institutions, academic/research libraries, art, law, and medical libraries, and other specialized information centers. The volume also includes descriptions of 1,275 recently awarded grants.

April 1995 / ISBN 0-87954-605-0 / $95

NATIONAL GUIDE TO FUNDING IN RELIGION, 3rd Edition

With the 3rd Edition of this volume, fundraisers who work for nonprofits affiliated with religious organizations have access to information on over 4,200 foundations and corporate direct-giving programs that have demonstrated or stated an interest in funding churches, missionary societies, religious welfare and education programs, and many other types of projects and institutions. The volume also includes descriptions of more than 5,300 recently awarded grants.

May 1995 / ISBN 0-87954-606-9 / $135

NATIONAL GUIDE TO FUNDING IN SUBSTANCE ABUSE, 1st Edition

The first edition of this volume contains essential facts on more than 600 foundations and corporate direct-giving programs interested in funding counseling services, preventive education, treatment, medical research, residential care and halfway houses, and projects addressing alcohol and drug abuse, smoking addiction, and drunk driving. The volume also includes descriptions of some 695 recently awarded grants.

April 1995 / ISBN 0-87954-602-6 / $95

NATIONAL GUIDE TO FUNDING FOR WOMEN AND GIRLS, 3rd Edition

The 3rd Edition of this volume covers some 1,000 foundations and corporate direct-giving programs with an interest in funding such projects as education scholarships, shelters for abused women, girls' clubs, health clinics, employment centers, and other diverse programs. The volume also provides descriptions of more than 4,000 recently awarded grants.

May 1995 / ISBN 0-87954-608-5 / $95

GRANT DIRECTORIES

GRANT GUIDES

Designed for fundraisers who work within defined fields of nonprofit development, this series of guides lists actual foundation grants of $10,000 or more in 30 key areas of grantmaking.

Each title in the series affords immediate access to the names, addresses, and giving limitations of the foundations listed. The grant descriptions provide fundraisers with the grant recipient's name and location; the amount of the grant; the date the grant was authorized; and a description of the grant's intended use.

In addition, each *Grant Guide* includes three indexes, which help fundraisers target possible sources of funding by the type of organization generally funded by the grantmaker, the subject focus of the foundation's grants, and the geographic area in which the foundation has already funded projects.

Each *Grant Guide* also includes a concise overview of the foundation spending patterns within the specified field. The introduction uses a series of statistical tables to document such important findings as (1) the 25 top funders in your area of interest (by total dollar amount of grants); (2) the 15 largest grants reported; (3) the total dollar amount and number of grants awarded for specific types of support, recipient organization type, and population group; and (4) the total grant dollars received in each U.S. state and many foreign countries.

The *Grant Guide* series gives fundraisers the data they need to target foundations making grants in their field, to network with organizations that share their goals, and to tailor their grant applications to the specific concerns of grantmakers as expressed by the grants they have already made.

Series published annually in October / 1996/1997 Editions / $75 each

THE FOUNDATION GRANTS INDEX, 1997 Edition

A foundation's recently awarded grants offer the best indication of its future funding priorities. The all-new 1996 (24th) Edition of *The Foundation Grants Index*—the volume fundraisers have relied upon since 1970—is the most current and accurate source of information on recent grantmaker awards. The *Grants Index* has steadily expanded its coverage since the 1st Edition: it now covers the grantmaking programs of over 1,000 of the largest independent, corporate, and community foundations in the U.S. and includes more than 72,000 grant descriptions in all.

The new 1997 Edition of the *Grants Index* is designed for fast and easy grants-based research. Grant descriptions are divided into 28 broad subject areas such as health, higher education, and arts and culture. Within each of these broad fields, the grant descriptions are listed geographically by state and alphabetically by the name of the foundation, an arrangement that helps fund-raisers find prospective funders who share their program interests and fund projects within their geographic region.

November 1996/ ISBN 0-87954-701-4 / $160

THE FOUNDATION GRANTS INDEX QUARTERLY

This unique subscription service gives fundraisers the most up-to-date information available, providing important new information on foundation funding every three months. Each issue of the *Quarterly* delivers descriptions of more than 5,000 recent foundation grants, arranged by state and indexed by subjects and recipients. This enables fundraisers to zero in on grants made in their subject area and within their geographic region. The *Quarterly* also contains helpful updates on grantmakers noting changes in foundation address, personnel, program interests, and application procedures, as well as a list of grantmakers' recent publications such as annual reports, information brochures, grants lists, and newsletters.

Annual subscription $95 / 4 issues ISSN 0735-2522

WHO GETS GRANTS / WHO GIVES GRANTS: Nonprofit Organizations and the Foundation Grants They Received, 3rd Edition

With the publication of the 3rd Edition of this directory, fundraisers can easily answer a crucial question: From which foundations do other nonprofits receive their funding? *Who Gets Grants* provides direct access to grant recipient information on more than 19,000 nonprofit organizations and more than 58,000 grants, an excellent way to find out who is awarding grants to organizations like yours.

Who Gets Grants helps fundraisers conduct their research by allowing them to target the funders of specific nonprofits, which are conveniently listed in the front of the book. Because the book is divided into 19 different subject headings, fundraisers can also scan through grants recently awarded within their field to generate lists of grant prospects. Within each subject area the grant recipients are listed by geographic area, an arrangement that helps fundraisers discover which foundations favor their state.

The grant recipient entries feature grant descriptions that include the grant amount, its duration and use, and the name of the grantmaker, while an index lists all the grants made by each foundation covered, the best way to determine a grantmaker's larger funding priorities.

February 1995 / ISBN 0-87954-596-8 / $95

GUIDEBOOKS, MANUALS, AND REPORTS

AIDS FUNDRAISING

Published in conjunction with Funders Concerned About AIDS, this guide helps nonprofit groups plan a strategy for raising money. *AIDS Fundraising* covers a vast array of money-generating initiatives, from membership drives to special events, direct mail, and grant applications.

July 1991 / ISBN 0-87954-390-6 / $10

ARTS FUNDING

This study, commissioned by Grantmakers in the Arts, provides a framework for understanding recent trends in foundation funding for arts and culture. The report analyzes grants awarded in the 1980s and also includes profiles of over 60 top foundation and corporate grantmakers.

April 1993 / ISBN 0-87594-448-1 / $40

ARTS FUNDING REVISITED

Arts Funding Revisited focuses on grantmaking in 1992, updating the original study by three years. It analyzes over 9,500 grants awarded in that year by over 800 of the major U.S. arts and culture grantmakers, providing a current picture of giving priorities in the field.

July 1995 / ISBN 0-87594-650-6 / $14.95

THE FOUNDATION CENTER'S GRANTS CLASSIFICATION SYSTEM INDEXING MANUAL WITH THESAURUS, Revised Edition

A complete "how-to" guide, the *Grants Classification Manual* provides an essential resource for any organization that wants to classify foundation grants or their recipients. The *Manual* includes a complete set of all classification codes to facilitate precise tracking of grants and recipients by subject, recipient type, and population categories. It also features a completely revised thesaurus to help identify the "official" terms and codes that represent thousands of subject areas and recipient types in the Center's system of grants classification.

May 1995 / ISBN 0-87954-644-1 / $95

THE FOUNDATION CENTER'S USER-FRIENDLY GUIDE: A Grantseeker's Guide to Resources, 4th Edition

This helpful book answers the most commonly asked questions about grantseeking in an upbeat, easy-to-read style. Specifically designed for novice grantseekers, the *User-Friendly Guide* leads the reader through the maze of unfamiliar jargon and wide range of research guides used successfully by professional fundraisers every day. Whether a grantseeker needs $100 or $100,000 for his or her project or organization, *The Foundation Center's User-Friendly Guide* offers an excellent first step in the fundraising process.

July 1996 / ISBN 0-87954-662-2 / $14.95

FOUNDATION FUNDAMENTALS: A Guide for Grantseekers, 5th Edition

This comprehensive, easy-to-read guidebook presents the facts you need to identify foundation funding sources for your organization. Illustrations take you step-by-step through the funding research process, and worksheets and checklists are provided to help you get started in your search for funding. Comprehensive bibliographies, detailed research examples, and an index are also supplied.

June 1994 / ISBN 0-87954-543-7 / $24.95

FOUNDATION GIVING: Yearbook of Facts and Figures on Private, Corporate and Community Foundations, 1996 Edition

Foundation Giving provides a comprehensive overview of the latest trends in foundation giving in the U.S. This volume uses a range of statistical tables to chart foundation giving by subject area and type of support, to categorize foundations by asset and giving amount, and to document other noteworthy data such as the breakdown of grants awarded by the 100 largest foundations.

July 1996 / ISBN 0-87954-667-0 / $24.95

THE FOUNDATION CENTER'S GUIDE TO PROPOSAL WRITING

The Foundation Center now offers its own comprehensive guide to the strategic thinking and mechanics of proposal writing. The *Guide to Proposal Writing* guides fundraisers through each step of the process, from pre-proposal planning to the writing itself to the essential post-grant follow-up. The book features many extracts from actual grant proposals and also includes candid advice from grantmakers on the "do's and don't's" of proposal writing. Written by professional fundraisers who have themselves been creating successful proposals for more than 25 years, *The Foundation Center's Guide to Proposal Writing* offers the kind of valuable tips and in-depth, practical instruction that no other source provides.

August 1993 / ISBN 0-87954-492-9 / $29.95

PROGRAM-RELATED INVESTMENTS: A GUIDE TO FUNDERS AND TRENDS

While most foundations make grants to support their programmatic interests, some funders have developed an alternative financing approach for supplying capital to the nonprofit sector known as program-related investing. This type of investment has been used to support community revitalization, low-income housing, microenterprise development, historic preservation, human services, and more.

Where can you learn about this unique funding tool? The Foundation Center's new *Program-Related Investments: A Guide to Funders and Trends* offers a wealth of information on this little-understood field, including current perspectives from providers and recipients; essays by experts in the field; strategies for success; and a directory of over 100 leading PRI providers. A truly comprehensive report, *Program Related Investments* gathers all the information you need to understand the in and outs of charitable investing.

April 1995 / ISBN 0-87954-558-5 / $45

SOUTHEASTERN FOUNDATIONS

This report provides a comprehensive picture of foundations in the Southeastern states—Alabama, Arkansas, Florida, Georgia, Kentucky, Louisiana, Mississippi, North Carolina, South Carolina, Tennessee, Virginia, and West Virginia. The report examines the size and scope of the foundation community in the region and in each separate state. It also provides a detailed analysis of funding patterns by subject, type of support, recipient type, and beneficiary group, and compares Southeastern trends with all U.S. funders.

October 1994 / ISBN 0-87954-556-9 / $14.95

BIBLIOGRAPHIES

THE LITERATURE OF THE NONPROFIT SECTOR: A Bibliography with Abstracts, Volumes I–VII

This bibliographical series helps fundraisers and other researchers tap into the vast and growing body of literature on philanthropy and voluntarism by listing the best references on fundraising, foundations, corporate giving, nonprofit management, and much more. Designed to help fundraisers access the books and articles they need quickly and easily, each volume is divided into twelve broad subject fields and includes a subject, title, and author index to help speed your research. Whether readers are searching for a manual that outlines development strategies for museums, an article that considers philanthropic responses to rural poverty in the 1970s, or a book that tackles the interplay of federal tax policy and charitable giving, *The Literature of the Nonprofit Sector* will prove to be an invaluable resource. The 8th volume expands series coverage to more than 13,000 titles.

Volume VIII, December 1996 / ISBN 0-87954-702-2 / $45
Volume VII, December 1995 / ISBN 0-87954-649-2 / $45
Volume VI, December 1994 / ISBN 0-87954-561-5 / $45
Volume V, November 1993 / ISBN 0-87954-509-7 / $45
Volume IV, September 1992 / ISBN 0-87954-447-3 / $45
Volume III, September 1991 / ISBN 0-87954-386-8 / $45
Volume II, July 1990 / ISBN 0-87954-343-4 / $45
Volume I, August 1989 / ISBN 0-87954-287-X / $55
Volumes I–VIII Set / $255

OTHER PUBLICATIONS

AMERICA'S NONPROFIT SECTOR: A Primer

by Lester M. Salamon

In this fascinating and informative book, Lester M. Salamon tackles "the widespread lack of knowledge about America's nonprofit sector and the role it plays in our social welfare system." Illustrated with numerous charts and tables that clearly explain various aspects of the nonprofit world, Salamon's book is an easy-to-understand primer for government officials, journalists, and students—in short, for anyone who wants to comprehend the makeup of America's nonprofit sector. It is also an invaluable resource for officials in Eastern Europe and other parts of the world who increasingly are seeking to learn from America's mixed system of social welfare.

August 1992 / ISBN 0-87954-451-1 / $14.95

THE BOARD MEMBER'S BOOK, 2nd Edition

by Brian O'Connell, President-Emeritus,
INDEPENDENT SECTOR

Based on his extensive experience working with and on the boards of voluntary organizations, Brian O'Connell has developed this practical guide to the essential functions of voluntary boards. O'Connell offers practical advice on how to be a more effective board member as well as on how board members can help their organizations make a difference, and also provides an extensive reading list. *The Board Member's Book* is an invaluable instructional and inspirational tool for anyone who works on or with a voluntary board.

October 1993 / ISBN 0-87954-502-X / $24.95

CAREERS FOR DREAMERS AND DOERS: A Guide to Management Careers in the Nonprofit Sector

by Lilly Cohen and Dennis R.Young

A comprehensive guide to management positions in the nonprofit world. *Careers for Dreamers and Doers* offers practical advice for starting a job search and suggests strategies used by successful managers throughout the voluntary sector. The book draws from experience of established professionals, providing career histories of nonprofit CEOs, development officers, and foundation officials who rose to top management positions in the field. the book also covers compensation patterns in the field, the fundamentals of resume writing and interviewing, and nonprofit management programs at colleges and universities.

November 1989 / ISBN 0-87954-294-2 / $24.95

ECONOMICS FOR NONPROFIT MANAGERS

by Dennis R. Young and Richard Steinberg

Economics for Nonprofit Managers is a complete course in the economic issues faced by America's nonprofit decision-makers. Young and Sternberg treat micro-economic analysis as an indispensable skill for nonprofit managers, they introduce and explain concepts such as opportunity cost, analysis at the margin, market equilibrium, market failure, and cost-benefit analysis. This volume also focuses on issues of particular concern to nonprofits, such as the economics of fundraising and volunteer recruiting, the regulatory environment, the impact of competition on nonprofit performance, interactions among sources of revenue, and much more.

July 1995 / ISBN 0-87954-610-7 / $34.95

HANDBOOK ON PRIVATE FOUNDATIONS

by David F. Freeman and the Council on Foundations

This publication, a completely revised edition of the classic *Handbook* published more than ten years ago, provides a thorough and up-to-date look at the issues facing the staff and boards of private foundations in the U.S. In this revised edition, sponsored by the Council on Foundations, author David F. Freeman offers sound advice on establishing, staffing, and governing foundations and provides insights into legal and tax guidelines as well. Each chapter concludes with a useful annotated bibliography. The *Handbook* is an excellent "how-to" guide for those who work in private foundations or serve on their boards.

September 1991
Softbound: ISBN 0-87954-404-X / $29.95
Hardbound: ISBN 0-87954-403-1 / $39.95

MANAGING FOUNDATION ASSETS: An Analysis of Foundation Investment and Payout Procedures and Performance

by Lester M. Salamon and Kenneth P. Voytek

In their study, Salamon and Voytek address critical questions on foundation investing and payout procedures, including: how do foundations manage the immense wealth in their control?, how does the payout requirement affect foundation investment operations?, and what impact has the change in the payout requirement of 1981 had on both the investment and payout performance of foundations? After addressing these questions, the authors offer insights into such key topics as the process foundations use to make their payout decisions and manage their investments, the rate of return they have achieved, and the payout rates foundations have adopted.

March 1989 / ISBN 0-87954-283-7 / $19.95

THE NONPROFIT ENTREPRENEUR: Creating Ventures to Earn Income

Edited by Edward Skloot

In a well-organized topic-by-topic approach to nonprofit venturing, nonprofit consultant and entrepreneur Edward Skloot demonstrates how nonprofits can launch successful earned-income enterprises without compromising their missions. Skloot has compiled a collection of writings by the nation's top practitioners and advisors in nonprofit enterprise. Topics covered include legal issues, marketing techniques, business planning, avoiding the pitfalls of venturing for smaller nonprofits, and a special section on museums and their retail operations.

September 1988 / ISBN 0-87954-239-X / $19.95

A NONPROFIT ORGANIZATION OPERATING MANUAL: Planning for Survival and Growth

by Arnold J. Olenick and Philip R. Olenick

This straightforward, all-inclusive desk manual for nonprofit executives covers all aspects of starting and managing a nonprofit. The authors discuss legal problems, obtaining tax exemption, organizational planning and development, and board relations; operational, proposal, cash, and capital budgeting; marketing, grant proposals, fundraising, and for-profit ventures; computerization; and tax planning and compliance.

July 1991 / ISBN 0-87954-293-4 / $29.95

PEOPLE POWER: SERVICE, ADVOCACY, EMPOWERMENT

by Brian O'Connell

Throughout his career, Brian O'Connell has broadened the impact of his own nonprofit work with thoughtful essays, speeches, and op-ed articles. *People Power,* a selection of O'Connell's most powerful writings, provides thought-provoking commentary on the nonprofit world. The 25+ essays included in this volume range from keen analyses of the role of voluntarism in American life, to sound advice for nonprofit managers, to suggestions for developing and strengthening the nonprofit sector of the future. Anyone involved in the nonprofit world will appreciate O'Connell's penetrating insights.

October 1994 / ISBN 0-87954-563-1 / $24.95

PROMOTING ISSUES AND IDEAS: A Guide to Public Relations for Nonprofit Organizations, Revised edition

by M Booth & Associates

In this newly revised edition, M Booth & Associates, specialists in promoting the issues and ideas of nonprofit groups, presents proven strategies that will put your organization on the map and attract the interest of the people you wish to influence and inform. Included are the "nuts-and-bolts" of advertising, publicity, speech-making, lobbying, and special events; how to write and produce informational literature that leaps off the page; public relations on a shoe-string budget; how to plan and evaluate PR efforts; the use of rapidly evolving communication technologies; and a new chapter on crisis management.

December 1995 / ISBN 0-87954-594-1 / $29.95

RAISE MORE MONEY FOR YOUR NONPROFIT ORGANIZATION: A Guide to Evaluating and Improving Your Fundraising

by Anne L. New

In *Raise More Money,* Anne New sets guidelines for a fundraising program that will benefit the incipient as well as the established nonprofit organization. The author divides her text into three sections: "The Basics," which delineates the necessary steps a nonprofit must take before launching a development campaign; "Fundraising Methods," which encourages organizational self-analysis and points the way to an effective program involving many sources of funding; and "Fundraising Resources," a 20-page bibliography that highlights the most useful research and funding directories available.

January 1991 / ISBN 0-87954-388-4 / $14.95

SECURING YOUR ORGANIZATION'S FUTURE: A Complete Guide to Fundraising Strategies

by Michael Seltzer

Michael Seltzer acts as your personal fundraising consultant. Beginners get bottom-line facts and easy-to-follow worksheets; veteran fundraisers receive a complete review of the basics plus new money-making ideas. Seltzer supplements his text with an extensive bibliography of selected readings and resource organizations. Highly recommended for use as a text in nonprofit management programs at colleges and universities.

March 1987 / ISBN 0-87954-190-3 / $24.95

SUCCEEDING WITH CONSULTANTS: Self-Assessment for the Changing Nonprofit

by Barbara Kibbe and Fred Setterberg

Succeeding with Consultants provides practical advice for nonprofit executives eager to improve their organization's performance. This inspirational book, written by Barbara Kibbe and Fred Setterberg and supported by the David and Lucile Packard Foundation, guides nonprofits through the process of selecting and utilizing consultants to strengthen their organization's operations. *Succeeding with Consultants* identifies the areas that could benefit from a consultant's advice and suggests ways to find, select, and hire the right consultant. The book emphasizes self assessment tools and covers six different areas in which a nonprofit organization might benefit from a consultant's advice: governance, planning, fund development, financial management, public relations and marketing, and quality assurance.

April 1992 / ISBN 0-87954-450-3 / $19.95

THE 21ST CENTURY NONPROFIT

by Paul B. Firstenberg

In *The 21st Century Nonprofit,* Paul B. Firstenberg provides nonprofit managers with the know-how to make their organizations effective agents of change. Drawing on his extensive experience in both the for-profit and non-profit sectors, he develops in this new book a systematic plan for organizational governance that draws on the latest management techniques. *The 21st Century Nonprofit* helps nonprofits become more vital social and cultural forces by encouraging managers to adopt strategies developed by the for-profit sector in recent years, including expanding their revenue base by diversifying grant sources, exploiting the possibilities of for-profit enterprises, developing human resources by learning how to attract and retain talented people, and exploring the nature of leadership through short profiles of three non-profit CEOs.

July 1996 / Softcover / ISBN 0-87954-672-7 / $34.95
Hardcover / ISBN 0-87594-652-2 / $39.95

MEMBERSHIP PROGRAM

ASSOCIATES PROGRAM
Direct Line to Fundraising Information

The Associates Program puts important facts and figures on your desk through a toll-free telephone reference service, helping you to:

- identify potential sources of foundation funding for your organization; and

- gather important information to use in targeting and presenting your proposals effectively.

Your annual membership in the Associates Program gives you vital information on a timely basis, saving you hundreds of hours of research time.

- Membership in the Associates Program entitles you to important funding information, including information from:
  - — foundation and corporate annual reports, brochures, press releases, grants lists, and other announcements
  - — IRS 990-PF information returns for all 37,500 active grantmaking U.S. foundations—often the only source of information on small foundations
  - — books and periodicals on the grantmaking field, including regulation and nonprofit management
- The Associates Program places this vital information at your fingertips via a toll-free telephone number. The annual fee of $495 for the Associates Program entitles you to 10 free calls of 15 minutes each, or 2½ hours worth of answers per month.
- Membership in the Associates Program allows you to request custom searches of the Foundation Center's computerized databases, which contain information on some 40,000 U.S. foundations and corporate givers. There is an additional cost for this service.
- Associates Program members may request photocopies of key documents. Important information from 990-PFs, annual reports, application guidelines, and other resources can be copied and either mailed or faxed to your office. The fee for this service, available only to Associate Members, is $2.00 for the first page of material and $1.00 for each additional page. Fax service is available at an additional charge.
- All Associates Program members receive the Associates Program quarterly newsletter, which provides news and information about new foundations, changes in boards of directors, new programs, and publications from both the Foundation Center and other publishers in the field.

Thousands of professional fundraisers find it extremely cost-effective to rely on the Center's Associates Program. Put our staff of experts to work for your fundraising program. For more information call 1-800-424-9836.

FOUNDATION CENTER DATABASES

Foundation and Grants Information Online

As the only nonprofit organization whose sole purpose is to provide information on grantmaking and grantseeking activity, the Foundation Center offers two important databases online. Perhaps the most flexible way to take advantage of the Foundation Center's vast resources, computer access lets you design your own search for the foundations and corporate givers most likely to support your nonprofit organization. Online retrieval provides vital information on funding sources, philanthropic giving, grant application guidelines, and the financial status of foundations to nonprofit organizations seeking funds, grantmaking institutions, corporate contributors, researchers, journalists, and legislators.

Searches of the Center's databases can provide comprehensive and timely answers to such questions as . . .

- Which New York foundations support urban projects? Who are their officers and trustees?
- What are the program interests of the ten largest corporate foundations? Which ones publish annual reports?
- Which foundations gave in excess of $100,000 in the past two years for continuing education for women?
- What are the ten largest foundations in Philadelphia by annual giving?
- What are the names and addresses of smaller foundations in the 441 zip code range?

The Center's up-to-date and authoritative data is available online through Knight-Ridder Information Services. For further information on accessing the Center's databases directly, contact Knight-Ridder at 1-800-334-2564.

DIALOG User Manual and Thesaurus, Revised Edition

To facilitate your foundation and corporate giving research in these powerful and flexible databases, the Center now offers a revised edition of its *User Manual and Thesaurus,* a comprehensive guide that will help you retrieve essential fundraising facts quickly and easily.

November 1995 / ISBN 0-87954-595-X/ $50

FOUNDATION CENTER COOPERATING COLLECTIONS

FREE FUNDING INFORMATION CENTERS

The Foundation Center is an independent national service organization established by foundations to provide an authoritative source of information on foundation and corporate giving. The New York, Washington, D.C., Atlanta, Cleveland, and San Francisco reference collections operated by the Foundation Center offer a wide variety of services and comprehensive collections of information on foundations and grants. Cooperating Collections are libraries, community foundations, and other nonprofit agencies that provide a core collection of Foundation Center publications and a variety of supplementary materials and services in areas useful to grantseekers. The core collection consists of:

THE FOUNDATION DIRECTORY 1 AND 2, AND SUPPLEMENT
THE FOUNDATION 1000
FOUNDATION FUNDAMENTALS
FOUNDATION GIVING
THE FOUNDATION GRANTS INDEX
THE FOUNDATION GRANTS INDEX QUARTERLY
FOUNDATION GRANTS TO INDIVIDUALS
GUIDE TO U.S. FOUNDATIONS, THEIR TRUSTEES, OFFICERS, AND DONORS
THE FOUNDATION CENTER'S GUIDE TO PROPOSAL WRITING
THE LITERATURE OF THE NONPROFIT SECTOR
NATIONAL DIRECTORY OF CORPORATE GIVING
NATIONAL DIRECTORY OF GRANTMAKING PUBLIC CHARITIES
NATIONAL GUIDE TO FUNDING IN. . . . (SERIES)
USER-FRIENDLY GUIDE

Many of the network members make available for public use sets of private foundation information returns (IRS Form 990-PF) for their state and/or neighboring states. A complete set of U.S. foundation returns can be found at the New York and Washington, D.C., offices of the Foundation Center. The Atlanta, Cleveland, and San Francisco offices contain IRS Form 990-PF returns for the southeastern, midwestern, and western states, respectively. Because the collections vary in their hours, materials, and services, ***it is recommended that you call the collection in advance.*** To check on new locations or current information, call toll-free 1-800-424-9836, or visit our Web site at http://fdncenter.org/library/library.html.

Symbols: ✱ sets of private foundation information returns for state and/or neighboring states available
✣ *FC Search: The Foundation Center's Database on CD-ROM* available for public use

REFERENCE COLLECTIONS OPERATED BY THE FOUNDATION CENTER

THE FOUNDATION CENTER
8th Floor
79 Fifth Avenue
New York, NY 10003
(212) 620-4230

THE FOUNDATION CENTER
312 Sutter St., Rm. 312
San Francisco, CA 94108
(415) 397-0902

THE FOUNDATION CENTER
1001 Connecticut Ave., NW
Washington, DC 20036
(202) 331-1400

THE FOUNDATION CENTER
Kent H. Smith Library
1422 Euclid, Suite 1356
Cleveland, OH 44115
(216) 861-1933

THE FOUNDATION CENTER
Suite 150, Grand Lobby
Hurt Bldg., 50 Hurt Plaza
Atlanta, GA 30303
(404) 880-0094

ALABAMA

BIRMINGHAM PUBLIC LIBRARY ✱
Government Documents
2100 Park Place
Birmingham 35203
(205) 226-3600

HUNTSVILLE PUBLIC LIBRARY
915 Monroe St.
Huntsville 35801
(205) 532-5940

UNIVERSITY OF SOUTH ALABAMA ✱
Library Building
Mobile 36688
(334) 460-7025

AUBURN UNIVERSITY AT MONTGOMERY LIBRARY ✱ ✣
7300 University Drive
Montgomery 36117-3596
(334) 244-3653

ALASKA

UNIVERSITY OF ALASKA AT ANCHORAGE ✱ ✣
Library
3211 Providence Drive
Anchorage 99508
(907) 786-1847

JUNEAU PUBLIC LIBRARY
Reference
292 Marine Way
Juneau 99801
(907) 586-5267

ARIZONA

PHOENIX PUBLIC LIBRARY ✱ ✣
Information Services Department
1221 N. Central
Phoenix 85004
(602) 262-4636

TUCSON PIMA LIBRARY ✱ ✣
101 N. Stone Ave.
Tucson 87501
(520) 791-4010

ARKANSAS

WESTARK COMMUNITY COLLEGE—BORHAM LIBRARY ✱
5210 Grand Avenue
Ft. Smith 72913
(501) 788-7200

CENTRAL ARKANSAS LIBRARY SYSTEM ✱ ✣
700 Louisiana
Little Rock 72201
(501) 370-5952

PINE BLUFF-JEFFERSON COUNTY LIBRARY SYSTEM
200 E. Eighth
Pine Bluff 71601
(501) 534-2159

CALIFORNIA

HUMBOLDT AREA FOUNDATION ✱ ✣
P.O. Box 99
Bayside 95524
(707) 442-2993

VENTURA COUNTY COMMUNITY FOUNDATION ✱
Funding and Information Resource Center
1355 Del Norte Rd.
Camarillo 93010
(805) 988-0196

CALIFORNIA COMMUNITY FOUNDATION ✱ ✣
Funding Information Center
606 S. Olive St., Suite 2400
Los Angeles 90014-1526
(213) 413-4042

OAKLAND NONPROFIT RESOURCE CENTER ✣
1203 Preservation Pkwy., Suite 100
Oakland 94612
(510) 834-1010

GRANT & RESOURCE CENTER OF NORTHERN CALIFORNIA ✱ ✣
Building C, Suite A
2280 Benton Dr.
Redding 96003
(916) 244-1219

LOS ANGELES PUBLIC LIBRARY ✣
West Valley Regional Branch Library
19036 Van Owen St.
Reseda 91335
(818) 345-4393

RIVERSIDE CITY & COUNTY PUBLIC LIBRARY ✣
3021 Franklin Ave.
Riverside 92502
(714) 782-5201

NONPROFIT RESOURCE CENTER ✣
Sacramento Public Library
828 I Street, 2nd Floor
Sacramento 95814
(916) 264-2772

SAN DIEGO COMMUNITY FOUNDATION ✱ ✣
Funding Information Center
101 West Broadway, Suite 1120
San Diego 92101
(619) 239-8815

NONPROFIT DEVELOPMENT CENTER ✣
Library
1922 The Alameda, Suite 212
San Jose 95126
(408) 248-9505

PENINSULA COMMUNITY FOUNDATION ✱
Funding Information Library
1700 S. El Camino Real, R301
San Mateo 94402-3049
(415) 358-9392

LOS ANGELES PUBLIC LIBRARY ✣
San Pedro Regional Branch
9131 S. Gaffey St.
San Pedro 90731
(310) 548-7779

VOLUNTEER CENTER OF GREATER ORANGE COUNTY ✣
Nonprofit Management Assistance Center
1901 E. 4th St., Ste. 100
Santa Ana 92705
(714) 953-1655

SANTA BARBARA PUBLIC LIBRARY ✣
40 E. Anapamu St.
Santa Barbara 93101
(805) 962-7653

SANTA MONICA PUBLIC LIBRARY ✣
1343 Sixth St.
Santa Monica 90401-1603
(310) 458-8600

SONOMA COUNTY LIBRARY
3rd & E Streets
Santa Rosa 95404
(707) 545-0831

SEASIDE BRANCH LIBRARY ✣
550 Harcourt St.
Seaside 93955
(408) 899-8131

COLORADO

EL POMAR NONPROFIT RESOURCE CENTER
1661 Mesa Ave.
Colorado Springs 80906
(800) 554-7711

DENVER PUBLIC LIBRARY ✱
General Reference
10 West 14th Ave. Pkwy.
Denver 80204
(303) 640-6200

CONNECTICUT

DANBURY PUBLIC LIBRARY
170 Main St.
Danbury 06810
(203) 797-4527

GREENWICH LIBRARY ✱ ✣
101 West Putnam Ave.
Greenwich 06830
(203) 622-7910

HARTFORD PUBLIC LIBRARY ✱ ✣
500 Main St.
Hartford 06103
(860) 543-8656

DELAWARE

UNIVERSITY OF DELAWARE ✱ ✣
Hugh Morris Library
Newark 19717-5267
(302) 831-2432

FLORIDA

VOLUSIA COUNTY LIBRARY CENTER ✣
City Island
Daytona Beach 32014-4484
(904) 257-6036

NOVA SOUTHEASTERN UNIVERSITY ✱ ✣
Einstein Library
3301 College Ave.
Fort Lauderdale 33314
(305) 475-7050

INDIAN RIVER COMMUNITY COLLEGE ✣
Charles S. Miley Learning Resource Center
3209 Virginia Ave.
Fort Pierce 34981-5599
(561) 462-4757

JACKSONVILLE PUBLIC LIBRARIES ✱ ✣
Grants Resource Center
122 N. Ocean St.
Jacksonville 32202
(904) 630-2665

MIAMI-DADE PUBLIC LIBRARY ✱ ✣
Humanities/Social Science
101 W. Flagler St.
Miami 33130
(305) 375-5575

ORLANDO PUBLIC LIBRARY ✱
Social Sciences Department
101 E. Central Blvd.
Orlando 32801
(407) 425-4694

SELBY PUBLIC LIBRARY
Reference
1001 Blvd. of the Arts
Sarasota 34236
(941) 951-5501

TAMPA-HILLSBOROUGH COUNTY PUBLIC LIBRARY ✱ ✣
900 N. Ashley Drive
Tampa 33602
(813) 273-3628

COMMUNITY FOUNDATION OF PALM BEACH & MARTIN COUNTIES ✱ ✣
324 Datura St., Suite 340
West Palm Beach 33401
(407) 659-6800

GEORGIA

ATLANTA-FULTON PUBLIC LIBRARY ✱
Foundation Collection—Ivan Allen Department
1 Margaret Mitchell Square
Atlanta 30303-1089
(404) 730-1900

UNITED WAY OF GEORGIA ✱ ✣
Community Resource Center
301 Mulberry St., Suite 301
Macon 31201
(912) 745-4732

THOMAS COUNTY PUBLIC LIBRARY ✱ ✣
201 N. Madison St.
Thomasville, GA 31792
(912) 225-5252

HAWAII

UNIVERSITY OF HAWAII ✱ ✣
Hamilton Library
2550 The Mall
Honolulu 96822
(808) 956-7214

HAWAII COMMUNITY FOUNDATION RESOURCE LIBRARY ✣
900 Fort St., Suite 1300
Honolulu 96813
(808) 537-6333

IDAHO

BOISE PUBLIC LIBRARY ✱ ✣
715 S. Capitol Blvd.
Boise 83702
(208) 384-4024

CALDWELL PUBLIC LIBRARY ✱ ✣
1010 Dearborn St.
Caldwell 83605
(208) 459-3242

ILLINOIS

DONORS FORUM OF CHICAGO ✱ ✣
208 South LaSalle, Suite 740
Chicago 60604
(312) 431-0265

EVANSTON PUBLIC LIBRARY ✱ ✣
1703 Orrington Ave.
Evanston 60201
(708) 866-0305

ROCK ISLAND PUBLIC LIBRARY ✣
401 - 19th St.
Rock Island 61201
(309) 788-7627

UNIVERSITY OF ILLINOIS AT SPRINGFIELD ✱ ✣
Brookens Library
Shepherd Road
Springfield 62794-9243
(217) 786-6633

INDIANA

ALLEN COUNTY PUBLIC LIBRARY ✱ ✣
900 Webster St.
Ft. Wayne 46802
(219) 424-0544

INDIANA UNIVERSITY NORTHWEST LIBRARY
3400 Broadway
Gary 46408
(219) 980-6582

INDIANAPOLIS–MARION COUNTY PUBLIC LIBRARY ✱ ✣
Social Sciences
40 E. St. Clair
Indianapolis 46206
(317) 269-1733

IOWA

CEDAR RAPIDS PUBLIC LIBRARY ✱
Foundation Center Collection
500 First St., SE
Cedar Rapids 52401
(319) 398-5123

SOUTHWESTERN COMMUNITY COLLEGE ✱
Learning Resource Center
1501 W. Townline Rd.
Creston 50801
(515) 782-7081

PUBLIC LIBRARY OF DES MOINES ✱ ✣
100 Locust
Des Moines 50309-1791
(515) 283-4152

SIOUX CITY PUBLIC LIBRARY ✱ ✣
529 Pierce St.
Sioux City 51101-1202
(712) 252-5669

KANSAS

DODGE CITY PUBLIC LIBRARY ✱ ✣
1001 2nd Ave.
Dodge City 67801
(316) 225-0248

TOPEKA AND SHAWNEE COUNTY PUBLIC LIBRARY ✱ ✣
1515 SW 10th Ave.
Topeka 66604-1374
(913) 233-2040

WICHITA PUBLIC LIBRARY ✱ ✣
223 S. Main St.
Wichita 67202
(316) 262-0611

KENTUCKY

WESTERN KENTUCKY UNIVERSITY ✣
Helm-Cravens Library
Bowling Green 42101-3576
(502) 745-6125

LEXINGTON PUBLIC LIBRARY ✱
140 E. Main St.
Lexington 40507-1376
(606) 231-5520

LOUISVILLE FREE PUBLIC LIBRARY ✱ ✣
301 York Street
Louisville 40203
(502) 574-1611

LOUISIANA

EAST BATON ROUGE PARISH LIBRARY ✱ ✣
Centroplex Branch Grants Collection
120 St. Louis
Baton Rouge 70802
(504) 389-4960

BEAUREGARD PARISH LIBRARY ✱ ✣
205 S. Washington Ave.
De Ridder 70634
(318) 463-6217

NEW ORLEANS PUBLIC LIBRARY ✱
Business & Science Division
219 Loyola Ave.
New Orleans 70140
(504) 596-2580

SHREVE MEMORIAL LIBRARY ✱ ✣
424 Texas St.
Shreveport 71120-1523
(318) 226-5894

MAINE

MAINE GRANTS INFORMATION CENTER ✱ ✣
University of Southern Maine
P. O. Box 9301, 314 Forrest Ave.
Portland 04104-9301
(207) 780-5029

MARYLAND

ENOCH PRATT FREE LIBRARY ✱ ✣
Social Science & History
400 Cathedral St.
Baltimore 21201
(410) 396-5430

MASSACHUSETTS

ASSOCIATED GRANTMAKERS OF MASSACHUSETTS ✱ ✣
294 Washington St., Suite 840
Boston 02108
(617) 426-2606

BOSTON PUBLIC LIBRARY ✱
Soc. Sci. Reference
666 Boylston St
Boston 02117
(617) 536-5400

WESTERN MASSACHUSETTS FUNDING RESOURCE CENTER ✣
65 Elliot St.
Springfield 01101-1730
(413) 732-3175

WORCESTER PUBLIC LIBRARY ✱ ✣
Grants Resource Center
Salem Square
Worcester 01608
(508) 799-1655

MICHIGAN

ALPENA COUNTY LIBRARY ✱ ✣
211 N. First St.
Alpena 49707
(517) 356-6188

UNIVERSITY OF MICHIGAN–ANN ARBOR ✱
Graduate Library
Reference & Research Services Department
Ann Arbor 48109-1205
(313) 764-9373

WILLARD PUBLIC LIBRARY ✱ ✣
7 W. Van Buren St.
Battle Creek 49017
(616) 968-8166

HENRY FORD CENTENNIAL LIBRARY ✱ ✣
Adult Services
16301 Michigan Ave.
Dearborn 48126
(313) 943-2330

WAYNE STATE UNIVERSITY ✱ ✣
Purdy/Kresge Library
5265 Cass Avenue
Detroit 48202
(313) 577-6424

MICHIGAN STATE UNIVERSITY LIBRARIES ✱ ✣
Social Sciences/Humanities
Main Library
East Lansing 48824-1048
(517) 353-8818

FARMINGTON COMMUNITY LIBRARY ✱ ✣
32737 West 12 Mile Rd.
Farmington Hills 48018
(810) 553-0300

UNIVERSITY OF MICHIGAN—FLINT ✱
Library
Flint 48502-2186
(810) 762-3408

GRAND RAPIDS PUBLIC LIBRARY ✱ ✣
Business Dept.—3rd Floor
60 Library Plaza NE
Grand Rapids 49503-3093
(616) 456-3600

MICHIGAN TECHNOLOGICAL UNIVERSITY
Van Pelt Library
1400 Townsend Dr.
Houghton 49931
(906) 487-2507

MAUD PRESTON PALENSKE MEMORIAL LIBRARY
500 Market St.
Saint Joseph 49085
(616) 983-7167

SAULT STE. MARIE AREA PUBLIC SCHOOLS
Office of Compensatory Education
460 W. Spruce St.
Sault Ste. Marie 49783-1874
(906) 635-6618

NORTHWESTERN MICHIGAN COLLEGE ✱ ✣
Mark & Helen Osterin Library
1701 E. Front St.
Traverse City 49684
(616) 922-1060

MINNESOTA

DULUTH PUBLIC LIBRARY ✱
520 W. Superior St.
Duluth 55802
(218) 723-3802

SOUTHWEST STATE UNIVERSITY ✱ ✣
University Library
Marshall 56258
(507) 537-6176

MINNEAPOLIS PUBLIC LIBRARY ✱ ✣
Sociology Department
300 Nicollet Mall
Minneapolis 55401
(612) 372-6555

ROCHESTER PUBLIC LIBRARY
101 2nd St. SE
Rochester 55904-3776
(507) 285-8002

ST. PAUL PUBLIC LIBRARY
90 W. Fourth St.
St. Paul 55102
(612) 292-6307

MISSISSIPPI

JACKSON/HINDS LIBRARY SYSTEM ✱
300 N. State St.
Jackson 39201
(601) 968-5803

MISSOURI

CLEARINGHOUSE FOR MIDCONTINENT FOUNDATIONS ✱ ✣
University of Missouri
5110 Cherry, Suite 310
Kansas City 64110
(816) 235-1176

KANSAS CITY PUBLIC LIBRARY ✱
311 E. 12th St.
Kansas City 64106
(816) 221-9650

METROPOLITAN ASSOCIATION FOR PHILANTHROPY, INC. ✱ ✣
5615 Pershing Avenue, Suite 20
St. Louis 63112
(314) 361-3900

SPRINGFIELD-GREENE COUNTY LIBRARY ✱ ✣
397 E. Central
Springfield 65802
(417) 837-5000

MONTANA

MONTANA STATE UNIVERSITY—BILLINGS ✱ ✣
Library—Special Collections
1500 North 30th St.
Billings 59101-0298
(406) 657-1662

BOZEMAN PUBLIC LIBRARY ✱
220 E. Lamme
Bozeman 59715
(406) 582-2402

MONTANA STATE LIBRARY ✱ ✣
Library Services
1515 E. 6th Ave.
Helena 59620
(406) 444-3004

UNIVERSITY OF MONTANA ✱ ✣
Maureen & Mike Mansfield Library
Missoula 59812-1195
(406) 243-6800

NEBRASKA

UNIVERSITY OF NEBRASKA—LINCOLN ✱ ✣
Love Library
14th & R Streets
Lincoln 68588-0410
(402) 472-2848

W. DALE CLARK LIBRARY ✱ ✣
Social Sciences Department
215 S. 15th St.
Omaha 68102
(402) 444-4826

NEVADA

LAS VEGAS–CLARK COUNTY LIBRARY DISTRICT ✱ ✣
1401 E. Flamingo
Las Vegas 89119
(702) 733-3642

WASHOE COUNTY LIBRARY ✱ ✣
301 S. Center St.
Reno 89501
(702) 785-4010

NEW HAMPSHIRE

NEW HAMPSHIRE CHARITABLE FDN. ✱ ✣
37 Pleasant St.
Concord 03301-4005
(603) 225-6641

PLYMOUTH STATE COLLEGE ✱ ✣
Herbert H. Lamson Library
Plymouth 03264
(603) 535-2258

NEW JERSEY

CUMBERLAND COUNTY LIBRARY ✣
800 E. Commerce St.
Bridgeton 08302
(609) 453-2210

FREE PUBLIC LIBRARY OF ELIZABETH ✱
11 S. Broad St.
Elizabeth 07202
(908) 354-6060

COUNTY COLLEGE OF MORRIS ✱ ✣
Learning Resource Center
214 Center Grove Rd.
Randolph 07869
(201) 328-5296

NEW JERSEY STATE LIBRARY ✱ ✣
Governmental Reference Services
185 W. State St.
Trenton 08625-0520
(609) 292-6220

NEW MEXICO

ALBUQUERQUE COMMUNITY FOUNDATION ✱
3301 Menual NE, Ste. 30
Albuquerque 87176-6960
(505) 883-6240

NEW MEXICO STATE LIBRARY ✱ ✣
Information Services
325 Don Gaspar
Santa Fe 87501-2777
(505) 827-3824

NEW YORK

NEW YORK STATE LIBRARY ✱ ✣
Humanities Reference
Cultural Education Center
Empire State Plaza
Albany 12230
(518) 474-5355

SUFFOLK COOPERATIVE LIBRARY SYSTEM ✣
627 N. Sunrise Service Rd.
Bellport 11713
(516) 286-1600

NEW YORK PUBLIC LIBRARY
Bronx Reference Center
Fordham Branch
2556 Bainbridge Ave.
Bronx 10458
(718) 220-6575

BROOKLYN IN TOUCH INFORMATION CENTER, INC. ✣
One Hanson Place—Room 2504
Brooklyn 11243
(718) 230-3200

BROOKLYN PUBLIC LIBRARY ✣
Social Sciences Division
Grand Army Plaza
Brooklyn 11238
(718) 780-7700

BUFFALO & ERIE COUNTY PUBLIC LIBRARY ✱ ✣
Business & Labor Dept.
Lafayette Square
Buffalo 14203
(716) 858-7097

HUNTINGTON PUBLIC LIBRARY
338 Main St.
Huntington 11743
(516) 427-5165

QUEENS BOROUGH PUBLIC LIBRARY ✣
Social Sciences Division
89-11 Merrick Blvd.
Jamaica 11432
(718) 990-0761

LEVITTOWN PUBLIC LIBRARY ✱
1 Bluegrass Lane
Levittown 11756
(516) 731-5728

NEW YORK PUBLIC LIBRARY
Countee Cullen Branch Library
104 W. 136th St.
New York 10030
(212) 491-2070

PLATTSBURGH PUBLIC LIBRARY ✣
19 Oak St.
Plattsburgh 12901
(518) 563-0921

ADRIANCE MEMORIAL LIBRARY ✣
Special Services Department
93 Market St.
Poughkeepsie 12601
(914) 485-3445

ROCHESTER PUBLIC LIBRARY ✱ ✣
Business, Economics & Law
115 South Ave.
Rochester 14604
(716) 428-7328

ONONDAGA COUNTY PUBLIC LIBRARY ✣
447 S. Salina St.
Syracuse 13202-2494
(315) 435-1800

UTICA PUBLIC LIBRARY ✣
303 Genesee St.
Utica 13501
(315) 735-2279

WHITE PLAINS PUBLIC LIBRARY ✣
100 Martine Ave.
White Plains 10601
(914) 422-1480

NORTH CAROLINA

COMMUNITY FDN. OF WESTERN NORTH CAROLINA ✱ ✣
Learning Resources Center
14 College St.
P.O. Box 1888
Asheville 28801
(704) 254-4960

THE DUKE ENDOWMENT ✱ ✣
100 N. Tryon St., Suite 3500
Charlotte 28202
(704) 376-0291

DURHAM COUNTY PUBLIC LIBRARY
301 North Roxboro
Durham 27702
(919) 560-0110

STATE LIBRARY OF NORTH CAROLINA ✱ ✣
Government and Business Services
Archives Bldg., 109 E. Jones St.
Raleigh 27601
(919) 733-3270

FORSYTH COUNTY PUBLIC LIBRARY ✱ ✣
660 W. 5th St.
Winston-Salem 27101
(910) 727-2680

NORTH DAKOTA

BISMARCK PUBLIC LIBRARY ✱
515 N. Fifth St.
Bismarck 58501
(701) 222-6410

FARGO PUBLIC LIBRARY ✱ ✣
102 N. 3rd St.
Fargo 58102
(701) 241-1491

OHIO

STARK COUNTY DISTRICT LIBRARY ✣
Humanities
715 Market Ave. N.
Canton 44702
(330) 452-0665

PUBLIC LIBRARY OF CINCINNATI & HAMILTON COUNTY ✱ ✣
Grants Resource Center
800 Vine St.—Library Square
Cincinnati 45202-2071
(513) 369-6940

COLUMBUS METROPOLITAN LIBRARY ✣
Business and Technology
96 S. Grant Ave.
Columbus 43215
(614) 645-2590

DAYTON & MONTGOMERY COUNTY PUBLIC LIBRARY ✱ ✣
Grants Resource Center
215 E. Third St.
Dayton 45402
(513) 227-9500 x211

MANSFIELD/RICHLAND COUNTY PUBLIC LIBRARY ✱ ✣
42 W. 3rd St.
Mansfield 44902
(419) 521-3110

TOLEDO–LUCAS COUNTY PUBLIC LIBRARY ✱ ✣
Social Sciences Department
325 Michigan St.
Toledo 43624-1614
(419) 259-5245

PUBLIC LIBRARY OF YOUNGSTOWN & MAHONING COUNTY ✱ ✣
305 Wick Ave.
Youngstown 44503
(216) 744-8636

MUSKINGUM COUNTY LIBRARY
220 N. 5th St.
Zanesville 43701
(614) 453-0391

OKLAHOMA

OKLAHOMA CITY UNIVERSITY ✱ ✣
Dulaney Browne Library
2501 N. Blackwelder
Oklahoma City 73106
(405) 521-5822

TULSA CITY–COUNTY LIBRARY ✱ ✣
400 Civic Center
Tulsa 74103
(918) 596-7944

OREGON

OREGON INSTITUTE OF TECHNOLOGY ✣
Library
3201 Campus Dr.
Klamath Falls 97601-8801
(503) 885-1773

PACIFIC NON-PROFIT NETWORK ✱ ✣
Grantsmanship Resource Library
33 N. Central, Suite 211
Medford 97501
(503) 779-6044

MULTNOMAH COUNTY LIBRARY ✣
Government Documents
801 SW Tenth Ave.
Portland 97205
(503) 248-5123

OREGON STATE LIBRARY ✱ ✣
State Library Building
Salem 97310
(503) 378-4277

PENNSYLVANIA

NORTHAMPTON COMMUNITY COLLEGE
Learning Resources Center
3835 Green Pond Rd.
Bethlehem 18017
(610) 861-5360

ERIE COUNTY LIBRARY SYSTEM ✣
27 S. Park Row
Erie 16501
(814) 451-6927

DAUPHIN COUNTY LIBRARY SYSTEM ✤
Central Library
101 Walnut St.
Harrisburg 17101
(717) 234-4976

LANCASTER COUNTY PUBLIC LIBRARY
125 N. Duke St.
Lancaster 17602
(717) 394-2651

FREE LIBRARY OF PHILADELPHIA ✱ ✤
Regional Foundation Center
Logan Square
Philadelphia 19103
(215) 686-5423

CARNEGIE LIBRARY OF PITTSBURGH ✱ ✤
Foundation Collection
4400 Forbes Ave.
Pittsburgh 15213-4080
(412) 622-1917

POCONO NORTHEAST DEVELOPMENT FUND ✤
James Pettinger Memorial Library
1151 Oak St.
Pittston 18640-3795
(717) 655-5581

READING PUBLIC LIBRARY
100 South Fifth St.
Reading 19602
(610) 655-6355

MARTIN LIBRARY ✱ ✤
159 Market St.
York 17401
(717) 846-5300

RHODE ISLAND

PROVIDENCE PUBLIC LIBRARY ✱ ✤
225 Washington St.
Providence 02906
(401) 455-8088

SOUTH CAROLINA

ANDERSON COUNTY LIBRARY ✱ ✤
202 East Greenville St.
Anderson 29621
(864) 260-4500

CHARLESTON COUNTY LIBRARY ✱ ✤
404 King St.
Charleston 29403
(803) 723-1645

SOUTH CAROLINA STATE LIBRARY ✱ ✤
1500 Senate St.
Columbia 29211
(803) 734-8666

SOUTH DAKOTA

SOUTH DAKOTA STATE LIBRARY ✱ ✤
800 Governors Drive
Pierre 57501-2294
(605) 773-5070
(800) 592-1841 (SD residents)

NONPROFIT GRANTS ASSISTANCE CENTER ✤
Dakota State University
Business and Education Institute
3534 Southwestern Ave.
Sioux Falls 57105
(605) 367-5380

SIOUXLAND LIBRARIES ✱
201 N. Main Ave.
Sioux Falls 57102-1132
(605) 367-7081

TENNESSEE

KNOX COUNTY PUBLIC LIBRARY ✱ ✤
500 W. Church Ave.
Knoxville 37902
(423) 544-5700

MEMPHIS & SHELBY COUNTY PUBLIC LIBRARY ✱
1850 Peabody Ave.
Memphis 38104
(901) 725-8877

NASHVILLE PUBLIC LIBRARY ✱ ✤
Business Information Division
225 Polk Ave.
Nashville 37203
(615) 862-5843

TEXAS

ABILENE CENTER FOR NONPROFIT MANAGEMENT ✤
Funding Information Library
500 N. Chestnut, Suite 1511
Abilene 79604
(915) 677-8166

AMARILLO AREA FOUNDATION ✱
700 First National Place
801 S. Fillmore
Amarillo 79101
(806) 376-4521

HOGG FOUNDATION FOR MENTAL HEALTH ✱
3001 Lake Austin Blvd.
Austin 78703
(512) 471-5041

TEXAS A & M UNIVERSITY AT CORPUS CHRISTI ✤
Bell Library
Reference Dept.
6300 Ocean Dr.
Corpus Christi 78412
(512) 994-5961

DALLAS PUBLIC LIBRARY ✱ ✤
Urban Information
1515 Young St.
Dallas 75201
(214) 670-1487

EL PASO COMMUNITY FOUNDATION
201 E. Main St., Suite 1616
El Paso 79901
(915) 533-4020

FUNDING INFORMATION CENTER OF FORT WORTH ✱ ✤
Texas Christian University Library
2800 S. University Dr.
Ft. Worth 76129
(817) 921-7664

HOUSTON PUBLIC LIBRARY ✱
Bibliographic Information Center
500 McKinney
Houston 77002
(713) 236-1313

LONGVIEW PUBLIC LIBRARY ✱
222 W. Cotton St.
Longview 75601
(903) 237-1352

LUBBOCK AREA FOUNDATION, INC. ✤
1655 Main St., Suite 209
Lubbock 79401
(806) 762-8061

NONPROFIT RESOURCE CENTER OF TEXAS ✱ ✤
11 Soledad, Suite 601
San Antonio 78205
(210) 227-4333

WACO-MCLENNAN COUNTY LIBRARY ✱ ✤
1717 Austin Ave.
Waco 76701
(817) 750-5944

NORTH TEXAS CENTER FOR NONPROFIT MANAGEMENT ✱ ✤
624 Indiana, Suite 307
Wichita Falls 76301
(817) 322-4961

UTAH

SALT LAKE CITY PUBLIC LIBRARY ✱
209 East 500 South
Salt Lake City 84111
(801) 524-8200

VERMONT

VERMONT DEPT. OF LIBRARIES ✱ ✤
Reference & Law Info. Services
109 State St.
Montpelier 05609
(802) 828-3268

VIRGINIA

HAMPTON PUBLIC LIBRARY ✤
4207 Victoria Blvd.
Hampton 23669
(804) 727-1312

RICHMOND PUBLIC LIBRARY ✱ ✤
Business, Science & Technology
101 East Franklin St.
Richmond 23219
(804) 780-8223

ROANOKE CITY PUBLIC LIBRARY SYSTEM ✱
Central Library
706 S. Jefferson St.
Roanoke 24016
(703) 981-2477

WASHINGTON

MID-COLUMBIA LIBRARY ✱
405 South Dayton
Kennewick 99336
(509)586-3156

SEATTLE PUBLIC LIBRARY ✱ ✤
Science, Social Science
1000 Fourth Ave.
Seattle 98104
(206) 386-4620

SPOKANE PUBLIC LIBRARY ✱
Funding Information Center
West 811 Main Ave.
Spokane 99201
(509) 626-5347

UNITED WAY OF PIERCE COUNTY ✱ ✤
Center for Nonprofit Development
1501 Pacific Ave., Suite 400
P.O. Box 2215
Tacoma 98401
(206) 272-4263

GREATER WENATCHEE COMMUNITY FOUNDATION AT THE WENATCHEE PUBLIC LIBRARY
310 Douglas St.
Wenatchee 98807
(509) 662-5021

WEST VIRGINIA

KANAWHA COUNTY PUBLIC LIBRARY ✱ ✤
123 Capitol St.
Charleston 25301
(304) 343-4646

WISCONSIN

UNIVERSITY OF WISCONSIN–MADISON ✱ ✤
Memorial Library
728 State St.
Madison 53706
(608) 262-3242

MARQUETTE UNIVERSITY MEMORIAL LIBRARY ✱ ✤
Funding Information Center
1415 W. Wisconsin Ave.
Milwaukee 53201-3141
(414) 288-1515

UNIVERSITY OF WISCONSIN—STEVENS POINT ✱ ✤
Library—Foundation Collection
99 Reserve St.
Stevens Point 54481-3897
(715) 346-4204

WYOMING

NATRONA COUNTY PUBLIC LIBRARY ✱ ✤
307 E. 2nd St.
Casper 82601-2598
(307) 237-4935

LARAMIE COUNTY COMMUNITY COLLEGE ✱ ✤
Instructional Resource Center
1400 E. College Dr.
Cheyenne 82007-3299
(307) 778-1206

CAMPBELL COUNTY PUBLIC LIBRARY ✱ ✤
2101 4-J Road
Gillette 82716
(307) 682-3223

TETON COUNTY LIBRARY ✱ ✤
320 S. King St.
Jackson 83001
(307) 733-2164

ROCK SPRINGS LIBRARY
400 C St.
Rock Springs 82901
(307) 352-6667

PUERTO RICO

UNIVERSITY OF PUERTO RICO ✤
Ponce Technological College Library
Box 7186
Ponce 00732
(809) 844-8181

UNIVERSIDAD DEL SAGRADO CORAZON
M.M.T. Guevara Library
Santurce 00914
(809) 728-1515 x 4357

Participants in the Foundation Center's Cooperating Collections network are libraries or nonprofit information centers that provide fundraising information and other funding-related technical assistance in their communities. Cooperating Collections agree to provide free public access to a basic collection of Foundation Center publications during a regular schedule of hours, offering free funding research guidance to all visitors. Many also provide a variety of services for local nonprofit organizations, using staff or volunteers to prepare special materials, organize workshops, or conduct orientations.

The Foundation Center welcomes inquiries from libraries or information centers in the U.S. interested in providing this type of public information service. If you are interested in establishing a funding information library for the use of nonprofit organizations in your area or in learning more about the program, please write to: Rich Romeo, Coordinator of Cooperating Collections, The Foundation Center, 79 Fifth Avenue, New York, NY 10003-3076.

SECTION I:
DESCRIPTIVE DIRECTORY OF GRANTMAKERS

DESCRIPTIVE DIRECTORY OF GRANTMAKERS

In 1994, more than 38,500 active private and community foundations awarded an estimated $11 billion in grants to nonprofit organizations across the country. Studies of foundation grantmaking patterns by the Foundation Center indicate that just under one percent of these grant dollars were directed toward programs that benefitted the elderly, in such areas as health and medical care, general welfare, education and community services, employment and pension issues, housing, recreation, volunteer services, social research, and advocacy and legal rights. Although foundation funds represent but a tiny fraction when compared to government spending for the elderly, they are still a key source of support for many nonprofit organizations.

This volume is intended as a starting point for grantseekers looking for foundation, corporate and other charitable support for programs, services, or research related to the elderly. This section includes 1,073 foundations, public charities, and corporate giving programs that have expressed an interest in the elderly as part of their stated purpose or through actual grants reported to the Foundation Center through mid-1996.

A review of the grants for the aged reported to the Foundation Center in 1994 and 1995 by 346 foundations reveals the funding trends shown in Tables 1 and 2, below.

Each entry in the *Guide* was carefully evaluated by Foundation Center staff to ensure that the grantmaker possesses a sufficient interest in the aged, either stated or demonstrated. Often, a grantmaker claims interest not only in programs related to the field of aging but in dozens of widely diverse fields. To determine if inclusion in this *Guide* is warranted in such cases, consideration is given to the grantmaker's purpose statement, giving limitations, and, if they exist, subject-related grants. Grantseekers should be aware that inclusion does not imply that these grantmakers will consider all programs serving the elderly.

Keep in mind that some grantmakers support particular programs because of their interest in a specific community or organization. Others may do so because the program relates to a highly specific subject interest of the grantmaker, such as housing for the elderly, senior centers, or geriatric research. Still others are interested in building the capacity of nonprofit institutions by providing specific types of support such as operating costs or challenge grants. Grantseekers are therefore urged to read each foundation and corporate giving program description carefully to determine the nature of the grantmaker's interests and to note any restrictions on giving that would prevent the grantmaker from considering their proposal.

MORE PRECISE INDEXING

Since 1989 the Foundation Center has used a Grants Classification System (GCS) based on the National Taxonomy of Exempt Entities (NTEE), a comprehensive organizational coding scheme developed by the National Center for Charitable Statistics (NCCS) that was adopted

TABLE 1

	Dollar Value of Grants 1994		Number of Grants 1994	
Subject	**Amount***	**%**	**No.**	**%**
Arts and culture	$3	0.0	2	0.3
Education	102	0.4	4	0.7
Environment and animals	0	0.0	0	0.0
Health	12,346	44.3	260	42.8
Human services	15,243	54.7	326	53.7
International affairs, development and peace	3	0.0	1	0.2
Public/society benefit	154	0.6	10	1.6
Science and technology	14	0.0	3	0.5
Social science	15	0.1	1	0.2
Religion	0	0.0	0	0.0
Other	0	0.0	0	0.0
Total	**$27,880**	**100.0**	**607**	**100.0**

* Dollar figures expressed in thousands; due to rounding, figures may not add up.

TABLE 2

	Dollar Value of Grants 1995		Number of Grants 1995	
Subject	**Amount***	**%**	**No.**	**%**
Arts and culture	$58	0.1	6	0.8
Education	370	0.8	6	0.8
Environment and animals	15	0.0	1	0.1
Health	28,866	62.4	271	38.1
Human services	16,098	34.8	395	55.6
International affairs, development and peace	0	0.0	0	0.0
Public/society benefit	543	1.2	17	2.4
Science and technology	35	0.1	1	0.1
Social science	250	0.5	8	1.1
Religion	44	0.1	4	0.6
Other	18	0.0	2	0.3
Total	**$46,296**	**100.0**	**711**	**100.0**

* Dollar figures expressed in thousands; due to rounding, figures may not add up.

[1] This volume also includes 14 grants reported for fiscal year 1996 that totaled $1,130,000. There were 2 grants (14.3%) in the Health category totaling $125,000 and 12 grants (85.7%) in the Human Services category totaling $1,005,000. Due to rounding, figures may not add up.

by the IRS in 1995. The GCS builds on the NTEE and is used by the Center to provide subject, types of support, and other grants information both online through two DIALOG files (a product of Knight-Ridder Information Services) and in print through *The Foundation Grants Index* and related publications.

This edition of *Funding in Aging: A Guide to Giving by Foundations, Corporations, and Charitable Organizations* represents, in part, the culmination of a major project to utilize the more comprehensive and precise GCS terminology across all Foundation Center publications and files. This process has resulted in the Center maintaining a more unified system of classification. The enhancements to this *Guide* resulting from the implementation of unified indexing terms include:

1. A new section in grantmaker descriptive entries identifying any international giving interests of an organization. Because of the conversion to the GCS terminology, the number of index terms describing the countries, continents, and regions in which grantmakers have giving interests has expanded from a few dozen to over 200, providing a much greater level of specificity.

2. The full scope of the terminology used to describe a grantmaker's areas of interests has also expanded following the conversion to unified GCS subject terms. The "Fields of Interest" section of each grantmaker descriptive entry will now include all indexed subject terms for the organization, rather than listing only its primary areas of giving. The "Purpose and Activities" section contains a more general statement of foundation funding priorities.

WHAT IS A FOUNDATION?

The Foundation Center defines a foundation as a nongovernmental, nonprofit organization with its own funds (usually derived from a single source, either an individual, family, or corporation) and a program managed by its own trustees and directors, which was established to maintain or aid educational, social, charitable, or other activities serving the common welfare, primarily by making grants to other nonprofit organizations.

The Internal Revenue Service code defines the category of "private foundation" only by exclusion of other nonprofit organizations, a circumstance that has led to some confusion. David Freedman, former president of the Council on Foundations, explains the Code's definition in his book *The Handbook on Private Foundations:*

> Starting with the universe of voluntary organizations described in section 501(c)(3), the Code excludes broad groups, e.g., churches, schools, hospitals, governmental units, publicly supported charities and their affiliates. Publicly supported charities are those which derive much of their general support from the public and reach out in other ways to a public constituency. All of the above kinds of excluded organizations are commonly referred to as 'public charities.' Section 501(c)(3) organizations remaining after these exclusions are, without more precise definition, 'private foundations.' One important result: organizations are included in the remainder as private foundations that are not really grantmaking foundations at all. These may include museums, homes for the aged, and libraries, among others, if they, while serving the public, happen to have been endowed by an individual or single family, or if they were established as public charities and lose that status by failing to prove they have received ongoing financial support from the general public.

A private **independent foundation** most commonly derives its assets from an individual, family, or group of individuals. The foundation may function under the voluntary direction of family members, or may bear a family name but have independent boards of trustees and professional staffs. Typically, independent foundations have broad charters which allow a range of giving activities, but in practice most limit their giving to a few specific fields of interest and to a specific geographic area.

Operating foundations are also private foundations under tax laws, but their primary purpose is to operate research, social welfare, or other charitable programs determined by the donor or governing body. Some grants may be made outside the foundation, but the majority of the foundation's funds are expended on its own programs.

Corporations contribute through foundations, direct giving programs, or both:

Corporate or **company-sponsored** foundations are created and funded by business corporations for the purpose of making grants and performing other philanthropic activities. Legally, they are separate from the sponsoring corporation and are governed by the same federal rules and regulations as independent foundations. Company-sponsored foundations are generally managed by a board of directors that includes corporate officials but may also include individuals with no corporate affiliation. Giving programs often focus on communities where the company has operations, and on research and education in fields related to company activities.

Direct corporate giving refers to all other giving by a company, that is, money not turned over to a foundation to administer. Direct giving programs are unregulated and restricted only by the limit of taxable earnings allowed as charitable deductions. In addition to cash contributions, corporate giving may include non-cash gifts of goods and services referred to as "in-kind" giving. Donations of company products, supplies, and equipment—from computers to food—is the most common form of in-kind giving. Other types of support include technical assistance and use of office space. Direct giving programs and foundations often share the same staff, although some companies keep these functions administratively separate.

Public charities, in general, are organizations that are tax-exempt under code section 501(c)(3) and are classified by the IRS as a public charity and not a private foundation. Public charities typically derive their funding or support substantially from the general public in carrying out their social, educational, religious, or other charitable activities serving the common welfare. Some public charities engage in grantmaking activities, although most engage in direct service or other tax-exempt activities. Public charities are eligible for maximum income tax-deductible contributions from the public and are not subject to the same rules and restrictions as private foundations. Some are also referred to as "public foundations" or "publicly supported foundations" and may use the term "foundation" in their names.

Community foundations are public charities supported by and operated for a specific community or region. They receive their funds from a variety of donors; in fact, their endowments are frequently composed of a number of different trust funds, some of which bear their donors' names. Their grantmaking activities are administered by a governing body or distribution committee representative of community interests. Although community foundations may support a wide range of activities, their grants are generally restricted to charitable organizations in their city or region.

Grantseekers should be aware that an increasing number of for-profit business have also adopted "foundation" as part of their name to promote their activities. While there are no legal restrictions on the use of the word "foundation," it is important for grantseekers to understand that many of these groups do not make grants and are not governed by the same rules and regulations as private foundations or nonprofit groups.

GRANTSEEKING FROM FOUNDATIONS

Foundations receive many thousands of worthy requests each year. Most of these requests are declined because there are not enough funds to go around or because the application clearly falls outside the foundation's fields of interest. Some of the applications denied are poorly prepared and do not reflect a careful analysis of the applicant organization's needs, its credibility, or its capacity to carry out the proposed project. Sometimes the qualifications of the organization's staff are not well established; the budget or the means of evaluating the project may not be presented convincingly; or the organization may not have asked itself whether it is especially suited to make a contribution to the solution of the problem, whether it can provide the service proposed, or whether others are not already effectively engaged in the same activity.

The first step in researching foundation funding support is to analyze your own program and organization to determine the need you plan to address, the audience you will serve, and the amount and type of support you need. Become familiar with the basic facts about foundations in general and how they operate. Consider other sources of funding, such as individual contributors, government grants, earned income possibilities, and so on. Although foundations are an important source of support for nonprofit organizations, their giving represents a relatively small percentage of the total philanthropic dollars contributed annually, and an even smaller percentage of the total when government grants and earned income are included. If you are new to grantseeking, we strongly urge you to visit one of the Foundation Center's many Cooperating Collections. They provide free access to a core collection of Foundation Center publications, as well as other materials on funding sources, program planning, and fundraising.

Once you have determined the amount and type of foundation support you need and the reasons why you are seeking support, this *Guide* can help you develop an initial list of foundations that might be interested in funding your project. In determining whether or not it is appropriate to approach a particular foundation with a grant request, keep in mind the following questions:

1. Does the foundation's interest in the field of aging include the specific type of service or program you are proposing?
2. Does it seem likely that the foundation will make a grant in your geographic area?
3. Does the amount of money you are requesting fit within the foundation's grant range?
4. Does the foundation have any policy prohibiting grants for the type of support you are requesting?
5. Does the foundation prefer to make grants that cover the full cost of a project or do they favor projects where other foundations or funding sources share the cost?
6. What types of organizations does the foundation tend to support?
7. Does the foundation have specific application deadlines and procedures or does it review proposals continuously?

Some of these questions can be answered from the information provided in this *Guide*, but grantseekers will almost always want to consult a few additional resources before submitting a request for funding. If the foundation issues an annual report, application guidelines, or other printed materials describing its program, it is advisable to obtain copies and study them carefully before preparing your proposal. The foundation's annual information return (Form 990-PF) includes a list of all grants paid by the foundation in addition to basic data about its finances, officers, and giving policies. Copies of these returns are available for examination at most of the Foundation Center's cooperating libraries.

The foundations listed in this *Guide* by no means represent all of the possible foundation funding sources for programs related to higher education. There are a number of foundations, including some 405 community foundations across the country, that support a wide variety of programs within a specific community or region. Grantseekers should learn as much as possible about the foundations in their own area, particularly when they are seeking relatively small grants for projects with purely local impact. Be sure to check any local or state directories of which the Foundation Center is currently aware. Copies of these directories are almost always available for use at your local Foundation Center cooperating library.

The Foundation Center publishes several national directories on an annual basis. *The Foundation Directory* describes foundations with assets of $2 million or more or annual giving of at least $200,000. *The Foundation Directory Part 2* provides information on the second tier of foundations, those with assets between $1 million and $2 million, or annual grantmaking between $50,000 and $200,000. Both the *Directory* and the *Directory Part 2* entries include a list of selected grants whenever available, providing concrete examples of a foundation's giving. The *Directory* and *Directory Part 2* are arranged by state and include a geographic index to help you identify foundations located or interested in your specific community. The Foundation Center also publishes the *Guide to U.S. Foundations, Their Trustees, Officers, and Donors,* which provides basic address and financial information on all the approximately 38,500 active grantmaking foundations in the United States, as well as fully indexed listings to all foundation trustees/directors, officers, and donors. The *Guide to U.S. Foundations* is arranged alphabetically by state. Within states, foundations are listed in descending order by annual giving amount.

For those who want more detailed information on how to identify appropriate foundation funding sources, the Center also publishes *Foundation Fundamentals.* This guide takes you step-by-step through the research strategies developed and taught by the Foundation Center, describing in the process how to gather the facts you need to best approach foundations for funding. All Foundation Center publications can be examined free of charge at Foundation Center libraries.

GRANTSEEKING FROM CORPORATIONS

The research process for corporate funding is similar to other institutional grantseeking: identifying companies that might be interested in an organization's mission and program, learning as much as possible about those companies, determining the best method of approach, and articulating program objectives so as to be in line with the company's giving rationale. It differs from researching other institutional funders, however, in that it is often more difficult to uncover the needed information. There is great diversity in method and style of giving among corporations, and companies are often looking for a quid pro quo for their giving. Because many corporations see their giving not in terms of altruism but as a responsibility or simply good business, corporate philanthropy is often considered something of an oxymoron. Soliciting support from corporations, therefore, often requires a shift in perspective, from appealing to a company's benevolence to promoting its self-interest.

Identifying corporations to approach is accomplished in several ways. Directories such as the *National Directory of Corporate Giving* describe companies with known corporate giving programs. These guides can help you identify a corporation's subject interests, geographical giving patterns, and/or the benefits it hopes to derive from its giving. General business directories aid in the search, as do the books and guides listed in the bibliography. Staff members, your organization's board, and volunteers often know or work for companies that ultimately may be able to provide funds. The telephone book is another good resource for tracking down local businesses.

After a list of likely prospects is compiled, you should continue your efforts to locate additional information about the company, its primary and secondary business activities, its officers, giving history, and any details helpful in understanding its giving rationale. Understanding why a company gives is essential, as it may point to a match of the grantseeker's programmatic goals and the corporation's giving goals. Although determining the reasons a company makes contributions can be difficult, it can be accomplished through careful research, including studying annual reports and the materials issued by other organizations the company has supported, as well as by speaking directly with company officials whenever possible.

This kind of research usually uncovers the best method for approaching a company with a request for support. Companies with formal giving programs may have guidelines and application procedures and require a written proposal, while companies with informal giving programs may be better approached through personal contacts made by board members or volunteers. Once the approach is determined, however, a written or oral presentation that articulates how your organization's programs fit into the company's giving rationale should be prepared.

Ultimately, the more you know about a company, the better your chance of obtaining support. A company should not be approached without some knowledge of its business activities or past giving history, as that may jeopardize your chances of receiving funding. This does not mean that corporations without a record of grantmaking should be ignored. Creative fundraisers have found ways of encouraging companies of all sizes, from small businesses to large corporations, to assist in their activities. Success in acquiring such support, however, is usually the result of good research and good contacts. The job of the corporate fundraiser is to be imaginative and thorough, calling on all the knowledge, people, and ideas available. It means learning where to ask, how to ask, and what to ask.

SOURCES OF INFORMATION

Foundation Center publications examine giving interests in two broad ways: what the grantmaker states as its purpose and what can be observed from a listing of its actual grants. In preparing *Funding in Aging: A Guide to Giving by Foundations, Corporations, and Charitable Organizations* we drew on five important tools to identify grantmakers with a specific interest in programs serving the elderly in addition to those that make contributions for related projects as part of a broader giving program:

1. *The Foundation Directory* provides descriptions of the nation's largest foundations (those with assets of $2 million or more or annual giving of at least $200,000). The statements of purpose for each foundation listed in the *Directory* are drawn from the descriptions provided by foundations in their annual reports, informational brochures or other publications, responses to our annual questionnaire mailings, and a broad analysis of the foundation's grantmaking program over the last three years. Although some of these statements provide very specific information about the foundation's giving interests, many were developed to last for substantial periods of time and, thus, left purposely broad to allow for future shifts in emphasis. To illustrate a foundation's giving pattern, lists of up to ten selected grants are included, whenever available, for foundations with annual giving of at least $50,000.

2. *The Foundation Directory Part 2* provides information on the second tier of U.S. grantmaking foundations, those with assets between $1 million and $2 million, or annual grantmaking between $50,000 and $200,000. Like the *Directory*, the *Directory Part 2* provides lists of up to ten selected grants whenever available.

3. The *National Directory of Corporate Giving* is the source of information on corporate grantmakers. The fourth edition of the directory, published in 1995, profiles 2,256 companies making contributions to nonprofit organizations. It includes entries describing 669 direct corporate giving programs and 1,972 corporate foundations. The most comprehensive directory on corporate giving available, it lists only corporations that provided information to the Center or for which public documents on giving were available.

4. The Center's *Foundation Grants Index* database, which records actual grants of $10,000 or more reported to the Center by approximately 1,020 major foundations, provides a more detailed picture of foundation giving interests. Each grant record includes the name and location of the organization receiving the grant, the amount of money awarded, and a brief description of the purpose for which the grant was made. Center staff analyze and index each grant by subject focus, type of organization receiving the grant, the type of support provided, and the special population group, if any, to be served by the program.

5. *The National Directory of Grantmaking Public Charities* contains information on over 800 public charities, including 450 community foundations, all of which offer some form of financial support to nonprofit organizations or individuals, whether it be grants, scholarships, fellowships, loans, or in-kind gifts. To qualify as a public charity an organization must meet IRS requirements of receiving at least 30 percent of its income from public sources related to its exempt purpose, and receiving no more than 30 percent of support from investments and unrelated business income. The grantmaking status of each public charity was verified by questionnaire, telephone, or other reliable public sources. The directory also includes, whenever available, descriptions of up to 25 selected grants which provide an indication of giving interests.

In addition to these sources, separate mail and telephone surveys were conducted, in particular to solicit information on the publicly supported organizations included in this edition.

DESCRIPTIVE DIRECTORY OF GRANTMAKERS

ALABAMA

1
Anna & Seymour Gitenstein Foundation
P.O. Box 327
Florala 36442

Established in 1963 in AL.
Donor(s): Seymour Gitenstein.
Financial data (yr. ended 03/31/94): Assets, $147,543 (M); expenditures, $448,514; qualifying distributions, $405,241, including $384,420 for 61 grants (high: $100,000; low: $10).
Purpose and activities: Giving primarily in the area of medical research, especially for Alzheimer's disease; support also for education, including higher education.
Fields of interest: Music; Higher education; Education; Medical research; Aging, centers & services; Aging.
Types of support: Research.
Limitations: Applications not accepted. Giving primarily in the eastern U.S. No grants to individuals.
Application information: Contributes only to pre-selected organizations.
Officer: Seymour Gitenstein, Chair. and Mgr.
EIN: 636045533
Grants for Aging:
University of Alabama, Department of Neurology, Birmingham, AL, $100,000. For Alzheimer's disease research. 94.
University of Florida Foundation, College of Medicine, Gainesville, FL, $42,000. For Alzheimer's disease research. 94.

2
Hill Crest Foundation, Inc.
310 North 19th St.
Bessemer 35020 (205) 425-5800
Contact: Jack G. Paden, Chair.

Established in 1967 in AL.
Financial data (yr. ended 06/30/94): Assets, $23,904,773 (M); expenditures, $1,405,064; qualifying distributions, $1,180,851, including $1,112,690 for 57 grants (high: $150,000; low: $1,000).
Purpose and activities: Priorities given to psychiatry and the field of mental health. Giving primarily for higher education, especially the psychiatry department of a university, and health, including mental and other health services, pharmacology, and hospitals; support also for the aged, arts and culture, a community fund, community development, and a youth organization.
Fields of interest: Arts/cultural programs; Higher education; Hospitals (general); Pharmacology; Health care; Substance abuse, services; Mental health, treatment; Mental health/crisis services; Alcoholism; Health organizations; Youth, services; Aging, centers & services; Community development; Federated giving programs; Aging.
Types of support: Capital campaigns, building/renovation, equipment, endowment funds, program development, professorships, publication, seed money, scholarship funds, research, technical assistance, matching funds.
Limitations: Giving limited to AL. No grants to individuals.
Publications: 990-PF.
Application information: Application form not required.
Initial approach: Letter
Copies of proposal: 8
Deadline(s): None
Board meeting date(s): Quarterly
Officers and Trustees:* Jack G. Paden,* Chair.; Charles R. Terry, Sr.,* Vice-Chair.; F. Brooks Yielding III,* Secy.; Hugh W. Agricola, Peter G. Cowin, Stanley E. Graham, Willard L. Hurley.
Number of staff: 2 full-time professional.
EIN: 630516927
Grants for Aging:
Methodist Home for the Aging, Birmingham, AL, $50,000. 94.

3
Terry W. Johnson and Sheron B. Johnson Charitable Trust
3900 Montclair Rd., Suite 301
Birmingham 35213
Contact: Terry W. Johnson, Trustee

Established in 1988 in AL.
Donor(s): Terry W. Johnson.
Financial data (yr. ended 12/31/93): Assets, $492,937 (M); gifts received, $2,485; expenditures, $63,984; qualifying distributions, $63,984, including $56,779 for 12 grants (high: $25,004; low: $100).
Fields of interest: Education; Children & youth, services; Youth, services; Aging, centers & services; Aging.
Limitations: Giving primarily in Birmingham, AL. No grants to individuals.
Application information: Application form required.
Deadline(s): None
Final notification: Within 2 months
Trustees: Terry W. Johnson, Jean Morris.
EIN: 570884953

4
Abraham A. Mitchell Charitable Foundation
P.O. Box 16006
Mobile 36616
Contact: Abraham A. Mitchell, Pres.

Established in 1986 in AL.
Donor(s): Abraham A. Mitchell.
Financial data (yr. ended 12/31/93): Assets, $593,142 (M); expenditures, $3,384; qualifying distributions, $2,837, including $2,837 for 5 grants (high: $2,500; low: $50).
Fields of interest: Theological school/education; Health associations; Medical research; Aging, centers & services; Jewish agencies & temples; Aging.
Limitations: Applications not accepted. Giving primarily in AL. No grants to individuals.
Application information: Contributes only to pre-selected organizations.
Officers: Abraham A. Mitchell, Pres.; Mayer Mitchell, V.P.; Jay Weber, Secy.-Treas.
EIN: 630935457

5
Carol W. & Myron J. Rothschild Fund
c/o First Alabama Bank
P.O. Box 511
Montgomery 36101

Donor(s): Carol W. Rothschild.
Financial data (yr. ended 12/31/92): Assets, $883,114 (M); gifts received, $47,657; expenditures, $24,134; qualifying distributions, $18,400.
Fields of interest: Arts/cultural programs; Education; Aging, centers & services; Jewish agencies & temples; Aging; General charitable giving.
Limitations: Applications not accepted. Giving primarily in Montgomery, AL.
Application information: Contributes only to pre-selected organizations.
Trustee: First Alabama Bank.
Advisory Director: Carol W. Rothschild.
EIN: 636050756

ARIZONA

6
The Howard Bendalin Charitable Foundation Trust
4246 West Dunlap Ave.
Phoenix 85051-3654 (602) 934-9642
Contact: Howard Bendalin

Established in 1986 in AZ.
Financial data (yr. ended 02/28/95): Assets, $50,527 (M); expenditures, $3,129; qualifying distributions, $2,650, including $2,650 for grants.
Fields of interest: Jewish agencies & temples; Aging.
Types of support: Scholarship funds.
Limitations: Giving primarily in Phoenix, AZ. No grants to individuals.
Application information:
Initial approach: Letter
Deadline(s): None
Trustees: Norman Fuchs, Ron Maceyko.
EIN: 860508479

7
The Charles and Gertrude Gordon Foundation
33 North Stone Ave., No. 2100
Tucson 85701-1415 (520) 624-9983
Contact: Gerald B. Hirsch, Pres.

Established in 1988 in AZ.
Financial data (yr. ended 03/31/95): Assets, $1,705,641 (M); gifts received, $1,000; expenditures, $134,191; qualifying distributions, $102,675, including $95,275 for 25 grants (high: $20,000; low: $100).
Purpose and activities: Giving primarily to local public hospitals and public nursing homes in the Tucson, AZ, area.
Fields of interest: Hospitals (general); Nursing home/convalescent facility; Human services; Children & youth, services; Hospices.
Types of support: General/operating support, capital campaigns.
Limitations: Giving limited to the Tucson, AZ, area. No grants to individuals.
Application information: Application form not required.
Deadline(s): None
Final notification: 2 months
Officers: Gerald B. Hirsch, Pres.; Marlene P. Hirsch, V.P.; David W. Richter, Secy.; Paul J. Rachbach, Treas.
EIN: 860554595

8
Frances Moynihan Huger Foundation, Inc.
P.O. Box 34350
Phoenix 85067-4350

Established in 1994 in AZ.
Donor(s): Huger Family Trust.
Foundation type: Operating
Financial data (yr. ended 06/30/95): Assets, $372,544 (M); gifts received, $398,535; expenditures, $409,107; qualifying distributions, $396,346, including $350,000 for 1 grant, $5,902 for 2 grants to individuals (high: $5,000; low: $902) and $40,444 for 2 foundation-administered programs.
Purpose and activities: A private operating foundation; provides direct support for a resident care home for victims of Alzheimer's Disease, including payment of patients' medical bills.
Fields of interest: Alzheimer's disease.
Types of support: Grants to individuals.
Limitations: Applications not accepted. Giving limited to Phoenix, AZ.
Application information: Unsolicited requests for funds not considered.
Officers and Directors:* John J. O'Brien,* Pres.; Karmen Lee,* V.P.; Jeffrey Bray,* Secy.; Dennis Landauer,* Treas.; Ray Huger.
EIN: 860763890

ARKANSAS

9
Wal-Mart Foundation
702 S.W. Eighth St.
Bentonville 72716-8071
Contact: Ginger Sanders, Dir.

Established in 1979 in AR.
Donor(s): Wal-Mart Stores, Inc.
Foundation type: Company-sponsored
Financial data (yr. ended 01/31/94): Assets, $24,071,464 (M); gifts received, $19,124,628; expenditures, $18,292,147; qualifying distributions, $18,278,445, including $18,260,749 for grants.
Purpose and activities: Giving for health and welfare, higher education, community funds, and youth. Foundation administers two scholarship programs: 1) to high school seniors graduating from schools in towns that patronize a Wal-Mart store, and 2) to associates of Wal-Mart or their children.
Fields of interest: Higher education; Adult education—literacy & basic skills; Reading; Education; Environment; Health care; Substance abuse, services; Alcoholism; Health organizations; Food services; Safety/disasters; Children & youth, services; Youth, services; Aging, centers & services; Minorities/immigrants, centers & services; Community development; Federated giving programs; Minorities; Aging.
Types of support: Scholarship funds, scholarships—to individuals, matching funds.
Limitations: Giving primarily in areas of company operations.
Publications: Informational brochure.
Application information: Application forms for community scholarships available at high schools, and from local store managers for associate scholarships.
Deadline(s): Mar. 1 for Associate Scholarship and Walton Foundation Scholarship Programs; contact high school counselors for application dates for Community Scholarship Program
Board meeting date(s): Mar., May, Aug., and Nov.
Trustees: David D. Glass, Don Soderquist, S. Robson Walton.
Number of staff: 1 full-time professional; 4 full-time support.
EIN: 716107283

10
Windgate Charitable Foundation, Inc.
c/o Sandlin, Parham & Anderson, Ltd.
1852 East Joyce
Fayetteville 72703
Contact: John E. Brown III, Exec. Dir.
Application address: P.O. Box 1527, Bentonville, AR 72712; Tel.: (501) 273-1502

Established in 1993 in AR.
Donor(s): Dorothea W. Hutcheson.
Financial data (yr. ended 12/31/93): Assets, $31,600,132 (M); gifts received, $37,996,489; expenditures, $468,360; qualifying distributions, $463,529, including $409,960 for 4 grants (high: $225,000; low: $4,960).
Fields of interest: Arts education; Elementary/secondary education; Recreation, community facilities; Children, day care; Family services; Christian agencies & churches; Aging.
Types of support: Program development, seed money, matching funds.
Limitations: No grants to individuals, or for endowments, undesignated annual funds, debt retirement, completed projects, or group travel for performance or competition.
Publications: Application guidelines.
Application information: Application form required.
Initial approach: Proposal
Copies of proposal: 1
Deadline(s): None
Board meeting date(s): Varies
Officer: John E. Brown III, Exec. Dir.
Directors: Robyn Horn, Karen Hutcheson, Mary E. Hutcheson, Richard Hutcheson, William L. Hutcheson.
Number of staff: 1 part-time professional; 1 part-time support.
EIN: 710723781

CALIFORNIA

11
Allgemeiner Deutscher Frauen-Hilfsverein
(also known as German Ladies General Benevolent Society)
P.O. Box 27101
San Francisco 94127 (415) 391-9947
Contact: Inge G. Byrnes, Secy.-Treas.

Established in 1881 in CA.
Foundation type: Operating
Financial data (yr. ended 12/31/95): Assets, $1,698,629 (M); gifts received, $26,644; expenditures, $109,515; qualifying distributions, $79,341, including $61,436 for grants to individuals.
Purpose and activities: Provides temporary assistance to needy women and children of

German descent residing in the San Francisco Bay Area, CA.
Fields of interest: Adult/continuing education; Human services; Children & youth, services; Aging, centers & services; Women, centers & services; Aging; Women; Economically disadvantaged.
Types of support: Emergency funds.
Limitations: Giving limited to the San Francisco Bay Area, CA.
Publications: Annual report.
Application information: Application form required.
Copies of proposal: 1
Deadline(s): None
Board meeting date(s): 2nd Tuesday of each month
Officers and Directors:* Christel von Rogov,* Pres.; Sigrid Jarrett,* 1st V.P.; Sigrid Heidenreich,* 2nd V.P.; Inge Byrnes,* Secy.-Treas.; Christel Anderson, Gisela Brugger, Elke Bullock, and 8 additional directors.
Number of staff: 1 part-time support.
EIN: 941528193

12
Apple Computer, Inc. Corporate Giving Program
20525 Mariani Ave., MS:38J
Cupertino 95014 (408) 974-2105

Financial data (yr. ended 12/31/95): Total giving, $6,600,000, including $600,000 for grants and $6,000,000 for in-kind gifts.
Purpose and activities: The Nonprofit Grants program gives computer grants to support collaborative efforts that involve 20 to 100 agencies. Proposals are submitted by a lead agency, which is a national or regional 501(c)(3) nonprofit that commits to support the computer-related activities of the group and that also has a history of working with the intended participants of the project. Nonprofit grants encourage collaborations and build bridges among nonprofits working on a common issue. They are intended to solve problems that cannot be approached as effective individually and that address community problems in new ways with technology. The Education Grants Program supports educational projects that use microcomputers to create new ways of learning and teaching, with a particular interest in K-12 programs for at-risk youth. The goal is to create examples of how microcomputer technology can be used to enhance instruction in ways that are difficult to do with traditional media. Collaborations between pre-school through high school grades in public and private schools across the U.S., colleges, universities, or nonprofit organizations will be considered. Recipients are tying computer technology to teaching and learning in the major curriculum areas—mathematics, science, writing, social studies, and the arts—with some incorporating interdisciplinary approaches to teaching traditional subjects. Several projects are designed to enhance the learning experience for students with special needs. Overall, the goal of the Education Grants program is to support teachers who integrate computers into the educational process in creative ways.
Fields of interest: Performing arts; Arts/cultural programs; Education; Environment; Health care; AIDS; Health organizations; AIDS research; Human services; Youth, services; Aging, centers & services; Engineering & technology; Science; Social sciences; Disabled; Aging.
Types of support: Employee volunteer services, donated equipment, in-kind gifts.
Limitations: Giving primarily in areas of company operations. No support for political, religious, discriminatory, or parent-supported organizations. No grants to individuals, or for auctions, raffles, or for athletic events.
Publications: Corporate giving report, informational brochure, application guidelines, newsletter.
Application information: Application form required.
Initial approach: Call for application and guidelines
Deadline(s): Call to find out latest deadlines
Final notification: 8 to 10 weeks after complete application is submitted
Administrators: Fred Silverman, Mgr., Community Affairs; Andrea Gooden, Prog. Mgr., Education Grants; Beverly Long, Prog. Mgr., Nonprofit Grants; Donna Mar, Prog. Mgr., Bay Area Initiative Grants; Anne McMullin, Prog. Mgr., Regional and International Progs.; Diana Henneberry, Oper. Analyst; John Statton, Community Affairs Specialist; Cristiana Mendoza, Prog. Coord.; Beatrice Socher, Areas Assoc.
Number of staff: 4 full-time professional; 4 full-time support.

13
ARCO Foundation
515 South Flower St., AP-50
Los Angeles 90071 (213) 486-3342
Contact: S.J. Giovanisci, Pres.

Incorporated in 1963 in NY.
Donor(s): Atlantic Richfield Co.
Foundation type: Company-sponsored
Financial data (yr. ended 12/31/95): Assets, $2,621,009 (M); gifts received, $4,983,999; expenditures, $10,000,000; qualifying distributions, $10,000,000, including $4,234,121 for 444 grants (high: $50,000; low: $2,500) and $5,765,879 for 15,371 employee matching gifts.
Purpose and activities: Giving primarily to programs that address the underlying causes of educational, social, and cultural disparity in American life. Early involvement in "root-cause" issues allows the foundation to test innovative models, build leadership and leverage its investments to generate the greatest return to ARCO and the society. Support largely for higher and pre-collegiate education, including minority retention programs in science and engineering; community programs, especially for low income groups, including job creation and job training programs, community economic development, neighborhood revitalization, and youth agencies; aging programs; access to the humanities and the arts; public information organizations; and environmental programs.
Fields of interest: Arts education; Performing arts; Arts/cultural programs; Higher education; Business school/education; Engineering school/education; Education, reform; Environment; Employment; Human services; Youth, services; Aging, centers & services; Community development; Engineering; Public policy, research; Minorities; Aging.
Types of support: General/operating support, equipment, land acquisition, program development, seed money, technical assistance, matching funds.
Limitations: Giving limited to areas of company operations, especially Anchorage, AK, Dallas, TX, and Los Angeles, CA. No support for sectarian religious organizations, professional associations, specialized health organizations, professional schools of art, academic art programs, university art museums, individual high school or college performing groups, or military or veterans' organizations. No grants to individuals, or for performances at colleges or universities, campus performance halls, endowment funds, annual campaigns, deficit financing, hospital or university operating funds, research, publications, building programs (except for economic revitalization in a deteriorating urban neighborhood), or conferences; no loans.
Publications: Annual report (including application guidelines), application guidelines.
Application information: Application form not required.
Initial approach: Proposal limited to 5 pages
Copies of proposal: 1
Deadline(s): None
Board meeting date(s): June and Dec.
Final notification: 4 to 6 months
Officers and Directors:* Mike R. Bowlin,* Chair.; Stephen J. Giovanisci,* Pres.; Russel G. Sakaguchi, Secy. and Exec. Dir; George S. Davis, Treas.; Ronald J. Arnault, Lodwrick M. Cook, Kenneth R. Dickerson, Anthony G. Fernandes, William E. Wade.
Staff: Annette M. Morales, Prog. Officer.
Number of staff: 2 full-time professional; 1 full-time support.
EIN: 953222292

14
Atkinson Foundation
1100 Grundy Ln., Suite 140
San Bruno 94066 (415) 876-0222
Contact: Elizabeth H. Curtis, Administrator

Incorporated in 1939 in CA.
Donor(s): George H. Atkinson,‡ Mildred M. Atkinson.‡
Financial data (yr. ended 12/31/95): Assets, $15,644,590 (M); expenditures, $809,229; qualifying distributions, $716,911, including $636,857 for 121 grants (high: $30,000; low: $500; average: $2,000-$10,000).
Purpose and activities: Primary areas of interest include the disadvantaged and the homeless, child welfare, family planning, and the handicapped. Broad purposes are to help people reach their highest potential in their spiritual and economic life and to reach self-sufficiency. Giving for social services, including youth and the aged, education, AIDS programs, the United Methodist Church and other church activities, and international development programs.

Fields of interest: Child development, education; Secondary school/education; Vocational education; Higher education; Medical school/education; Adult education—literacy & basic skills; Family planning; Substance abuse, services; Mental health/crisis services; AIDS; Alcoholism; Delinquency prevention/services; Food services; Human services; Children & youth, services; Child development, services; Family services; Hospices; Aging, centers & services; Women, centers & services; Minorities/immigrants, centers & services; Homeless, human services; International economic development; Protestant agencies & churches; Minorities; Disabled; Women; Economically disadvantaged; Africa; Latin America.
Types of support: General/operating support, continuing support, program development, seed money, scholarship funds, technical assistance.
Limitations: Giving primarily in San Mateo County, CA, for social welfare, secondary schools, and colleges; northern CA for United Methodist churches and church activities; and international grantmaking primarily in Latin America and Africa for technical assistance, population issues, and development. No support for doctoral study, elementary schools, sports groups, or national or statewide umbrella organizations. No grants to individuals directly (including scholarships), or for research, annual campaigns, travel to conferences or events, media presentations, or fundraising events; no loans.
Publications: Annual report (including application guidelines), application guidelines.
Application information: Application Cover Sheet required. Application form not required.
Initial approach: Telephone or letter
Copies of proposal: 1
Deadline(s): Mar. 31 and Aug. 31 for international grants; no set deadline for other grants
Board meeting date(s): Mar., June, Sept., and Dec.
Final notification: Within 3 months
Officers and Directors:* Duane E. Atkinson,* Pres.; Ray N. Atkinson,* V.P.; Thomas J. Henderson,* V.P.; James C. Ingwersen,* Secy.; John E. Herrell,* Treas.; Elizabeth H. Curtis,* Administrator; Lavina M. Atkinson, Linda L. Lanier, Lawrence A. Wright.
Number of staff: 1 full-time professional.
EIN: 946075613

15
The Legler Benbough Foundation

2550 Fifth Ave., Suite 132
San Diego 92103-6622 (619) 235-8099
Contact: Thomas E. Cisco, Treas.

Established in 1985 in CA.
Donor(s): Legler Benbough.
Financial data (yr. ended 12/31/94): Assets, $4,658,515 (M); gifts received, $12,000; expenditures, $253,418; qualifying distributions, $242,555, including $222,235 for 18 grants (high: $85,000; low: $17).
Purpose and activities: Giving limited to San Diego County, CA, for health associations and health care, and museums; some support for community development and facilities, and education.
Fields of interest: Museums; Elementary school/education; Education; Hospitals (general); Health care; Substance abuse, services; Health associations; Cancer; Health organizations; Cancer research; Crime/law enforcement; Children & youth, services; Hospices; Aging, centers & services; Community development; Minorities; Disabled; Aging; General charitable giving.
Types of support: Building/renovation, equipment, endowment funds, program development, scholarship funds, research.
Limitations: Giving limited the San Diego County, CA, area. No grants to individuals.
Publications: Informational brochure (including application guidelines).
Application information: Application form not required.
Initial approach: Letter
Deadline(s): Sept. 30
Board meeting date(s): Nov.
Officers and Directors:* Legler Benbough,* Pres.; Peter K. Ellsworth,* V.P. and Secy.; Thomas E. Cisco,* Treas.; Miles A. Pelky.
Number of staff: 1 part-time support.
EIN: 330105049
Grants for Aging:
Meals on Wheels, San Diego, CA, $1,356. 94.

16
The Aaron and Marie Blackman Foundation, Inc.

100 Spear St., Suite 1800
San Francisco 94105-1528 (415) 777-3001
Contact: Milton Jacobs, Dir.

Established in 1989 in CA.
Donor(s): Marie Blackman.
Financial data (yr. ended 12/31/94): Assets, $3,668,840 (M); expenditures, $236,529; qualifying distributions, $232,166, including $226,500 for 11 grants (high: $200,000; low: $500).
Fields of interest: Higher education; Nursing home/convalescent facility; Human services; Children & youth, services; Aging, centers & services; Jewish agencies & temples; Israel.
Limitations: Giving primarily in CA and Israel. No grants to individuals.
Application information: Application form not required.
Deadline(s): None
Officer and Directors:* Marie Blackman,* Pres.; Milton Jacobs, Elizabeth Landers, Herb Meiberger, Matook Nissim, Ron Solomon, Stuart Weinstein.
EIN: 943105905
Grants for Aging:
Jewish Home for the Aged, San Francisco, CA, $200,000. 94.

17
The Borinstein Family Foundation

1010 Westwood Blvd.
Los Angeles 90024-2912

Established in 1977 in CA.
Donor(s): Manuel A. Borinstein.‡
Financial data (yr. ended 12/31/95): Assets, $699 (M); gifts received, $40,000; expenditures, $40,640; qualifying distributions, $40,640, including $40,000 for 2 grants (high: $35,000; low: $5,000).
Fields of interest: Nursing home/convalescent facility; Jewish federated giving programs; Jewish agencies & temples.
Limitations: Applications not accepted. Giving primarily in CA. No grants to individuals.
Application information: Contributes only to pre-selected organizations.
Officers and Trustees:* Pearl A. Borinstein,* Pres.; Joan N. Borinstein,* V.P.; Albert Fink,* Secy.-Treas.
EIN: 953190689

18
The Bothin Foundation

P.O. Box 29906
San Francisco 94729 (415) 561-6540
Contact: Lyman H. Casey, Exec. Dir.
FAX: (415) 561-6477

Incorporated in 1917 in CA.
Donor(s): Henry E. Bothin,‡ Ellen Chabot Bothin,‡ Genevieve Bothin de Limur.‡
Financial data (yr. ended 12/31/95): Assets, $16,282,490 (M); expenditures, $1,171,919; qualifying distributions, $747,279, including $747,279 for 81 grants (high: $50,000; low: $1,000; average: $1,000-$25,000).
Purpose and activities: Giving primarily for youth, the elderly, disabled, including the learning disabled, health care, community human services and the environment; grants to arts groups are limited to those serving youth. The foundation prefers to make grants for capital or building and equipment needs.
Fields of interest: Environment; Human services; Youth, services; Child development, services; Family services; Aging, centers & services; Homeless, human services; Disabled.
Types of support: Capital campaigns, building/renovation, equipment.
Limitations: Giving primarily in CA, with emphasis on San Francisco, Marin, Sonoma, San Mateo, and Santa Barbara counties. No support for religious organizations, medical research, educational institutions (except those directly aiding the developmentally or learning disabled), or for production or distribution of films or other media presentations. No grants to individuals, or for general operating funds, endowment funds, program support, scholarships, fellowships, or conferences; no loans.
Publications: Biennial report (including application guidelines).
Application information: Application form not required.
Initial approach: Letter containing a brief outline of the project
Copies of proposal: 1
Deadline(s): 12 weeks prior to meeting
Board meeting date(s): Early to mid-Feb., June, and Oct.
Final notification: 2 to 3 months
Officers and Directors:* Genevieve Di San Faustino,* Pres.; Edmona Lyman Mansell,* 1st V.P.; A. Michael Casey,* 2nd V.P. and Corp.

Secy.; Stephanie P. MacColl, Robert L. Miller, Rhoda W. Schultz.
Number of staff: None.
EIN: 941196182

19
Briggs Foundation
6106 La Flecha, No. 205
P.O. Box 1510
Rancho Santa Fe 92067-1510
Contact: Blaine A. Briggs, Trustee

Established in 1985 in CA.
Donor(s): Blaine A. Briggs, James M. Briggs, Robert B. Briggs, Victoria L. Briggs, Thomas C. Hansch, Ruth Hempelman.
Financial data (yr. ended 07/31/95): Assets, $1,389,109 (M); gifts received, $34,587; expenditures, $89,805; qualifying distributions, $85,788, including $76,019 for 115 grants (high: $29,140; low: $25).
Purpose and activities: Support only for organizations in which the trustees are personally involved or interested.
Fields of interest: Secondary school/education; Domestic violence prevention; Reproductive rights; Federated giving programs; Protestant agencies & churches; Disabled; Aging; Women; Economically disadvantaged; Homeless.
Limitations: Applications not accepted. Giving primarily in San Diego County, CA. No grants to individuals.
Application information: Contributes only to pre-selected organizations.
Trustees: Blaine A. Briggs, LaVerne S. Briggs.
Number of staff: 1 part-time support.
EIN: 330119350
Grants for Aging:
Foster Grandparents Program, San Diego, CA, $100. 95.
Senior Adult Services, San Diego, CA, $100. 95.
Senior Community Centers of San Diego, San Diego, CA, $125. 95.

20
Alix Brotman Foundation
16830 Ventura Blvd., Suite 236
Encino 91436
Contact: Robert Hartford, Treas.

Financial data (yr. ended 12/31/94): Assets, $324,277 (M); expenditures, $24,594; qualifying distributions, $21,337, including $15,000 for 1 grant.
Fields of interest: Alzheimer's disease research.
Limitations: Giving primarily in Southern CA.
Application information:
Initial approach: Proposal
Deadline(s): None
Officers and Directors:* Michael B. Sherman,* Pres.; Lowell Marks,* Secy.; Robert Hartford,* Treas.; Toni Brotman.
EIN: 952589230

21
Byer Foundation
66 Potero Ave.
San Francisco 94103
Contact: Allan G. Byer, Trustee

Established in 1995 in CA.
Donor(s): Allan G. Byer.
Financial data (yr. ended 12/31/95): Assets, $359,621 (M); gifts received, $500,000; expenditures, $145,370; qualifying distributions, $145,370, including $144,850 for 16 grants (high: $129,500; low: $250).
Fields of interest: Aging, centers & services; Jewish agencies & temples.
Limitations: No grants to individuals.
Application information:
Initial approach: Letter
Deadline(s): None
Trustees: Allan G. Byer, Marian Byer.
EIN: 943216991
Grants for Aging:
Jewish Home for the Aged, San Francisco, CA, $129,500. 95.

22
California Community Foundation
606 South Olive St., Suite 2400
Los Angeles 90014 (213) 413-4042
Contact: Sr. Prog. Secy.
FAX: (213) 383-2046

Established in 1915 in CA by bank resolution.
Foundation type: Community
Financial data (yr. ended 06/30/95): Assets, $171,092,879 (M); gifts received, $50,367,611; expenditures, $18,030,879, including $12,633,499 for grants (high: $1,048,250; low: $100; average: $1,500-$5,000), $527,543 for 247 grants to individuals (high: $15,000; low: $100; average: $100-$15,000), $6,152 for 32 employee matching gifts and $723,261 for 75 program-related investments.
Purpose and activities: Giving in the areas of arts and culture, civic affairs, community education, health and medicine, human services, children and youth, community development, animal welfare, and the environment.
Fields of interest: Arts/cultural programs; Education; Environment; Animal welfare; Health care; AIDS; AIDS research; Domestic violence prevention; Housing/shelter, development; Human services; Children & youth, services; Youth, services; Aging, centers & services; Race/intergroup relations; Community development; Public affairs; Asians/Pacific Islanders; African Americans; Latinos; Native Americans; Disabled; Aging; Women; People with AIDS (PWAs); Gays/lesbians; Immigrants/refugees; Economically disadvantaged; Homeless.
Types of support: Emergency funds, program development, seed money, technical assistance, program-related investments/loans, matching funds.
Limitations: Giving limited to the greater Los Angeles County, CA, area. No support for sectarian purposes. No grants for building funds, annual campaigns, equipment, endowment funds, debt reduction, operating budgets, scholarships, fellowships, films, conferences, dinners, or special events.
Publications: Annual report (including application guidelines), application guidelines, informational brochure, newsletter.
Application information: Application form required.
Initial approach: Request for application form
Copies of proposal: 1
Deadline(s): Sept. 1 or Mar. 1 for Community Development, Human Services, and Children, Youth and Families; Dec. 1 and June 1 for most other programs
Board meeting date(s): Quarterly
Final notification: 5 months after application deadline
Officers: Jack Shakely, Pres.; Linda Shestock, Exec. V.P. and C.F.O.; Joe Lumarda, V.P., Development and Communications; Judith A. Spiegel, V.P., Progs.
Board of Governors: David A. Peters, Chair.; Linda Griego, Nini Moore Horn, Paul C. Hudson, Vilma S. Martinez, Carl N. McKinzie, Olivia E. Mitchell, Ki Suh Park, William F. Podlich, Bruce M. Ramer, Virgil P. Roberts, Richard J. Sadowski, Tony M. Salazar, John C. Siciliano, Jean French Smith, Andrea Van de Kamp, Daniel L. Villanueva, Esther Wachtell, Ruth K. Watanabe.
Staff: Terri Jones, Dir., Special Projects; Ken Gregorio, Sr. Prog. Officer; Cheryl Mendoza, Prog. Officer; Virginia Victorin, Prog. Officer; Juana Kennedy, Prog. Consultant.
Number of staff: 13 full-time professional; 2 part-time professional; 11 full-time support.
EIN: 953510055
Grants for Aging:
California Advocates for Nursing Home Reform, San Francisco, CA, $29,065. To promote access for Los Angeles residents to pre-placement services helping elderly and families obtain appropriate nursing home services and improve quality of care received by elderly. 95.
Gordon Street Neighborhood Coalition, Pomona, CA, $25,000. For community garden, neighborhood watch program, activities for senior citizens and children and housing rehabilitation. 95.

23
The Callison Foundation
1493 Beach Park Blvd., No. 295
Foster City 94404
Contact: Gerald Hing, Secy.

Established in 1965 in CA.
Donor(s): Ferd W. Callison.‡
Financial data (yr. ended 12/31/94): Assets, $5,434,493 (M); gifts received, $457,864; expenditures, $353,999; qualifying distributions, $285,870, including $285,870 for 24 grants (high: $30,000; low: $5,000).
Fields of interest: Arts/cultural programs; Hospitals (general); Human services; Youth, services; Aging, centers & services; Roman Catholic agencies & churches; Disabled; Aging.
Types of support: General/operating support.
Limitations: Giving primarily in San Francisco, CA. No grants to individuals.
Publications: 990-PF.

Application information: Application form required.
Initial approach: Proposal
Deadline(s): Aug. 1
Board meeting date(s): Varies
Officers and Directors:* Mort Pactor,* Pres.; Gerald Hing,* Secy.; Peter O'Hara,* Treas.; Ward Ingersoll, Frances M. Smith.
Number of staff: None.
EIN: 946127962

24
Coast Federal Bank Giving Program

1000 Wilshire Blvd.
Los Angeles 90017-2457 (213) 362-2136
Contact: David W. Porges, V.P. and Dir., Public Affairs

Established in 1935 in Los Angeles, CA.
Financial data (yr. ended 12/31/94): Total giving, $300,000, including $300,000 for 300 grants (high: $25,000; low: $50).
Purpose and activities: Supports the elderly, children, and low-income housing issues.
Fields of interest: Housing/shelter, development; Children, services; Aging, centers & services; Aging.
Types of support: Annual campaigns, capital campaigns, building/renovation, emergency funds, employee volunteer services, loaned talent, public relations services.
Limitations: Giving limited to CA.
Publications: Corporate report.
Application information: Public Affairs Department handles giving. Application form not required.
Initial approach: Letter of inquiry only; send requests to headquarters
Copies of proposal: 1
Deadline(s): None
Board meeting date(s): Varies

25
Coastal Community Foundation

P.O. Box 230415
Encinitas 92023-0415 (619) 942-9245
Contact: Sharon Omahen, Exec. Dir.

Established in 1986 in CA.
Foundation type: Community
Financial data (yr. ended 06/30/95): Assets, $71,801 (L); gifts received, $32,945; expenditures, $36,199, including $15,271 for grants (high: $500; low: $75; average: $50-$1,000).
Fields of interest: Visual arts; Performing arts; Theater; Historic preservation/historical societies; Arts/cultural programs; Elementary/secondary education; Environment; Mental health/crisis services; Human services; Children & youth, services; Family services; Homeless, human services; Aging; General charitable giving.
Types of support: General/operating support, continuing support, annual campaigns, equipment, program development, seed money, curriculum development, scholarship funds, matching funds.
Limitations: Giving limited to the north coastal San Diego County, CA, area, including Del Mar, Solana Beach, Encinitas, Rancho Santa Fe, La Costa, and Carmel Valley. No grants to individuals.
Publications: Informational brochure, grants list, financial statement, 990-PF, newsletter.
Application information: Application form required.
Initial approach: Letter or telephone
Copies of proposal: 3
Deadline(s): None
Board meeting date(s): Bi-monthly
Officers and Directors:* Lou Aspell,* Pres.; Sue Hartley,* V.P.; Veronica Seay,* Secy.; Helmut Kiffman,* Treas.; Sharon Omahen, Exec. Dir.; Jim Baumann, Carolyn Cope, Bill Dean, Pastor Bill Harman, Sandy Munroe, Jeanne Orphan, Dee Rich, Michele Riley.
Number of staff: 1 part-time professional.
EIN: 330216692

26
Community Advantage Foundation

23092 Mill Creek Rd.
Laguna Hills 92653

Financial data (yr. ended 12/31/92): Assets, $2,417 (M); expenditures, $59,490; qualifying distributions, $36,000, including $36,000 for 1 grant.
Fields of interest: Aging, centers & services; Aging.
Limitations: Applications not accepted.
Application information: Contributes only to pre-selected organizations.
Officers: Don Bomeisler, Pres.; Bill Von Gremp, Secy.
EIN: 953135255

27
Consolidated Freightways Corporate Contributions Program

3240 Hillview Ave.
Palo Alto 94304 (415) 494-2900
Contact: Henry A. Schmitt, Asst. V.P. and Dir., Corp. Rels.

Purpose and activities: Company primarily supports health and human services. Support also for higher education, including scholarships, civic and community affairs, and culture and the arts.
Fields of interest: Arts/cultural programs; Higher education; Hospitals (general); Health care; Health organizations; Human services; Youth, services; Aging, centers & services; Government/public administration; Disabled; Aging.
Types of support: General/operating support, program development, matching funds.
Limitations: No support for political, religious, veterans', labor, fraternal, atheletic and social clubs and organizations or for recipients of United Way funds. No grants to individuals or for endowment funds, capital programs except for pre-selected locations with major operating areas, fundraising events, advertising or travel.
Publications: Application guidelines.
Application information:
Initial approach: Letter or proposal
Deadline(s): Applications accepted throughout the year
Board meeting date(s): Quarterly
Final notification: 3 months

28
James S. Copley Foundation

7776 Ivanhoe Ave.
P.O. Box 1530
La Jolla 92038-1530 (619) 454-0411
Contact: Anita A. Baumgardner, Secy.

Incorporated in 1953 in CA.
Donor(s): The Copley Press, Inc.
Foundation type: Company-sponsored
Financial data (yr. ended 12/31/95): Assets, $22,650,285 (M); gifts received, $13,857; expenditures, $1,315,484; qualifying distributions, $1,212,885, including $1,172,025 for 123 grants (average: $500-$10,000) and $40,860 for 188 employee matching gifts.
Purpose and activities: Support for higher and secondary education, including an employee matching gift program, performing arts groups and other cultural programs, community funds, journalism, social services, hospices and hospitals, the aged, and youth and child development.
Fields of interest: Journalism & publishing; Museums; Performing arts; Dance; Theater; Music; Arts/cultural programs; Child development, education; Elementary school/education; Secondary school/education; Higher education; Adult education—literacy & basic skills; Libraries/library science; Reading; Education; Hospitals (general); Health care; Substance abuse, services; AIDS; Health organizations; Recreation; Human services; Youth, services; Child development, services; Hospices; Aging, centers & services; Homeless, human services; Federated giving programs; Aging; Homeless.
Types of support: Capital campaigns, building/renovation, equipment, land acquisition, endowment funds, scholarship funds, employee matching gifts.
Limitations: Giving primarily in immediate circulation areas of company newspapers: San Diego, Torrance, San Pedro, and Santa Monica in CA; and Aurora, Elgin, Joliet, Springfield, Lincoln, Naperville, Plainfield, and Waukegan in IL. No support for religious, fraternal, or athletic organizations, government agencies, local chapters of national organizations, or public elementary or secondary schools. No grants to individuals, or for research, publications, conferences, unrestricted purposes, operating budgets, or large campaigns; no loans.
Publications: Informational brochure (including application guidelines).
Application information: Application form not required.
Initial approach: Letter
Copies of proposal: 1
Deadline(s): Delivered by Jan. 2 for Feb. meeting
Board meeting date(s): Feb. and as required
Final notification: 2 to 3 weeks
Officers and Directors:* Helen K. Copley,* Chair.; David C. Copley,* Pres.; Robert F. Crouch, V.P.; Alex De Bakcsy,* V.P.; Karl ZoBell, V.P.; Anita A. Baumgardner,* Secy.; Charles F. Patrick,* Treas.

Number of staff: None.
EIN: 956051770

29
Danish Cheer Committee, Inc.
1557 Lakewood Way
Upland 91786

Financial data (yr. ended 12/31/94): Assets, $146,239 (M); gifts received, $6,130; expenditures, $7,964; qualifying distributions, $7,964, including $2,000 for 1 grant and $3,077 for 69 grants to individuals (high: $100; low: $10).
Fields of interest: Aging; Economically disadvantaged.
Types of support: Grants to individuals.
Limitations: Giving primarily in CA.
Application information:
Initial approach: Letter
Deadline(s): None
Officers: Kate Krake Nielsen, Pres.; Carlo Christensen, 1st V.P.; Karl Duus, 2nd V.P.; Lillian Mathiesen, Secy.; Svend Ingerslev, Treas.
EIN: 956066174

30
Carrie Estelle Doheny Foundation
911 Wilshire Blvd., Suite 1750
Los Angeles 90017 (213) 488-1122
Contact: Robert A. Smith III, Pres., Carrie Estelle Doheny Foundation Corp.
FAX: (213) 488-1544

Trust established in 1949 in CA.
Donor(s): Mrs. Edward L. Doheny.‡
Financial data (yr. ended 12/31/94): Assets, $103,947,209 (M); expenditures, $6,344,142; qualifying distributions, $5,527,106, including $5,392,704 for 118 grants (high: $1,507,360; low: $1,500; average: $2,500-$10,000).
Purpose and activities: The foundation was established for the "advancement of education, medicine, religion, science; the improvement of the health and welfare of infants, children, adults, families, and the aged; the help and care of the sick, aged, and incapacitated; and the aid of the needy."
Fields of interest: Elementary/secondary education; Higher education; Hospitals (general); Eye disease; Medical research; Eye research; Children & youth, services; Family services; Aging, centers & services; Roman Catholic agencies & churches; Religion; Disabled; Aging.
Types of support: General/operating support.
Limitations: Giving primarily in the Los Angeles, CA, area. No support for tax-supported organizations or radio or television programs. No grants to individuals, or for endowment funds, publications, travel, advertising, or scholarships.
Publications: Annual report (including application guidelines).
Application information: Application form not required.
Initial approach: Letter
Copies of proposal: 1
Deadline(s): None
Board meeting date(s): Monthly
Final notification: 1 to 3 months
Trustee: Carrie Estelle Doheny Foundation Corp.
Officers and Directors:* Robert A. Smith III,* Pres.; Arthur E. Thunell, Secy.-Treas.; Robert F. Erburu, Austin F. Gavin, George Gibbs, Joseph Nally, Rev. F. David Pansini, C.M., Mrs. Terry Seidler.
Staff: Shirley M. Bernard, Grants Coord.
Number of staff: 1 full-time professional; 1 part-time support.
EIN: 952051633
Grants for Aging:
Hospitaller Foundation of California, Los Angeles, CA, $25,000. 94.
Nazareth House, Los Angeles, CA, $10,000. 94.
Saint Josephs Convalescent Hospital, Ojai, CA, $22,500. 94.
Saint Vincent Senior Citizen Nutrition Program, Los Angeles, CA, $10,000. 94.

31
The Richard F. Dwyer and Eleanor W. Dwyer Fund for Excellence
(Formerly American Foundation for Oceanography)
c/o Allan Lasher
321 Las Casas
Pacific Palisades 90272

Established in 1953.
Donor(s): Darlene Lasher, Allan Lasher, Richard F. Dwyer.
Financial data (yr. ended 06/30/95): Assets, $4,319,837 (M); gifts received, $2,242; expenditures, $233,650; qualifying distributions, $218,800, including $218,800 for 26 grants (high: $50,000; low: $1,000).
Fields of interest: Orchestra (symphony); Mental health, treatment; Cancer research; Housing/shelter, homeless; Aging; Women; Economically disadvantaged; Homeless.
Limitations: Applications not accepted. Giving primarily in CA. No grants to individuals.
Application information: Contributes only to pre-selected organizations.
Officers and Directors:* Carole Greene,* Pres.; Allan Lasher,* V.P. and Secy.; Michael Parker,* Treas.
EIN: 956027788

32
Lucius & Eva Eastman Fund, Inc.
5926 Fiddletown Place
San Jose 95120 (408) 924-2401
Contact: Lucius R. Eastman, Jr., Pres.
For East Coast contact: Jennifer Eastman, 48 Lakeshore Dr., Westwood, MA 02090; Tel.: (617) 326-7922; FAX: for West Coast (408) 268-2083

Established in 1946 in NY.
Donor(s): Eva Hills Eastman,‡ Lucius R. Eastman.‡
Financial data (yr. ended 12/31/94): Assets, $2,233,851 (M); gifts received, $423,514; expenditures, $132,402; qualifying distributions, $112,940, including $91,300 for 42 grants (high: $4,000; low: $500).
Fields of interest: Media/communications; Film/video; Theater; Aging, centers & services; Women, centers & services; Aging; Women.
Types of support: Seed money, matching funds.
Limitations: No grants to individuals.
Application information: Application form not required.
Deadline(s): None
Board meeting date(s): Quarterly
Officer: Lucius R. Eastman, Jr., Pres.
Number of staff: None.
EIN: 131958483

33
Elks of Los Angeles Foundation Fund
c/o Wells Fargo Bank, N.A.
333 South Grand
Los Angeles 90071
Contact: Lee S. Linden, Pres.
Mailing address: 5013 Dobkin Ave., Tarzana, CA 91356

Established in 1929 in CA.
Donor(s): Louis J. Christopher Trust, members of the Hirsch Family.
Financial data (yr. ended 12/31/94): Assets, $2,783,069 (M); gifts received, $70,394; expenditures, $227,250; qualifying distributions, $188,159, including $188,159 for 46 grants (high: $9,000; low: $2,500).
Purpose and activities: Giving limited to community-based charities in the greater Los Angeles, CA, area.
Fields of interest: Medical research; Children & youth, services; Youth, services; Child development, services; Family services; Aging, centers & services; Homeless, human services.
Limitations: Applications not accepted. Giving limited to Los Angeles, CA. No grants to individuals.
Application information: Contributions limited to local charities already known to the foundation; requests for funds from ineligible organizations not considered.
Officer: Lee S. Linden, Pres.
Trustee: Wells Fargo Bank, N.A.
EIN: 956019849

34
Max Factor Family Foundation
9777 Wilshire Blvd., Suite 1015
Beverly Hills 90212 (310) 274-8193
Contact: Barbara Factor Bentley, Trustee

Trust established in 1941 in CA.
Donor(s): Members of the Factor family.
Financial data (yr. ended 12/31/95): Assets, $11,989,878 (M); expenditures, $771,076; qualifying distributions, $781,791, including $721,500 for 22 grants (high: $237,500; low: $1,000; average: $1,000-$50,000).
Fields of interest: Medicine/medical care, fund raising; Hospitals (general); Eye disease; Jewish federated giving programs; Aging.
Types of support: General/operating support, continuing support, building/renovation, scholarship funds, research.
Limitations: Giving primarily in Southern CA. No grants to individuals.
Application information:
Initial approach: Letter
Deadline(s): None
Board meeting date(s): Monthly

Trustees: Barbara Factor Bentley, Gerald Factor, Max Factor III.
Number of staff: 3 part-time professional.
EIN: 956030779
Grants for Aging:
Jewish Home for the Aged, Los Angeles, CA, $60,000. 95.
Jewish Homes for the Aging of Greater Los Angeles, Reseda, CA, $30,000. 94.

35
Freeman E. Fairfield Foundation
3610 Long Beach Blvd.
P.O. Box 7798
Long Beach 90807 (310) 427-7219
Contact: Edna E. Sellers, Trustee

Established in 1969 in CA.
Donor(s): Freeman E. Fairfield.‡
Financial data (yr. ended 12/31/95): Assets, $4,510,274 (M); expenditures, $284,078; qualifying distributions, $245,423, including $213,925 for 19 grants (high: $35,000; low: $1,000; average: $3,250-$37,500).
Purpose and activities: Primary areas of interest include the elderly and child development, especially day nursery programs and boys and girls clubs.
Fields of interest: Performing arts; Child development, education; Dental care; Health care; Mental health, treatment; Cancer; Alcoholism; Cancer research; Youth development, centers & clubs; Human services; Youth, services; Child development, services; Hospices; Aging, centers & services; Disabled; Aging.
Types of support: General/operating support, building/renovation, equipment, program development, matching funds.
Limitations: Giving limited to Long Beach and Signal Hill, CA. No support for religious purposes. No grants to individuals, or for endowment funds, unrestricted operating costs, deficit financing, intermediary funding agencies, or general fundraising drives.
Publications: Program policy statement, application guidelines, 990-PF (including application guidelines).
Application information: Application form required.
Initial approach: Proposal
Copies of proposal: 3
Deadline(s): May 1
Board meeting date(s): As required
Final notification: July 1
Trustees: Pierre E. Auw, Glenn J. Conway, Edna E. Sellers.
Number of staff: 1 part-time support.
EIN: 237055338

36
FHP Foundation
401 East Ocean Blvd., Suite 206
Long Beach 90802-4933 (310) 590-8655
Contact: Mary Ellen Courtright, Prog. Officer
FAX: (310) 495-0317

Established in 1985 in CA.
Financial data (yr. ended 06/30/94): Assets, $69,587,229; gifts received, $15,516,703; expenditures, $2,703,811; qualifying distributions, $2,307,599, including $1,911,534 for grants.
Purpose and activities: Support for direct delivery of health care services including health education programs, programs for the elderly and chronically ill, primary care projects in underserved areas, and for educational and research activities.
Fields of interest: Education; Health care; Aging, centers & services; Aging.
Types of support: Program development, technical assistance.
Limitations: Giving limited to Southern CA, with the exception of occasional specific program requests that are solicited by the foundation. No support for biomedical research or programs that solely provide or distribute food. No grants to individuals, or for capital expenditures, "bricks and mortar" or building campaigns.
Publications: Annual report, application guidelines, newsletter, occasional report, informational brochure (including application guidelines).
Application information: Inquiries by FAX not accepted. Application form not required.
Initial approach: Letter of inquiry (no more than 10 pages)
Copies of proposal: 1
Deadline(s): July 15
Board meeting date(s): Mar., June, Sept., and Dec.
Final notification: After board meetings
Officers and Directors:* John T. Knox,* Chair.; Joseph F. Prevratil,* C.E.O. and Pres.; Len Hughes Andrus, M.D., Robert C. Maxson, J. W. Peltason, Westcott W. Price III, Renee B. Simon, Harriett M. Wieder.
Staff: Mary Ellen Courtright, Prog. Officer; Sandra Lund Gavin, Dir., Special Projects.
Number of staff: 3 full-time professional; 1 full-time support; 1 part-time support.
EIN: 330133359

37
Fireman's Fund Foundation
(Formerly Fireman's Fund Insurance Company Foundation)
777 San Marin Dr.
P.O. Box 777
Novato 94998-1406 (415) 899-2757
Contact: Barbara B. Friede, Dir.

Incorporated in 1953 in CA.
Donor(s): Fireman's Fund Insurance Co., and subsidiaries.
Foundation type: Company-sponsored
Financial data (yr. ended 12/31/94): Assets, $106,335 (M); gifts received, $999,999; expenditures, $1,010,269; qualifying distributions, $1,098,636, including $857,996 for 633 grants (high: $30,000; low: $100; average: $5,000-$10,000), $140,640 for 505 employee matching gifts and $100,000 for in-kind gifts.
Purpose and activities: Giving primarily to human service agencies, including the aged, the disabled, substance abuse programs, rehabilitation, and youth groups; and civic and cultural activities. Grants also for United Way campaigns nationwide in cities where principal company offices are located. Giving for education is done via the employee gift matching program only.
Fields of interest: Visual arts; Museums; Performing arts; Dance; Theater; Music; Arts/cultural programs; Child development, education; Substance abuse, services; Human services; Children & youth, services; Youth, services; Child development, services; Family services; Hospices; Aging, centers & services; Women, centers & services; Homeless, human services; Voluntarism promotion; Disabled; Aging; Women; Economically disadvantaged; Homeless.
Types of support: Equipment, program development, employee matching gifts.
Limitations: Giving primarily in the counties of San Francisco, Marin, and Sonoma, CA. No support for religious organizations for religious purposes, fraternal, veterans', sectarian, health, or national organizations, or other grantmaking bodies. No grants to individuals, or for scholarships, capital campaigns, endowment funds, medical research, travel, benefit events, video or film production, or operating expenses; no loans.
Publications: Informational brochure (including application guidelines).
Application information: Application form not required.
Initial approach: Letter
Copies of proposal: 1
Deadline(s): None
Board meeting date(s): Mar. and Dec.; distribution committee meets 4 times a year
Final notification: 3 months
Officers and Directors:* John Meyer,* Chair.; Gary E. Black,* Pres.; Barbara B. Friede,* Secy.; Harold Marsh, Treas.; Timothy Koo, Kathryn Murrell, David Pollard, Thomas E. Rowe, Joe Stinnette, Thomas A. Swanson.
Number of staff: 1 full-time professional; 1 full-time support.
EIN: 946078025

38
First Myrtle Fund
275 Battery St., Suite 960
San Francisco 94111-3332

Established in 1965 in CA.
Financial data (yr. ended 12/31/95): Assets, $523,712 (M); expenditures, $49,943; qualifying distributions, $45,000, including $45,000 for 1 grant.
Fields of interest: Humanities; History & archaeology; Arts/cultural programs; Higher education; Youth, services; Aging, centers & services; Federated giving programs; Aging.
Types of support: General/operating support.
Limitations: Applications not accepted. Giving primarily in the San Francisco Bay Area, CA. No grants to individuals.
Application information: Contributes only to pre-selected organizations.
Trustee: Fred Drexler.
EIN: 946122151

39
Myrtle V. Fitschen Charitable Trust
25 Van Ness Ave., Suite 200
San Francisco 94102
Contact: Richard Livingston, Exec. Dir.

Established about 1982 in CA.
Donor(s): Myrtle V. Fitschen.‡
Financial data (yr. ended 11/30/94): Assets, $1,242,710 (M); expenditures, $129,879; qualifying distributions, $89,510, including $89,000 for 13 grants (high: $12,000; low: $1,500).
Purpose and activities: Support for health and related services for the elderly residents of San Francisco, including medical, dental, hospital, psychological, educational, and social assistance.
Fields of interest: Health care; Human services; Aging, centers & services; Aging.
Limitations: Giving limited to San Francisco and San Francisco County, CA. No grants to individuals.
Application information: Application form not required.
Initial approach: Proposal
Copies of proposal: 1
Deadline(s): Sept. 1
Directors: Richard Livingston, Exec. Dir.; Allan D. Bonapart, Robert Gamble, Nancy C. Lenuin, Linda Lucero, Haig G. Mardikian, Barbara Turner.
Trustee: Ricardo Hernandez.
EIN: 946551204
Grants for Aging:
Bernal Heights Frail Elderly Services Coalition, San Francisco, CA, $3,500. 94.
Centro Latino de San Francisco, San Francisco, CA, $1,500. 94.
North of Market Senior Services, San Francisco, CA, $7,500. 94.
Self Help for the Elderly, San Francisco, CA, $8,000. 94.

40
Samuel H. French III and Katharine Weaver French Fund
c/o Wells Fargo Private Banking Group
101 West Broadway, Suite 301
San Diego 92101 (619) 238-6504
Contact: Rebecca A. Cowlishaw

Established in 1986 in CA.
Financial data (yr. ended 05/31/95): Assets, $7,625,949 (M); expenditures, $445,782; qualifying distributions, $383,270, including $375,925 for 60 grants (high: $20,000; low: $1,000).
Purpose and activities: Support for a hospital, health organizations, child welfare and youth services, and the elderly.
Fields of interest: Hospitals (general); Health associations; Children & youth, services; Aging, centers & services; Aging.
Limitations: Giving limited to San Diego County, CA. No grants to individuals or for salaries.
Application information: Application form not required.
Initial approach: Letter
Copies of proposal: 1
Deadline(s): None
Board meeting date(s): Mar., June, Sept., and Dec.
Trustee: Wells Fargo Private Banking Group.
Number of staff: None.
EIN: 954111082
Grants for Aging:
Alzheimers Family Center, San Diego, CA, $2,800. 94.
Clairemont Friendship Senior Center, $2,500. 94.

41
Furthur Foundation
P.O. Box 1688
Glen Ellen 95442

Established in 1988 in CA.
Donor(s): Robert H. Weir.
Financial data (yr. ended 01/31/95): Assets, $707,129 (M); gifts received, $103,135; expenditures, $60,936; qualifying distributions, $59,503, including $55,200 for 20 grants (high: $7,500; low: $1,000).
Fields of interest: Elementary/secondary education; Education; Natural resource conservation & protection; Environment; Homeless, human services; Aging; Women; Economically disadvantaged; Homeless.
Limitations: Giving primarily in CA and OR.
Publications: Grants list, informational brochure (including application guidelines).
Application information: Application form required.
Initial approach: Letter requesting application
Copies of proposal: 1
Deadline(s): Jan. 31
Board meeting date(s): Spring
Officers and Directors:* Robert H. Weir,* Pres.; Barbara Whitestone,* Secy.-Treas.; Andre Carothers, Ram Dass, Carolyn Garcia.
Number of staff: None.
EIN: 680177715

42
John Jewett & H. Chandler Garland Foundation
P.O. Box 550
Pasadena 91102-0550
Contact: G.E. Morrow, Mgr.

Trust established in 1959 in CA.
Donor(s): Members of the Garland family.
Financial data (yr. ended 12/31/94): Assets, $238,773 (M); expenditures, $1,318,502; qualifying distributions, $1,318,259, including $1,270,540 for grants.
Purpose and activities: Support primarily for cultural and historical programs, secondary and higher education, social services, especially for the elderly, youth agencies, hospitals, and health services.
Fields of interest: Historic preservation/historical societies; Arts/cultural programs; Education; Hospitals (general); Health care; Human services; Youth, services; Aging, centers & services; Homeless, human services; Aging; Homeless.
Limitations: Giving primarily in CA, with emphasis on Southern CA. No grants to individuals, or for seed money.
Application information: Application form not required.
Initial approach: Letter only; no telephone inquiries
Copies of proposal: 1
Deadline(s): None
Board meeting date(s): 3 times per year
Final notification: After each meeting
Officer and Trustees:* G.E. Morrow,* Mgr.; Ann Kelsey Babcock, Gwendolyn Garland Babcock, John Carlile Babcock, Sarah Garland Babcock, Susan Hinman Babcock, William May Garland III, Hillary Garland Ritcheson.
Number of staff: None.
EIN: 956023587

43
The Carl Gellert and Celia Berta Gellert Foundation
(Formerly The Carl Gellert Foundation)
1169 Market St., Suite 808
San Francisco 94103 (415) 255-2829
Contact: Peter J. Brusati, Secy.

Incorporated in 1958 in CA.
Donor(s): Carl Gellert,‡ Gertrude E. Gellert,‡ Celia Berta Gellert, Atlas Realty Co., Pacific Coast Construction Co.
Financial data (yr. ended 11/30/95): Assets, $11,471,647 (M); expenditures, $882,502; qualifying distributions, $842,942, including $784,785 for 110 grants (high: $73,025; low: $760; average: $1,000-$10,000).
Purpose and activities: Support for the aged, medical research, drug abuse programs, and hospitals; grants also for Roman Catholic church support; higher, secondary, and elementary education, including engineering and scholarship funds; and community development programs and social service agencies, including family planning.
Fields of interest: Elementary school/education; Secondary school/education; Higher education; Engineering school/education; Education; Hospitals (general); Family planning; Substance abuse, services; Medical research; Human services; Aging, centers & services; Community development; Engineering; Roman Catholic agencies & churches; Aging; General charitable giving.
Types of support: General/operating support, continuing support, annual campaigns, capital campaigns, building/renovation, equipment, endowment funds, debt reduction, program development, publication, scholarship funds, research.
Limitations: Giving limited to the nine counties of the greater San Francisco Bay Area, CA. No grants to individuals, or for seed money, emergency funds, land acquisition, matching gifts, or conferences; no loans.
Publications: 990-PF, program policy statement, application guidelines.
Application information: Application form not required.
Initial approach: Proposal
Copies of proposal: 1
Deadline(s): Submit proposal preferably in Aug.; deadline Oct. 1
Board meeting date(s): Apr. and Nov.
Final notification: Nov. 30, positive responses only

Officers and Directors:* Fred R. Bahrt,* Pres.; Robert L. Pauly,* V.P.; Peter J. Brusati,* Secy.; Robert J. Grassilli,* Treas.; Andrew A. Cresci.
Number of staff: 1 full-time professional; 1 full-time support.
EIN: 946062858
Grants for Aging:
Independent Living Resource Center, San Francisco, CA, $2,500. For Elder Independence program. 95.

44
The Fred Gellert Foundation
One Embarcadero Ctr., Suite 2480
San Francisco 94111-5994 (415) 433-6174
Contact: Fred Gellert, Jr., Chair.
Environmental funding inquiries: contact Jacqueline Young, Charitable Contribs. Consultant; Tel.: (415) 668-1119

Established in 1958 in CA.
Donor(s): Fred Gellert, Sr.‡
Financial data (yr. ended 11/30/95): Assets, $11,324,559 (M); expenditures, $1,036,111; qualifying distributions, $925,036, including $883,050 for 122 grants (high: $50,000; low: $1,000; average: $1,000-$5,000).
Purpose and activities: "Support for programs in the following categories: health care, the disabled, social services, community services, education, arts, youth and senior services. The trustees have allocated one quarter of funds for local and national groups organized to find solutions for a healthy planet. Of particular interest are environmental organizations working to balance human numbers with the earth's resources and organizations forming coalitions to make environmental quality a national priority."
Fields of interest: Arts/cultural programs; Education; Natural resource conservation & protection; Environment; Hospitals (general); Family planning; Health care; Mental health/crisis services; Human services; Youth, services; Family services; Aging, centers & services; Community development; Disabled; Economically disadvantaged.
Types of support: General/operating support, continuing support, building/renovation, equipment, program development, curriculum development, research.
Limitations: Giving primarily in San Francisco, San Mateo, and Marin counties, CA; giving on a local and national level for environmental grants. No grants to individuals, or for annual campaigns; no loans.
Publications: Application guidelines, financial statement, grants list.
Application information: Telephone inquiries regarding status of request are discouraged. Application form not required.
Initial approach: 1- to 3-page letter or summary
Copies of proposal: 1
Deadline(s): Feb. 1 for education, environment and population; Aug. 1 for health, youth and families.
Board meeting date(s): Apr. and Nov.
Final notification: Apr. 30 and Nov. 30
Officers and Directors:* Fred Gellert, Jr.,* Chair.; John D. Howard,* Secy.-Treas.; Annette Gellert, Lori R. Thomas.
Number of staff: 2 part-time professional.
EIN: 946062859
Grants for Aging:
Little Brothers Friends of the Elderly, $1,000. 95.

45
The William G. Gilmore Foundation
120 Montgomery St., Suite 1880
San Francisco 94104 (415) 546-1400
Contact: Faye Wilson, Secy.

Incorporated in 1953 in CA.
Donor(s): William G. Gilmore,‡ Mrs. William G. Gilmore.‡
Financial data (yr. ended 12/31/95): Assets, $15,758,964 (M); expenditures, $1,385,474; qualifying distributions, $1,284,627, including $1,194,125 for 194 grants (high: $40,000; low: $250; average: $500-$5,000).
Purpose and activities: Grants largely for community-based organizations, including development and urban affairs, family and social services, the elderly, child welfare and development, health services, medical education, AIDS programs, conservation, and the arts.
Fields of interest: Arts/cultural programs; Child development, education; Medical school/education; Education; Natural resource conservation & protection; Health care; Mental health/crisis services; AIDS; Human services; Children & youth, services; Child development, services; Family services; Hospices; Aging, centers & services; Homeless, human services; Community development; Public affairs; Disabled; Aging; People with AIDS (PWAs); Economically disadvantaged; Homeless.
Types of support: General/operating support, continuing support, annual campaigns, emergency funds, scholarship funds.
Limitations: Giving primarily in northern CA and OR. No grants to individuals.
Publications: Application guidelines.
Application information: Application form not required.
Initial approach: Proposal
Copies of proposal: 1
Deadline(s): May 1 and Nov. 1
Board meeting date(s): June and Dec.
Final notification: 2 months
Officers and Trustees:* Robert C. Harris,* Pres.; Lee Emerson,* V.P., and Treas.; William R. Mackey,* V.P.; Faye Wilson, Secy.; Thomas B. Boklund, V. Neil Fulton.
Number of staff: 1 part-time support.
EIN: 946079493
Grants for Aging:
Project Open Hand, San Francisco, CA, $30,000. 94.

46
Paul F. Glenn Foundation for Medical Research, Inc.
1250 Coast Village Rd., Suite K
Santa Barbara 93108 (805) 565-3363
Contact: Mark R. Collins, Exec. V.P.
URL: http://www.glenn.deco.net

Established in 1966 in NY; reincorporated in 1992 in AZ.
Financial data (yr. ended 09/30/95): Assets, $11,875,690 (M); gifts received, $3,754,210; expenditures, $457,076; qualifying distributions, $376,546, including $292,000 for 18 grants (high: $100,000; low: $3,000; average: $7,000) and $20,000 for 2 grants to individuals of $10,000 each.
Purpose and activities: "Grants and awards to encourage and accelerate research in molecular and cellular gerontology with the objective of delaying or preventing the onset of disease and prolonging the healthful productive years of life."
Fields of interest: Medical research; Aging, centers & services; Biological sciences; Aging.
Types of support: Conferences/seminars, fellowships, research.
Limitations: Applications not accepted. No support for sociological, as opposed to biological, aging projects.
Publications: Grants list, informational brochure, program policy statement.
Application information: The foundation does not consider unsolicited grant applications or fellowship nominations.
Officers and Directors:* Paul F. Glenn,* Chair., Pres., and Treas.; Mark R. Collins, Exec. V.P. and Secy.; Brian D. Frenzel, Jack N. Rudel.
Number of staff: 3 part-time professional.
EIN: 860710305
Grants for Aging:
American Federation for Aging Research (AFAR), NYC, NY, $50,000. For research. 94.
Institute for Advanced Studies in Immunology and Aging, DC, $1,000. For conference. 94.
Linas Pauling Institute of Science and Medicine, Palo Alto, CA, $2,000. For Therapeutical Potential of Biological Antioxidants symposium. 94.
Louisana State University, Department of Biochemistry and Molecular Biology, Baton Rouge, LA, $10,000. For aging research. 94.
Lovelace Medical Center, Albuquerque, NM, $6,000. For summer fellowships on aging. 94.
National Heart, Lung, and Blood Institute, Gerontology Society of America, Bethesda, MD, $20,000. For Glenn Award. 94.
National Institute on Aging, Bethesda, MD, $60,000. For workshop. 94.
Oklahoma Medical Research Foundation, Free Radical Biology and Aging Research, Oklahoma City, OK, $1,500. For summer aging fellowship. 94.
University of Oklahoma, Norman, OK, $10,000. For aging research. 94.

47
Richard and Rhoda Goldman Fund
One Lombard St., Suite 303
San Francisco 94111 (415) 788-1090
Contact: Duane Silverstein, Exec. Dir.
FAX: (415) 788-7890

Incorporated in 1951 in CA.
Donor(s): Rhoda H. Goldman,‡ Richard N. Goldman.
Financial data (yr. ended 12/31/95): Assets, $160,236,332 (M); expenditures, $8,920,324; qualifying distributions, $7,907,233, including $7,491,833 for grants (average: $2,500-$50,000).
Purpose and activities: Giving primarily to "programs that will have a significant positive

impact in an array of fields, including: environment, population, Jewish affairs, children and youth, and the elderly."
Fields of interest: Adult education—literacy & basic skills; Environment; Family planning; Health care; Health organizations; Children & youth, services; Youth, services; Aging, centers & services; Population studies; Jewish agencies & temples; Aging; Israel.
Types of support: Continuing support, capital campaigns, program development, seed money.
Limitations: Giving primarily in the San Francisco Bay Area, CA. No support for unsolicited proposals from arts organizations, or from primary, secondary, or higher educational institutions. No grants to individuals, or for deficit budgets, endowment funds, documentary films, conferences, research, scholarships, fellowships, matching gifts, or general operating budgets of established organizations; no loans.
Publications: Annual report (including application guidelines).
Application information: Application form not required.
Initial approach: 2-page letter
Copies of proposal: 1
Deadline(s): None
Board meeting date(s): Mar., June, Sept., and Dec.
Officers and Directors:* Richard N. Goldman,* Pres.; Duane Silverstein,* Exec. Dir.; Michael C. Gelman, Susan R. Gelman, Douglas E. Goldman, John D. Goldman, Marcia L. Goldman.
Staff: Brenda Jackson Drake, Assoc. Dir.; Amy Lyons, Prog. Exec.; Lise Miller, Communications.
Number of staff: 2 full-time professional; 2 full-time support.
EIN: 946064502
Grants for Aging:

Alzheimers Disease and Related Disorders Association of Palo Alto, Palo Alto, CA, $25,000. For Family Connections Program, providing support services to families. 94.

California Advocates for Nursing Home Reform, San Francisco, CA, $30,000. For Bay Area Consumer Information and Outreach Program, to provide training and written materials to consumers and service provides on changes in medicaid laws related to long-term care for elderly. 94.

Center for Elderly Suicide Prevention and Grief Related Services, San Francisco, CA, $24,000. For Minority Volunteer Recruitment Project, to increase number of minority volunteers for hotline, telephone outreach and visiting services for elderly. 94.

Family Caregiver Alliance, San Francisco, CA, $15,000. For Second Family Volunteer Respite Caregiver Program, to recruit and train volunteers to care for minimally brain impaired adults to allow family members needed respite. 94.

Friends for Youth, Redwood City, CA, $10,000. For expansion and diversification of volunteer base for mentoring program for at-risk youth in San Mateo County. 94.

Jewish Home for the Aged, San Francisco, CA, $75,000. To construct Howard A. Friedman Nursing Pavilion, nursing facility for frail and chronically ill residents. 94.

Meals on Wheels of San Francisco, San Francisco, CA, $75,000. For capital campaign to purchase and renovate new kitchen and administrative headquarters. 94.

Northern California Community Services Council, San Francisco, CA, $20,000. For Planning for Elders in Central City's Senior Survival School, multi-lingual program to educate seniors and caregivers on ways to access available services and resources. 94.

On Lok Senior Health Services, San Francisco, CA, $50,000. For capital campaign for Dr. William L. Gee Center, which provides housing and two adult day health centers for frail elderly and offices for On Lok's administrative staff. 94.

San Francisco Food Bank, San Francisco, CA, $10,000. For general support. 94.

Tenderloin Senior Organizing Project, San Francisco, CA, $10,000. For general support. 94.

Toward Utility Rate Normalization, San Francisco, CA, $25,000. For Energy Utility Advocacy Trainings, educating organizations serving elderly on how to advocate for better utility services. 94.

48
The Leslie and Susan Gonda Foundation

1999 Ave. of the Stars, 39th Fl.
Los Angeles 90067

Established in 1988 in CA.
Donor(s): Leslie Gonda, Susan Gonda.
Financial data (yr. ended 12/31/95): Assets, $1,552 (M); gifts received, $52,011; expenditures, $52,868; qualifying distributions, $52,868, including $41,352 for 17 grants (high: $8,800; low: $100).
Purpose and activities: Giving primarily for health associations and medical research; support also for Jewish organizations, including welfare funds and support for Israel.
Fields of interest: Medical school/education; Health associations; Human services; Jewish federated giving programs; Jewish agencies & temples; Israel; Aging.
Types of support: Capital campaigns, endowment funds, scholarship funds, research.
Limitations: Applications not accepted. Giving primarily in CA. No grants to individuals.
Application information: Contributes only to pre-selected organizations.
Officers and Directors:* Leslie Gonda,* Pres.; Larry Heller, Secy.; Alan Lund, C.F.O.; Susan Gonda.
Staff: Cheryl Zoller, Foundation Manager.
Number of staff: 1 full-time professional.
EIN: 954197904

49
Gould Family Foundation, Inc.

12067 MacDonald Dr.
Ojai 93023
Contact: Richard S. Gould, M.D., Secy.

Established in 1974 in NY.
Donor(s): Leon Gould, Mildred Gould.‡
Financial data (yr. ended 12/31/94): Assets, $1,230,906 (M); expenditures, $57,167; qualifying distributions, $57,167, including $50,260 for grants (high: $10,000; average: $500-$5,000).
Purpose and activities: Giving primarily for specific disease associations.
Fields of interest: Arts/cultural programs; Medical school/education; Education; Health associations; Medical research; Engineering & technology; Science; Aging.
Types of support: General/operating support, annual campaigns, emergency funds, seed money, research, program-related investments/loans.
Limitations: Giving primarily in CA. No grants to individuals.
Publications: Informational brochure.
Application information: Application form required for scholarships; contributions to organizations are pre-selected.
Initial approach: Letter
Copies of proposal: 1
Board meeting date(s): Jan.
Officers and Directors:* A.M. Gould,* Pres.; Richard S. Gould, M.D.,* Secy.
Number of staff: None.
EIN: 237259693

50
Stella B. Gross Charitable Trust

c/o Bank of the West
P.O. Box 1121
San Jose 95108 (408) 998-6856
Contact: Lori C. Stetzenmeyer, Trust Officer, Bank of the West
Application address: c/o Louis O'Neal, Esq., 96 North Third St., No. 620, San Jose, CA 95112; Tel.: (408) 999-5678

Trust established in 1966 in CA.
Donor(s): Stella B. Gross.‡
Financial data (yr. ended 06/30/95): Assets, $6,840,474 (M); expenditures, $309,795; qualifying distributions, $253,473, including $206,581 for 53 grants (high: $20,000; low: $500; average: $1,000-$10,000).
Fields of interest: Visual arts; Museums; Performing arts; Arts/cultural programs; Child development, education; Elementary school/education; Higher education; Education; Hospitals (general); Health care; Health associations; Cancer; Heart/circulatory disease; Cancer research; Heart/circulatory research; Human services; Children & youth, services; Child development, services; Hospices; Aging, centers & services; Roman Catholic federated giving programs; Government/public administration; Disabled; Aging.
Types of support: General/operating support, continuing support, program development, seed money.
Limitations: Giving limited to Santa Clara County, CA. No grants to individuals.
Publications: Annual report, 990-PF.
Application information: Application form not required.
Deadline(s): None
Board meeting date(s): June and Dec.
Advisors: Hon. Thomas P. Hansen, Arthur K. Lund, Louis O'Neal.
Trustee: Bank of the West.
Number of staff: None.
EIN: 237142181
Grants for Aging:

Villa Siena, Mountain View, CA, $5,000. 95.

51
The Grove Foundation

P.O. Box 645
Los Altos 94023-0645

Established in 1986 in CA.
Donor(s): Andrew S. Grove, Eva K. Grove.
Financial data (yr. ended 09/30/95): Assets, $925,169 (M); gifts received, $650,000; expenditures, $243,049; qualifying distributions, $239,542, including $237,578 for 33 grants (high: $25,500; low: $500).
Purpose and activities: Giving primarily for family planning and other social services, vocational or professional education, Jewish welfare, international refugee assistance, and the performing arts.
Fields of interest: Performing arts; Higher education; Family planning; Homeless, human services; International relief; Civil rights, advocacy; Reproductive rights; Aging; Women; Immigrants/refugees; Economically disadvantaged; Homeless.
Limitations: Applications not accepted. Giving primarily in CA. No grants to individuals.
Application information: Unsolicited requests not considered; funds are fully committed.
Officers: Andrew S. Grove, Pres.; Eva K. Grove, Secy.
Number of staff: None.
EIN: 770108124
Grants for Aging:
Project Match, San Jose, CA, $2,000. 95.

52
Evelyn and Walter Haas, Jr. Fund

One Lombard St., Suite 305
San Francisco 94111 (415) 398-3744
Contact: Lisa Arnold, Grant Administrator
FAX: (415) 986-4779

Incorporated in 1953 in CA.
Donor(s): Walter A. Haas, Jr.,‡ Evelyn D. Haas.
Financial data (yr. ended 12/31/95): Assets, $287,669,519 (M); expenditures, $9,368,441; qualifying distributions, $8,466,897, including $7,168,400 for 309 grants (high: $500,000; low: $100; average: $5,000-$75,000) and $4,805 for 18 employee matching gifts.
Purpose and activities: Emphasis on strengthening children, youth, families, and the elderly; strengthening neighborhoods and communities; reducing hunger and homelessness; and encouraging volunteer service, philanthropy, and nonprofit management assistance.
Fields of interest: Food services; Children & youth, services; Family services; Aging, centers & services; Youth development, services; Community development, neighborhood development; Economic development; Philanthropy/voluntarism; Homeless.
Types of support: General/operating support, program development, seed money, technical assistance.
Limitations: Giving primarily in San Francisco and Alameda counties, CA. No support for private foundations, consumer or professional groups, labor or trade associations, research centers, or religious organizations. No grants to individuals, or for deficit or emergency financing, workshops, major equipment, scholarships, direct mail campaigns, fundraising events, annual appeals, conferences, publications, capital or endowment campaigns, films or videos, or basic research.
Publications: Annual report (including application guidelines).
Application information: Grants in the areas of arts and education are initiated by the trustees. Application form not required.
Initial approach: 2- to 3-page letter
Copies of proposal: 1
Deadline(s): None
Board meeting date(s): 3 to 4 times a year
Final notification: Within 4 months
Officers and Trustees:* Evelyn D. Haas,* Co-Chair.; Walter J. Haas,* Co-Chair.; Ira S. Hirschfield,* Pres.; Elizabeth Haas Eisenhardt,* Secy.; Robert D. Haas,* Treas.
Number of staff: 6 full-time professional; 2 full-time support; 1 part-time support.
EIN: 946068932
Grants for Aging:
Alzheimers Disease and Related Disorders Association, San Francisco, CA, $35,000. To expand and deepen services to Bay Area Family caregivers. 94.
Alzheimers Services of the East Bay, Berkeley, CA, $75,000. For program expansion and to attract new donors. 94.
California Advocates for Nursing Home Reform, San Francisco, CA, $30,000. For general support to monitor quality of care in California nursing homes and to educate residents and their families about long-term care. 94.
Center for Elders Independence, Oakland, CA, $50,000. To start second site. 94.
Center for Elders Independence, Oakland, CA, $12,500. For coordinated system of community-based, long-term care services for frail elderly in Oakland. 94.
Congregation Emanu-El, San Francisco, CA, $100,000. For Community Service Program, range of community and congregation-based programs for people with AIDS, homeless, at-risk youth, seniors and families. 94.
Episcopal Community Service of San Francisco, San Francisco, CA, $10,000. For general support of shelter and other services ranging from transitional housing to senior services. 94.
Grandparents Who Care, San Francisco, CA, $15,000. For program coordinator to assist grandparents who are caretakers for their grandchildren. 94.
Independent Living Resource Center, San Francisco, CA, $10,000. For general support services, information and advocacy on behalf of disabled and elderly populations. 94.
Jewish Home for the Aged, San Francisco, CA, $62,500. For construction of Howard A. Friedman Pavilion. 94.
LifePlan Center, San Francisco, CA, $10,000. For start-up support for center to help people in mid-life make transition from workforce to retirement. 94.
Meals on Wheels of San Francisco, San Francisco, CA, $50,000. For capital support to purchase and renovate new headquarters. 94.
On Lok Senior Health Services, San Francisco, CA, $250,000. For capital campaign to purchase and renovate Dr. William Gee House providing low-income and frail elderly with non-institutional, community-based, long-term care services. 94.
On Lok Senior Health Services, San Francisco, CA, $11,400. For Program of All-Inclusive Care for the Elderly, technical assistance program for On Lok replication projects. 94.
Over Sixty Health Center, Oakland, CA, $25,000. For capacity-building in preparation for managed care. 94.
Planning for Elders in the Central City, San Francisco, CA, $15,000. For project to reform In-Home Supportive Services system in San Francisco. 94.
San Francisco Adult Day Health Network, San Francisco, CA, $30,000. For advocacy work. 94.
San Francisco Food Bank, San Francisco, CA, $25,000. For operating support. 94.
San Francisco Senior Action Network, San Francisco, CA, $15,000. For advocacy work. 94.
Senior Net Tri-City Community Coalition for Independent Elders, Fremont, CA, $10,000. To address the needs of southern Alameda County's elders. 94.

53
Crescent Porter Hale Foundation

220 Bush St., Suite 1069
San Francisco 94104 (415) 986-5177
Contact: Ulla Davis, Consultant

Incorporated in 1961 in CA.
Donor(s): Elwyn C. Hale,‡ M. Eugenie Hale.‡
Financial data (yr. ended 12/31/94): Assets, $21,796,669 (M); expenditures, $1,024,057; qualifying distributions, $946,517, including $822,565 for 101 grants (high: $50,000; low: $1,000; average: $10,000).
Fields of interest: Education, fund raising; Higher education; Education; AIDS; AIDS research; Children & youth, services; Aging, centers & services; Roman Catholic agencies & churches; Minorities; Aging.
Types of support: General/operating support, capital campaigns, equipment, program development, scholarship funds.
Limitations: Giving primarily in the San Francisco Bay Area, CA. No grants to individuals, or for research.
Publications: Application guidelines, program policy statement.
Application information: Application form not required.
Initial approach: Letter of intent
Deadline(s): Given after letter of intent is received
Board meeting date(s): 3 times a year
Final notification: After board meeting
Officers: L.E. Alford, Pres.; Thomas J. Mellon, Jr., V.P.; A.L. Ballard, Secy.-Treas.
Directors: Eugene E. Bleck, M.D., Joan Withers Dinner, Rev. Charles Dullea, S.J., Ephraim P. Engleman, M.D., Elfreda Hale, E. William Swanson.
Number of staff: 1 full-time professional; 1 part-time support.
EIN: 946093385

54
Harden Foundation

P.O. Box 779
Salinas 93902-0779 (408) 442-3005
Contact: Joseph C. Grainger, Exec. Dir.
Application address: 17 East Gabilan St., Salinas, CA 93901

Established in 1963 in CA.
Donor(s): Eugene E. Harden,‡ Ercia E. Harden.‡
Financial data (yr. ended 02/28/95): Assets, $46,619,948 (M); expenditures, $3,006,137; qualifying distributions, $1,612,830, including $1,337,490 for 81 grants (high: $60,000; low: $1,000; average: $10,000-$50,000).
Purpose and activities: The foundation supports projects that improve the well-being of young people; strengthen the family; develop individual self-reliance and health; prevent inappropriate institutionalization of individuals; improve the quality of life through cultural activities; encourage more humane treatment of animals; and eliminate duplication and improve coordination of social and community services.
Fields of interest: Arts/cultural programs; Higher education; Animal welfare; Health care; Mental health, treatment; Agriculture; Human services; Children & youth, services; Family services; Aging, centers & services.
Types of support: General/operating support, capital campaigns, seed money, matching funds.
Limitations: Giving limited to Monterey County, with emphasis on the Salinas Valley, CA, area. No support for sectarian religious programs, non-agricultural related educational programs; operating foundations, or associations established for the benefit of organizations receiving substantial tax support. No grants for endowments, annual campaigns, conferences, or fundraising events.
Publications: Application guidelines, annual report (including application guidelines).
Application information: Application form required.
Initial approach: Letter
Copies of proposal: 2
Deadline(s): Mar. 1 and Sept. 1
Board meeting date(s): June and Dec.
Officers and Directors:* Ralph L. Kokjer,* Pres.; C. Bill Elliot,* V.P.; Thomas Merrill,* V.P.; Patricia Tynan-Chapman,* Secy.; Frank Ferrasci, Treas.; Joseph C. Grainger, Exec. Dir.
Number of staff: 1 full-time professional; 2 part-time professional; 2 full-time support.
EIN: 946098887

55
The John Randolph Haynes and Dora Haynes Foundation

888 West Sixth St., Suite 1150
Los Angeles 90017-2737 (213) 623-9151
Contact: Diane D. Cornwell, Admin. Dir.

Trust established in 1926 in CA.
Donor(s): John Randolph Haynes,‡ Mrs. John Randolph Haynes.‡
Financial data (yr. ended 08/31/95): Assets, $42,248,188 (M); expenditures, $2,856,106; qualifying distributions, $2,540,214, including $2,540,214 for 45 grants (high: $546,000; low: $1,000; average: $60,000-$200,000).
Purpose and activities: "Promoting the well-being of mankind" by making grants for study and research in the social sciences — economics, history, government, and sociology; emphasis is placed on education, the environment, immigration and public policy. The foundation also provides undergraduate scholarships, graduate fellowships, and fellowships for faculty members in the social sciences in selected colleges and universities. Grants made only through local colleges and universities or other nonprofit institutions.
Fields of interest: History & archaeology; Education, research; Elementary school/education; Higher education; Education; Environment; Crime/law enforcement; Labor unions/organizations; Employment; Housing/shelter, development; Youth development, citizenship; Aging, centers & services; Minorities/immigrants, centers & services; Homeless, human services; Race/intergroup relations; Urban/community development; Community development; Social sciences; Anthropology & sociology; Economics; Political science; Population studies; Public policy, research; Government/public administration; Public affairs, citizen participation; Transportation; Public affairs; Minorities; Aging; Immigrants/refugees; Homeless.
Types of support: Fellowships, internships, scholarship funds, research.
Limitations: Giving limited to the greater Los Angeles, CA, area. No grants to individuals, or for building or endowment funds or operating budgets.
Publications: Informational brochure (including application guidelines).
Application information: Application form not required.
Initial approach: Letter or telephone
Copies of proposal: 20
Deadline(s): Several weeks before board meetings
Board meeting date(s): Quarterly
Final notification: 1 to 2 weeks
Officers and Trustees:* F. Haynes Lindley, Jr.,* Pres. and Secy.-Treas.; Robert R. Dockson,* 1st V.P.; Jack K. Horton,* 2nd V.P.; Philip M. Hawley, Daniel A. Mazmanian, Chauncey J. Medberry III, Donn B. Miller, Jane G. Pisano, Gilbert T. Ray.
Number of staff: 1 full-time professional; 1 part-time support.
EIN: 951644020

56
W. E. Helbling Fund

c/o Pacific Bell
2600 Camino Ramon, Rm. 2W000V
San Ramon 94583 (510) 823-6118
Application address: c/o Prudential Asset Management Co., P.O. 5340, Scranton, PA 18505-5340; Tel.: (800) 435-2435

Established in 1989 in CA.
Financial data (yr. ended 12/31/95): Assets, $1,750,766 (M); expenditures, $104,494; qualifying distributions, $82,306, including $82,306 for 42 grants to individuals (high: $8,819; low: $100).
Purpose and activities: Provides financial assistance to retirees of Pacific Telesis Group or one of its affiliates.
Fields of interest: Aging, centers & services; Aging.
Types of support: Grants to individuals.
Limitations: Giving primarily in CA.
Application information: Application form required.
Initial approach: Letter or telephone
Deadline(s): None
Officers: Chuck Maley, Pres.; J.K. Beck, Secy.; G.V. Koch, Treas.
EIN: 943096823

57
Mildred Hitchcock Huff Charitable Trust

P.O. Box LAW
Monterey 93940 (408) 649-1100
Contact: George R. Walker, Trustee

Financial data (yr. ended 06/30/95): Assets, $989,337 (M); expenditures, $63,837; qualifying distributions, $51,835, including $43,500 for grants.
Fields of interest: History & archaeology; Historic preservation/historical societies; Early childhood education; Higher education; Law school/education; Libraries/library science; Education; Animal welfare; Legal services; Youth, services; Aging, centers & services; Aging; General charitable giving.
Types of support: Annual campaigns, capital campaigns, building/renovation, equipment.
Limitations: Giving primarily in the Monterey Peninsula, CA, area. No grants to individuals.
Application information:
Initial approach: Letter
Deadline(s): May 15
Trustee: George R. Walker.
EIN: 770031703

58
The Lauralie Irvine Foundation

95 Robles Del Rio
Carmel Valley 93924 (408) 659-4490
Contact: J.J. Irvine, Pres.

Established in 1976.
Financial data (yr. ended 12/31/95): Assets, $1,144,628 (M); expenditures, $61,361; qualifying distributions, $57,050, including $57,050 for 35 grants (high: $5,000; low: $300; average: $500-$6,700).
Purpose and activities: Primary areas of interest include child welfare and development, family services, the elderly, and health services.
Fields of interest: Arts/cultural programs; Child development, education; Education; Hospitals (general); Family planning; Health care; Substance abuse, services; Health associations; AIDS; Alcoholism; AIDS research; Delinquency prevention/services; Human services; Children & youth, services; Child development, services; Family services; Aging, centers & services; Aging.
Types of support: Continuing support, capital campaigns, building/renovation, scholarship funds.

Limitations: Giving limited to Monterey and San Benito counties, CA. No support for schools or religious associations.
Publications: 990-PF, grants list, application guidelines.
Application information: Application form not required.
Initial approach: Letter
Copies of proposal: 1
Deadline(s): June 30 and Nov. 30
Board meeting date(s): July and Dec.
Final notification: Following board meetings
Officers: J.J. Irvine, Pres.; J.J. Rudolph, V.P.
Director: J.M. Merrill.
Number of staff: None.
EIN: 510159257
Grants for Aging:
Alliance on Aging, Monterey, CA, $1,000. 95.
Legal Services for Seniors, Pacific Grove, CA, $500. 95.

59
Irvine Health Foundation
18301 Von Karman Ave., Suite 440
Irvine 92715-1009 (714) 253-2959
Contact: Edward B. Kacic, Exec. Dir.
FAX: (714) 253-2962; E-mail: 102336.2265@compuserve.com;
URL: http://www.ihf.org

Established in 1985 in CA.
Donor(s): Irvine Medical Center, Inc.
Financial data (yr. ended 06/30/94): Assets, $20,709,188 (M); expenditures, $1,561,730; qualifying distributions, $1,305,473, including $890,275 for 37 grants (high: $175,000; low: $500).
Purpose and activities: Emphasis on community health care, including support for basic and applied medical research, research on health care systems and programs, and health promotion programs and clinics, including a senior care center and a drug abuse program; support also for educational therapy for learning-disabled children, and for prevention of child abuse.
Fields of interest: Child development, education; Health care; Substance abuse, services; Mental health/crisis services; AIDS; Alcoholism; Biomedicine; Health organizations; Medical research; Nutrition; Youth, services; Child development, services; Hospices; Aging, centers & services; Women, centers & services; Women; Homeless.
Types of support: Program development, seed money, research, matching funds.
Limitations: Giving limited to Orange County, CA. No support for religious organizations for religious purposes. No grants to individuals.
Publications: Multi-year report (including application guidelines), informational brochure (including application guidelines).
Application information: Application form not required.
Initial approach: Letter
Board meeting date(s): Regularly
Officers and Directors:* David G. Sills,* Chair.; Timothy L. Strader,* Vice-Chair.; Carol A. Hoffman,* Secy.; John C. Gaffney,* Treas.; Edward B. Kacic, Exec. Dir.; Gary H. Hunt, Jack W. Peltason, Ph.D., Gerald B. Sinykin, M.D.
Staff: Patricia A. Cruz, Prog. Dir.; Linda L. Wasserman, Prog. Secy.
Number of staff: 2 full-time professional; 1 part-time support.
EIN: 330141599
Grants for Aging:
Irvine Adult Day Health Service, Senior Center, Irvine, CA, $200,000. 94.

60
Italian-American Community Services Agency
(Formerly Italian Welfare Agency, Inc.)
678 Green St.
San Francisco 94133-3896

Established in 1916 in CA; classified as a private operating foundation in 1972.
Donor(s): Marini Family Trust.
Foundation type: Operating
Financial data (yr. ended 12/31/95): Assets, $2,178,882 (M); gifts received, $263,418; expenditures, $415,507; qualifying distributions, $554,586, including $166,607 for grants to individuals and $387,979 for foundation-administered programs.
Purpose and activities: Awards grants to indigent individuals, including senior citizens; support also for direct charitable programs.
Fields of interest: Aging; Economically disadvantaged.
Types of support: Grants to individuals.
Officers and Directors:* Anthony A. Barbieri,* Pres.; Donald G. Parachini,* V.P.; David T. Giannini,* Secy.; Raymond V. Beccio,* C.F.O.
EIN: 941196199

61
Jewish Federation Foundation
3801 East Willow St.
Long Beach 90815-1791 (310) 426-7601
Contact: Sandi Goldstein, Exec. Dir.

Established in 1972.
Financial data (yr. ended 03/31/95): Assets, $1,333,778 (M); gifts received, $491,176; expenditures, $324,904; qualifying distributions, $316,158, including $309,961 for grants (high: $107,200; low: $50).
Purpose and activities: Giving to programs that will benefit the Jewish community of greater Long Beach and West Orange County, CA.
Fields of interest: Higher education; Aging, centers & services; Jewish federated giving programs; Jewish agencies & temples.
Types of support: Endowment funds.
Limitations: Giving primarily in Limited to the greater Long Beach and West Orange County, CA, area. Generally no grants to individuals.
Application information: Application form required.
Deadline(s): None
Officers: Stanley Goldin, Pres.; Alex Britton, V.P.; Joseph E. Lessin, Secy.; Shirley Ross, Treas.
Directors: Ravenna Auguston, Jean Blakey, Eva Cooper, Bernard Cooperman, Miriam Lapid, Richard Lipeles, Louis Meltzer, Arthur Miller, Donna Punim, Charles Samuel, Eugene Schlesinger, Mort Stuhlbarg.
Number of staff: None.
EIN: 237397882

62
Kawaguchi-Kihara Memorial Foundation
1324-1327 East 15th St.
Los Angeles 90021
Contact: Mrs. Mitsuko Kawaguchi, Pres.

Established in 1979 in CA.
Donor(s): Fishking Processors, Inc.
Financial data (yr. ended 03/31/96): Assets, $20,404 (M); expenditures, $6,930; qualifying distributions, $6,930, including $6,850 for grants.
Purpose and activities: Support for Japanese organizations, including Buddhist temples, education, culture, and human services.
Fields of interest: Arts/cultural programs; Education; Human services; Aging, centers & services; Religion; Aging; Japan.
Limitations: Giving primarily in CA. No grants to individuals.
Application information: Application form not required.
Deadline(s): Apr. 1
Officers: Mitsuko Kawaguchi, Pres.; Norman Furukawa, V.P.; Gary Kawaguchi, Secy.; Kiyoshi Kawaguchi, Treas.
Number of staff: 1 part-time professional; 1 part-time support.
EIN: 953397616
Grants for Aging:
Keiro Nursing Home, Los Angeles, CA, $5,000. For Vision for Keiro Campaign. 94.
Keiro Services, Los Angeles, CA, $20,000. 94.

63
The King's Daughter Home Foundation
2361 East 29th St.
Oakland 94606
Contact: Exec. Dir.

Established in 1984 in CA.
Donor(s): Florence French Trust.
Financial data (yr. ended 05/31/95): Assets, $77,148 (M); gifts received, $42,502; expenditures, $92,746; qualifying distributions, $92,770, including $90,002 for 8 grants (high: $42,502; low: $2,500).
Purpose and activities: Supports various religious or charitable organizations and hospitals providing care for the sick, indigent, or elderly persons.
Fields of interest: Health care; Alzheimer's disease; Human services; Aging, centers & services; Aging.
Types of support: General/operating support, equipment, emergency funds.
Limitations: Giving limited to Alameda County, CA. No grants to individuals, or for building funds or capital campaigns.
Application information: Telephone calls are not considered. Application form required.
Initial approach: Proposal
Copies of proposal: 1
Deadline(s): 6 weeks prior to board meetings
Board meeting date(s): Semiannually, usually June and Jan.

Officers: Alice Smetts, Pres.; Naomi Viez, Secy.; Elizabeth Hussey, Treas.
Number of staff: 1
EIN: 941167407
Grants for Aging:
Alzheimer Frail Elderly, $5,000. 95.
Alzheimers Services of the East Bay, Berkeley, CA, $20,375. 94.
Alzheimers Services of the East Bay, Berkeley, CA, $10,000. 95.
Center for Elders Independence, Oakland, CA, $15,000. 94.
Coordinated Association of United Seniors, Fremont, CA, $2,500. 95.
Over 60 Health Center, Berkeley, CA, $15,000. 94.
Saint Marys Center, Oakland, CA, $5,000. For senior advocacy program. 95.
Saint Peters Community Adult Day Care Center, San Leandro, CA, $10,000. 95.

64
The Karl Kirchgessner Foundation
c/o Greenberg, Glusker, Fields, Claman & Machtinger
1900 Ave. of the Stars, Suite 2200
Los Angeles 90067 (213) 553-3610
Contact: Martin H. Webster, Pres.

Established in 1977 in CA.
Donor(s): Karl Kramer,‡ Nina Kramer.‡
Financial data (yr. ended 06/30/95): Assets, $15,220,382 (M); gifts received, $469,320; expenditures, $619,585; qualifying distributions, $516,161, including $473,629 for 19 grants (high: $134,129; low: $500; average: $10,000-$50,000).
Purpose and activities: "For the advancement of medical research and for the provision of medical and clinical services to disadvantaged persons, particularly the elderly, the young and handicapped." Applicants should be involved with research and/or clinical programs connected with eyesight, eye care, or helping the blind and partially-sighted to be more self-sufficient.
Fields of interest: Medical research; Youth, services; Aging, centers & services; Disabled; Aging.
Types of support: General/operating support, continuing support, equipment, endowment funds, program development, professorships, publication, seed money, scholarship funds, research, technical assistance, matching funds.
Limitations: Giving limited to the Southern CA area; geographical restriction may be broadened in the future. No grants to individuals, or for fundraising campaigns.
Publications: Informational brochure, application guidelines.
Application information: Application form not required.
Initial approach: Brief letter of intent
Copies of proposal: 1
Deadline(s): Jan. 1 for preliminary applications
Board meeting date(s): Grants made once a year, generally on or about June 30
Final notification: Before June 30
Officers and Directors:* Martin H. Webster,* Pres.; Amelia Louise Mills,* V.P.; Lewis Whitney,* Secy.; Karl Kramer, Jr., C.F.O.; Rev. Patrick Cahalan, Jr.
Number of staff: None.
EIN: 953439716

65
Eugene and Rose Kleiner Family Foundation
(Formerly Kleiner Family Foundation)
One Alexis Court
Menlo Park 94025-6624
Contact: Eugene Kleiner, Trustee

Established in 1985 in CA.
Financial data (yr. ended 12/31/94): Assets, $1,476,689 (M); expenditures, $122,712; qualifying distributions, $120,925, including $120,000 for 9 grants (high: $80,000; low: $400).
Fields of interest: Higher education; Health care; Health organizations; Human services; Aging, centers & services; International affairs; Jewish federated giving programs; Aging.
Limitations: Applications not accepted. Giving primarily in CA.
Trustees: Lisa Kleiner Chanoff, Eugene Kleiner, Robert Kleiner, Rose Kleiner.
Number of staff: None.
EIN: 770080746

66
Koret Foundation
33 New Montgomery St., Suite 1090
San Francisco 94105-4509 (415) 882-7740
Contact: Michael A. Papo, Exec. Dir.
FAX: (415) 882-7775

Established in 1966 in CA.
Donor(s): Joseph Koret,‡ Stephanie Koret.‡
Financial data (yr. ended 12/31/94): Assets, $184,762,451 (M); gifts received, $135,529; expenditures, $17,029,402; qualifying distributions, $11,521,253, including $10,251,382 for 315 grants (high: $714,000; low: $1,000; average: $10,000-$125,000).
Purpose and activities: Seeks to alleviate suffering and misfortune, build community, and enhance human life in the Jewish and general communities of the San Francisco Bay Area and in Israel.
Fields of interest: Higher education; Youth development, services; Aging, centers & services; Homeless, human services; Voluntarism promotion; Public policy, research; Jewish agencies & temples; Israel.
Types of support: General/operating support, continuing support, building/renovation, program development, seed money, fellowships, consulting services.
Limitations: Giving limited to the Bay Area counties of San Francisco, Alameda, Contra Costa, Marin, Santa Clara, and San Mateo, CA, and Israel. No support for private foundations, or veterans', fraternal, military, religious, or sectarian organizations whose principal activity is for the benefit of their own membership. No grants to individuals, or for general fundraising campaigns, scholarships, endowment funds, equipment funds, deficit financing, or emergency funds; no loans.
Publications: Application guidelines, annual report (including application guidelines).
Application information: Application form not required.
Initial approach: Letter of inquiry
Copies of proposal: 1
Board meeting date(s): 5 times per year
Final notification: 2 to 6 months
Officers and Directors:* Susan Koret,* Chair.; Eugene L. Friend,* Vice-Chair.; Thaddeus N. Taube,* Pres.; Michael A. Papo, C.E.O. and Exec. Dir.; Jack R. Curley, C.F.O and Admin. Officer; Michael J. Boskin, William K. Coblentz, Richard L. Greene, Stanley Herzstein.
Staff: Sandra Edwards, Prog. Officer; Michael Kesselman, Prog. Officer; Joseph Walsh, Prog. Officer; Cynthia Ernest, Grants Information Officer; Helen Ring, Prog. Assoc.
Number of staff: 6 full-time professional; 1 part-time professional; 4 full-time support; 1 part-time support.
EIN: 941624987
Grants for Aging:
Alzheimers Services of the East Bay, Berkeley Center, Berkeley, CA, $25,000. For expansion of services. 94.
Bread and Roses, Mill Valley, CA, $22,000. To maintain and expand San Francisco Program. 94.
Edgewood Childrens Center and Day Treatment Program, San Francisco, CA, $10,000. For general operating support for Grandparents Who Care Program. 94.
Fromm Institute for Lifelong Learning, Friends of the, San Francisco, CA, $15,000. For general operating support. 94.
Hospice of the Valley, San Jose, CA, $25,000. For expansion of hospice care and case management services to terminally ill elders. 94.
Meals on Wheels of San Francisco, San Francisco, CA, $100,000. For purchase and renovation of new kitchen. 94.
Pleasure Endeavors Projects, San Francisco, CA, $10,000. For general operating support. 94.
San Francisco Food Bank, San Francisco, CA, $15,000. For food and shelter program over holiday season. 94.

67
George S. Ladd Memorial Fund
c/o Wells Fargo Bank, N.A., Trust Tax Dept.
P.O. Box 63954
San Francisco 94163
Application address: c/o Prudential Asset Management Co., P.O. Box 5340, Scranton, PA 18505-5340; Tel.: (800) 435-2435

Established in 1915 in CA; reincorporated in 1986 in CA.
Financial data (yr. ended 12/31/94): Assets, $508,749 (M); gifts received, $320; expenditures, $34,104; qualifying distributions, $23,729, including $23,729 for 23 grants to individuals (high: $5,227; low: $125).
Purpose and activities: Grants to financially needy elderly and retired employees of Pacific Bell, Nevada Bell, and Pacific Northwest Bell.
Fields of interest: Aging.
Types of support: Grants to individuals.
Limitations: Giving limited to NV and CA.
Application information: Application form required.
Deadline(s): None

Trustee: L.L. Christensen.
EIN: 946070933

68
Herbert & Gertrude Latkin Charitable Foundation

c/o Santa Barbara Bank and Trust
P.O. Box 2340
Santa Barbara 93120 (805) 899-8407
Contact: John Berryhill, Trustee and Terease Cann, Trustee
Application address: 820 State St., Santa Barbara, CA 93101

Established in 1992 in CA.
Donor(s): Herbert and Gertrude Latkin Trust.
Financial data (yr. ended 12/31/94): Assets, $3,664,441 (M); expenditures, $263,662; qualifying distributions, $193,901, including $186,500 for 30 grants (high: $12,500; low: $1,000; average: $1,000-$10,000).
Purpose and activities: Giving primarily to "provide assistance to and promote the welfare and health of the aged, prevent cruelty to animals, provide educational scholarships for deserving students enrolled in institutions of higher learning, provide medical assistance, supplies, and equipment for persons suffering as a result of calamity or disaster, prevent child abuse, and provide assistance to the needy."
Fields of interest: Human services; Family services; Aging, centers & services; Roman Catholic federated giving programs; Aging.
Types of support: General/operating support, scholarship funds.
Limitations: Giving primarily in Santa Barbara County, CA.
Application information: Application form required.
Initial approach: Letter
Copies of proposal: 1
Deadline(s): Apr. 1 and Oct. 1
Trustees: John Berryhill, Terease Cann.
EIN: 776070540
Grants for Aging:
Alzheimers Disease and Related Disorders Association, Santa Barbara, CA, $10,000. 94.
Friendship Center of Santa Barbara, Santa Barbara, CA, $5,000. For senior day-care. 94.
Valley Haven, Solvang, CA, $5,000. 94.

69
Bertha Russ Lytel Foundation

P.O. Box 893
Ferndale 95536
Contact: George Hindley, Mgr.

Established in 1974 in CA.
Donor(s): Bertha Russ Lytel,‡ L.D. O'Rourke.‡
Financial data (yr. ended 09/30/95): Assets, $12,413,857 (M); expenditures, $542,650; qualifying distributions, $414,801, including $390,457 for 37 grants (high: $53,000; low: $100).
Purpose and activities: Giving primarily to social service agencies for the aged and handicapped, civic and cultural programs, including libraries and museums, elementary and higher education, health associations, including hospitals and hospices, and agricultural and nursing scholarship funds.
Fields of interest: Museums; Arts/cultural programs; Elementary school/education; Higher education; Libraries/library science; Education; Hospitals (general); Substance abuse, services; Health associations; Human services; Hospices; Aging, centers & services; Government/public administration; Disabled; Aging.
Types of support: General/operating support, continuing support, building/renovation, equipment, seed money, scholarship funds, matching funds.
Limitations: Giving limited to Humboldt County, CA. No grants to individuals, or for annual campaigns, emergency or endowment funds, deficit financing, land acquisition, renovations, research, demonstration projects, or publications; no loans.
Publications: Application guidelines, 990-PF.
Application information: Application form required.
Initial approach: Letter
Copies of proposal: 8
Deadline(s): 1st Thursday of each month
Board meeting date(s): Monthly
Final notification: 30 to 60 days
Officers and Directors:* Charles M. Lawrence,* Pres.; Gerald Becker,* V.P. and Treas.; James K. Morrison,* Secy.; George Hindley, Mgr.; Betty Diehl, Charles Lakin, Jack Russ, Jack Smith.
Number of staff: 1 part-time professional.
EIN: 942271250
Grants for Aging:
Humboldt Senior Resource Center, Eureka, CA, $50,000. 94.
Humboldt Senior Resource Center, Eureka, CA, $50,000. 95.
Redwoods United, Arcata, CA, $53,000. For homemakers for the elderly. 94.
Redwoods United, Arcata, CA, $53,000. For financial aid to homemakers for elderly. 95.

70
The Marguerite Home Association

555 Capitol Mall, Suite 200
Sacramento 95814-4557

Established in 1884 in CA.
Donor(s): Margaret Crocker.‡
Financial data (yr. ended 06/30/95): Assets, $1,044,065 (M); expenditures, $62,901; qualifying distributions, $62,253, including $54,350 for 22 grants to individuals (high: $4,200; low: $600).
Purpose and activities: Support limited to financial assistance to needy, elderly single women in the Sacramento, CA, area.
Fields of interest: Aging; Women; Economically disadvantaged.
Types of support: Grants to individuals.
Limitations: Applications not accepted. Giving primarily in the Sacramento, CA, area.
Application information: Contributes only to pre-selected individuals.
Officers and Directors:* Lawrence A. Schei,* Pres.; Gene Pendergast,* V.P.; William H. Schaw,* V.P.; Carl E. Spilman,* Secy.; Thomas R. Bolton,* Treas.
Number of staff: 2 part-time support.
EIN: 946065622

71
Marin Community Foundation

17 East Sir Francis Drake Blvd., Suite 200
Larkspur 94939 (415) 461-3333
Contact: Stephen M. Dobbs, Pres. and C.E.O.
FAX: (415) 461-3386

Incorporated in 1986 in CA; the Leonard and Beryl Buck Foundation, its original donor, was established in 1973 and administered by the San Francisco Foundation through 1986.
Foundation type: Community
Financial data (yr. ended 06/30/95): Assets, $620,118,000 (M); gifts received, $5,314,000; expenditures, $35,129,000, including $32,562,000 for 507 grants and $1,038,000 for 3 loans.
Purpose and activities: The Marin Community Foundation is a tax-exempt charity that administers private funds for public purposes. It was established in 1986 to help improve the human condition and enhance the quality of life for all residents of the community. The foundation supports a broad array of programs, projects, and services, including fund development and management for individuals and organizations who place their philanthropic funds in its care. The foundation accepts applications for funding in seven program areas: Human Needs, Community Development, Community Recognition Awards, Education and Training, Religion, Environment, and Arts.
Fields of interest: Arts/cultural programs; Adult education—literacy & basic skills; Education; Environment; AIDS; Legal services; Employment; Housing/shelter, development; Human services; Community development; Religion; Homeless; Disabled; Aging.
Types of support: General/operating support, continuing support, building/renovation, equipment, land acquisition, emergency funds, program development, seed money, technical assistance, program-related investments/loans, employee matching gifts, matching funds.
Limitations: Giving from the Buck Trust is limited to Marin County, CA. No grants to individuals, or for planning initiatives, research, or generally for capital projects (except those meeting criteria specified in the funding guidelines). Other limitations specific to each program area are outlined in the funding guidelines.
Publications: Annual report, application guidelines, newsletter, informational brochure.
Application information: Application form not required.
Initial approach: Request funding policies and application guidelines
Copies of proposal: 2
Board meeting date(s): Every 6 weeks (except July and Aug.)
Final notification: 3 months minimum
Officers: Stephen Mark Dobbs, Ph.D., Pres. and C.E.O.; Stephen M. Jackson, V.P., Fund Development; Sid Hartman, V.P., Administration & Finance and C.I.O.; Barbara H. Kehrer, Ph.D., V.P., Progs.; Pamela R. Lynch, Corp. Secy.
Trustees: Shirley A. Thornton, Ed.D., Chair.; David Werderger, M.D., Vice-Chair.; Kathleen Foote, William L. Hamilton, Grace Hughes, Joanne Saxe, Karin Uranhart.
Staff: Michael Groza, Dir., Community Progs.; Stephen Barton, Prog. Officer; Carolyn Evans,

Prog. Officer; Bettie Hodges, Prog. Officer; Donald Jen, Prog. Officer; Lourdes Martinez, Prog. Officer; Sallyanne Wilson, Prog. Officer.
Number of staff: 15 full-time professional; 2 part-time professional; 9 full-time support; 4 part-time support.
EIN: 943007979
Grants for Aging:
Ecumenical Association for Housing, San Rafael, CA, $20,000. For preliminary feasibility analysis of proposed senior housing project at Hamilton Air Force Base. 96.
Love Is The Answer, Novato, CA, $60,000. For programs to improve lives of elderly persons in senior care facilities. 96.
Marin Senior Coordinating Council, San Rafael, CA, $312,000. For operating support. 96.
Senior Access, San Anselmo, CA, $240,000. For adult day health care and care management programs. 96.

72
MCA Foundation, Ltd.
100 Universal City Plaza
Universal City 91608 (818) 777-1208
Contact: Helen Yatsko Giambrone, Administrator

Incorporated in 1956 in CA.
Donor(s): MCA, Inc.
Foundation type: Company-sponsored
Financial data (yr. ended 12/31/94): Assets, $12,535,588 (M); gifts received, $2,026,000; expenditures, $3,864,877; qualifying distributions, $3,847,010, including $3,847,000 for 52 grants (high: $3,000,000; low: $2,000; average: $5,000-$10,000).
Purpose and activities: Grants largely for health and welfare, including support for minorities, cultural programs, higher and other education, child and youth agencies, and women.
Fields of interest: Performing arts; Arts/cultural programs; Higher education; Medical school/education; Education; Health care; AIDS; Health organizations; AIDS research; Gun control; Domestic violence prevention; Children & youth, services; Youth, services; Women, centers & services; Minorities/immigrants, centers & services; Civil rights, minorities; Civil rights, disabled; Civil rights, women; Civil rights, aging; Civil rights, gays/lesbians; Minorities; Asians/Pacific Islanders; African Americans; Latinos; Native Americans; Disabled; Aging; Women; People with AIDS (PWAs); Gays/lesbians; Economically disadvantaged; Homeless.
Types of support: General/operating support, annual campaigns, capital campaigns, building/renovation, endowment funds, program development, seed money, fellowships, scholarship funds, employee matching gifts.
Limitations: Giving primarily in the Los Angeles, CA, and New York, NY, areas. No grants to individuals, or for film, video, or television projects.
Publications: Application guidelines.
Application information: Application form not required.
Initial approach: Proposal (not exceeding 3 pages)
Copies of proposal: 1
Deadline(s): None
Officers and Directors:* Sidney J. Sheinberg,* Pres.; Richard Baker,* V.P. and C.F.O.; Thomas Wertheimer,* V.P.; Michael Samuel, Secy.
Number of staff: 2 full-time professional.
EIN: 136096061

73
The McConnell Foundation
P.O. Box 991870
Redding 96099-1870 (916) 222-0696
Contact: Lee W. Salter, C.E.O. and Pres.

Established in 1964 in CA.
Donor(s): Carl R. McConnell,‡ Leah F. McConnell.‡
Financial data (yr. ended 12/31/95): Assets, $195,776,232 (M); gifts received, $99,209,790; expenditures, $2,534,249; qualifying distributions, $3,816,280, including $1,523,479 for 29 grants (high: $435,037; low: $838; average: $500-$550,000) and $18,386 for 2 in-kind gifts.
Purpose and activities: Primary interests include the environment, environmental education, and recreation; projects that benefit the working poor; projects for the larger public good; and the promotion of volunteerism.
Fields of interest: Museums; Performing arts; Historical activities; Arts/cultural programs; Secondary school/education; Adult education—literacy & basic skills; Reading; Environment; Health care; Recreation; Aging, centers & services; Voluntarism promotion.
Types of support: Equipment, scholarship funds, matching funds.
Limitations: Giving primarily in Shasta and Siskiyou counties, CA. No support for sectarian religious purposes. No grants to individuals, or for endowment funds, annual fund drives, budget deficits, or purchase or construction of buildings.
Publications: Application guidelines, annual report.
Application information: Application form required.
Initial approach: Letter of intent
Copies of proposal: 1
Deadline(s): Feb. 15
Board meeting date(s): Feb., Mar., July, and Oct.
Final notification: July 31
Officers and Directors:* Doreeta Domke,* Chair.; Lee W. Salter,* C.E.O. and Pres.; John A. Mancasola,* Exec. V.P. and Secy.-Treas.; Leonard B. Nelson, William B. Nystrom.
Staff: Karen S. Bennett, Sr. Prog. Officer; Shannon E. Phillips, Prog. Officer.
Number of staff: 3 full-time professional; 4 part-time professional; 2 part-time support.
EIN: 946102700

74
Henry J. Mello Foundation
32 White Rd.
Watsonville 95076
Application address: P.O. Box 32, Watsonville, CA 95077

Established in 1990 in CA.
Donor(s): Henry J. Mello.
Financial data (yr. ended 12/31/95): Assets, $102,297 (M); expenditures, $6,515; qualifying distributions, $5,500, including $5,500 for 4 grants (high: $2,000; low: $750).
Purpose and activities: Support only for organizations benefitting senior citizens or children.
Fields of interest: Youth, services; Aging, centers & services; Aging.
Limitations: Giving primarily in Watsonville, CA. No grants to individuals.
Application information:
Deadline(s): None
Officers and Directors:* Henry J. Mello,* Pres.; Helen A. Mello,* V.P.; John Mello, Michael Mello, Stephen Mello, Timothy Mello, Thomas Skillicorn.
EIN: 770238728

75
Mericos Foundation
625 Fair Oaks Ave., Suite 360
South Pasadena 91030-2630 (818) 441-5188
Contact: Linda J. Blinkenberg, Secy.

Established in 1980 in CA.
Donor(s): Donald W. Whittier Charitable Trust.
Financial data (yr. ended 12/31/95): Assets, $26,606,439 (M); expenditures, $668,500; qualifying distributions, $541,764, including $437,250 for 15 grants (high: $114,000; low: $10,000; average: $10,000-$100,000).
Purpose and activities: Primarily giving for cultural programs, the aged, and medical research.
Fields of interest: Arts/cultural programs; Child development, education; Higher education; Education; Medical research; Children & youth, services; Child development, services; Aging, centers & services; Aging.
Types of support: Building/renovation, equipment, endowment funds, program development, fellowships, matching funds.
Limitations: Giving limited to Santa Barbara, CA. No grants to individuals; no loans.
Application information: Grants generally initiated by foundation. Application form not required.
Initial approach: 1- to 2-page letter of inquiry
Deadline(s): None
Officers: Joanne W. Blokker, Pres.; Michael J. Casey, V.P.; Linda J. Blinkenberg, Secy.; Arlo G. Sorensen, Treas.
Number of staff: 2 full-time professional.
EIN: 953500491

76
National Metal and Steel Foundation
11755 Wilshire Blvd., Suite 2150
Los Angeles 90025-1528

Established in 1974 in CA.
Donor(s): Clean Steel, Inc.
Foundation type: Company-sponsored
Financial data (yr. ended 02/28/95): Assets, $954,912 (M); expenditures, $46,871; qualifying distributions, $45,375, including $45,375 for 40 grants (high: $2,500; low: $200).
Fields of interest: Arts/cultural programs; Education; Health care; Human services; Youth, services; Aging, centers & services; Jewish agencies & temples; Aging.
Types of support: General/operating support.

Limitations: Applications not accepted. Giving primarily in CA. No grants to individuals.
Application information: Contributes only to pre-selected organizations.
Officers: Harry Faversham, Pres.; Jack Garret, V.P.
EIN: 237424802

77
New Horizons Foundation
c/o Gifford & Dearing
700 South Flower St., Suite 1222
Los Angeles 90017-4160 (213) 626-4481
Contact: G. Grant Gifford, Pres.

Financial data (yr. ended 05/31/95): Assets, $419,614 (M); expenditures, $32,508; qualifying distributions, $28,643, including $22,962 for 8 grants to individuals (high: $6,000; low: $162).
Purpose and activities: Provides assistance to elderly Christian Scientists in need who have exhausted all conventional means of support.
Fields of interest: Aging, centers & services; Christian agencies & churches; Aging; Economically disadvantaged.
Types of support: Grants to individuals.
Limitations: Giving limited to Los Angeles County, CA.
Application information: To be eligible for grant, the applicant must satisfy the following general requirements: 1) be a member in The Mother Church or an authorized branch thereof; 2) be at least 65 years of age; and 3) demonstrate financial need. Application form not required.
Initial approach: Letter or telephone
Deadline(s): None
Officers and Directors:* G. Grant Gifford,* Pres.; Henry H. Dearing,* Secy.
EIN: 956031571

78
The Oakland Athletics Community Fund
Oakland-Alameda County Coliseum
Oakland 94621
Contact: Dave Perron, Trustee

Established in 1981 in CA.
Financial data (yr. ended 12/31/94): Assets, $179,715 (M); gifts received, $181,559; expenditures, $178,709; qualifying distributions, $178,709, including $138,310 for grants.
Purpose and activities: "To enable individuals to attend Oakland A's baseball games, who might otherwise be unable to afford tickets; to provide recreational activity for the elderly, disabled and children; to provide organizations with a medium for providing awards for achievement in school or special learning programs; and to provide disaster relief assistance."
Fields of interest: Education; Housing/shelter; Recreation; Youth, services; Aging, centers & services; Aging.
Limitations: Giving primarily in CA. No grants to individuals.
Application information: Application form not required.
Deadline(s): None
Trustees: Walter J. Haas, Dave Perron.
EIN: 942826655

79
Offer-Scult Family Foundation
(Formerly Offer Family Foundation)
11677 San Vicente Blvd., No. 307
Los Angeles 90049

Established in 1961.
Donor(s): Charles S. Offer, Sr.‡
Financial data (yr. ended 12/31/94): Assets, $705,640 (M); expenditures, $26,077; qualifying distributions, $20,575, including $20,500 for 19 grants (high: $5,600; low: $100).
Fields of interest: Museums; Higher education; Hospitals (general); Human services; Jewish federated giving programs; Jewish agencies & temples; General charitable giving; Aging.
Limitations: Applications not accepted. Giving limited to Phoenix, AZ, Los Angeles and San Diego, CA, Boston, MA, and HI.
Officers: Arlene Scult, Pres.; Charles S. Offer, Jr., V.P.; Morton Scult, V.P.
EIN: 956027953

80
The Parker Foundation
4365 Executive Dr., Suite 1600
San Diego 92121-2189 (619) 677-1431
Contact: Robbin C. Powell, Asst. Secy.

Trust established in 1971 in CA; incorporated in 1975.
Donor(s): Gerald T. Parker,‡ Inez Grant Parker.‡
Financial data (yr. ended 09/30/95): Assets, $17,485,425 (M); gifts received, $6,545; expenditures, $978,736; qualifying distributions, $832,882, including $771,323 for 73 grants (high: $100,000; low: $500; average: $5,000-$15,000).
Purpose and activities: Equal emphasis on cultural programs, health and welfare, including medical support and research, adult services, and youth agencies; grants also for education and community activities. Giving largely in the form of partial seed money and matching or challenge grants; generally no support that would make an organization dependent on the foundation.
Fields of interest: Arts/cultural programs; Education; Health care; Youth, services; Aging, centers & services; Community development.
Types of support: General/operating support, continuing support, annual campaigns, building/renovation, equipment, land acquisition, emergency funds, program development, publication, seed money, research, program-related investments/loans, matching funds.
Limitations: Giving limited to San Diego County, CA. No support for sectarian religious purposes. No grants to individuals, or for endowment funds, scholarships, or fellowships; no loans.
Publications: Annual report, informational brochure (including application guidelines).
Application information: Application form not required.
Initial approach: Letter
Copies of proposal: 10
Deadline(s): None
Board meeting date(s): Monthly
Final notification: 2 months
Officers and Directors:* William E. Beamer,* Pres.; Judy McDonald,* V.P. and General Counsel; Paul Mosher,* Secy.-Treas.; Sandra Pay, Sylvia Rios, Mark Trotter.
Number of staff: None.
EIN: 510141231

81
The Ralph M. Parsons Foundation
1055 Wilshire Blvd., Suite 1701
Los Angeles 90017 (213) 482-3185
Contact: Christine Sisley, Exec. Dir.

Incorporated in 1961 in CA.
Donor(s): Ralph M. Parsons.‡
Financial data (yr. ended 12/31/94): Assets, $187,133,616 (M); expenditures, $10,180,459; qualifying distributions, $9,300,662, including $8,350,514 for 197 grants (high: $400,000; low: $500; average: $10,000-$75,000).
Purpose and activities: Giving for higher and pre-collegiate education, with emphasis on engineering, technology, science and medicine; and for social impact areas, including assistance to children, women, families, and seniors; grants also for cultural and civic projects, and health services for disadvantaged populations.
Fields of interest: Performing arts; Arts/cultural programs; Early childhood education; Secondary school/education; Higher education; Engineering school/education; Education; Hospitals (general); Health care; AIDS; Legal services; Housing/shelter, development; Human services; Children & youth, services; Youth, services; Family services; Aging, centers & services; Homeless, human services; Community development; Engineering & technology; Computer science; Engineering; Science; Aging; Economically disadvantaged; Homeless.
Types of support: General/operating support, capital campaigns, building/renovation, equipment, program development, seed money, fellowships, internships, scholarship funds, research, matching funds.
Limitations: Giving limited to Los Angeles County, CA, with the exception of some grants for higher education. No support for sectarian, religious, or fraternal purposes, or for programs for which substantial support from government or other sources is readily available. No grants to individuals, or for continuing support, annual campaigns, federated fundraising appeals, emergency or endowment funds, land acquisition, workshops, exhibits, surveys, or conferences.
Publications: Annual report.
Application information: Application form not required.
Initial approach: Letter
Copies of proposal: 1
Deadline(s): None
Board meeting date(s): Bimonthly beginning in Jan.
Final notification: 6 months
Officers and Directors:* Joseph G. Hurley,* Pres.; Albert A. Dorskind,* V.P. and C.F.O.; Leroy B. Houghton,* V.P.; Edgar R. Jackson,* V.P.; Everett B. Laybourne,* V.P.; Christine Sisley,

Exec. Dir.; Robert F. Erburu, Paul T. Hartung, James A. Thomas, Franklin E. Ulf, Francis M. Wheat.
Staff: Wendy Garen, Prog. Dir.; Nancy Berglass, Prog. Officer; Ricardo Lima, Grants Administrator.
Number of staff: 3 full-time professional; 3 full-time support.
EIN: 956085895
Grants for Aging:
AltaMed Health Services, Los Angeles, CA, $50,000. For specialized medical and rehabilitation equipment for new Adult Day Health Care Center in East Los Angeles serving frail and elderly Latino population. 94.
California P.E.O. Home, Alhambra, CA, $100,000. Toward demolition and rebuilding of Robbins Hall, retirement residence for P.E.O members. 94.
Hospital of the Good Samaritan, Los Angeles, CA, $50,000. For Respite Care and Case Management Program, which offers health and social services to low-income, frail elderly. 94.
Jewish Family Service of Los Angeles, North Hollywood, CA, $53,032. For expansion of Adult Day Health Care Program, serving physically disabled young adults. 94.
Jewish Homes for the Aging of Greater Los Angeles, Reseda, CA, $50,000. For repair of earthquake-damaged campuses that provide residential care to fragile elderly. 94.
Motion Picture and Television Fund, Woodland Hills, CA, $25,000. For special care unit providing long-term care for victims of Alzheimer's disease and other forms of dementia. 94.
Saint Vincent Senior Citizen Nutrition Program, Los Angeles, CA, $40,000. For vans to be used for delivery of meals to low-income, homebound seniors. 94.

82
Pasadena Foundation

16 North Marengo Ave., Suite 302
Pasadena 91101 (818) 796-2097
Contact: Virginia C. Krueger, Exec. Dir.
FAX: (818) 583-4738

Established in 1953 in CA by resolution and declaration of trust.
Donor(s): Louis A. Webb,‡ Marion L. Webb,‡ Helen B. Lockett,‡ Dorothy I. Stewart,‡ Rebecca R. Anthony,‡ Lucille Crumb.‡
Foundation type: Community
Financial data (yr. ended 12/31/95): Assets, $12,732,643 (M); gifts received, $799,307; expenditures, $1,234,551, including $1,099,021 for 281 grants (average: $100-$50,000).
Purpose and activities: Grants for capital improvements to established local agencies, with emphasis on child welfare and development, youth agencies, minorities, the handicapped, health services, and senior citizen welfare; support also for alcohol and drug abuse programs, family planning and services, hospitals, hospices, mental health, and medical research.
Fields of interest: Education, association; Child development, education; Libraries/library science; Animal welfare; Hospitals (general); Family planning; Health care; Substance abuse, services; Mental health/crisis services; Health associations; Cancer; AIDS; Alcoholism; Biomedicine; Medical research; Cancer research; AIDS research; Children & youth, services; Youth, services; Child development, services; Family services; Hospices; Aging, centers & services; Homeless, human services; Minorities; Disabled; Aging; Homeless.
Types of support: Capital campaigns, building/renovation, equipment, research, matching funds.
Limitations: Giving limited to the Pasadena, CA, area. No support for sports programs or organizations, or religious organizations for religious purposes. No grants to individuals, or for operating budgets, continuing support, annual campaigns, emergency funds, seed money, deficit financing, land acquisition, endowment funds, special projects, publications, conferences, consulting services, scholarships, or fellowships; no loans.
Publications: Annual report, application guidelines, informational brochure, newsletter.
Application information: Application form required.
Initial approach: Letter
Copies of proposal: 1
Deadline(s): Oct. 1
Board meeting date(s): Quarterly
Final notification: After Dec. meeting
Officers and Advisory Board:* James M. King, Sr.,* Chair.; Harriman L. Cronk,* Vice-Chair.; Virginia C. Krueger,* Exec. Dir.; Guillermina Gutierrez Byrne, Donald R. Cameron, Fred H. Felberg, Bernard J. Johnson, Peggy Phelps, Gloria S. Pitzer, David A. Werbelow, Marjorie Wyatt.
Trustees: Bank of America, Citizens Business, Sanwa Bank California.
Number of staff: 1 full-time professional; 1 part-time support.
EIN: 956047660

83
The Patron Saints Foundation

P.O. Box 40706
Pasadena 91114-7706 (818) 797-2303
Contact: Jacquie Fennessy, Dir.

Established in 1986 in CA.
Financial data (yr. ended 06/30/95): Assets, $3,821,096 (M); expenditures, $190,235; qualifying distributions, $165,623, including $143,306 for 18 grants (high: $16,000; low: $5,000).
Purpose and activities: Giving primarily for medical and other professional health care programs, including community health education and services, community outreach programs, hospitals, and medical research.
Fields of interest: Hospitals (general); Medical care, rehabilitation; Health care; Substance abuse, services; Mental health/crisis services; Health associations; Alcoholism; Medical research; Human services; Children & youth, services; Family services; Aging, centers & services; Aging; Economically disadvantaged.
Types of support: Continuing support, capital campaigns, building/renovation, equipment, program development, seed money, research.
Limitations: Giving limited to the San Gabriel Valley, CA, area. No grants to individuals, or for endowment funds, conferences, seminars, workshops, exhibits, travel, or surveys.
Publications: Application guidelines.
Application information: Application form required.
Copies of proposal: 10
Deadline(s): Early Mar. and early Oct.
Board meeting date(s): Mid-May and early Dec.
Final notification: May and Dec.
Officers and Directors:* Dorothy Shea,* Pres.; James W. Graunke,* Secy.; Debra J. Spiegal,* Treas.; Michael Costello, W. Allan Edmiston, M.D., Jacquie Fennessy, Margaret Landry, James R. Lee, Albert Lowe, Robert Nesbitt, Victor Petrone, David K. Robinson, Sally Sims, Christine Sisley, Jacqueline Stiff, Melinda Thompson, Sharon Thralls.
Number of staff: 1 part-time professional.
EIN: 953484257
Grants for Aging:
Pasadena Senior Center, Pasadena, CA, $5,500. For TLC program. 95.
Pasadena Senior Center, Pasadena, CA, $5,000. For caregiver referral service. 94.
Scripps Home, Altadena, CA, $8,906. For Wander Guard System. 95.

84
Peninsula Community Foundation

1700 South El Camino Real, No. 300
San Mateo 94402-3049 (415) 358-9369
Contact: Sterling K. Speirn, Exec. Dir.
FAX: (415) 358-9817

Established as a trust in 1964 in CA; incorporated in 1981.
Foundation type: Community
Financial data (yr. ended 12/31/95): Assets, $112,019,436 (M); gifts received, $19,087,562; expenditures, $9,371,943, including $7,944,574 for 942 grants (high: $250,000; low: $23; average: $25,000), $106,400 for 67 grants to individuals (high: $5,000; low: $200; average: $1,000), $3,123 for 16 employee matching gifts, $353,403 for 2 foundation-administered programs and $150,000 for 2 loans.
Purpose and activities: To support local cultural, educational, social service, and health programs. Primary areas of interest include homelessness and housing, children and youth, adult services, social services, and education, including programs for minorities, the disadvantaged, and early childhood education; other interests include the environment, arts and culture, senior citizens and the needs of the aging, the disabled, civic concerns, and recreation; provides counseling services for local fund seekers. Giving includes grants to individuals as student aid, emergency assistance, and grants to local artists.
Fields of interest: Arts/cultural programs; Early childhood education; Child development, education; Education; Environment; Health care; Health organizations; Housing/shelter, development; Recreation; Human services; Children & youth, services; Youth, services; Child development, services; Aging, centers & services; Homeless, human services; Government/public administration; Minorities;

Disabled; Aging; Economically disadvantaged; Homeless.
Types of support: Continuing support, emergency funds, program development, conferences/seminars, seed money, curriculum development, internships, scholarship funds, technical assistance, consulting services, scholarships—to individuals, matching funds.
Limitations: Giving limited to San Mateo County and northern Santa Clara County, CA. No grants for endowment funds, annual campaigns, building funds, deficit financing, land acquisition, or research.
Publications: Annual report, application guidelines, informational brochure, newsletter, grants list, financial statement.
Application information: Application form not required.
Initial approach: Letter of inquiry
Copies of proposal: 1
Deadline(s): None
Board meeting date(s): Distribution committee meets in Jan., Mar., May, July, Sept., and Nov.
Final notification: 2 to 3 months
Officers and Directors:* Robert Kirkwood,* Chair.; William Wilson III,* Vice-Chair.; Sterling K. Speirn, Secy. and Exec. Dir.; Tom Bailard,* Treas.; Hugh C. Burroughs, John Clinton, Susan Ford, Thomas M. Jenkins, Charles B. Johnson, Olivia G. Martinez, Karen Van Hoesen Olson, Gordon Russell, Donald H. Seiler, Rosemary Young.
Staff: Christina Sutherland, Prog. Officer; Jeanne Friedman, Dir., Development; Vera Bennett, Dir., Finance and Administration.
Number of staff: 7 full-time professional; 7 full-time support; 2 part-time support.
EIN: 942746687
Grants for Aging:
Mid-Peninsula Hospice Foundation, Menlo Park, CA, $10,000. For coordinator for Nursing Home Project. 94.

85
Pete P. Peters Foundation
4170 South Fowler
Fresno 93725-9326

Established in 1980.
Donor(s): Pete P. Peters.
Financial data (yr. ended 11/30/94): Assets, $1,510,138 (M); gifts received, $20,000; expenditures, $82,840; qualifying distributions, $81,582, including $80,340 for 20 grants (high: $25,250; low: $50).
Fields of interest: Media/communications; Arts/cultural programs; Higher education; Health care; Health organizations; Human services; Aging, centers & services; Aging.
Limitations: Applications not accepted. Giving primarily in Fresno, CA. No grants to individuals.
Application information: Contributes only to pre-selected organizations.
Officers: Pete P. Peters, Pres.; Ronald D. Peters, Secy.-Treas.
EIN: 942738016

86
Mary Pickford Foundation
9171 Wilshire Blvd., Suite 512
Beverly Hills 90210
Contact: Edward G. Stotsenberg, Pres.

Established in 1968.
Donor(s): Mary Pickford Rogers.‡
Financial data (yr. ended 05/31/95): Assets, $9,708,075 (M); expenditures, $863,521; qualifying distributions, $677,719, including $644,038 for 125 grants (high: $60,000; low: $175).
Purpose and activities: Grants largely for scholarship funds at colleges and universities, and for "well-established medical or community service organizations," including performing arts programs, museums, and agencies serving the elderly and other disadvantaged groups.
Fields of interest: Film/video; Museums; Theater; Arts/cultural programs; Higher education; Business school/education; Education; Hospitals (general); Health associations; Human services; Aging, centers & services; Community development; Aging; Economically disadvantaged; Canada.
Types of support: General/operating support, endowment funds, scholarship funds.
Limitations: Giving primarily in CA. No support for drug rehabilitation or medical research. No grants to individuals, or for building funds or land acquisition.
Application information: Application form not required.
Initial approach: Letter or telephone
Deadline(s): None
Officers and Director:* Edward G. Stotsenberg,* Pres. and C.E.O.; Sull Lawrence, Secy.; Charles B. Rogers, Treas.
Number of staff: None.
EIN: 956093487
Grants for Aging:
Senior Gleaners, North Highlands, CA, $1,000. 95.
University of Southern California, School of Gerontology, Los Angeles, CA, $25,000. For scholarship fund. 94.

87
Margaret Pillsbury Foundation
c/o Bilter
425 California St., No. 2200
San Francisco 94104
Contact: John Cocherell, V.P.
Application address: 621 West Line St., Bishop, CA 93514-3320; Tel.: (619) 872-4431

Established in 1989 in CA.
Donor(s): Margaret P. Sorbello.
Financial data (yr. ended 12/31/95): Assets, $950,928 (M); expenditures, $50,887; qualifying distributions, $43,014, including $37,000 for grants.
Fields of interest: Medical care, in-patient care; Geriatrics; American Red Cross; Human services; Roman Catholic agencies & churches.
Application information:
Initial approach: Letter
Deadline(s): None
Officers: Judith Rawlings, Pres.; John Cocherell, V.P.; D. Keith Bilter, Secy.-Treas.
EIN: 943103001

88
The Roberts Foundation
Presidio Bldg. 1016, Suite 300
Torney Ave. and Lincoln Blvd., P.O. Box 29906
San Francisco 94129-0906 (415) 561-6540
Contact: Lyman H. Casey, Exec. Dir.
FAX: (415) 561-6477

Established in 1985 in CA.
Donor(s): George R. Roberts, Leanne B. Roberts.
Financial data (yr. ended 12/31/94): Assets, $11,152,629 (M); gifts received, $1,830,000; expenditures, $3,749,291; qualifying distributions, $3,695,948, including $3,285,524 for 95 grants (high: $833,333; low: $1,300; average: $5,000-$25,000).
Purpose and activities: Giving primarily to children, youth, and families, education, environmental issues, and wildlife preservation and animal welfare. Within the field of education, the foundation prefers to fund programs for the learning disabled and disadvantaged youth. The foundation places a high priority on social service projects of an entrepreneurial nature that enable individuals to move from positions of dependency to independence and self-reliance.
Fields of interest: Education, special; Vocational education; Education; Natural resource conservation & protection; Environment; Animal welfare; Wildlife preservation & protection; Health care; Youth, services; Family services; Aging, centers & services; Homeless, human services; Economic development; Economically disadvantaged; Homeless.
Types of support: Program development.
Limitations: Giving limited to northern CA, with emphasis on San Francisco County and adjacent counties; limited funding for organizations in Marin, Alameda, and Contra Costa counties. No support for religious organizations. No grants to individuals, or for medical research, endowment funds, or annual or year end appeals.
Publications: Biennial report, application guidelines.
Application information:
Initial approach: Written proposal
Copies of proposal: 1
Deadline(s): 12 weeks prior to the board meeting
Board meeting date(s): Spring and fall
Final notification: Following board meeting
Officers and Directors:* Leanne B. Roberts,* Pres. and C.E.O.; George R. Roberts, V.P., Secy.-Treas., and C.F.O.; Lyman H. Casey,* V.P. and Exec. Dir.
Staff: Jed Emerson, Prog. Dir., Homeless Economic Development Fund.
EIN: 942967074
Grants for Aging:
Jewish Home for the Aged, San Francisco, CA, $50,000. 94.
Meals on Wheels of San Francisco, San Francisco, CA, $10,000. 94.

89
Sacramento Regional Foundation
2180 Harvard St., Suite 255
Sacramento 95815 (916) 927-2241
Contact: Lauren Wolkov, Exec. Dir.
FAX: (916) 927-0110

Incorporated in 1983 in CA.
Foundation type: Community
Financial data (yr. ended 12/31/94): Assets, $8,790,745 (M); gifts received, $1,708,893; expenditures, $1,558,681, including $1,260,234 for grants (average: $1,000-$7,500).
Purpose and activities: Primary areas of interest include the arts and humanities, education, community development, health, human services, and the environment.
Fields of interest: Museums; Performing arts; Theater; Humanities; Historic preservation/historical societies; Arts/cultural programs; Child development, education; Elementary school/education; Higher education; Adult education—literacy & basic skills; Reading; Education; Natural resource conservation & protection; Environment; Health care; Mental health/crisis services; AIDS; Alcoholism; Health organizations; Legal services; Food services; Housing/shelter, development; Youth development, services; Human services; Youth, services; Child development, services; Family services; Hospices; Aging, centers & services; Minorities/immigrants, centers & services; Homeless, human services; Urban/community development; Community development; Voluntarism promotion; Social sciences; Public policy, research; Government/public administration; Leadership development; Minorities; Disabled; Aging; Economically disadvantaged; Homeless.
Types of support: Equipment, emergency funds, program development, conferences/seminars, publication, seed money, scholarship funds, technical assistance, scholarships—to individuals.
Limitations: Giving limited to organizations within or those offering services to Sacramento, Yolo, Placer, and El Dorado counties, CA. No support for sectarian purposes or private foundations. No grants to individuals (except scholarships through designated funds, and through Artists in Crisis Fund), or for annual campaigns, operating funds, capital campaigns, endowments, building funds, continuing support, deficit financing, foundation-managed projects, research, or land acquisition; no loans.
Publications: Annual report, financial statement, grants list, application guidelines.
Application information: Grantseekers forum held in Oct. explaining parameters of grantmaking program. Application form required.
Copies of proposal: 10
Deadline(s): Dec. 12
Board meeting date(s): Jan., Mar., May, July, Sept., and Nov.
Final notification: After board meeting in Mar.
Officers and Directors:* Malcolm Weintraub,* Pres.; Forrest A. Plant, Sr.,* V.P.; Melina Ose,* Secy.; Gerald Bays,* Treas.; Lauren Wolkov, Exec. Dir.; and 17 additional directors.
Number of staff: 2 full-time professional; 1 full-time support.
EIN: 942891517

90
Safeway Inc.
(Formerly Safeway Stores Corporate Giving Program)
201 Fourth St.
Oakland 94660 (510) 891-3000
Contact: Debra Lambert, Corp. Dir., Public Affairs
Application addresses: Seattle Div., 1121 124 Ave. N.E., Bellevue, WA 98005-0990; Portland Div., 16300 S.E. Evelyn St., Clackamas, OR 97015; Northern California Div., 47400 Kato Rd., Fremont, CA 94538; Denver Div., 6900 South Yosemite, Englewood, CO 80112-1412; Eastern Div., 4551 Forbes Blvd., Lanham, MD 20706; Phoenix Div., 2750 South Priest Dr., Tempe, AZ 85282

Established in 1926.
Purpose and activities: "Safeway's contributions program is confined to organizations which directly serve the residents in communities where we have stores." Each of Safeway's 6 independent U.S. retail divisions sets its own funding priorities, has its own giving budget and contributions committee. Types of support generally include donations of food to food banks and employee volunteerism. Safeway generally supports programs for youth, the aged, minorities, athletics, health and welfare, civic concerns, and the arts and culture. Funding is limited, however, and primarily occurs at the individual store level.
Fields of interest: Arts/cultural programs; Human services; Youth, services; Aging, centers & services; Minorities.
Types of support: General/operating support, donated products.
Limitations: Giving primarily in major operating locations. No support for organizations outside operating areas. National organizations can only receive support from central office. No grants to individuals, United Way recipients, capital campaigns, building funds, endowments, scholarships or fellowships.
Publications: including application guidelines.
Application information: Send all requests to the nearest operating retail division. Applications not accepted at headquarters.
Deadline(s): Applications accepted throughout the year. For events, send requests at least 3 weeks before function date
Board meeting date(s): Applications reviewed on a case by case basis

91
San Diego Community Foundation
Wells Fargo Bank Bldg.
101 West Broadway, Suite 1120
San Diego 92101 (619) 239-8815
Contact: Robert A. Kelly, C.E.O.
FAX: (619) 239-1710

Established in 1975 in CA.
Foundation type: Community
Financial data (yr. ended 06/30/94): Assets, $113,226,033 (M); gifts received, $39,639,675; expenditures, $8,158,405, including $4,922,817 for 383 grants (high: $246,410; low: $31; average: $2,000-$15,000).
Purpose and activities: Giving to social service agencies with emphasis on children, youth, and families, cultural activities, education, health, civic affairs, and recreational activities.
Fields of interest: Visual arts; Museums; Performing arts; Dance; Theater; Music; Arts/cultural programs; Early childhood education; Child development, education; Elementary school/education; Secondary school/education; Vocational education; Higher education; Adult education—literacy & basic skills; Reading; Education; Environment; Animal welfare; Family planning; Health care; Substance abuse, services; Mental health/crisis services; AIDS; Alcoholism; Health organizations; Medical research; AIDS research; Delinquency prevention/services; Housing/shelter, development; Recreation; Human services; Children & youth, services; Youth, services; Child development, services; Family services; Hospices; Aging, centers & services; Women, centers & services; Homeless, human services; Community development; Voluntarism promotion; Federated giving programs; Government/public administration; Public affairs; Minorities; Disabled; Aging; Women; Economically disadvantaged; Homeless.
Types of support: General/operating support, building/renovation, equipment, program development, publication, seed money, scholarship funds, technical assistance, employee matching gifts, matching funds.
Limitations: Giving limited to San Diego County, CA. No support for political or religious organizations. No grants to individuals, or for annual or capital fund campaigns, endowment funds, conferences, travel, or to underwrite fundraising events and performances; no loans.
Publications: Annual report, informational brochure (including application guidelines), newsletter.
Application information: Application form required.
Initial approach: Telephone
Copies of proposal: 1
Deadline(s): Quarterly; call for details
Board meeting date(s): Bimonthly beginning in Jan.
Final notification: 3 months
Officers and Board of Governors:* Ann Parode,* Chair.; Susan A. Maddox,* Vice-Chair.; Robert A. Kelly, C.E.O.; Frank Ault,* V.P., Finance and Treas.; Philip C. Blair,* V.P., Distribs.; John D. Messner,* V.P., Investments; Thomas B. Robertson,* V.P., Marketing; Elsie Weston,* V.P., Development; Michel Anderson, Ron Blair, Hon. Federico Castro, Paul Ecke, Jr., Howard Goldfeder, Anita S. Harbert, Daniel Herde, Jerome Katzin, Hon. Judith Keep, Art Madrid, Robert McRann, Sandra Fleet Mooers, Thomas Murphy, Gail Stoorza-Gill, Albert Trepte, Barbara Walbridge, Mary Walshok, Su-Mei Yu.
Staff: Reed Morgan, Prog. Dir.; Jill Houska, Prog. Officer; Becky Obayashi, Prog. Officer; Tonette M. Dease, Grants Administrator.
Number of staff: 6 full-time professional; 2 part-time professional; 7 full-time support.
EIN: 952942582
Grants for Aging:
Mamas Kitchen, San Diego, CA, $130,992. 95.
Saint Pauls Retirement Homes Foundation, San Diego, CA, $16,244. 95.
Special Delivery, San Diego, CA, $11,500. 95.

92
San Francisco Family Foundation
1750 Montgomery St.
San Francisco 94111 (415) 922-4091
Contact: Beryle Kaye, Exec. Dir.

Established in 1990 in CA as partial successor to Foster Charitable Trust.
Financial data (yr. ended 12/31/93): Assets, $1,183,884 (M); expenditures, $73,423; qualifying distributions, $63,526, including $38,364 for 24 grants to individuals (high: $3,000; low: $500; average: $500-$3,000).
Purpose and activities: Provides goods, clothing, rent, home care, and medical supplies reimbursement for elderly individuals through social service agencies. Applicants must have during their life time helped others, and who now find themselves in need.
Fields of interest: Aging, centers & services; Aging.
Types of support: Grants to individuals.
Limitations: Giving limited to residents of San Francisco Bay Area, CA.
Application information: Application form required.
Initial approach: Write or call for application form
Copies of proposal: 1
Deadline(s): None
Officers: H. Roy Gordon, Chair.; Gail F. Gordon, Pres.; Beryl Kay, Secy. and Exec. Dir.; Malcolm Stroud, Treas.
EIN: 680217117

93
The San Francisco Foundation
685 Market St., Suite 910
San Francisco 94105-9716 (415) 495-3100
Contact: Robert M. Fisher, Dir.
Additional tel.: (510) 436-3100

Established in 1948 in CA by resolution and declaration of trust.
Foundation type: Community
Financial data (yr. ended 06/30/95): Assets, $325,268,333 (M); gifts received, $39,677,683; expenditures, $31,118,917, including $28,756,355 for 2,226 grants (high: $500,000; low: $10; average: $5,000-$50,000), $6,021 for 62 employee matching gifts and $400,000 for 2 program-related investments.
Purpose and activities: Grants principally in six categories: the arts and humanities, community health, education, environment, neighborhood and community development, and social services. Technical assistance grants also made, primarily to current recipients. The foundation serves five counties of the Bay Area.
Fields of interest: Media/communications; Performing arts; Dance; Humanities; Arts/cultural programs; Early childhood education; Child development, education; Elementary school/education; Adult education—literacy & basic skills; Reading; Education; Natural resource conservation & protection; Environment; Family planning; Health care; Substance abuse, services; Mental health/crisis services; Cancer; AIDS; Alcoholism; Health organizations; Cancer research; AIDS research; Delinquency prevention/services; Legal services; Employment; Housing/shelter, development; Youth development, services; Human services; Children & youth, services; Youth, services; Child development, services; Family services; Aging, centers & services; Homeless, human services; Human rights (international); Civil rights; Urban/community development; Community development; Voluntarism promotion; Public policy, research; Government/public administration; Leadership development; Public affairs; Minorities; Disabled; Aging; Immigrants/refugees; Economically disadvantaged; Homeless.
Types of support: General/operating support, program development, seed money, technical assistance, program-related investments/loans.
Limitations: Giving limited to the San Francisco Bay Area, CA, counties of Alameda, Contra Costa, Marin, San Francisco, and San Mateo. No support for religious purposes. No grants for annual campaigns, general fundraising campaigns, emergency or endowment funds, deficit financing, matching funds, or for scholarships or fellowships, except when so designated by donor.
Publications: Annual report, newsletter, application guidelines, program policy statement, informational brochure, grants list.
Application information: Application form required.
Initial approach: Letter of intent (no more than 3 pages)
Copies of proposal: 1
Deadline(s): Letters reviewed continuously; proposal closing dates available upon request
Board meeting date(s): Monthly except Aug., Jan., and Apr.; applications are reviewed 4 to 6 times each year
Final notification: 3 to 4 months
Director: Robert M. Fisher.
Board of Trustees: T.J. Saenger, Chair.; William J. Powers, C.F.O.; Lucille S. Abrahamson, F. Warren Hellman, Leslie Hume, Leonard E. Kingsley, Rolland C. Lowe, M.D., Stephanie C. MacColl, David Sanchez, Mary Lee Widener.
Staff: Joseph Brooks, Prog. Exec., Neighborhood and Comm. Dev.; John Kreidler, Sr., Prog. Exec., Arts and Humanities; Jane Rogers, Prog. Exec., Environment; Wendy Everett, Prog. Exec., Community Health; Eleanor Clement Glass, Prog. Exec., Education and Community Health; Carol Callen, Prog. Coord., The Lifeline Initiative; Elaine Lee, Prog. Coord., Koshland Awards; Robert Uyeki, Prog. Coord., Special Awards.
Number of staff: 24 full-time professional; 1 part-time professional; 8 full-time support; 7 part-time support.
EIN: 941101547
Grants for Aging:
Alzheimers Disease and Related Disorders Association of Palo Alto, Palo Alto, CA, $15,000. Toward expansion of model project supporting caregivers of Alzheimer's patients in Greater San Francisco Bay Area. 95.
Alzheimers Services of the East Bay, Berkeley, CA, $15,000. For expansion of adult day health care services for individuals with Alzheimer's disease and dementia-related disabilities in Alameda and Contra Costa Counties. 95.
Bay Area Community Services, Oakland, CA, $60,000. For seed grant to expand money management services provided by volunteers to elders. 95.
Center for Elders Independence, Oakland, CA, $50,000. To develop adult day health center in downtown Oakland's San Pablo Hotel to enable poor, frail elders to live independently. 95.
Meals on Wheels of San Francisco, San Francisco, CA, $66,000. For volunteer coordinator position. 95.
New Light Senior Center, Berkeley, CA, $10,000. For home visiting to homebound elderly residents of South and West Berkeley. 95.
Project Open Hand, San Francisco, CA, $18,000. To reorganize hot meal and grocery delivery system in Tenderloin for people with HIV/AIDS. 95.
Satellite Senior Homes, Oakland, CA, $15,000. To hire project manager for organizational capacity building. 95.

94
Frances Schermer Charitable Trust
c/o City National Bank
120 South Spalding Dr., P.O. Box 1141
Beverly Hills 90213
Contact: James L. Pazol, Trustee and Dr. Saul Friedman, Trustee
Application address: 21 North Wickliffe Circle, Youngstown, OH 44515; Tel.: (330) 792-6033

Trust established in 1980 in CA.
Donor(s): Charles I. Schermer,‡ Frances Schermer.‡
Financial data (yr. ended 06/30/95): Assets, $1,875,568 (M); expenditures, $163,657; qualifying distributions, $138,335, including $121,848 for 55 grants (high: $13,250; low: $231).
Purpose and activities: Giving to Jewish welfare funds and Israel, higher education, social service agencies, including aid to the handicapped, disadvantaged and aged, child welfare, inner city projects, and community funds.
Fields of interest: Higher education; Human services; Children & youth, services; Aging, centers & services; Federated giving programs; Jewish federated giving programs; Disabled; Aging; Economically disadvantaged; Israel.
Types of support: Capital campaigns, emergency funds, program development, curriculum development, matching funds.
Limitations: Giving primarily in CA and OH; giving also in Israel. No support for religious purposes. No grants to individuals.
Publications: Annual report.
Application information: Application form not required.
Initial approach: Letter and budget
Copies of proposal: 1
Deadline(s): None
Final notification: 90 days
Trustees: Saul Friedman, James L. Pazol, City National Bank.
Number of staff: 1 part-time support.
EIN: 956685749
Grants for Aging:
Senior Gleaners, North Highlands, CA, $1,000. 95.

95
The Schuman Foundation, Inc.
9777 Wilshire Blvd., Suite 816
Beverly Hills 90212-1884 (310) 275-6680
Contact: Sidney W. Schuman, Pres.

Established in 1949.
Donor(s): Edith C. Schuman, Sidney W. Schuman, Meyer Schuman Co.
Financial data (yr. ended 12/31/94): Assets, $711,664 (M); expenditures, $71,763; qualifying distributions, $69,400, including $69,400 for 132 grants (high: $25,100; low: $25).
Fields of interest: Hospitals (general); Health associations; Human services; Children & youth, services; Youth, services; Aging, centers & services; Jewish federated giving programs; Jewish agencies & temples; Aging.
Limitations: Giving primarily in Los Angeles, CA. No grants to individuals.
Application information:
Initial approach: Letter
Deadline(s): None
Officers: Sidney W. Schuman, Pres. and Treas.; Edith C. Schuman, V.P. and Secy.
EIN: 956029868
Grants for Aging:
Jewish Homes for the Aging of Greater Los Angeles, Reseda, CA, $25,100. 94.
Jewish Homes for the Aging of Greater Los Angeles, Reseda, CA, $5,250. 94.

96
The Schwab Family Foundation
c/o Claire M. Buckey
2233 Watt Ave., Suite 295
Sacramento 95825 (916) 484-0282

Established in 1992 in CA.
Donor(s): Barbara M. Schwab.‡
Financial data (yr. ended 12/31/94): Assets, $290,471 (M); gifts received, $245,000; expenditures, $215,041; qualifying distributions, $215,041, including $122,800 for 35 grants (high: $10,000; low: $500).
Purpose and activities: Primary areas of interest are children and family needs and hospice programs for the elderly.
Fields of interest: AIDS; Food services; Human services; Children & youth, services; Family services; Hospices; Roman Catholic agencies & churches; Aging; Economically disadvantaged; Homeless.
Limitations: Giving limited to northern CA.
Application information: Application form required.
Initial approach: Proposal
Deadline(s): None
Officers: Mary B. Schwab, Pres.; Claire M. Buckey, Secy.
EIN: 680264934
Grants for Aging:
Senior Gleaners, North Highlands, CA, $5,000. 94.

97
Serra Medical Hospital
999 West Taylor St., Suite B
San Jose 95126
Contact: Lawrence L. May, Pres.

Financial data (yr. ended 03/31/95): Assets, $8,015 (M); expenditures, $98,998; qualifying distributions, $97,500, including $97,500 for grants.
Purpose and activities: Giving to organizations that serve the aged, youth or physically handicapped and generally involving a medical related activity.
Fields of interest: Higher education; Human services; Youth, services; Hospices; Aging, centers & services; Disabled; Aging.
Limitations: Giving primarily in CA. No grants to individuals.
Application information:
Initial approach: Letter
Deadline(s): Dec. 31
Officers: Lawrence L. May, Pres.; Joseph Kirby, V.P.; Leo W. Ruth, Secy.
EIN: 941547001

98
Sierra Health Foundation
(Formerly The Sierra Foundation)
1321 Garden Hwy.
Sacramento 95833 (916) 922-4755
Contact: Nicole Caffo, Cont.

Established in 1984 in CA.
Donor(s): Foundation Health Plan of Sacramento, Americare Health Corp.
Financial data (yr. ended 06/30/95): Assets, $131,390,375 (M); expenditures, $4,573,094; qualifying distributions, $7,554,706, including $2,684,505 for grants (average: $15,000-$80,000) and $82,850 for 1 in-kind gift.
Purpose and activities: Giving for health-related programs that 1) will have a long-term impact on the general health of the population; 2) provide a positive change in health care systems; and 3) may cause a positive change in the use of health care resources. Support also for model projects that may be replicated by others. The foundation has an ongoing significant involvement in prenatal care, AIDS, youth, and the elderly.
Fields of interest: Child development, education; Hospitals (general); Family planning; Medical care, rehabilitation; Health care; Substance abuse, services; Mental health/crisis services; Health associations; Cancer; Heart/circulatory disease; Skin disorders; AIDS; Alcoholism; Biomedicine; Health organizations; Medical research; Cancer research; Heart/circulatory research; Skin research; AIDS research; Delinquency prevention/services; Nutrition; Human services; Children & youth, services; Youth, services; Child development, services; Family services; Aging, centers & services; Minorities/immigrants, centers & services; Community development; Minorities; Aging; Economically disadvantaged.
Types of support: Program development, conferences/seminars, seed money, technical assistance, consulting services, program-related investments/loans, employee matching gifts, matching funds.
Limitations: Giving limited to the following CA counties: Alpine, Amador, Butte, Calaveras, Colusa, El Dorado, Glenn, Lassen, Modoc, Mono, Nevada, Placer, Plumas, Sacramento, San Joaquin, Shasta, Sierra, Siskiyou, Solano (eastern), Stanislaus, Sutter, Tehama, Trinity, Tuolumne, Yolo, and Yuba. No support for programs, activities, or organizations that are not health-related. No grants to individuals, or for endowments or scholarships.
Publications: Grants list, newsletter, application guidelines, informational brochure (including application guidelines), occasional report.
Application information: Application form not required.
Initial approach: Letter of intent
Copies of proposal: 1
Deadline(s): None
Board meeting date(s): Quarterly
Officers and Directors:* J. Rod Eason,* Chair.; Len McCandliss,* Pres.; Dorothy Meehan, V.P.; Rev. Leo McAllister, Byron Demorest, M.D., George Deubel, Wendy Everett, Albert R. Jonsen, Robert Petersen, Gordon D. Schaber, James Schubert, M.D.
Number of staff: 8 full-time professional; 9 full-time support; 2 part-time support.
EIN: 680050036

99
Will C. Silliman Memorial
3354 Pershing Ave.
San Bernardino 92405 (909) 882-3596
Contact: Dicta S. Faber, Pres.

Financial data (yr. ended 12/31/95): Assets, $56,066 (M); expenditures, $12,061; qualifying distributions, $9,814, including $1,040 for 3 grants to individuals (high: $440; low: $300).
Fields of interest: Aging, centers & services; Aging.
Types of support: Scholarships—to individuals.
Limitations: Giving limited to residents of San Bernadino County, CA.
Application information: Application form required.
Deadline(s): Apr. 1
Final notification: June 30
Officers and Directors:* Dicta S. Faber,* Pres. and Treas.; Eleanor Taylor,* V.P.; Mary Seels,* Secy.; Jack Carver, Margaret Griffiths, Eleanor Kelly.
EIN: 952223145

100
The May and Stanley Smith Trust
49 Geary St., Suite 244
San Francisco 94108 (415) 391-0292
Contact: N. Dale Matheny, Trustee

Established in 1977 in CA.
Donor(s): May Smith.
Financial data (yr. ended 12/31/95): Assets, $6,007,696 (M); expenditures, $215,881; qualifying distributions, $197,857, including $195,850 for 54 grants (high: $6,000; low: $300).
Purpose and activities: Giving primarily for the visually impaired and other disabilities, the aged, children, and the disadvantaged; support also for social service agencies.

Fields of interest: Education; Human services; Children & youth, services; Aging, centers & services; Disabled; Aging; Economically disadvantaged; Canada.
Types of support: General/operating support, scholarship funds.
Limitations: Giving primarily in North America, with emphasis on the San Francisco Bay Area, CA, and in Canada. No grants to individuals.
Publications: Application guidelines.
Application information: Application form not required.
Initial approach: Letter
Copies of proposal: 1
Deadline(s): Sept. 30; consideration begins Apr. 15
Board meeting date(s): Late fall
Final notification: Notification when approved; payment made in early Dec.
Trustees: John P. Collins, Jr., J.R. Gibbs, N. Dale Matheny.
Number of staff: None.
EIN: 946435244
Grants for Aging:
Saint Francis Lutheran Church, San Francisco, $6,000. For Senior Outreach program. 95.
San Francisco Food Bank, San Francisco, CA, $6,000. For Brown Bag program. 94.

101
Y. & H. Soda Foundation
Two Theatre Sq., Suite 211
Orinda 94563-3346 (510) 253-2630
Contact: Judith Murphy, Exec. V.P. and C.E.O.

Established in 1964.
Donor(s): Y. Charles Soda Trust, Y. Charles Soda,‡ Helen C. Soda.‡
Financial data (yr. ended 11/30/95): Assets, $81,234,069 (M); expenditures, $1,687,799; qualifying distributions, $928,476, including $393,280 for 78 grants (high: $21,765; low: $50; average: $500-$20,000) and $150 for 2 employee matching gifts.
Purpose and activities: Support for education, health, human services, youth development, and religious organizations (primarily Catholic).
Fields of interest: Early childhood education; Child development, education; Elementary school/education; Vocational education; Higher education; Food services; Youth development, services; Human services; Children & youth, services; Family services; Aging, centers & services; Women, centers & services; Homeless, human services; Community development; Roman Catholic agencies & churches; Religion; Minorities; Disabled; Aging; Women; Economically disadvantaged; Homeless.
Types of support: General/operating support, building/renovation, equipment, program development, seed money, in-kind gifts, matching funds.
Limitations: Giving primarily in Alameda and Contra Costa counties, CA. No support for animal welfare, the arts, environmental causes, private foundations, national medical research organizations, or political organizations. No grants to individuals, or for annual fundraising campaigns, faculty chairs, or operating expenses.
Publications: Application guidelines.
Application information: Application form not required.
Initial approach: Letter
Copies of proposal: 1
Deadline(s): Mar. 1, June 1, Sept. 1, and Dec. 1
Board meeting date(s): 2nd Wednesday of the month
Officers and Directors:* Alfred Dossa, Pres.; Judith Murphy,* Exec. V.P. and C.E.O.; Rosemary Soda-Maricic, V.P.; James Dye, Secy.; Alan Holloway,* Treas. and C.F.O.
Number of staff: 2 full-time professional; 1 part-time professional; 1 full-time support; 1 part-time support.
EIN: 941611668

102
The Sonoma County Community Foundation
(Formerly The Sonoma County Foundation)
3550 Round Barn Blvd., Suite 212
Santa Rosa 95403 (707) 579-4073
Contact: Kay Marquet, Exec. Dir.

Incorporated in 1983 in CA.
Foundation type: Community
Financial data (yr. ended 12/31/95): Assets, $23,414,000 (M); gifts received, $18,144,000; expenditures, $1,582,000, including $989,000 for grants (average: $500-$5,000), $41,000 for grants to individuals and $150,000 for 2 program-related investments.
Fields of interest: Journalism & publishing; Visual arts; Museums; Performing arts; Dance; Theater; Music; Humanities; Historic preservation/historical societies; Arts/cultural programs; Child development, education; Higher education; Business school/education; Medical school/education; Adult/continuing education; Adult education—literacy & basic skills; Reading; Education; Natural resource conservation & protection; Environment; Health care; Substance abuse, services; Mental health/crisis services; Health associations; AIDS; Alcoholism; Health organizations; AIDS research; Delinquency prevention/services; Agriculture; Food services; Youth development, services; Youth development, citizenship; Human services; Children & youth, services; Youth, services; Child development, services; Family services; Aging, centers & services; Minorities/immigrants, centers & services; Homeless, human services; International affairs, goodwill promotion; Race/intergroup relations; Rural development; Community development; Voluntarism promotion; Public affairs, citizen participation; Leadership development; Minorities; African Americans; Latinos; Native Americans; Disabled; Aging; Women; People with AIDS (PWAs); Economically disadvantaged; Homeless.
Types of support: General/operating support, building/renovation, equipment, program development, publication, seed money, scholarship funds, technical assistance, scholarships—to individuals, matching funds.
Limitations: Giving limited to Sonoma County, CA. No support for religious purposes or advocacy activities. No grants for special fundraising events, annual fund campaigns, or debt retirement.
Publications: Annual report, 990-PF, program policy statement, financial statement, grants list, newsletter, application guidelines, informational brochure.
Application information: 2 major funding periods each year in addition to Schulz mini-grants. Application form required.
Initial approach: Letter requesting application material
Deadline(s): Feb. and Aug.; June for Schulz mini-grants
Board meeting date(s): 2nd Tuesday of most months
Final notification: May and Nov.; Aug. for Schulz mini-grants
Officers and Directors:* Patrick K. Kilkenny,* Pres.; Rhoann Ponseti,* V.P.; Peggy J. Furth,* Secy.; Irwin S. Rothenberg,* Treas.; Kay Marquet, Exec. Dir.; and 16 additional directors.
Number of staff: 3 full-time professional; 2 full-time support; 1 part-time support.
EIN: 680003212

103
Sonora Area Foundation
Box 274
Sonora 95370 (209) 533-2596
Contact: Sue Ellen Harwood, Exec. Dir.

Established in 1989 in CA.
Donor(s): Elinor Brown,‡ Martha Barnes, Elaine Symons Baker,‡ Mother Lode Art Assn., El Capitan National Bank, Sonora 49er Rotary, Joseph Haratani, Amy Haratani.
Foundation type: Community
Financial data (yr. ended 12/31/95): Assets, $4,532,217 (L); gifts received, $526,204; expenditures, $189,447, including $86,665 for 25 grants (high: $5,000; low: $100; average: $600-$5,000) and $13,550 for 11 grants to individuals (high: $2,500; low: $100; average: $100-$2,500).
Fields of interest: Media/communications; Visual arts; Performing arts; Music; Arts/cultural programs; Early childhood education; Child development, education; Elementary school/education; Higher education; Adult/continuing education; Libraries/library science; Education; Environment; Animal welfare; Hospitals (general); Health care; Substance abuse, services; Mental health/crisis services; Alcoholism; Health organizations; Delinquency prevention/services; Legal services; Crime/law enforcement; Food services; Recreation; Human services; Children & youth, services; Youth, services; Child development, services; Family services; Hospices; Aging, centers & services; Women, centers & services; Voluntarism promotion; Federated giving programs; Government/public administration; Disabled; Aging; Women; Economically disadvantaged; Homeless.
Types of support: Equipment, program development, conferences/seminars, seed money, scholarship funds, consulting services, matching funds.
Limitations: Giving limited to Tuolumne County, CA. No support for sectarian purposes, private foundations, or political purposes. No grants for general operating support, annual or capital campaigns, endowment funds, or debt retirement.

Publications: Annual report, financial statement, grants list, application guidelines, informational brochure (including application guidelines).
Application information: Application form required.
Copies of proposal: 8
Deadline(s): Feb. 21
Board meeting date(s): 2nd Tuesday of each month
Final notification: Apr. 1
Officer: Sue Ellen Harwood, Exec. Dir.
Number of staff: 1 full-time professional; 1 part-time support.
EIN: 931023051

104
C. J. Stafford & Dot Stafford Memorial Trust
c/o First Interstate Bank of California
P.O. Box 129113
San Diego 92112-9113 (619) 557-3164
Contact: Lynn Powers, Trust Officer, First Interstate Bank of California

Established in 1984 in CA.
Donor(s): C.J. Stafford,‡ Dot Stafford.‡
Financial data (yr. ended 04/30/95): Assets, $1,415,105 (M); expenditures, $157,018; qualifying distributions, $132,542, including $119,049 for 37 grants (high: $10,000; low: $1,000).
Purpose and activities: Giving primarily for social services, including youth, the elderly, and the homeless; support also for hospitals, alcohol and drug abuse programs, medical research and health associations, vocational and other education, the fine and performing arts, community funds, and religion.
Fields of interest: Visual arts; Museums; Performing arts; Music; Vocational education; Education; Hospitals (general); Substance abuse, services; Health associations; Alcoholism; Medical research; Human services; Youth, services; Aging, centers & services; Homeless, human services; Federated giving programs; Religion; Aging; Homeless; General charitable giving.
Types of support: General/operating support, continuing support, capital campaigns, building/renovation, equipment, emergency funds, program development, matching funds.
Limitations: Giving limited to San Diego County, CA.
Publications: 990-PF, application guidelines.
Application information:
Initial approach: Letter
Copies of proposal: 6
Deadline(s): Apr. 1
Board meeting date(s): Quarterly - varies
Trustee: First Interstate Bank of California.
Number of staff: 1 full-time professional; 4 part-time professional; 1 full-time support.
EIN: 330085374
Grants for Aging:
Mamas Kitchen, San Diego, CA, $2,500. 95.
Senior Adult Services, San Diego, CA, $4,000. 94.

105
Swift Memorial Health Care Foundation
1355 Del Norte Rd.
Camarillo 93010 (805) 988-0196
Contact: Kate McLean, Administrator

Established in 1984 in CA.
Financial data (yr. ended 06/30/95): Assets, $2,624,844 (M); expenditures, $107,718; qualifying distributions, $98,835, including $87,835 for grants (high: $2,500; average: $2,000-$5,000), $6,000 for 6 grants to individuals of $1,000 each and $5,000 for 2 employee matching gifts.
Fields of interest: Medical school/education; Nursing school/education; Hospitals (general); Dental care; Family planning; Medical care, rehabilitation; Nursing care; Health care; Substance abuse, services; Mental health/crisis services; Health associations; Cancer; Eye disease; Heart/circulatory disease; AIDS; Alcoholism; Biomedicine; Health organizations; Medical research; Cancer research; Eye research; Heart/circulatory research; AIDS research; Human services; Hospices; Homeless, human services; Psychology/behavioral science; Disabled; Aging; Homeless.
Types of support: General/operating support, capital campaigns, building/renovation, equipment, emergency funds, internships, scholarship funds, research, scholarships—to individuals, matching funds.
Limitations: Giving limited to Ventura County, CA.
Publications: Occasional report, 990-PF, informational brochure (including application guidelines).
Application information: Application form required.
Initial approach: Letter
Copies of proposal: 1
Deadline(s): Apr. 30 and Oct. 31
Board meeting date(s): Bimonthly
Final notification: 2 months
Officers and Directors:* Frank Leiblien, Pres.; Jack Erbeck,* V.P.; Fred Buenger,* Secy.; Allen Camp, C. Flager Horn, Robert E. Jordan, M.D., Patty Lowthorp, R. Blinn Maxwell, Emma Mayer, Ray Swift, Jessie White.
Number of staff: 1 part-time professional.
EIN: 770132512
Grants for Aging:
Long-Term Care Ombudsman, Ventura, CA, $5,000. 94.

106
Mark Taper Foundation
12011 San Vicente Blvd., Suite 401
Los Angeles 90049 (310) 476-5413
Contact: Raymond F. Reisler, Exec. Dir.

Incorporated in 1952 in CA.
Donor(s): S. Mark Taper.‡
Financial data (yr. ended 06/30/95): Assets, $5,120,518 (M); expenditures, $837,477; qualifying distributions, $826,436, including $701,000 for 4 grants (high: $500,000; low: $1,000; average: $100,000-$500,000).
Purpose and activities: Currently undergoing an internal review and assessment in order to chart a course for future grantmaking.
Fields of interest: Arts/cultural programs; Child development, education; Education; Environment; Family planning; Nursing care; Health care; Mental health/crisis services; Cancer; Health organizations; Cancer research; Delinquency prevention/services; Food services; Youth development, services; Human services; Children & youth, services; Youth, services; Child development, services; Family services; Aging, centers & services; Women, centers & services; Urban/community development; Voluntarism promotion; Public policy, research; Government/public administration; Leadership development; Public affairs; Disabled; Aging; Women.
Types of support: General/operating support, building/renovation, program development.
Limitations: Giving primarily in CA. No grants to individuals.
Publications: Application guidelines.
Application information: Application form required.
Initial approach: Letter with brief background information is the sole means of initial approach. If appropriate, an application form will be sent
Deadline(s): None
Board meeting date(s): As required
Final notification: As needed
Officers and Directors:* Barry H. Taper,* V.P. and Secy.; Janice Taper Lazarof,* V.P. and Treas.
Number of staff: 1 full-time professional; 1 full-time support.
EIN: 956027846

107
S. Mark Taper Foundation
12011 San Vicente Blvd., Suite 400
Los Angeles 90049 (310) 476-5413
Contact: Raymond F. Reisler, Exec. Dir.

Incorporated in 1989 in CA.
Donor(s): S. Mark Taper.‡
Financial data (yr. ended 12/31/95): Assets, $104,213,425 (M); gifts received, $94,700,000; expenditures, $428,424; qualifying distributions, $279,612, including $279,612 for grants.
Fields of interest: Arts/cultural programs; Education; Environment; Domestic violence prevention; Housing/shelter, development; Human services; Youth, services; Family services; Homeless, human services; Reproductive rights; Disabled; Aging; Women; People with AIDS (PWAs); Economically disadvantaged; Homeless.
Types of support: General/operating support, annual campaigns, capital campaigns, building/renovation, equipment, emergency funds, program development, conferences/seminars, publication, seed money, scholarship funds, research, program-related investments/loans, matching funds.
Limitations: Giving primarily in CA. No grants to individuals.
Publications: Application guidelines.
Application information: Application form required.
Initial approach: Letter
Copies of proposal: 1

Deadline(s): None
Board meeting date(s): As required
Final notification: As needed
Officer and Director:* Janice Taper Lazarof,* Pres.
Number of staff: 2 full-time professional; 2 full-time support.
EIN: 954245076
Grants for Aging:
Saint Barnabas Senior Center, Los Angeles, CA, $7,500. 94.

108
Teichert Foundation

3500 American River Dr.
Sacramento 95864 (916) 484-3344
Contact: Frederick A. Teichert, Exec. Dir.

Established in 1990 in CA.
Donor(s): A. Teichert & Son, Inc.
Foundation type: Company-sponsored
Financial data (yr. ended 03/31/95): Assets, $376,428 (M); gifts received, $118,240; expenditures, $145,679; qualifying distributions, $145,679, including $145,679 for 63 grants (high: $10,000; low: $500; average: $500-$3,000).
Purpose and activities: Support for culture and the arts, education, youth and elderly, environmental planning and preservation, transportation planning, civic improvement and historical restoration, community and social services, and rehabilitation and health services.
Fields of interest: Historic preservation/historical societies; Arts/cultural programs; Education; Environment; Medical care, rehabilitation; Health care; Health organizations; Human services; Youth, services; Aging, centers & services; Federated giving programs; Government/public administration; Aging.
Limitations: Giving primarily in Sacramento and the Central Valley, CA. No support for religious, political, or fraternal organizations. No grants to individuals, or for national fundraising campaigns, or for courtesy advertising, benefits, and telephone solicitations.
Publications: Application guidelines.
Application information: Application form required.
Initial approach: Letter of inquiry
Copies of proposal: 3
Deadline(s): Mar.
Board meeting date(s): Quarterly
Final notification: Within 1 month
Officers and Directors* Anne S. Haslam, Secy.; Bruce E. Stimson, C.F.O.; Frederick A. Teichert,* Exec. Dir.; Thomas J. Hammer, Judson T. Riggs, Melita M. Teichert.
EIN: 680212355

109
Times Mirror Corporate Giving Program

c/o Times Mirror Co.
Times Mirror Sq.
Los Angeles 90053 (573) 237-3993
Contact: Cassandra Malry, Dir., Corp. Contribs.
Environmental Education Address: Consuelo Murtagh, Admin. Secy., 1705 De Sales St. NW, Suite 801, Washington, DC 20036; Tel.: (202) 467-4949. Additional addresses: Cindy Beyl, Public Rels. Mgr., The Times Orange County Edition, 1375 Sunflower Ave., Costa Mesa, CA 92626; Tel.: (714) 966-4627; Horst A. Bergmann, Chair., Pres., and C.E.O., Jeppesen Sanderson, 55 Inverness Dr. East, Englewood, CO 80112-5498; Tel.: (303) 799-9090; Gina Swearington, Dir., Mktg. and Communications, The Baltimore Sun Co., 501 North Calvert St., P.O. Box 1377, Baltimore, MD 21278-0001; Tel.: (410) 332-6245; John F. Dill, Chair., Pres., and C.E.O., Mosby-Year Book, Inc., 11830 Westline Industrial Dr., St. Louis, MO 63146; Tel.: (314) 453-4216; Kelly L. Scarpino, Exec. Secy. to the Pres., The Morning Call, 101 North Sixth St., P.O. Box 1260, Allentown, PA 18105; Tel.: (610) 820-6708

Financial data (yr. ended 12/31/94): Total giving, $5,665,081, including $4,588,617 for 143 grants, $76,104 for grants to individuals and $1,000,360 for employee matching gifts.
Purpose and activities: "As the charitable contributions programs of The Times Mirror Company and The Times Mirror Foundation have grown, so has our commitment to the communities in which we do business. We believe that one of the most important ways this commitment is demonstrated is through the community and charitable contributions programs of Times Mirror's operating units located across the country. Giving back to our communities is one of the wisest investments we can make." The Corporate Grants Program makes a limited number of national and industry-related grants, and may support fundraising events. The Matching Gifts Program matches gifts of employees, retirees, and their spouses to education, culture, hospitals, and conservation. The Scholarship Program grants scholarships to children of employees. Total giving figures for 1994 include charitable contributions by operating companies.
Fields of interest: Museums; Performing arts; Dance; Humanities; Arts/cultural programs; Early childhood education; Child development, education; Elementary school/education; Secondary school/education; Higher education; Adult education—literacy & basic skills; Reading; Education; Environment; Health care; AIDS; AIDS research; Employment; Housing/shelter, development; Human services; Child development, services; Family services; Aging, centers & services; Women, centers & services; Minorities/immigrants, centers & services; Homeless, human services; International affairs, goodwill promotion; Race/intergroup relations; Community development; Government/public administration; Minorities; Aging; Women; Economically disadvantaged; Homeless.
Types of support: General/operating support, continuing support, capital campaigns, building/renovation, program development, scholarship funds, technical assistance, employee volunteer services, use of facilities, employee matching gifts, matching funds.
Limitations: Giving primarily in Southern CA, and communities served by the subsidiaries. No support for religious or fraternal groups. No grants to individuals, or for films, videos, or television programs, publications, or conferences; no more than one request every twelve months from an organization desired.
Publications: Corporate giving report (including application guidelines), corporate report.
Application information: Nonprofit organizations located in Long Island, NY, should forward requests to New York Newsday. Application form not required.
Initial approach: Letter to nearest operating unit
Copies of proposal: 1
Deadline(s): At least 8 weeks before meetings
Board meeting date(s): Apr. 1 and Oct. 1
Final notification: 2 to 3 weeks following each meeting
Number of staff: 1 full-time professional; 1 full-time support.

110
The Valley Foundation

16450 Los Gatos Blvd., Suite 210
Los Gatos 95032 (408) 358-4545
Contact: Ms. Ervie L. Smith, Exec. Dir.
FAX: (408) 358-4548

Established in 1984 in CA.
Financial data (yr. ended 09/30/95): Assets, $50,625,915 (M); expenditures, $2,712,572; qualifying distributions, $2,265,996, including $2,152,917 for 60 grants (high: $100,000; low: $10,000; average: $10,000-$100,000).
Purpose and activities: Support primarily for medical services and health care for lower income households within Santa Clara County and for research, social services, and education. Support also for youth, the arts, senior citizens, education, and general medical areas.
Fields of interest: Arts/cultural programs; Education; Health care; Medical research; Human services; Youth, services; Aging, centers & services; Aging; Economically disadvantaged.
Types of support: General/operating support, continuing support, equipment, program development, seed money, research, matching funds.
Limitations: Giving limited to Santa Clara County, CA. No support for religious purposes. No grants to individuals.
Publications: Annual report, grants list, 990-PF, informational brochure (including application guidelines).
Application information: Application form required.
Initial approach: Letter of intent
Copies of proposal: 1
Deadline(s): Nov. 1, Feb. 1, June 1, and Aug. 1
Board meeting date(s): Quarterly
Officers and Directors:* Phillip R. Boyce,* Chair.; Ralph Ross,* Vice-Chair.; Richard Sieve, M.D., Secy.; Sidney Resnick, Treas. and C.F.O.; Ervie L. Smith, Exec. Dir.; Herbert Kain, M.D., Edgar G. La Veque, M.D., Michael Rubenstein, Walter Silberman, M.D.
Number of staff: 1 part-time professional; 1 part-time support.
EIN: 941584547
Grants for Aging:
Live Oak Adult Day Care Services, Los Gatos, CA, $40,000. Toward ongoing operating support. 94.

Project Match, San Jose, CA, $17,500. For Bridges to Independence Program and to hire case manager. 94.
Respite and Research for Alzheimers Disease, Mountain View, CA, $50,000. Toward construction of residential facility. 94.
Salvation Army of Santa Clara County, San Jose, CA, $30,000. For mini-bus to transport senior citizens to and from senior program. 94.

111
Wolf Family Foundation
12100 Wilshire Blvd., Suite 1030
Los Angeles 90025

Established in 1990.
Financial data (yr. ended 12/31/94): Assets, $1,293,428 (M); expenditures, $69,381; qualifying distributions, $59,300, including $59,300 for 19 grants (high: $25,600; low: $50).
Fields of interest: Human services; Aging, centers & services; Jewish federated giving programs; Jewish agencies & temples.
Limitations: Applications not accepted. Giving primarily in Southern CA. No grants to individuals.
Application information: Contributes only to pre-selected organizations.
Trustees: Susan W. Kozberg, Bennett L. Wolf, Donald S. Wolf.
EIN: 954279254
Grants for Aging:
Jewish Homes for the Aging of Greater Los Angeles, Reseda, CA, $7,500. 94.

112
The Women's Foundation
340 Pine St., 3rd Floor
San Francisco 94105 (415) 431-1290
Contact: Patti Chang, Exec. Dir.
FAX: (415) 864-7287;
E-mail: womensfoun@igc.apc.org

Founded in 1981 in CA.
Financial data (yr. ended 06/30/94): Assets, $2,039,083 (M); gifts received, $723,085; expenditures, $872,462; qualifying distributions, $643,464, including $249,340 for grants.
Purpose and activities: To create environments in which low-income women and girls empower themselves.
Fields of interest: Arts/cultural programs; Health care; Health organizations; Human services; Children & youth, services; Aging, centers & services; Women, centers & services; Minorities/immigrants, centers & services; Homeless, human services; Minorities; Aging; Women; Gays/lesbians; Economically disadvantaged; Homeless.
Types of support: General/operating support, conferences/seminars, scholarship funds, scholarships—to individuals.
Limitations: Giving limited to San Francisco and northern CA.
Publications: Annual report.
Officers and Directors:* Willa Seldon,* Pres.; Patricia Chang,* Exec. Dir.; Tangerine Brigham, Adriana Cardenas, Mary Cosper, Mary Daddio, Katie Deamer, Lillian Johnson, Tara Kelly, Luz Vega Marquis, Mary Ann Massenburg, Raeann Rivera, Barbara Weiss.

113
Henry B. Woo Foundation
c/o Bessie K. Woo
1750 Taylor St., Suite 1903
San Francisco 94133

Financial data (yr. ended 03/31/95): Assets, $197,830 (M); expenditures, $12,913; qualifying distributions, $12,500, including $12,500 for 5 grants (high: $5,000; low: $1,000).
Fields of interest: Arts/cultural programs; Aging, centers & services; Aging.
Limitations: Applications not accepted. Giving primarily in San Francisco, CA.
Application information: Contributes only to pre-selected organizations.
Officers: Bessie K. Woo, C.E.O.; Karen W. Chin, Secy.; Russell D. Woo, C.F.O.
EIN: 942922498

COLORADO

114
The Anschutz Family Foundation
555 17th St., Suite 2400
Denver 80202 (303) 293-2338
Contact: Sue Anschutz-Rodgers, Pres.

Established in 1982 in CO.
Donor(s): Fred B. Anschutz,‡ Sue Anschutz-Rodgers.
Financial data (yr. ended 11/30/95): Assets, $4,426,023 (M); expenditures, $1,104,252; qualifying distributions, $893,221, including $893,221 for 211 grants (high: $20,000; low: $200; average: $1,000-$10,000).
Purpose and activities: "The foundation's mission is to support efforts to assist the elderly, the young, and the economically disadvantaged. The foundation expresses special interest in endeavors that promote community development which emphasizes self-sufficiency. Further, the foundation encourages strengthening the family and their values to become responsible citizens of society. The foundation's goal in philanthropy is to help people help themselves while preserving their self-respect."
Fields of interest: Arts/cultural programs; Education; Health care; Mental health/crisis services; Food services; Housing/shelter, temporary shelter; Human services; Children & youth, services; Family services; Human services, self-help groups; Aging, centers & services; Community development, neighborhood development; Aging; Economically disadvantaged.
Types of support: General/operating support.
Limitations: Giving primarily in CO, with emphasis on Denver. No support for programs within educational or research institutions, or religious organizations for religious purposes. No grants to individuals, or for capital or building funds, deficit financing, endowment funds, special events or promotions, scholarships, fellowships, conferences, or graduate or post-graduate research.
Publications: Annual report (including application guidelines).
Application information: Organizations receiving successive support for 2 years are ineligible to apply the following year. Only 1 proposal per organization per 12-month funding cycle will be considered. Application form not required.
Initial approach: 2-to 3-page letter
Copies of proposal: 1
Deadline(s): Submit proposal before Mar. 1 and Sept. 1
Board meeting date(s): May and Nov.
Final notification: By Nov. 30
Officers and Directors:* Sue Anschutz-Rodgers,* Pres. and Exec. Dir.; Nancy P. Anschutz,* V.P.; Philip F. Anschutz,* V.P.; Hugh C. Braly,* Secy.; Susan A. Spindler,* Treas.; Sarah Anschutz, Melinda Rodgers Couzens, Melissa Rodgers Padgett, Susan E. Rodgers.
Number of staff: 2 full-time professional; 1 full-time support.
EIN: 742132676
Grants for Aging:
Denver Inner City Parish, Denver, CO, $8,500. For Parish Pals program. 95.
Meals on Wheels of Greeley, Greeley, CO, $3,500. 95.
Senior Support Services, Denver, CO, $5,000. 95.

115
The Aristek Foundation, Inc.
1400 South Colorado Blvd., Suite 410
Denver 80222
Contact: Craig M. Bollman, Jr., Dir.

Financial data (yr. ended 11/30/94): Assets, $32,533 (M); gifts received, $5,000; expenditures, $969; qualifying distributions, $214.
Fields of interest: Education; Aging, centers & services; Aging.
Limitations: Giving primarily in AZ and CO. No grants to individuals.
Application information: No grants paid in fiscal 1994.
Initial approach: Letter
Deadline(s): None
Director: Craig M. Bollman, Jr.
EIN: 841008697

116
Margaret McDonald Boss Living Trust
4704 Harlan St., Suite 685
Denver 80212-7420
Contact: Richard D. Casey, Trustee

Financial data (yr. ended 02/28/95): Assets, $499,480 (M); expenditures, $44,211; qualifying distributions, $33,483, including $24,860 for 153 grants (high: $750; low: $50).
Fields of interest: Arts/cultural programs; Education; Health care; Hospices; Aging, centers & services; Government/public administration; Christian agencies & churches; Aging.
Limitations: Giving primarily in CO.
Application information:
Initial approach: Letter
Deadline(s): None
Trustee: Richard D. Casey.
EIN: 846076742

117
Nathan B. & Florence R. Burt Foundation, Inc.

1600 Lincoln St., Suite 2750
Denver 80264 (303) 863-8400
Contact: Harry L. Arkin, Pres.

Established in 1984.
Donor(s): N.B. Burt,‡ F.R. Burt.‡
Financial data (yr. ended 09/30/95): Assets, $1,805,716 (M); gifts received, $102,712; expenditures, $105,154; qualifying distributions, $79,360, including $60,456 for 34 grants (high: $3,500; low: $500).
Fields of interest: Health care; Geriatrics; Children & youth, services.
Limitations: Giving primarily in CO. No grants to individuals.
Publications: 990-PF, application guidelines.
Application information: Application form required.
Copies of proposal: 1
Deadline(s): Apr. and Oct.
Board meeting date(s): May and Nov.
Officers: Harry L. Arkin, Pres.; John C. Baker, V.P.; Harrison F. Hayes, M.D., Secy.; Bruce M. Heider, Treas.
Directors: Ramon Burt, Bruce W. Jafek, M.D., Natalie Meyer.
Number of staff: 1 part-time professional; 1 part-time support.
EIN: 840972203
Grants for Aging:
Association for Senior Citizens, Denver, CO, $2,500. 94.

118
Colorado Springs Community Trust Fund

90 South Cascade, Suite 1000
Colorado Springs 80903 (719) 475-7730
Contact: Jack W. Foutch

Established in 1928 in CO by declaration of trust.
Foundation type: Community
Financial data (yr. ended 12/31/94): Assets, $3,530,471 (M); expenditures, $175,132, including $109,863 for 39 grants (high: $7,576; low: $300; average: $5,000-$10,000).
Purpose and activities: Emphasis on community funds, youth agencies, health, and child welfare.
Fields of interest: Visual arts; Museums; Performing arts; Historic preservation/historical societies; Arts/cultural programs; Education, research; Child development, education; Elementary school/education; Higher education; Adult education—literacy & basic skills; Reading; Education; Hospitals (general); Medical care, rehabilitation; Nursing care; Health care; Substance abuse, services; Mental health/crisis services; Health associations; Alcoholism; Delinquency prevention/services; Crime/law enforcement; Food services; Recreation; Human services; Children & youth, services; Child development, services; Family services; Hospices; Aging, centers & services; Women, centers & services; Minorities/immigrants, centers & services; International relief; Human rights (international); Community development; Voluntarism promotion; Federated giving programs; Social sciences; Government/public administration; Minorities; Disabled; Aging; Women; Economically disadvantaged.
Types of support: Continuing support, annual campaigns, building/renovation, equipment, emergency funds, program development, seed money.
Limitations: Giving primarily in CO, with emphasis on El Paso County. No grants to individuals, or for operating budgets, deficit financing, endowment funds, matching gifts, scholarships, fellowships, research, demonstration projects, publications, or conferences; no loans.
Publications: Annual report, informational brochure (including application guidelines).
Application information: Application form not required.
Initial approach: Letter
Copies of proposal: 1
Deadline(s): None
Board meeting date(s): 4 times a year
Final notification: 1 week
Trustees: Casey Brady, Charles F. Emmer, Donald R. Sall.
Director: Wilton Cogswell III.
Number of staff: 1 part-time support.
EIN: 510217708

119
Comprecare Foundation, Inc.

1390 Logan St., Suite 402
Denver 80203 (303) 832-1005
Contact: J.R. Gilsdorf, Exec. Dir.

Established in 1986 in CO.
Financial data (yr. ended 12/31/95): Assets, $5,098,176 (M); gifts received, $50,000; expenditures, $316,965; qualifying distributions, $214,239, including $214,239 for grants.
Purpose and activities: "To encourage, aid or assist specific health related programs and to support the activities of organizations and individuals who advance and promote health care education, the delivery of health care services, and the improvement of community health and welfare."
Fields of interest: Health care; Mental health/crisis services; Health associations; Alcoholism; Health organizations; Children & youth, services; Aging, centers & services; Aging.
Types of support: Program development, conferences/seminars, seed money, research.
Limitations: Giving limited to CO. No grants to individuals, or for fellowships, scholarships, operating expenses, debt reduction, land acquisition, fundraising events, or testimonial dinners or promotions.
Publications: Annual report.
Application information: Application form not required.
Initial approach: Letter (1 to 2 pages)
Copies of proposal: 1
Deadline(s): Aug. 15 for following calendar year
Board meeting date(s): Monthly
Final notification: Following board meeting
Officers and Directors:* Joseph P. Natale,* Chair.; Marcus B. Bond, M.D.,* Vice-Chair.; Richard F. Negri,* Secy.-Treas.; Bradford L. Darling, D.O., Raymond C. Delisle, Ellen J. Mangione, M.D., Stephen T. O'Dell, M. Eugene Sherman, M.D., Eric D. Sipf.
Number of staff: 1 part-time professional; 1 part-time support.
EIN: 840641406
Grants for Aging:
Grand Valley Senior Daybreak, Grand Junction, CO, $10,600. 94.
Senior Hub, Federal Heights, CO, $500. 94.

120
George W. Doering Family Foundation

14495 WCR 64
Greeley 80631

Established in 1990 in CO.
Donor(s): George W. Doering.
Financial data (yr. ended 12/31/94): Assets, $817,900 (M); gifts received, $552,859; expenditures, $45,904; qualifying distributions, $45,000, including $45,000 for grants.
Fields of interest: Education; Human services; Aging.
Limitations: Applications not accepted. Giving primarily in CO and TX.
Application information: Contributes only to pre-selected organizations.
Officers: George W. Doering, Pres.; Gayle E. Doering, Secy.
Directors: Christopher Doering, Elisabeth J. Reeves.
EIN: 841158147

121
The Joseph Henry Edmondson Foundation

810 Holly Sugar Bldg.
Colorado Springs 80903
Contact: Robert H. Ramsay, Pres.

Established in 1987 in CO.
Financial data (yr. ended 07/31/95): Assets, $7,660,986 (M); gifts received, $21,586; expenditures, $411,656; qualifying distributions, $376,304, including $361,875 for 26 grants (high: $50,000; low: $500).
Purpose and activities: Giving limited to the welfare of children, the ill, and the elderly, the preservation and improvement of the environment, historic and folk art museums, medical research, and outreach programs administered by the United Church of Christ.
Fields of interest: Museums; Environment; Health care; Medical research; Children & youth, services; Family services; Aging, centers & services; Homeless, human services.
Types of support: Continuing support, capital campaigns, building/renovation, emergency funds, program development, seed money.
Limitations: Applications not accepted. Giving limited to the Colorado Springs, CO, area. No grants to individuals.
Officers and Directors:* Robert H. Ramsay,* Pres. and Treas.; Ruth Rouss,* V.P. and Secy.; Bruce T. Buell, Christopher Bruce Duff, Susan Gould.
Number of staff: None.
EIN: 841090456
Grants for Aging:
Pikes Peak Seniors, Colorado Springs, CO, $15,000. 94.

Silver Key Senior Services, Colorado Springs, CO, $2,000. 94.

122
El Pomar Foundation
Ten Lake Circle
Colorado Springs 80906 (719) 633-7733
Contact: William J. Hybl, Chair.
Application address: P.O. Box 158, Colorado Springs, CO 80901

Incorporated in 1937 in CO.
Donor(s): Spencer Penrose,‡ Mrs. Spencer Penrose.‡
Financial data (yr. ended 12/31/94): Assets, $289,230,720 (M); expenditures, $13,548,191; qualifying distributions, $13,021,345, including $10,453,092 for 184 grants (high: $10,000,000; low: $500), $1,700 for 4 employee matching gifts, $1,029,037 for 1 program-related investment and $70,213 for 1 in-kind gift.
Purpose and activities: Grants only to nonprofit organizations for public, educational, arts and humanities, health, and welfare purposes, including child welfare, the disadvantaged, and housing; municipalities may request funds for specific projects.
Fields of interest: Media/communications; Visual arts; Museums; Performing arts; Theater; Music; Humanities; Historic preservation/historical societies; Arts/cultural programs; Child development, education; Elementary school/education; Secondary school/education; Vocational education; Higher education; Adult/continuing education; Adult education—literacy & basic skills; Libraries/library science; Reading; Education; Natural resource conservation & protection; Environment; Hospitals (general); Pharmacology; Health care; Substance abuse, services; Health organizations; Employment; Food services; Nutrition; Housing/shelter, development; Recreation; Human services; Children & youth, services; Child development, services; Family services; Hospices; Aging, centers & services; Homeless, human services; Community development; Voluntarism promotion; Federated giving programs; Transportation; Minorities; Disabled; Aging; Economically disadvantaged; Homeless.
Types of support: General/operating support, continuing support, capital campaigns, building/renovation, equipment, land acquisition, emergency funds, program development, scholarship funds, program-related investments/loans, employee matching gifts.
Limitations: Giving limited to CO. No support for organizations that distribute funds to other grantees, or for camps or seasonal facilities. No grants to individuals, or for annual campaigns, travel, film or other media projects, conferences, deficit financing, endowment funds, research, matching gifts, seed money, or publications.
Publications: Annual report (including application guidelines), application guidelines, grants list, informational brochure.
Application information: Application form not required.
Initial approach: Proposal
Copies of proposal: 1
Deadline(s): None
Board meeting date(s): 6 to 8 times a year
Final notification: 90 days
Officers and Trustees:* William J. Hybl,* Chair. and C.E.O.; Karl E. Eitel, Chair., Exec. Comm.; R. Thayer Tutt, Jr.,* Pres. and C.I.O.; Robert J. Hilbert,* V.P., Administration and Secy.-Treas.; David J. Palenchar, V.P., Progs.; Kent O. Olin.
Number of staff: 18 full-time professional; 12 full-time support; 3 part-time support.
EIN: 846002373
Grants for Aging:
Montrose County Senior Transportation, Montrose, CO, $10,000. For minivan. 94.
Pueblo Senior Citizen Resource Development and Coordinating Agency, Pueblo, CO, $100,000. For kitchen equipment and furniture. 94.
Sisters of Charity of Cincinnati, Colorado Springs, CO, $50,000. For conferences and maintenance of retirement center. 94.
West Routt Rural Health Council, Hayden, CO, $10,000. For Senior Assisted Living Center. 94.

123
Gates Foundation
3200 Cherry Creek South Dr., Suite 630
Denver 80209-3247 (303) 722-1881
Contact: Thomas Stokes, Exec. Dir.

Incorporated in 1946 in CO.
Donor(s): Charles C. Gates, Sr.,‡ Hazel Gates,‡ John Gates.‡
Financial data (yr. ended 12/31/95): Assets, $150,222,785 (M); expenditures, $7,169,337; qualifying distributions, $6,334,774, including $5,682,197 for 97 grants (high: $500,000; low: $750; average: $5,000-$100,000).
Purpose and activities: To promote the health, welfare, and broad education of mankind whether by means of research, grants, publications, the foundation's own agencies and activities, or through cooperation with agencies and institutions already in existence. Grants primarily for education and youth services, including leadership development; public policy; historic preservation, humanities, and cultural affairs; health care, including cost reduction; and human services.
Fields of interest: Visual arts; Museums; Performing arts; Dance; Theater; Music; Humanities; Historic preservation/historical societies; Arts/cultural programs; Education, association; Education, fund raising; Elementary school/education; Secondary school/education; Higher education; Adult/continuing education; Adult education—literacy & basic skills; Libraries/library science; Reading; Education; Natural resource conservation & protection; Recreation; Youth development, services; Human services; Youth, services; Aging, centers & services; Economics; Public policy, research; Government/public administration; Leadership development; Aging.
Types of support: General/operating support, continuing support, capital campaigns, building/renovation, equipment, land acquisition, endowment funds, program development, publication, fellowships, matching funds.
Limitations: Giving limited to CO, especially the Denver area, except for foundation-initiated grants. No support for private foundations, medical facilities, or individual public schools of public school districts. No grants to individuals, or for operating budgets, medical research, annual campaigns, emergency funds, deficit financing, purchase of tickets for fundraising dinners, parties, balls, or other social fundraising events, purchase of vehicles or office equipment, research, or scholarships; no loans.
Publications: Annual report (including application guidelines), grants list.
Application information: Application form not required.
Initial approach: Telephone call or short summary proposal
Copies of proposal: 1
Deadline(s): Jan. 15, Apr. 1, July 15, and Oct. 1
Board meeting date(s): Approximately Apr. 1, June 15, Oct. 1, and Dec. 15
Final notification: 2 weeks following meetings
Officers and Trustees:* Charles C. Gates,* Pres.; Diane Gates Wallach,* V.P.; Thomas C. Stokes, Secy.-Treas. and Exec. Dir.; George B. Beardsley, Charles G. Cannon, F. Charles Froelicher, William W. Grant III, Mike Wilfley.
Staff: Ellen K. Fisher, Prog. Officer.
Number of staff: 3 full-time professional; 2 full-time support.
EIN: 840474837
Grants for Aging:
Pueblo Senior Citizen Resource Development and Coordinating Agency, Pueblo, CO, $50,000. For kitchen equipment and furniture in new senior center. 94.

124
HealthONE
(Formerly Presbyterian/St. Luke's Community Foundation)
600 South Cherry St., Suite 217
Denver 80222 (303) 322-3515
Contact: Mary Anstine, Pres. and C.E.O.
FAX: (303) 322-4576

Established in 1979 in CO; current name adopted in 1994 following merger with Swedish Medical Center Foundation.
Donor(s): Gerald H. Phipps, Inc., Hensel-Phelps Construction Co.
Foundation type: Community
Financial data (yr. ended 08/31/95): Assets, $29,347,912 (M); gifts received, $1,021,447; expenditures, $2,830,153, including $1,981,759 for grants.
Purpose and activities: To promote health care services, research, and education that improve the quality of human lives within the Rocky Mountain region. Interests include addressing health care and social needs of the elderly, women, children, organ transplant patients, and cancer patients; support also for public and health professions education. HealthONE is in the process of revising its purpose statement.
Fields of interest: Public health school/education; Health sciences school/education; Medicine/medical care, community health systems; Health care; Health associations; Medical research; Aging, centers & services.
Types of support: Program development, seed money, research.
Limitations: Giving limited to the Front Range, CO, area. No grants to individuals.

Publications: Annual report, newsletter, application guidelines.
Application information: Application form required.
Initial approach: Telephone
Copies of proposal: 3
Deadline(s): First Friday in Oct., Jan., Apr., and July
Board meeting date(s): Quarterly
Officers and Directors:* Robert B. Sawyer, M.D.,* Chair.; Jean C. Jones,* Vice-Chair.; Mary Anstine, Pres. and C.E.O.; Carol Spies, M.D.,* Secy.; Lewis Douglas, Jr., Treas.; Sue Baird, and 19 additional directors.
Staff: Katherine E. Gibson, Network Analyst; Khanh T.T. Nguyen, Grants Administrator; Leslie Strate, Prog. Coord.
Number of staff: None.
EIN: 742568941

125
A. V. Hunter Trust, Inc.

55 Madison St., Suite 225
Denver 80206 (303) 399-5450
Contact: Sharon Siddons, Secy.

Trust established in 1927; incorporated in 1937 in CO.
Donor(s): A.V. Hunter.‡
Financial data (yr. ended 12/31/95): Assets, $39,482,000 (M); expenditures, $2,202,793; qualifying distributions, $1,847,824, including $1,469,955 for 125 grants (high: $90,000; low: $2,000; average: $5,000-$10,000) and $290,401 for 1,354 grants to individuals.
Purpose and activities: Distributions to organizations who give aid, comfort, support, or assistance to children, aged persons, indigent adults, or the needy; no direct grant payments made to individuals. Special interest in prevention programs targeting child abuse, domestic violence, gangs, teenage pregnancy, and senior services.
Fields of interest: Human services; Children & youth, services; Disabled; Aging; Economically disadvantaged; Homeless.
Types of support: General/operating support.
Limitations: Giving limited to CO. No support for tax-supported institutions. No grants to individuals directly, or for scholarships, capital improvements, or acquisitions; no loans.
Publications: Annual report, informational brochure (including application guidelines).
Application information: Application form required for grants to individuals; accepts Common Grant Application form. Application form required.
Initial approach: Letter
Copies of proposal: 1
Deadline(s): Mar. 1, June 1, and Aug. 1
Board meeting date(s): May., Aug., and Nov. and as required
Final notification: Within 20 days after meeting
Officers and Trustees:* William K. Coors,* Pres.; George Gibson,* V.P.; Sharon Siddons, Secy.; Allan B. Adams,* Treas.; W. Robert Alexander, Mary Anstine.
Number of staff: 3 full-time professional.
EIN: 840461332
Grants for Aging:
Association of Senior Citizens, Denver, CO, $10,000. 94.
Brothers Redevelopment, Denver, CO, $20,000. 94.
Hilltop Foundation, Grand Junction, CO, $30,000. For Senior Services program. 94.
Seniors, Denver, CO, $10,000. 94.
Visiting Nurse Association of the Denver Area, Denver, CO, $20,000. For Senior Services program. 94.

126
Helen K. and Arthur E. Johnson Foundation

1700 Broadway, Rm. 2302
Denver 80290 (303) 861-4127
Contact: Stan Kamprath, Exec. Dir.
FAX: (303) 861-0607

Incorporated in 1948 in CO.
Donor(s): Arthur E. Johnson,‡ Helen K. Johnson.‡
Financial data (yr. ended 12/31/95): Assets, $89,188,567 (M); expenditures, $6,133,367; qualifying distributions, $4,635,186, including $4,507,048 for 164 grants (high: $500,000; low: $250; average: $5,000-$30,000).
Purpose and activities: "To solve human problems and enrich the quality of human life." Emphasis on operational and capital support for community and social services, education, youth, senior citizens, health, and civic and cultural affairs.
Fields of interest: Arts/cultural programs; Education; Health care; Youth, services; Community development; Aging.
Types of support: General/operating support, continuing support, annual campaigns, capital campaigns, building/renovation, equipment, land acquisition, program development, seed money, scholarship funds, research, technical assistance, matching funds.
Limitations: Giving limited to CO. No grants to individuals, or for endowment funds, conferences, or purchase of blocks of tickets; no loans.
Publications: Annual report (including application guidelines).
Application information: Application form not required.
Initial approach: Letter or preliminary proposal (no more than 2 pages)
Copies of proposal: 1
Deadline(s): Jan. 1, Apr. 1, July 1, and Oct. 1
Board meeting date(s): Mar., June, Sept., and Dec.
Final notification: 2 weeks after board meeting
Officers and Trustees:* Mrs. James R. Hartley,* Pres.; Lynn H. Campion, V.P. and Treas.; Stan Kamprath, V.P. and Exec. Dir.; Gerald R. Hillyard, Jr.,* Secy.; Thomas B. Campion, Jr., Charles R. Hazelrigg, Roger D. Knight, Jr., Ronald L. Lehr, Stanley D. Neeleman.
Staff: Brigit A. Davis, Prog. Officer.
Number of staff: 1 full-time professional; 2 full-time support; 1 part-time support.
EIN: 846020702
Grants for Aging:
Alzheimers Disease and Related Disorders Association, Denver, CO, $30,000. For general support. 94.
Bonell Good Samaritan Center, Greeley, CO, $10,000. For Alzheimer's Care Unit. 94.
Brothers Redevelopment, Denver, CO, $20,000. For Volunteer Home Repair Program. 94.
Christian Living Campus at University Hills, Denver, CO, $380,000. For expansion project. 94.
Elderhaus, Adult Program, Fort Collins, CO, $10,000. For Eagles Club. 94.
Grand County Council on Aging, Granby, CO, $15,000. For van. 94.
Grand Valley Senior Daybreak, Grand Junction, CO, $16,000. For facility renovations. 94.
Hospice of Metro Denver, Denver, CO, $25,000. For home services. 94.
Pikes Peak Seniors, Colorado Springs, CO, $30,000. For Child Care Program. 94.
Seniors, Denver, CO, $15,000. For Money Management Program. 94.

127
The Carl W. and Carrie Mae Joslyn Charitable Trust

c/o Bank One, Colorado Springs, N.A.
P.O. Box 1699, Trust Dept.
Colorado Springs 80942 (719) 471-5125

Trust established in 1971 in CO.
Donor(s): Carl W. Joslyn,‡ Carrie Mae Joslyn.‡
Financial data (yr. ended 12/31/95): Assets, $2,186,362 (M); expenditures, $86,217; qualifying distributions, $80,599, including $76,480 for 12 grants (high: $34,900; low: $950).
Fields of interest: Education; Medical care, rehabilitation; Children & youth, services; Aging, centers & services; Disabled; Aging.
Types of support: General/operating support, annual campaigns, building/renovation, equipment, endowment funds, program development.
Limitations: Giving limited to El Paso County, CO. No grants to individuals, or for research, scholarships, fellowships, or matching gifts; no loans.
Publications: Application guidelines, 990-PF.
Application information: Application form not required.
Initial approach: Letter
Copies of proposal: 1
Deadline(s): Submit proposal preferably in Apr. or Oct.; deadlines Apr. 30 and Oct. 31
Board meeting date(s): May and Nov.
Final notification: July 1 and Dec. 1
Trustee: Bank One, Colorado Springs, N.A.
Number of staff: None.
EIN: 237135817
Grants for Aging:
Silver Key Senior Services, Colorado Springs, CO, $34,900. 95.

128
The KBK Foundation

(Formerly The Kavadas Foundation)
c/o Judson W. Detrick
1700 Lincoln, Suite 4100
Denver 80203 (303) 861-7000
Contact: Paul D. Holleman, Trustee

Established in 1991 in CO.
Donor(s): Kathryn B. Kavadas.

Financial data (yr. ended 12/31/95): Assets, $471,479 (M); gifts received, $97,000; expenditures, $103,008; qualifying distributions, $95,800, including $95,800 for 10 grants (high: $25,000; low: $1,000; average: $1,000-$25,000).
Fields of interest: Museums; Elementary/secondary education; Higher education; Senior continuing care community; Aging.
Limitations: Applications not accepted. Giving primarily in the greater Boston, MA, area. No grants to individuals.
Application information: Contributes only to pre-selected organizations.
Officer and Trustees:* Kathryn B. Kavadas,* Mgr.; Judson W. Detrick, Paul D. Holleman, Thomas A. Richardson.
EIN: 841186316

129
Kitzmiller-Bales Trust
P.O. Box 96
Wray 80758 (303) 332-4824
Contact: Robert U. Hansen, Trustee
Additional tel.: (303) 332-4406

Established in 1984 in CO.
Donor(s): Edna B. Kitzmiller.‡
Financial data (yr. ended 12/31/93): Assets, $5,635,944 (M); expenditures, $359,862; qualifying distributions, $335,963, including $334,582 for 16 grants (high: $117,000; low: $400).
Fields of interest: Historic preservation/historical societies; Arts/cultural programs; Education, fund raising; Libraries/library science; Education; Hospitals (general); Medical care, rehabilitation; Health care; Health organizations; Recreation; Aging, centers & services; Community development; Federated giving programs; Government/public administration; Aging.
Types of support: Continuing support, capital campaigns, building/renovation, equipment, program development, matching funds.
Limitations: Giving limited to projects benefiting the area of East Yuma County School District, RJ-2, CO.
Application information: Application form not required.
Initial approach: Letter
Copies of proposal: 1
Deadline(s): None
Board meeting date(s): Monthly
Final notification: Following board meetings
Trustees: Duard Fix, Robert U. Hansen, Farmers State Bank, Brush.
Number of staff: None.
EIN: 846178085

130
The Raphael Levy Memorial Foundation, Inc.
P.O. Box 100217
Denver 80250
Contact: Barbara Goldburg, Pres.

Incorporated in 1944 in CO.
Financial data (yr. ended 12/31/95): Assets, $3,707,585 (M); expenditures, $216,635; qualifying distributions, $181,413, including $172,717 for 88 grants (high: $50,000; low: $200; average: $200-$50,000).
Purpose and activities: Primary areas of giving include hospitals, Jewish organizations, education, the environment, music, and community welfare.
Fields of interest: Museums; Performing arts; Music; Arts/cultural programs; Education; Natural resource conservation & protection; Environment; Wildlife preservation & protection; Hospitals (general); Health care; Mental health/crisis services; Health associations; AIDS; AIDS research; Recreation; Human services; Children & youth, services; Family services; Hospices; Aging, centers & services; Women, centers & services; Homeless, human services; Peace; Human rights (international); Race/intergroup relations; Civil rights; Federated giving programs; Jewish agencies & temples; Disabled; Aging; Women; Gays/lesbians; Homeless.
Limitations: Giving primarily in CO. No grants to individuals.
Application information: Application form not required.
Copies of proposal: 1
Deadline(s): None
Board meeting date(s): As required
Officers and Directors:* Barbara Goldburg,* Pres.; John Levy,* V.P. and Treas.; Edward Levy.
Number of staff: 1 part-time support.
EIN: 846022586

131
The Neusteter Colorado Company
2552 East Alameda Ave., Rm. 119
Denver 80209-3325

Established in 1945 in CO.
Financial data (yr. ended 12/31/94): Assets, $795,625 (M); expenditures, $37,330; qualifying distributions, $33,817, including $30,955 for 35 grants (high: $10,075; low: $25).
Fields of interest: Arts/cultural programs; Nursing home/convalescent facility; Health organizations; Human services; Jewish agencies & temples.
Limitations: Applications not accepted. Giving primarily in Denver, CO. No grants to individuals.
Application information: Contributes only to pre-selected organizations.
Officers: Shirley R. Neusteter, Pres.; Nancy R. Neusteter, V.P. and Secy.-Treas.; Cynthia N. Auer, V.P. and Mgr.; Myron David Neusteter, Jr., V.P.
Trustee: Myron D. Neusteter.
EIN: 846021735

132
Public Service Company of Colorado Corporate Contributions Program
P.O. Box 840
Denver 80201-0840 (303) 294-8212
Contact: Marilyn Gerdes, Community Rels. Assoc.
FAX: (303) 294-8120

Established in 1866 in CO.
Financial data (yr. ended 12/31/93): Total giving, $2,799,504, including $2,767,504 for 598 grants (high: $1,000,000; low: $500; average: $500-$2,750) and $32,000 for employee matching gifts.
Purpose and activities: "Public Service Company is committed to helping solve community problems. Each year, PSCo selects targeted populations or programs for corporate support. The Charitable Contributions program has several dimensions, including: in-kind donations, employee volunteerism and board involvement, special event sponsorship, and direct contributions. These services are offered in areas of the state where Public Service Company is active in providing energy services."
Fields of interest: Education; Environment, pollution control; Environment, waste management; Natural resource conservation & protection; Environment; Employment, services; Civil rights, aging.
Types of support: Annual campaigns, program development, scholarship funds, technical assistance, cause-related marketing, consulting services, employee volunteer services, loaned talent, public relations services, use of facilities, sponsorships, employee matching gifts, employee-related scholarships, donated equipment, donated products, in-kind gifts, matching funds.
Limitations: Giving primarily in CO, and areas of company operations. No support for religious or political organizations, or non-tax exempt organizations. No grants to individuals, or for video or research projects, multi-year pledges or commitments, or consecutive year funding.
Publications: Corporate report, informational brochure (including application guidelines).
Application information: The company has a contributions staff. Application form required.
Initial approach: Request current guidelines by telephone or letter to headquarters
Copies of proposal: 1
Deadline(s): Mar. 15, June 15, Sept. 15, and Nov. 15
Final notification: 2 to 6 weeks after deadlines
Administrator: Dan Danbom, Mgr., Community Rels., and Employee Communications.
Number of staff: 3 full-time professional; 1 part-time support.

133
Harry W. Rabb Foundation
6242 South Elmira Circle
Englewood 80111
Contact: Richard A. Zarlengo, Secy.-Treas.

Established in 1960.
Donor(s): Harry W. Rabb.‡
Financial data (yr. ended 06/30/95): Assets, $1,677,848 (M); expenditures, $143,753; qualifying distributions, $129,750, including $128,850 for 48 grants (high: $25,000; low: $200).
Fields of interest: Hospitals (general); AIDS; AIDS research; Human services; Hospices; Aging, centers & services; Jewish federated giving programs; Aging; General charitable giving.
Types of support: Annual campaigns.

Limitations: Giving limited to CO, with emphasis on Denver. No support for religious or parochial schools, or religious organizations for religious purposes, or to organizations which discriminate for reasons of race, sex, national origin, physical handicap, or sexual orientation. No grants to individuals, or for travel, conferences, conventions, meetings, or seminars.
Application information: No telephone calls. Application form not required.
Initial approach: Letter (1 to 2 pages)
Copies of proposal: 1
Deadline(s): None
Board meeting date(s): Approximately every 2 months
Officers and Trustees:* Bernard Maiman,* Pres.; Miles Dolan,* V.P.; Richard A. Zarlengo,* Secy.-Treas.
Number of staff: 1 part-time professional.
EIN: 237236149
Grants for Aging:
Seniors, Denver, CO, $2,200. 95.

134
The Summit Foundation
P.O. Box 4000
Breckenridge 80424 (970) 453-5970
Contact: Debra Edwards, Exec. Dir.
Additional address for non-U.S. mail deliveries: 130 Ski Hill Rd., Suite 235, Breckenridge, CO 80424; FAX: (970) 453-1423

Established in 1984 in CO.
Foundation type: Community
Financial data (yr. ended 12/31/94): Assets, $316,401 (M); gifts received, $368,590; expenditures, $427,771, including $249,700 for 47 grants (high: $40,000; low: $500).
Purpose and activities: Giving primarily for arts and culture, health and human services, education, environment, sports, scholarships, and projects with measurable results.
Fields of interest: Film/video; Visual arts; Museums; Performing arts; Theater; Music; Historic preservation/historical societies; Arts/cultural programs; Early childhood education; Elementary school/education; Education; Natural resource conservation & protection; Environment; Health care; Mental health/crisis services; Health organizations; Recreation; Youth, services; Family services; Hospices; Aging, centers & services; Disabled.
Types of support: Continuing support, annual campaigns, capital campaigns, building/renovation, equipment, land acquisition, program development, conferences/seminars, seed money, curriculum development, scholarship funds, technical assistance, program-related investments/loans, scholarships—to individuals, exchange programs, matching funds.
Limitations: Giving limited to Summit County, CO. No support for religious organizations or political campaigns. No grants to individuals (except for designated scholarship program), or for operating budgets.
Publications: Multi-year report, 990-PF, grants list, newsletter, informational brochure, program policy statement, application guidelines.
Application information: Applications accepted during designated time periods only. Application form required.
Initial approach: Letter
Copies of proposal: 19
Deadline(s): Spring and fall, specific date established for each cycle
Board meeting date(s): 2nd Wednesday of each month
Final notification: Within 2 to 3 months
Officers and Directors:* Gordon Briner,* Pres.; Win Lockwood,* V.P.; Anne Stonington,* Secy.; Terie Roubos,* Treas.; Bill DeForrest, Marilyn Hogan, Rick Hum, Cleve Keller, Meg Lass, Gary Martinez, Ann McCrerey, Phil Noll, Jeff Paffrath, John Rutter, John Wood.
Number of staff: 2 full-time professional; 1 full-time support.
EIN: 742341399
Grants for Aging:
Summit County Senior Citizens, Frisco, CO, $8,000. 94.

135
True North Foundation
P.O. Box 271308
Fort Collins 80527 (303) 223-5285
Contact: Ms. K. Hoffman, Pres.
FAX: (303) 495-0892

Established in 1986 in CO.
Financial data (yr. ended 12/31/95): Assets, $12,019,409 (M); expenditures, $1,224,460; qualifying distributions, $1,073,782, including $1,073,782 for 79 grants (high: $75,000; low: $500).
Fields of interest: Natural resource conservation & protection; Environment; Wildlife preservation & protection; Health care, reproductive health; Family planning; Disabled; Aging.
Types of support: General/operating support, equipment, land acquisition, program development, conferences/seminars, seed money, research, technical assistance, consulting services, matching funds.
Limitations: Giving primarily in CA, with emphasis on the San Francisco Bay Area; some giving in the Pacific Northwest. No support for religious purposes. No grants to individuals.
Publications: Informational brochure (including application guidelines).
Application information: Application form required.
Initial approach: Letter
Copies of proposal: 1
Deadline(s): None
Board meeting date(s): Approximately bimonthly
Officer and Directors:* K. Hoffman,* Pres.; S. O'Hara, K.F. Stephens.
Number of staff: 2 part-time professional.
EIN: 742421528

CONNECTICUT

136
Adler Foundation, Inc.
534 East Putnam Ave.
Greenwich 06830 (203) 622-9069
Contact: John Adler, Pres.

Incorporated in 1951 in NY.
Donor(s): Morton M. Adler,‡ Helen R. Adler,‡ Harry Rosenthal.‡
Financial data (yr. ended 09/30/94): Assets, $7,058,369 (M); gifts received, $176,225; expenditures, $480,093; qualifying distributions, $407,810, including $335,450 for 12 grants (high: $75,000; low: $100) and $65,550 for 3 foundation-administered programs.
Purpose and activities: Grants limited to medical research in diabetes, leukemia, and Alzheimer's disease.
Fields of interest: Leukemia research; Alzheimer's disease research; Diabetes research.
Types of support: Conferences/seminars, seed money, research.
Limitations: No grants to individuals.
Application information: Application form not required.
Initial approach: Letter
Copies of proposal: 2
Deadline(s): None
Board meeting date(s): Late Apr.
Officers and Trustees:* John Adler,* Pres.; Joel I. Berson,* Secy.; Helen A. Potter,* Treas.; Katherine A. Astrove, William C. Felch, William G. Kuhns, Paul Leblang, Edmond V. Ledonne, Kenneth E. Quickel, Jr., Dennis J. Selkoe, Wylie Vale.
Number of staff: None.
EIN: 136087869

137
Aged & Indigent Women's Fund
(also known as David Lane Fund for Indigent Women)
c/o Bank of Boston Connecticut, Tax Dept.
P.O. Box 2210
Waterbury 06702

Financial data (yr. ended 12/31/94): Assets, $748,692 (M); expenditures, $40,900; qualifying distributions, $29,694, including $27,590 for 23 grants (high: $11,400; low: $250) and $1,700 for 4 grants to individuals (high: $600; low: $240).
Purpose and activities: Primarily supports aged, indigent women.
Fields of interest: Aging, centers & services; Women, centers & services; Aging; Women; Economically disadvantaged.
Types of support: General/operating support, grants to individuals.
Limitations: Giving limited to Ansonia, Derby, and Shelton, CT.
Application information: Request application forms from Team, Inc. or Connecticut Visiting Nurses Assn. Application form required.
Deadline(s): None
Trustee: Bank of Boston Connecticut.
EIN: 066038194

138
Harlan E. Anderson Foundation
P.O. Box 426
New Canaan 06840
Contact: Harlan E. Anderson, Trustee

Donor(s): Harlan E. Anderson.
Financial data (yr. ended 12/31/93): Assets, $873,106 (M); gifts received, $100,025;

expenditures, $31,451; qualifying distributions, $29,500.
Fields of interest: Historic preservation/historical societies; Aging, centers & services.
Limitations: Giving primarily in the New Canaan, CT, area. No grants to individuals.
Application information: Application form not required.
Deadline(s): None
Trustees: Harlan E. Anderson, Lois J. Anderson, Francis W. Dubreuil.
EIN: 237011480

139
Vernal W. & Florence H. Bates Foundation
c/o James O. Walsh
P.O. Box 1302
New Haven 06505-1302
Application address: 6503 29th Ave. West, Bradenton, FL 34209

Established in 1956 in CT.
Financial data (yr. ended 06/30/95): Assets, $913,057 (M); expenditures, $77,500; qualifying distributions, $58,415, including $48,800 for 7 grants (high: $25,000; low: $1,000).
Purpose and activities: Giving primarily for the purpose of assisting, whether by loan or grant, individuals seeking education, and/or for the purpose of establishing scholarships, fellowships, research projects, professorships, and for chairs of learning at preparatory schools, high schools, colleges, universities, and other institutions of learning, and for the care of the aged, retarded, and handicapped.
Fields of interest: Performing arts; Higher education; Education; Children & youth, services; Youth, services; Aging, centers & services; Disabled; Aging.
Types of support: Professorships, fellowships, scholarship funds, research.
Limitations: Giving primarily in CT and FL.
Application information:
Initial approach: Proposal
Deadline(s): May 1
Board meeting date(s): Between June 1 and July 31
Final notification: Within 5 months after deadline
Officers and Trustees:* Lois Flach,* Chair.; Donna F. George, Secy.; James O. Walsh.
EIN: 066034880

140
Bigelow Tea
201 Black Rock Tpke.
Fairfield 06432 (203) 334-1212
Contact: Cynthia Bigelow, Mgr., Purchasing and Customer Svc.

Purpose and activities: Bigelow's main giving focus is children in need and the elderly. The company makes product donations weekly, and Bigelow employees volunteer as tutors in local schools.
Fields of interest: Education; Children, services; Youth, services; Aging.
Types of support: Scholarship funds, employee volunteer services, donated products.
Limitations: Applications not accepted. Giving primarily in communities near company locations. No support for arts programs.

141
Bodenwein Public Benevolent Foundation
c/o Shawmut Bank, N.A.
250 State St.
New London 06320 (860) 447-6133
Contact: Mildred E. Devine, V.P., Shawmut Bank, N.A.
Application tel.: (860) 447-6155

Established in 1938 in CT.
Donor(s): The Day Trust, Theodore Bodenwein.‡
Financial data (yr. ended 12/31/94): Assets, $446,972 (M); gifts received, $278,145; expenditures, $323,265; qualifying distributions, $321,340, including $314,706 for 30 grants (high: $75,000; low: $500; average: $972-$25,000).
Purpose and activities: Giving to social service and health agencies, including AIDS support, the fine and performing arts and other cultural programs, youth and child welfare agencies, civic affairs and community development groups, education, and minority programs.
Fields of interest: Visual arts; Museums; Performing arts; Theater; Language & linguistics; Literature; Arts/cultural programs; Early childhood education; Child development, education; Adult/continuing education; Adult education—literacy & basic skills; Libraries/library science; Reading; Education; Environment; Animal welfare; Hospitals (general); Family planning; Medical care, rehabilitation; Health care; Substance abuse, services; Mental health/crisis services; Health associations; Cancer; AIDS; Alcoholism; Cancer research; AIDS research; Legal services; Youth development, services; Human services; Children & youth, services; Child development, services; Family services; Aging, centers & services; Women, centers & services; Minorities/immigrants, centers & services; Community development; Voluntarism promotion; Jewish federated giving programs; Engineering & technology; Science; Government/public administration; Transportation; Leadership development; Roman Catholic agencies & churches; Religion; Minorities; Aging; Women.
Types of support: Capital campaigns, building/renovation, equipment, program development, conferences/seminars, publication, seed money, scholarship funds, research, consulting services, matching funds.
Limitations: Giving limited to Lyme, Old Lyme, East Lyme, Waterford, New London, Montville, Groton, Ledyard, Stonington, North Stonington, and Salem, CT.
Publications: Informational brochure (including application guidelines), program policy statement.
Application information: An applicant is limited to submission of 1 grant application per calendar year. Application form required.
Initial approach: Telephone
Copies of proposal: 1
Deadline(s): May 15 and Nov. 15
Board meeting date(s): Jan. and July
Final notification: Feb. 1 and Aug. 1
Trustee: Shawmut Bank, N.A.
Number of staff: None.
EIN: 066030548

142
Bridgeport Ladies Charitable Trust
c/o The Chase Manhattan Bank of Connecticut, N.A.
999 Broad St.
Bridgeport 06604

Chartered in 1814 in CT.
Financial data (yr. ended 09/30/95): Assets, $851,737 (M); gifts received, $365; expenditures, $47,254; qualifying distributions, $38,445, including $38,445 for grants to individuals.
Fields of interest: Education; Health care; Health organizations; Children & youth, services; Youth, services; Family services; Aging, centers & services; Disabled; Aging.
Types of support: Emergency funds, grants to individuals.
Limitations: Applications not accepted. Giving limited to the greater Bridgeport, CT, area.
Publications: Informational brochure.
Application information: Grantees are referred from Emily Woodside Services or community agencies for needy cases requiring health and home assistance.
Officers: Elizabeth E. Shaw, Pres.; Mrs. Robert W. Winton, V.P.; Mrs. Samuel Gilliland, Corresponding Secy.; Mrs. David B. Smith, Recording Secy.; Mrs. Arthur C. Williams, Treas.
Trustee: The Chase Manhattan Bank of Connecticut, N.A.
EIN: 066068224

143
City Missionary Association of New Haven, Inc.
c/o Bank of Boston Connecticut, Tax Dept.
P.O. Box 2210
Waterbury 06722-2210 (203) 393-1562
Contact: Alan O. Dann, Pres.
Application address: 118 Seymour Rd., Woodbridge, CT 06798

Established in 1876 in CT.
Financial data (yr. ended 12/31/94): Assets, $1,068,445 (M); gifts received, $9,000; expenditures, $62,236; qualifying distributions, $49,772, including $49,295 for grants (high: $4,000).
Purpose and activities: Support for Protestant and ecumenical religious activities, public child welfare, Christian teaching, and maintenance of Christian values.
Fields of interest: Mental health/crisis services; AIDS; AIDS research; Food services; Food services, congregate meals; Housing/shelter, development; Camps; Youth, services; Aging, centers & services; Homeless, human services; Christian agencies & churches; Protestant agencies & churches; Aging; Homeless; General charitable giving.

Types of support: General/operating support, emergency funds, matching funds.
Limitations: Giving limited to the greater New Haven, CT, area.
Publications: Program policy statement, grants list.
Application information: Application form not required.
Initial approach: Proposal
Copies of proposal: 6
Deadline(s): Nov. 1
Board meeting date(s): Late Feb.
Final notification: Mar.
Officers: Alan O. Dann, Pres.; Bradford Gesler, V.P.; Georgia Erickson, Secy.; N.H. Borgerson, Jr., Treas.
Trustee: Bank of Boston Connecticut.
EIN: 066032939

144
The Community Foundation of Southeastern Connecticut

(Formerly The Pequot Community Foundation, Inc.)
302 State St.
P.O. Box 769
New London 06320 (860) 442-3572
Contact: Alice F. Fitzpatrick, Exec. Dir.
FAX: (860) 442-0584

Established in 1982 in CT.
Foundation type: Community
Financial data (yr. ended 12/31/95): Assets, $4,165,178 (L); expenditures, $451,797, including $281,453 for grants (average: $1,000-$2,000).
Purpose and activities: To promote learning, to advance scientific research, to provide care for the needy, sick, aged, or helpless, to secure the care of children, to encourage historical, literary, cultural and artistic endeavors, for environmental study, and to otherwise contribute to the general welfare.
Fields of interest: Museums; Historic preservation/historical societies; Arts/cultural programs; Higher education; Adult/continuing education; Adult education—literacy & basic skills; Libraries/library science; Reading; Education; Natural resource conservation & protection; Environment; Health care; Substance abuse, services; Mental health/crisis services; AIDS; Health organizations; Recreation; Human services; Children & youth, services; Youth, services; Family services; Aging, centers & services; Women, centers & services; Community development; Voluntarism promotion; Disabled; Aging; Women; Economically disadvantaged.
Types of support: Building/renovation, equipment, emergency funds, program development, conferences/seminars, publication, seed money, scholarship funds, scholarships—to individuals, in-kind gifts.
Limitations: Giving limited to southeastern CT, including East Lyme, Groton, Ledyard, Lyme, Montville, New London, North Stonington, Old Lyme, Salem, Stonington, and Waterford. No support for sectarian or religious programs. No grants to individuals (except for scholarships awarded by nomination only) or for endowment, memorial, or building funds, operating expenses, deficit financing, or annual campaigns; no loans.
Publications: Annual report, application guidelines, financial statement, grants list, newsletter.
Application information: Application form required.
Initial approach: Telephone or letter
Copies of proposal: 2
Deadline(s): Nov. 15; Apr. 1 for scholarship applications
Board meeting date(s): Mar., June, Sept., and Nov.
Final notification: Grants are distributed in Mar.; scholarships are awarded in June
Officers and Trustees:* Ann den Tex,* Pres.; Daniel Spring,* V.P.; Jeanette Hersey,* Secy.; Francis Pavetti,* Treas.; Alice F. Fitzpatrick, Exec. Dir.; and 26 additional trustees.
Number of staff: 1 full-time professional; 2 part-time support.
EIN: 061080097

145
Connecticut Natural Gas Corporate Contributions Program

100 Columbus Ave.
Hartford 06144-1500 (860) 727-3237
Contact: Frank H. Livingston, V.P., Office of the Chair.

Purpose and activities: Connecticut Natural Gas Corporation has an annual contribution budget of $175,000. Approximately $100,000 of that budget is allocated to the United Way campaigns in Hartford and Greenwich, CT. Other funds are divided into four categories: education, culture, health and human services, and civic and community affairs. Generally, grants of $100 and above are awarded.
Fields of interest: Humanities; Historic preservation/historical societies; Arts/cultural programs; Elementary school/education; Secondary school/education; Adult education—literacy & basic skills; Reading; Education; Natural resource conservation & protection; Energy; Environment; Hospitals (general); Substance abuse, services; Health associations; Crime/law enforcement; Food services; Housing/shelter, development; Safety/disasters; Youth development, services; Youth development, citizenship; Children & youth, services; Youth, services; Family services; Aging, centers & services; Women, centers & services; Minorities/immigrants, centers & services; Homeless, human services; Human rights (international); Civil rights; Urban/community development; Business & industry; Community development; Voluntarism promotion; Economics; Public policy, research; Government/public administration; Public affairs, citizen participation; Leadership development; Public affairs; Minorities; Aging; Women; Homeless.
Types of support: General/operating support, continuing support, annual campaigns, capital campaigns, building/renovation, equipment, conferences/seminars, publication, seed money, technical assistance, employee volunteer services, loaned talent, use of facilities, employee matching gifts, donated equipment, donated products, in-kind gifts.
Limitations: Giving primarily in Hartford, Greenwich, and New Britain, CT, CNG's service territory.
Publications: Corporate report.
Application information: Connecticut Natural Gas Board members must approve requests of $1,000 and above. Application form not required.
Initial approach: Letter to headquarters
Deadline(s): Quarterly
Board meeting date(s): Mar., June, Sept., and Dec.
Administrator: Frank H. Livingston, V.P., Office of the Chair.

146
The Daphne Seybolt Culpeper Memorial Foundation, Inc.

129 Musket Ridge Rd.
Norwalk 06850 (203) 762-3984
Contact: Nicholas J. Nardi, Secy.-Treas.
Application address: P.O. Box 206, Norwalk, CT 06852-0206

Established in 1983 in DE.
Donor(s): Daphne Seybolt Culpeper.‡
Financial data (yr. ended 12/31/95): Assets, $13,619,375 (M); expenditures, $663,204; qualifying distributions, $627,404, including $610,905 for 186 grants (high: $40,000; low: $250).
Fields of interest: Higher education; Medical school/education; Nursing school/education; Education; Hospitals (general); Health care; Health organizations; Domestic violence prevention; Food services; Human services; Children & youth, services; Hospices; Minorities; Native Americans; Disabled; Aging; Women; Economically disadvantaged; Homeless.
Types of support: General/operating support, annual campaigns, capital campaigns, equipment, program development, scholarship funds, matching funds.
Limitations: Giving limited to CT and FL. No grants to individuals.
Publications: Application guidelines.
Application information: Application form not required.
Initial approach: Letter
Copies of proposal: 1
Deadline(s): None
Board meeting date(s): Varies
Officers and Trustees:* Rodney S. Eielson,* Pres.; Nicholas J. Nardi,* Secy.-Treas.
Number of staff: 1 full-time professional.
EIN: 222478755

147
Eastern Connecticut Community Foundation

(Formerly Eastern Connecticut Foundation for Public Giving)
P.O. Box 303
53 Broadway
Norwich 06360 (860) 887-3303
Contact: Gregory P. Fessenden, Exec. Dir.

Incorporated in 1988 in CT.
Foundation type: Community

Financial data (yr. ended 12/31/94): Assets, $225,848 (M); expenditures, $44,597, including $8,750 for grants.
Fields of interest: Historic preservation/historical societies; Arts/cultural programs; Adult education—literacy & basic skills; Reading; Education; Environment; Health care; AIDS; Health organizations; AIDS research; Domestic violence prevention; Housing/shelter, development; Human services; Youth, services; Aging, centers & services; Women, centers & services; Engineering & technology; Science; Disabled; Aging; Women; Economically disadvantaged; Homeless.
Types of support: Seed money.
Limitations: Giving limited to eastern CT. No support for on-going operations, endowments, or memorial or building fund campaigns. No grants to individuals.
Publications: Annual report, informational brochure, financial statement, grants list, application guidelines.
Application information: Application form required.
Initial approach: Letter or telephone
Copies of proposal: 3
Deadline(s): Mar. 15
Board meeting date(s): Quarterly
Final notification: July 1
Officers and Directors:* Kathleen L. Chartier,* Pres.; Robert Sullivan,* V.P.; Philip G. James,* Secy.; Martin Botnick,* Treas.; Gregory P. Fessenden, Exec. Dir.; Elaine M. Coletti, Richard J. Duda, Myles J. Laffey, Marjorie Mandell, and 20 additional directors.
Number of staff: 1 part-time professional.
EIN: 222897455

148
EIS Foundation, Inc.
19 West Walk
Clinton 06413 (860) 669-5367
Contact: Maurice L. Schwarz, Pres.
Additional address (Oct. 15 to May 15): 6931 Queenferry Circle, Boca Raton, FL 33496; Tel.: (561) 852-6854

Incorporated in 1951 in CT.
Donor(s): Joseph W. Gilfix,‡ C.C. Weiss,‡ and members of the Weiss and Schwarz families.
Financial data (yr. ended 12/31/93): Assets, $2,569,778 (M); expenditures, $252,353; qualifying distributions, $244,150, including $277,650 for grants (high: $20,000; low: $250).
Purpose and activities: Grants largely for Jewish welfare funds, hospitals, higher education, care of the aged and physically handicapped, temple support, and Israel.
Fields of interest: Higher education; Hospitals (general); Human services; Children & youth, services; Aging, centers & services; Jewish federated giving programs; Jewish agencies & temples; Disabled; Aging; Israel.
Types of support: Continuing support, capital campaigns, emergency funds, scholarship funds.
Limitations: Giving primarily in CT, NY, and FL. No grants to individuals.
Application information: Application form not required.
Initial approach: Letter
Deadline(s): None
Board meeting date(s): Quarterly
Officers and Director:* Maurice L. Schwarz,* Pres. and Treas.; Bernard M. Schwarz, V.P. and Secy.-Treas.
Number of staff: None.
EIN: 066021896

149
Fisher Foundation, Inc.
36 Brookside Blvd.
West Hartford 06107 (860) 523-7247
Contact: Martha Newman, Exec. Dir.

Established in 1959.
Donor(s): Stanley D. Fisher Trust, FIP Corp.
Financial data (yr. ended 12/31/94): Assets, $40,448 (M); gifts received, $691,766; expenditures, $662,192; qualifying distributions, $662,192, including $640,746 for 120 grants (high: $75,000; low: $100; average: $100-$75,000).
Fields of interest: Early childhood education; Elementary school/education; Adult education—literacy & basic skills; Reading; Education; Health care; Employment; Housing/shelter, development; Human services; Children & youth, services; Aging, centers & services; Homeless, human services; Minorities; Aging; Economically disadvantaged.
Types of support: General/operating support, program development.
Limitations: Giving primarily in the greater Hartford, CT, area.
Publications: Application guidelines.
Application information: Application form required.
Initial approach: Proposal
Copies of proposal: 2
Deadline(s): Jan. 15, Apr. 15, and Sept. 15
Board meeting date(s): Mar., June, and Nov.
Officers and Directors:* Hinda N. Fisher,* Pres. and Treas.; Diane Fisher Bell,* V.P.; Lois Fisher Ruge,* V.P.; Martha S. Newman, Exec. Dir.; Michael Finkelstein.
Number of staff: 1 part-time professional.
EIN: 066039415

150
Pauline E. Fitzpatrick Charitable Trust
P.O. Box 411
Norwalk 06852 (203) 838-0665
Contact: John B. Devine, Trustee

Established in 1991 in CT.
Donor(s): Pauline E. Fitzpatrick.‡
Financial data (yr. ended 12/31/94): Assets, $776,641 (M); expenditures, $50,530; qualifying distributions, $48,698, including $41,000 for 17 grants (high: $9,500; low: $1,500).
Fields of interest: Human services; Roman Catholic agencies & churches; Aging.
Limitations: Giving limited to the greater Norwalk, CT, area.
Application information:
Initial approach: Proposal
Deadline(s): None
Trustee: John B. Devine.
EIN: 226538192

151
Maurice Goodman Foundation, Inc.
c/o The Chase Manhattan Bank of Connecticut
999 Broad St.
Bridgeport 06604
Contact: Kenneth M. Park, Pres.
Application address: c/o Lepofsky, Lepofsky & Lang, 7-9 Isaac St., Norwalk, CT 06852

Established about 1968 in CT.
Donor(s): Maurice Goodman.‡
Financial data (yr. ended 12/31/94): Assets, $1,418,343 (M); expenditures, $78,969; qualifying distributions, $66,000, including $66,000 for 30 grants (high: $10,000; low: $500).
Fields of interest: Historic preservation/historical societies; Hospitals (general); Human services; Aging, centers & services; Jewish agencies & temples; Aging.
Types of support: General/operating support, continuing support, annual campaigns, capital campaigns, program development, seed money.
Limitations: Giving primarily in the greater Norwalk, CT, area. No grants to individuals.
Application information: Application form not required.
Initial approach: Letter
Deadline(s): Nov. 1
Board meeting date(s): Nov.
Officers and Board Members:* Kenneth M. Park,* Pres.; Irma Lepofsky,* V.P.; Jules Lang,* Secy.; David Fite Waters,* Treas.
Number of staff: None.
EIN: 066100554
Grants for Aging:
Norwalk Congregate Homes for the Elderly, Norwalk, CT, $1,500. 94.

152
The Hartford Courant Foundation, Inc.
285 Broad St.
Hartford 06115 (860) 241-6472
Contact: Alexandrina M. Sergio, Exec. Dir.

Established in 1950 in CT as a corporate foundation; restructured in 1980 as a private, independent foundation.
Financial data (yr. ended 12/31/95): Assets, $10,877,693 (M); expenditures, $700,988; qualifying distributions, $699,090, including $639,065 for 81 grants (high: $70,000; low: $1,000; average: $3,000-$10,000) and $45,200 for 1 foundation-administered program.
Purpose and activities: Giving primarily for arts and cultural programs, education, health, social services, and community development agencies, and for emerging community needs; aid for Hispanic secondary school students through limited foundation-operated program.
Fields of interest: Journalism & publishing; Visual arts; Museums; Performing arts; Dance; Arts/cultural programs; Early childhood education; Child development, education; Secondary school/education; Higher education; Education; Health care; Substance abuse, services; Mental health/crisis services; AIDS; Health organizations; Domestic violence prevention; Housing/shelter, development; Human services; Youth, services; Child

development, services; Family services; Aging, centers & services; Homeless, human services; Community development; Minorities; Disabled; Aging; People with AIDS (PWAs); Economically disadvantaged; Homeless; General charitable giving.
Types of support: General/operating support, capital campaigns, building/renovation, equipment, land acquisition, program development, publication, seed money, technical assistance, matching funds.
Limitations: Giving limited to central CT, including Tolland, Hartford, and Middlesex counties. No support for religious organizations for sectarian purposes, veterans', fraternal, professional, or business associations, or private schools. No grants to individuals, or for continuing support, endowment or emergency funds, conferences, performances, or other short-term, one-time events; no loans.
Publications: Annual report, application guidelines, informational brochure (including application guidelines).
Application information: Application form required.
Initial approach: Telephone
Copies of proposal: 1
Deadline(s): Dec. 15, Mar. 15, June 15, and Sept. 15
Board meeting date(s): Feb., May, Sept., and Nov.
Final notification: 3 months
Officers and Trustees:* George A. Scott,* Pres.; Millard H. Pryor, Jr.,* V.P.; Alexandrina M. Sergio, Secy. and Exec. Dir.; Richard H. King,* Treas.; Eddie L. Davis, Luis Diez-Morales, Bernard Fox, Martha S. Newman, Marty Petty, Michael E. Waller, Donald Wright, Efrem Zimbalist III.
Number of staff: 1 full-time professional.
EIN: 060759107

153
Hartford Fire Insurance Corporate Giving Program

Hartford Plaza
Hartford 06115 (860) 547-3799
Contact: Richard Madden, Dir., Corp. Communications

Financial data (yr. ended 12/31/95): Total giving, $3,300,000, including $104,000 for employee matching gifts.
Purpose and activities: "ITT Hartford, through the corporation, makes grants in five program areas: Education and Equal Opportunity, Health and Human Services, Urban and Civic Affairs, Arts and Culture, and Mature Americans. Additionally, contributions are made to local nonprofit agencies and organizations in 44 field offices around the country through the General Managers Giving Program. A community service fund supports employees' volunteer efforts by providing grants between $25 and $350 to organizations to which employees volunteer their time." The company tries to respond to the shifting needs of community priorities by trying to best allocate human and financial resources.
Fields of interest: Higher education; Education; Health care; AIDS; Health organizations; AIDS research; Employment; Human services; Aging, centers & services; Community development; Voluntarism promotion; Public affairs; Aging; Economically disadvantaged.
Types of support: Capital campaigns, emergency funds, program development, employee volunteer services, use of facilities, employee matching gifts, donated equipment, in-kind gifts, matching funds.
Limitations: Giving limited to headquarters and company locations, mainly in Hartford, CT. Generally support for national fund drives and research programs is limited to those efforts with a clear relationship to the company's overall interest and only on an exception basis. No support for organizations receiving United Way funding, single disease organizations, programs benefiting only members of any one religious group, or international organizations. No grants to individuals, or for endowments, conferences or seminars, courtesy advertising, testimonial or fundraising dinners, or professional memberships.
Publications: Corporate report, corporate giving report (including application guidelines), program policy statement.
Application information: Community Affairs staff handles contributions. Application form required.
Initial approach: Write to General Manager in nearest regional office. Depending on size of the grant requested, manager may fund it or forward it to headquarters. Proposals received in Hartford from agencies outside Hartford will be referred to appropriate regional manager
Copies of proposal: 1
Deadline(s): None
Board meeting date(s): Quarterly
Contributions Committee: Edward L. Morgan, Jr., V.P. and Chair., Contribs. Comm.; Joseph Gareau, Exec. V.P.; Jerome E. Bartow, Sr. V.P.; Sandra A. Sharr, Dir., Community Affairs.
Administrators: Michael S. Wilder, Sr. V.P., Gen. Coun., and Secy.; William L. Harrison, Sr. V.P.; David M. Klein, Sr. V.P.
Number of staff: 1 full-time professional; 2 full-time support.

154
Hartford Foundation for Public Giving

85 Gillett St.
Hartford 06105 (860) 548-1888
Contact: Christopher H. Hall, Dir., Progs.
FAX: (860) 524-8346

Established in 1925 in CT by resolution and declaration of trust.
Foundation type: Community
Financial data (yr. ended 09/30/95): Assets, $296,105,899 (M); gifts received, $8,721,658; expenditures, $13,503,617, including $10,715,069 for 566 grants (high: $464,310; low: $73; average: $45,000-$55,000).
Purpose and activities: Giving for demonstration programs and capital purposes, with emphasis on community advancement, educational institutions, youth groups, hospitals, social services, including the aged, and cultural and civic endeavors.
Fields of interest: Arts/cultural programs; Education; Hospitals (general); Health care; AIDS; Health organizations; AIDS research; Human services; Youth, services; Aging, centers & services; Community development; Government/public administration; Aging.
Types of support: Capital campaigns, building/renovation, equipment, land acquisition, emergency funds, program development, seed money, scholarship funds, technical assistance, program-related investments/loans, matching funds.
Limitations: Giving limited to the greater Hartford, CT, area. No support for sectarian purposes or tax-supported agencies. No grants to individuals, or for operating budgets, continuing support, annual campaigns, deficit financing, endowment funds, research, publications, or conferences.
Publications: Annual report, application guidelines, program policy statement, newsletter, informational brochure.
Application information: Application form required.
Initial approach: Telephone
Copies of proposal: 3
Deadline(s): Education & youth, Jan. 30; Family, children, & early childhood, Mar. 30; Health care, July 30; Housing & economic development, Sept. 30; Arts & culture, Nov. 30; Summer program & camperships, Jan. 15; and general grants, May 30
Board meeting date(s): Monthly except Aug. and Feb.
Final notification: 60 to 90 days
Officers and Distribution Committee:* James F. English, Jr.,* Chair.; Sue Ann Shay,* Vice-Chair.; Brewster B. Perkins,* Treas.; Michael R. Bangser,* Exec. Dir.; John C. Brittain, James A. Crowley, Jon O. Newman, Nancy Rankin, Rosaida Morales Rosario, Wilson Wilde.
Trustee Banks: Bank of Boston Connecticut, Fleet Bank, N.A., Shawmut Bank, N.A., State Street Bank & Trust Co. of Connecticut, Trust Co. of Connecticut.
Staff: Christopher H. Hall, Dir., Progs.; Sylvia deHaas-Phillips, Prog. Officer; Adrianna Falcon-Trafford, Prog. Officer; Glee Ivory Holton, Prog. Officer; Judith L. Rozie-Battle, Prog. Officer; Michael E. Rosano, Grants Mgr.
Number of staff: 11 full-time professional; 1 part-time professional; 7 full-time support.
EIN: 060699252
Grants for Aging:
Big Brothers/Big Sisters, Nutmeg/Foster Grandparents, Hartford, CT, $200,000. For three-year plan to strengthen development efforts. 95.
Saint Francis Hospital and Medical Center, Hartford, CT, $315,000. For comprehensive center for senior health and wellness. 95.
Visiting Nurse and Home Care, Plainville, CT, $128,700. For pen-based computers for nurses, therapists and medical social workers to be used in field for compiling patient assessments and developing care plans. 95.

155
ITT Hartford Insurance Group Foundation, Inc.

(Formerly The Hartford Insurance Group Foundation, Inc.)
Hartford Plaza
Hartford 06115 (860) 547-5000

Contact: Dick Madden
Additional tel.: (860) 547-5816

Incorporated in 1966 in CT.
Donor(s): ITT Hartford Fire Insurance Co., and affiliates.
Foundation type: Company-sponsored
Financial data (yr. ended 12/31/94): Assets, $469,766 (M); gifts received, $2,200,000; expenditures, $1,858,221; qualifying distributions, $1,857,534, including $1,570,300 for 488 grants (high: $300,000; low: $50; average: $1,000-$10,000) and $287,234 for 1,834 employee matching gifts.
Purpose and activities: Giving primarily for higher education (including employee-related scholarships through the National Merit Scholarship Corporation and employee matching gifts), job training, community funds, health, urban and civic affairs, arts and culture, and the aged; also administers a community service fund that supports the efforts of its employees in community programs.
Fields of interest: Arts/cultural programs; Higher education; Business school/education; Education; Health care; Substance abuse, services; AIDS; Alcoholism; Health organizations; AIDS research; Employment; Food services; Housing/shelter, development; Human services; Aging, centers & services; Homeless, human services; Community development; Voluntarism promotion; Federated giving programs; Government/public administration; Public affairs; Minorities; Aging; Homeless.
Types of support: Annual campaigns, building/renovation, program development, scholarship funds, employee matching gifts, employee-related scholarships.
Limitations: Giving primarily in the Hartford, CT, area, and in communities where the company has a regional office. No support for political or religious purposes, disease-specific health organizations, student group trips or parades, United Way member agencies, international organizations, public educational organizations (except for matching gift program), or national fund drives or research programs not having a clear relationship to overall interests of the company and only on an exceptional basis. No grants to individuals, or for endowment funds, conferences, travel, testimonial or fundraising dinners, membership in business, professional and trade associations, courtesy advertising, or capital fund drives outside the Greater Hartford area.
Publications: Corporate giving report (including application guidelines), informational brochure.
Application information: Application form required.
Initial approach: Letter
Copies of proposal: 1
Deadline(s): None
Board meeting date(s): Quarterly
Officers and Directors:* Donald R. Frahm,* Pres.; Edward L. Morgan, Jr., V.P.; Michael S. Wilder,* V.P.; Michael O'Halloran, Secy.; J. Richard Garrett, Treas.; Joseph H. Gareau.
Number of staff: 1 full-time professional; 1 part-time support.
EIN: 066079761
Grants for Aging:
Center for Understanding Aging, Framingham, MA, $50,000. 94.
Christmas in April-Hartford, Hartford, CT, $10,000. 94.
Connecticut Senior Housing Improvement Program, Manchester, CT, $10,000. 94.

156
Irmgard Johanna Laszig Trust
c/o Union Trust Co.
P.O. Box 404
New Haven 06502 (203) 773-0500

Financial data (yr. ended 05/31/94): Assets, $866,127 (M); expenditures, $41,835; qualifying distributions, $34,000.
Purpose and activities: Supports only organizations that assist elderly residents of Ridgefield, CT.
Fields of interest: Human services; Aging, centers & services; Community development; Aging.
Types of support: General/operating support.
Limitations: Giving primarily in Ridgefield, CT. No grants to individuals.
Application information: Application form not required.
Deadline(s): May 31
Trustee: Union Trust Co.
EIN: 066235627

157
George A. and Grace L. Long Foundation
c/o Shawmut Bank, N.A.
777 Main St., MSN 242
Hartford 06115 (860) 986-4071
Contact: Maggie Willard, Trust Officer, Shawmut Bank, N.A.

Trust established in 1960 in CT.
Donor(s): George A. Long,‡ Grace L. Long.‡
Financial data (yr. ended 12/31/94): Assets, $6,654,245 (M); expenditures, $384,816; qualifying distributions, $328,047, including $283,375 for 89 grants (high: $15,000; low: $500).
Purpose and activities: Primary areas of interest include the arts, education, health services, community development, and family services.
Fields of interest: Arts/cultural programs; Education, fund raising; Early childhood education; Child development, education; Adult/continuing education; Education; Environment; Hospitals (general); Health care; Health associations; AIDS; AIDS research; Human services; Children & youth, services; Child development, services; Family services; Aging, centers & services; Community development; Federated giving programs; Minorities; Disabled; Aging.
Types of support: General/operating support, continuing support, building/renovation, program development, technical assistance.
Limitations: Giving primarily in the greater Hartford, CT, area. No grants to individuals, or for operating budgets or endowment funds; no loans.
Application information: Application form required.
Initial approach: Letter
Copies of proposal: 2
Deadline(s): Mar. 15 and Sept. 15
Board meeting date(s): Apr. and Oct.
Trustees: Charles R. Moore, Jr., Shawmut Bank, N.A.
EIN: 066030953

158
The John G. Martin Foundation
Two Batterson Park Rd.
Farmington 06032 (860) 677-4574
Contact: Daniel F. Flynn, Pres.
Application address: P.O. Box 338, Farmington, CT 06032

Established about 1958 as the Jane & John Martin Foundation.
Donor(s): John G. Martin.‡
Financial data (yr. ended 12/31/94): Assets, $7,056,550 (M); expenditures, $373,640; qualifying distributions, $307,149, including $247,150 for 28 grants (high: $35,500; low: $50).
Purpose and activities: Primary areas of interest include the elderly, the homeless, higher education, and the performing arts.
Fields of interest: Visual arts; Performing arts; Arts/cultural programs; Education, fund raising; Early childhood education; Elementary school/education; Secondary school/education; Higher education; Education; Health care; Health organizations; Human services; Children & youth, services; Youth, services; Aging, centers & services; Homeless, human services; Community development; Aging; Economically disadvantaged; Homeless; General charitable giving.
Types of support: Capital campaigns, building/renovation, matching funds.
Limitations: Giving primarily in the Hartford, CT, area.
Application information: Application form not required.
Initial approach: Letter
Copies of proposal: 1
Deadline(s): None
Board meeting date(s): Quarterly, and as needed
Officers and Directors:* Daniel F. Flynn,* Pres.; Frank M. Loehmann, Jr.,* V.P. and Treas.; Sandra Johnson,* V.P.; Donna B. Flamio, Secy.
Number of staff: 1 part-time support.
EIN: 066042495

159
Kathleen M. and Peter E. Naktenis Family Foundation
c/o Dr. Peter E. Naktenis
125 Adelaide Rd.
Manchester 06040
Contact: Peter E. Naktenis, Pres.

Established in 1986 in CT.
Financial data (yr. ended 12/31/95): Assets, $296,035 (M); expenditures, $18,725; qualifying distributions, $11,551, including $10,000 for 11 grants (high: $3,000; low: $500).
Fields of interest: Hospitals (general); Alzheimer's disease; General charitable giving.

Application information: Application form required.
Deadline(s): None
Officers and Directors:* Peter E. Naktenis,* Pres.; Kathleen M. Naktenis,* V.P.; Patricia E. Naktenis,* V.P.; J. Paul Harnois,* Secy.; Peter A. Naktenis,* Treas.; Dominic J. Squatrito.
Trustee: Fleet Bank, N.A.
EIN: 061186224

160
New Britain Foundation for Public Giving

29 Russell St.
New Britain 06052 (860) 229-6018
Contact: Mary-Ellen Powell, Exec. Dir.

Established in 1941 in CT.
Foundation type: Community
Financial data (yr. ended 12/31/95): Assets, $4,300,000 (M); gifts received, $155,795; expenditures, $351,865, including $207,818 for 16 grants (high: $50,000; low: $1,500), $6,900 for 12 grants to individuals (high: $1,000; low: $125) and $7,365 for 1 foundation-administered program.
Purpose and activities: "To meet the needs of the community through support of programs dedicated to health and human services, children, youth, education, rehabilitation services, arts, culture, and civic affairs."
Fields of interest: Arts/cultural programs; Child development, education; Secondary school/education; Libraries/library science; Education; Hospitals (general); Family planning; Health care; Substance abuse, services; Mental health/crisis services; Health organizations; Domestic violence prevention; Food services; Youth development, services; Human services; Children & youth, services; Youth, services; Child development, services; Family services; Aging, centers & services; Homeless, human services; Community development; Leadership development; African Americans; Latinos; Disabled; Aging; People with AIDS (PWAs); Economically disadvantaged; Homeless; General charitable giving.
Types of support: General/operating support, continuing support, capital campaigns, building/renovation, equipment, emergency funds, program development, conferences/seminars, seed money, curriculum development, scholarship funds, technical assistance, scholarships—to individuals, matching funds.
Limitations: Giving limited to central CT with emphasis on New Britain.
Publications: Annual report (including application guidelines), newsletter, financial statement, application guidelines.
Application information: Application form not required.
Initial approach: Contact foundation for application format
Copies of proposal: 18
Deadline(s): Feb. 1, May 1, Aug. 1, and Nov. 1
Board meeting date(s): Mar., June, Sept., and Dec.
Officers and Directors:* Charles Bauer,* Chair.; Bill McCue,* Treas.; Mary-Ellen Powell, Exec. Dir.; Diane Alverio, George Brusznicki, Connie Collins, Donald Davidson, Carol Gordon, Edward Januszewski, Nancy Judd, Peter Rosa, George Springer, Talcott Stanley, Linda Tatarczuch, Lindsley Wellman.
Number of staff: 1 full-time professional; 2 part-time professional; 1 full-time support.
EIN: 066036461

161
Henry Nias Foundation, Inc.

20 Carmen Rd.
Milford 06460
Contact: Charles D. Fleischman, V.P.

Incorporated in 1955 in NY.
Donor(s): Henry Nias.‡
Financial data (yr. ended 11/30/95): Assets, $18,800,227 (M); expenditures, $854,400; qualifying distributions, $705,500, including $705,500 for 56 grants (high: $30,000; low: $2,500; average: $5,000-$15,000).
Purpose and activities: Emphasis on medical sciences, including hospitals, aid to the handicapped, and medical school student loan funds; support also for education, cultural programs, child welfare and youth, the aged, and Jewish organizations, including welfare funds.
Fields of interest: Arts/cultural programs; Medical school/education; Education; Hospitals (general); Human services; Children & youth, services; Aging, centers & services; Jewish federated giving programs; Jewish agencies & temples; Disabled; Aging.
Types of support: Continuing support.
Limitations: Giving limited to the metropolitan New York, NY, area.
Application information: Applications by invitation only.
Deadline(s): Aug.
Board meeting date(s): Sept. and Oct.
Final notification: Grants paid in Nov.
Officers and Directors:* Stanley Edelman, M.D.,* Chair.; Albert J. Rosenberg,* Pres.; William F. Rosenberg,* V.P. and Secy.; Charles D. Fleischman,* V.P. and Treas.; Richard J. Edelman,* V.P.
Number of staff: None.
EIN: 136075785
Grants for Aging:
Jewish Association for Services for the Aged, NYC, NY, $25,000. 95.
Jewish Home and Hospital for Aged, NYC, NY, $30,000. 95.
Village Nursing Home, NYC, NY, $5,000. 95.

162
John H. and Ethel G. Noble Charitable Trust

c/o Bankers Trust Co. Connecticut, Ltd.
One Fawcett Place
Greenwich 06830 (203) 629-7120
Contact: Paul J. Bisset, V.P., Bankers Trust Co. Connecticut, Ltd.

Trust established in 1969 in CT.
Donor(s): Ethel G. Noble,‡ John H. Noble.‡
Financial data (yr. ended 05/31/95): Assets, $13,546,061 (M); expenditures, $748,508; qualifying distributions, $679,460, including $679,460 for 36 grants (high: $75,000; low: $1,500).
Purpose and activities: Grants for organizations that provide shelter or support to the aged and places for the care and treatment of crippled or handicapped children.
Fields of interest: Hospitals (general); Medical care, rehabilitation; Health care; Aging, centers & services; Disabled; Aging.
Limitations: Giving limited to CT, NY, and FL. No grants to individuals.
Application information: Application form not required.
Initial approach: Proposal
Copies of proposal: 1
Trustee: Bankers Trust Co. Connecticut, Ltd.
EIN: 136307313

163
Orange Foundation

P.O. Box 729
Orange 06477-0729 (203) 795-3716
Contact: Robert E. Archambault, Chair., Distribs. Comm.

Established in 1976 in CT.
Foundation type: Community
Financial data (yr. ended 12/31/94): Assets, $263,000 (M); gifts received, $6,300; expenditures, $15,147, including $3,147 for 4 grants (high: $1,600; low: $300) and $12,000 for 7 grants to individuals (high: $2,000; low: $500).
Fields of interest: Education; Recreation; Aging, centers & services; Community development; Aging.
Types of support: Seed money, scholarships—to individuals.
Limitations: Giving limited to Orange, CT.
Publications: Annual report, newsletter, informational brochure, application guidelines.
Application information: Application form required.
Initial approach: Letter
Copies of proposal: 1
Deadline(s): Aug. 1
Board meeting date(s): Quarterly
Final notification: Sept. 10
Officer and Distribution Committee:* Robert E. Archambault,* Chair.; Giulio Balestrino, Doris Burbaum, Ernest Dichele, Micheal Dorney, Augusta Downey, Eleanor Joyal, Linda Saffer, Katepalli Sreenivasan.
Executive Committee: Barbara Cronenberg, Barbara Rashba, Cheryl Serfilippi, Arthur B. Williams III, C.P.A.
Number of staff: None.
EIN: 060955006

164
The Frank Loomis Palmer Fund

c/o Shawmut Bank, N.A.
250 State St.
New London 06320 (860) 447-6133
Contact: Mildred E. Devine, V.P., Shawmut Bank, N.A.
Additional tel. for application information: (860) 447-6155

Trust established in 1936 in CT.
Donor(s): Virginia Palmer.‡

Financial data (yr. ended 07/31/95): Assets, $19,775,082 (M); gifts received, $20,000; expenditures, $949,995; qualifying distributions, $805,394, including $725,270 for 39 grants (high: $100,000; low: $429; average: $700-$174,000).
Purpose and activities: Grants to encourage new projects and to provide seed money, with emphasis on child welfare and family services, youth agencies, and higher and secondary education; support also for civic groups, cultural programs, social services, churches, and hospitals.
Fields of interest: Performing arts; Arts/cultural programs; Elementary school/education; Secondary school/education; Higher education; Adult/continuing education; Libraries/library science; Education; Natural resource conservation & protection; Environment; Hospitals (general); Family planning; Health care; AIDS; Alcoholism; Health organizations; AIDS research; Legal services; Safety/disasters; Children & youth, services; Family services; Hospices; Aging, centers & services; Minorities/immigrants, centers & services; Community development; Engineering & technology; Science; Government/public administration; Transportation; Roman Catholic agencies & churches; Jewish agencies & temples; Religion; Minorities; Aging.
Types of support: Capital campaigns, building/renovation, equipment, program development, conferences/seminars, publication, seed money, scholarship funds, research, consulting services, matching funds.
Limitations: Giving limited to New London, CT. No grants to individuals, or for endowment funds.
Publications: Informational brochure (including application guidelines).
Application information: Application form required.
Initial approach: Telephone
Copies of proposal: 1
Deadline(s): May 15 and Nov. 15
Board meeting date(s): Jan. and July
Final notification: Feb. 1 and Aug. 1
Trustee: Shawmut Bank, N.A.
Number of staff: None.
EIN: 066026043
Grants for Aging:
Retired Senior Volunteer Program (RSVP), New London, CT, $2,131. 94.

165
Adrianne B. Reilly Foundation
c/o Putnam Trust Co.
Ten Mason St.
Greenwich 06830
Contact: Adrianne B. Reilly, Trustee
Application address: 92 Rockwood Ln., Greenwich, CT 06830

Established in 1990 in CT.
Donor(s): Adrianne B. Reilly.
Financial data (yr. ended 12/31/95): Assets, $179,117 (M); gifts received, $50,000; expenditures, $87,870; qualifying distributions, $85,900, including $85,900 for 8 grants (high: $34,400; low: $500).
Fields of interest: Natural resource conservation & protection; Health care; Health associations; Human services; Aging, centers & services; Religious federated giving programs; Christian agencies & churches; Religion; Aging; General charitable giving.
Types of support: Program development.
Limitations: Giving primarily in CT. No grants to individuals.
Application information:
Initial approach: Proposal
Deadline(s): None
Trustees: Adrianne B. Reilly, Robert V. Taylor, John Winthrop, Putnam Trust Co.
EIN: 223109258

166
The Robert and Ruth Satter Charitable Trust
c/o Robert Satter
Capitol Place, 21 Oak St.
Hartford 06106-8002

Established in 1989 in CT.
Donor(s): Robert Satter, Ruth Satter, Helen and Milton Kimmelman Foundation.
Financial data (yr. ended 04/30/95): Assets, $116,716 (M); expenditures, $7,894; qualifying distributions, $6,000, including $6,000 for 7 grants (high: $1,500; low: $500).
Fields of interest: Performing arts; Education; Natural resource conservation & protection; Family planning; Cancer; Cancer research; Delinquency prevention/services; Crime/law enforcement; Human services; Aging, centers & services; Civil rights; Aging; Economically disadvantaged.
Types of support: General/operating support.
Limitations: Applications not accepted. Giving primarily in CT. No grants to individuals.
Application information: Contributes only to pre-selected organizations.
Board meeting date(s): Mid-Apr.
Trustee: Robert Satter.
Number of staff: None.
EIN: 222986191

167
Senior Services of Stamford, Inc.
600 Summer St.
Stamford 06901 (203) 324-6584
Contact: Roberta Ratcliff, Exec. Dir.

Established in 1909 in CT.
Financial data (yr. ended 02/28/95): Assets, $10,099,780 (M); gifts received, $9,816; expenditures, $599,391; qualifying distributions, $552,153, including $329,606 for grants (high: $123,767; low: $200).
Purpose and activities: Support for 1) social service organizations serving the elderly; 2) organizations that provide information and referral, counseling, advocacy, and emergency financial assistance to needy elderly; and 3) operation of a senior center. Focus on programs offering innovative solutions to problems of older persons, particularly in access to health care, housing, transportation, and isolation.
Fields of interest: Aging, centers & services; Aging.
Types of support: Endowment funds.
Limitations: Giving limited to Stamford, CT.
Publications: Informational brochure.
Application information: Application form required.
Initial approach: Letter
Copies of proposal: 1
Deadline(s): Oct. 15
Board meeting date(s): Mar., June, Sept., and Dec.
Final notification: Within 4 months
Officers and Directors:* Kate Adamson,* Pres.; Judith Davis,* V.P.; Joan Danoff,* Secy.; Robert J. Bromfield,* Treas.; Roberta Ratcliff, Exec. Dir.; and 16 additional directors.
Number of staff: 1 full-time professional; 2 part-time professional; 1 full-time support; 1 part-time support.
EIN: 060646916

168
Smith Memorial Fund, Inc.
(Formerly Smith Memorial Home, Inc.)
261 Williams St.
P.O. Box 1390
New London 06320 (860) 442-0150
Contact: Joseph A. Cipparone, Pres.

Established in 1884 in CT.
Donor(s): Seth Smith.‡
Financial data (yr. ended 09/30/95): Assets, $731,974 (M); expenditures, $42,973; qualifying distributions, $35,916, including $34,275 for grants.
Purpose and activities: Support to organizations that benefit elderly women of New London, CT.
Fields of interest: Aging, centers & services; Women, centers & services; Aging; Women.
Limitations: Giving limited to New London, CT.
Application information: Request application. Application form required.
Deadline(s): Sept. 1
Officer: Joseph A. Cipparone, Pres.
EIN: 060539600

169
The United Illuminating Company
(Formerly The United Illuminating Company Contributions Program)
157 Church St., P.O. Box 1564
Mail Stop 1-16
New Haven 06506-0901 (203) 499-2012
Contact: Maryann Ott, Special Projects Administrator

Established in 1986 in CT.
Financial data (yr. ended 12/31/94): Total giving, $30,000, including $25,000 for grants (high: $1,000; low: $100) and $5,000 for 40 employee matching gifts.
Purpose and activities: "In 1985 the officers of our company recognized that United Illuminating has an obligation to participate in the establishment and maintenance of a healthy physical and social environment in its service territory; that good citizenship is good business and essential to the future health and profitability of the company; that changes in operating conditions or corporate priorities do not diminish—in fact may increase—the company's need to maintain good relationships with the diverse public it serves." Support for arts and culture, environmental issues,

education, job training, housing, health, elderly, and urban needs.
Fields of interest: Arts/cultural programs; Education; Environment; Health care; Health organizations; Housing/shelter, development; Aging, centers & services; Urban/community development; Aging.
Types of support: Program development, technical assistance, consulting services, sponsorships, employee matching gifts, in-kind gifts.
Limitations: Giving primarily in the CT towns served by the company: New Haven, West Haven, Orange, Woodbridge, Hampden, North Haven, North Branford, East Haven, Bridgeport, Stratford, Trumbull, Easton, Fairfield, Milford, Derby, Ansonia, and Shelton.
Publications: Annual report.
Application information: Application form not required.
Initial approach: Send request in letter form to headquarters
Copies of proposal: 1
Deadline(s): None
Administrators: Maryann Ott, Special Projects Administrator; William F. Murphy, Asst. to Pres. and Dir., Corp. Community Rels.; Cathy Zezon, Community Rels.
Number of staff: 2 full-time professional; 1 part-time professional.

170
UST Corporate Giving Program

100 West Putnam Ave.
Greenwich 06830 (203) 622-3696
Contact: Geraldine K. Morgan, Mgr., Corp. Contribs. Comm.

Fields of interest: Visual arts; Museums; Performing arts; Theater; Humanities; Arts/cultural programs; Secondary school/education; Higher education; Engineering school/education; Adult education—literacy & basic skills; Reading; Education; Natural resource conservation & protection; Environment; Wildlife preservation & protection; Health care; Alcoholism; Health organizations; Medical research; Food services; Housing/shelter, development; Safety/disasters; Youth development, services; Human services; Youth, services; Aging, centers & services; Women, centers & services; Minorities/immigrants, centers & services; Homeless, human services; International relief; Community development; Voluntarism promotion; Marine science; Engineering; Government/public administration; Leadership development; Public affairs; Minorities; Native Americans; Aging; Women; Homeless; General charitable giving.
Types of support: General/operating support, capital campaigns, endowment funds, program development, employee matching gifts, employee-related scholarships, in-kind gifts.
Limitations: Giving primarily in headquarters city and major operating locations. No support for fraternal organizations, political or lobbying groups, or religious organizations. No grants to individuals, or for dinners, or goodwill advertising.
Publications: Corporate report, corporate giving report.
Application information: Company has a staff that only handles contributions. Application form not required.
Initial approach: Letter and proposal; send requests to headquarters
Copies of proposal: 1
Deadline(s): None
Board meeting date(s): Quarterly
Administrators: Harry W. Peter III, Chair., Corp. Contribs.; Geraldine K. Morgan, Mgr., Corp. Contribs.
Number of staff: 2 full-time professional; 1 full-time support.

171
The Waterbury Foundation

156 West Main St.
Waterbury 06702-1216 (203) 753-1315
Contact: Mrs. Ingrid Manning, Dir.

Incorporated in 1923 by special Act of the CT Legislature.
Donor(s): Katherine Pomeroy,‡ Edith Chase.‡
Foundation type: Community
Financial data (yr. ended 12/31/95): Assets, $15,200,000 (M); gifts received, $694,000; expenditures, $795,000, including $500,000 for 55 grants (high: $20,000; low: $40) and $69,000 for 100 grants to individuals (high: $2,000; low: $100; average: $100-$2,000).
Purpose and activities: Current priority areas of grantmaking are teenage growth and development and arts and humanities; emphasis on providing seed money and venture capital for new projects.
Fields of interest: Humanities; Historic preservation/historical societies; Arts/cultural programs; Early childhood education; Child development, education; Secondary school/education; Vocational education; Higher education; Adult/continuing education; Education; Health care; Substance abuse, services; Mental health/crisis services; Health associations; Heart/circulatory disease; AIDS; Housing/shelter, development; Recreation; Human services; Children & youth, services; Child development, services; Family services; Hospices; Aging, centers & services; Homeless, human services; Community development; Minorities; Disabled; Aging; Economically disadvantaged; Homeless; General charitable giving.
Types of support: Capital campaigns, building/renovation, equipment, endowment funds, emergency funds, program development, conferences/seminars, publication, seed money, scholarship funds, research, technical assistance, consulting services, scholarships—to individuals, matching funds.
Limitations: Giving limited to the greater Waterbury, CT, area. No support for sectarian or religious purposes. No grants to individuals (except for college scholarships), or for deficit financing, continuing support, or annual campaigns; no loans.
Publications: Annual report, newsletter, application guidelines.
Application information: Application form required.
Initial approach: Telephone or letter
Copies of proposal: 15
Deadline(s): Jan. for arts and historic preservation and summer programs requests; Apr. for teenage growth and development and education; and Sept. for all other requests
Board meeting date(s): Mar., June, and Nov.; grants committee meets twice, 6 weeks and 1 week prior to each board meeting
Final notification: 10 weeks
Officers and Trustees:* Charles W. Henry,* Pres.; James Emison,* V.P.; Patricia B. Sweet,* V.P.; W. Scott Peterson, M.D.,* Secy.; Walter F. Torrance, Jr.,* Treas.; Burton Albert, Dutch Barhydt, Lillian H. Brown, Conrad Fleisher, Lynn Franklin-Henry, Rev. Larry Green, Emily Littman, Marcia Managan, Isabel Romero, Michael E. Sendzimir, Ann Y. Smith.
Staff: Ingrid Manning, Dir.; Carol O'Donnell, Prog. Officer.
Number of staff: 1 full-time professional; 2 part-time professional; 1 full-time support; 1 part-time support.
EIN: 066038074
Grants for Aging:
Connecticut Community Care, Bristol, CT, $18,000. For volunteer training program, in collaboration with YWCA, for city teenagers to become companions to Waterbury's homebound elderly. 94.

172
The Xerox Foundation

800 Long Ridge Rd.
P.O. Box 1600
Stamford 06904 (203) 968-3445
Contact: Dr. Joseph M. Cahalan, V.P.

Incorporated in 1978 in DE as successor to Xerox Fund.
Donor(s): Xerox Corp.
Foundation type: Company-sponsored
Financial data (yr. ended 12/31/94): Assets, $64 (M); gifts received, $186,623; expenditures, $222,257; qualifying distributions, $220,736, including $185,379 for 46 grants (high: $35,379; low: $500; average: $1,000-$10,000).
Purpose and activities: Broad commitment in support of higher education to prepare qualified men and women for careers in business, government, and education; advance knowledge in science and technology; commitment also to enhance learning opportunities for minorities and the disadvantaged. Also operates employee matching gift program. Support additionally for social, civic, and cultural organizations including the United Way, providing broad-based programs and services in cities where Xerox employees live and work, organizations that foster debate on major national public policy issues, and worldwide, for leadership efforts around major social problems, education, employability, and student exchange.
Fields of interest: Performing arts; Dance; Theater; Arts/cultural programs; Education, research; Early childhood education; Secondary school/education; Higher education; Business school/education; Engineering school/education; Adult education—literacy & basic skills; Reading; Education; Substance abuse, services; Employment; Human services;

Children & youth, services; Family services; Minorities/immigrants, centers & services; Foreign policy; International affairs; Civil rights, immigrants; Civil rights, minorities; Civil rights, disabled; Civil rights, women; Civil rights, aging; Civil rights, gays/lesbians; Civil rights; Rural development; Community development; Federated giving programs; Engineering & technology; Computer science; Engineering; Science; Public policy, research; Government/public administration; Public affairs; Minorities; Asians/Pacific Islanders; African Americans; Latinos; Native Americans; Disabled; Aging; Women; People with AIDS (PWAs); Gays/lesbians; Immigrants/refugees; Economically disadvantaged; Homeless; Canada; Caribbean; United Kingdom; Latin America; Mexico; Venezuela; Asia; Middle East; Turkey; Japan.
Types of support: General/operating support, continuing support, annual campaigns, equipment, emergency funds, program development, professorships, publication, curriculum development, fellowships, internships, scholarship funds, research, technical assistance, program-related investments/loans, employee matching gifts, employee-related scholarships, exchange programs, in-kind gifts.
Limitations: Giving on a national and international basis. No support for community colleges, organizations supported by United Way, religious organizations, political organizations or candidates, or governmental agencies. No grants to individuals, or for capital or endowment funds.
Publications: Application guidelines, annual report, informational brochure (including application guidelines).
Application information: Application form not required.
Initial approach: Brief proposal
Copies of proposal: 1
Deadline(s): None
Board meeting date(s): Quarterly and as required
Final notification: 30 to 60 days
Officers and Trustees:* Paul A. Allaire,* Pres.; Joseph M. Cahalan, V.P.; Martin S. Wagner, Secy.; Allan E. Dugan, David E. Garnett, John A. Lopiano, Anne M. Mulcahy, Mark B. Myers, Addison B. Rand.
Number of staff: 1 full-time professional; 4 full-time support.
EIN: 060996443

DELAWARE

173
Borkee-Hagley Foundation, Inc.
P.O. Box 4590
Wilmington 19807 (302) 652-8616
Contact: Henry H. Silliman, Jr., Pres.

Incorporated in 1955 in DE.
Financial data (yr. ended 12/31/95): Assets, $6,892,438 (M); expenditures, $287,609; qualifying distributions, $283,128, including $281,100 for 46 grants (high: $40,100; low: $500).
Purpose and activities: "Principal purpose to provide financial assistance to local organizations engaged in caring for the elderly."
Fields of interest: Housing/shelter, development; Aging, centers & services; Aging.
Types of support: General/operating support, annual campaigns, capital campaigns, building/renovation, equipment, endowment funds, emergency funds, conferences/seminars.
Limitations: Giving primarily in DE. No support for specific churches or synagogues. No grants to individuals.
Publications: Application guidelines.
Application information:
Initial approach: Letter and proposal
Deadline(s): Nov. 1
Board meeting date(s): Early Dec.
Final notification: Within 2 weeks of annual meeting
Officers and Trustees:* Henry H. Silliman, Jr.,* Pres.; Robert M. Silliman,* V.P. and Treas.; John E. Silliman,* V.P.; Eleanor S. Maroney,* Secy.; Thomas F. Husbands, George A. Sandbach, Doris S. Stockly.
Number of staff: None.
EIN: 516011644

174
Crystal Trust
1088 DuPont Bldg.
Wilmington 19898 (302) 774-8421
Contact: Stephen C. Doberstein, Dir.

Trust established in 1947 in DE.
Donor(s): Irenee duPont.‡
Financial data (yr. ended 12/31/95): Assets, $91,854,208 (M); expenditures, $3,535,841; qualifying distributions, $3,474,916, including $3,355,200 for 67 grants (high: $250,000; low: $5,000; average: $10,000-$100,000).
Purpose and activities: Giving mainly for higher and secondary education and social and family services, including youth and child welfare agencies, family planning, and programs for the aged, the disadvantaged, and the homeless; support also for the arts and cultural programs, health and hospitals, conservation programs, and historical preservation. Needs of the State of Delaware have priority.
Fields of interest: Museums; Music; Arts/cultural programs; Secondary school/education; Higher education; Libraries/library science; Education; Natural resource conservation & protection; Hospitals (general); Family planning; Health care; Health organizations; Food services; Housing/shelter, development; Human services; Children & youth, services; Youth, services; Family services; Hospices; Aging, centers & services; Homeless, human services; Aging; Economically disadvantaged; Homeless.
Types of support: Capital campaigns, building/renovation, equipment, land acquisition, program development.
Limitations: Giving primarily in DE, especially Wilmington. No grants to individuals, or for endowment funds, research, scholarships, fellowships, or matching gifts.
Publications: Informational brochure (including application guidelines).
Application information: Application form not required.
Initial approach: Proposal
Copies of proposal: 1
Deadline(s): Sept. 30
Board meeting date(s): Nov.
Final notification: Dec. 15
Director: Stephen C. Doberstein.
Trustees: Irenee duPont, Jr., David Greenewalt, Eleanor S. Maroney.
Number of staff: 1 part-time professional; 1 part-time support.
EIN: 516015063
Grants for Aging:
Gilpin Hall, Wilmington, DE, $100,000. For capital campaign. 94.
Layton Home for Aged Persons, Wilmington, DE, $100,000. For capital campaign. 94.

175
Delmarva Power and Light Corporate Giving Program
P.O. Box 231
Wilmington 19899 (302) 429-3410
Contact: Richard H. Evans, Chair., Contribs. Comm.

Fields of interest: Media/communications; Arts/cultural programs; Business school/education; Adult education—literacy & basic skills; Reading; Natural resource conservation & protection; Energy; Mental health/crisis services; Cancer; Cancer research; Legal services; Crime/law enforcement; Employment; Youth development, services; Youth development, citizenship; Aging, centers & services; Minorities/immigrants, centers & services; Rural development; Business & industry; Community development; Voluntarism promotion; Engineering & technology; Computer science; Science; Economics; Public affairs, citizen participation; Leadership development; Minorities; Aging.
Types of support: General/operating support, annual campaigns, capital campaigns, building/renovation, conferences/seminars, scholarship funds, research.
Limitations: Giving primarily in the service territory of the corporation.
Publications: Informational brochure (including application guidelines).
Application information: Application form required.
Board meeting date(s): July and as necessary
Final notification: Within 30 days of application

176
Palmer Home, Inc.
P.O. Box 1751
Dover 19903-1751 (302) 678-3100
Contact: Frances Jean DeLeo, Pres.

Established in 1930.
Foundation type: Operating
Financial data (yr. ended 02/28/94): Assets, $2,981,592 (M); gifts received, $33,043; expenditures, $189,986; qualifying distributions, $166,983, including $123,500 for 15 grants (high: $20,000; low: $500).

Purpose and activities: Giving primarily to benefit the elderly.
Fields of interest: Aging, centers & services; Aging.
Limitations: Giving limited to Dover, DE. No grants to individuals.
Application information:
Initial approach: Letter
Deadline(s): Nov. 30
Officers and Directors:* Jean T. DeLeo,* Pres.; Carol Braverman,* V.P.; Eleanor Parker,* V.P.; Lillian Hamm,* Secy.-Treas.; Sylvia Cooper, Peg Edgell, Carol Ewing, Margaret Foard, Christine Hopkins, Ethel Loftus, Gertrude Lord, Annabell Lynch, Susan Rosello, Mary E. Wagner, Yvonne Whitman, Ann Zimmer.
EIN: 510066737

DISTRICT OF COLUMBIA

177
The Morris and Gwendolyn Cafritz Foundation
1825 K St., N.W., 14th Fl.
Washington 20006 (202) 223-3100
Contact: Anne Allen, Exec. Dir.

Incorporated in 1948 in DC.
Donor(s): Morris Cafritz,‡ Gwendolyn D. Cafritz.‡
Financial data (yr. ended 04/30/95): Assets, $160,356,581 (M); gifts received, $19,041,036; expenditures, $8,428,774; qualifying distributions, $6,943,151, including $6,323,957 for 226 grants (high: $333,333; low: $100; average: $10,000-$25,000).
Purpose and activities: Giving only for programs of direct assistance, with emphasis on community service, arts and humanities, education, and health.
Fields of interest: Museums; Performing arts; Dance; Theater; Music; Arts/cultural programs; Education, association; Early childhood education; Child development, education; Elementary school/education; Secondary school/education; Higher education; Medical school/education; Adult/continuing education; Adult education—literacy & basic skills; Reading; Education; Natural resource conservation & protection; Environment; Family planning; Medical care, rehabilitation; Health care; Substance abuse, services; Mental health/crisis services; AIDS; Health organizations; AIDS research; Crime/law enforcement; Housing/shelter, development; Human services; Children & youth, services; Youth, services; Child development, services; Family services; Hospices; Aging, centers & services; Women, centers & services; Homeless, human services; Civil rights, immigrants; Civil rights, minorities; Civil rights, women; Civil rights, aging; Reproductive rights; Civil rights; Community development; Voluntarism promotion; Minorities; Asians/Pacific Islanders; African Americans; Latinos; Disabled; Aging; Women; People with AIDS (PWAs); Immigrants/refugees; Economically disadvantaged; Homeless.
Types of support: General/operating support, continuing support, equipment, seed money, fellowships, scholarship funds, technical assistance, matching funds.
Limitations: Giving limited to the greater metropolitan Washington, DC, area. No grants to individuals, or for emergency funds, deficit financing, capital, endowment, or building funds, demonstration projects, or conferences; no loans.
Publications: Annual report, application guidelines.
Application information: Application form required.
Initial approach: Proposal
Copies of proposal: 1
Deadline(s): July 1, Nov. 1, and Mar. 1
Board meeting date(s): Generally 3 to 4 months after deadline dates
Officers and Directors:* Calvin Cafritz,* Chair., Pres., and Treas.; Roger A. Clark, Secy.; Anne Allen, Exec. Dir.; Martin Atlas, Daniel J. Boorstin, J. Carter Brown, William P. Rogers.
Number of staff: 4 full-time professional; 3 full-time support.
EIN: 526036989
Grants for Aging:
Christmas in April, DC, $15,000. For roofing project. 95.
Downtown Clusters Geriatric Day Care Center, DC, $30,000. For matching grant for therapeutic and supportive services program. 95.
Downtown Clusters Geriatric Day Care Center, DC, $25,000. For general support. 95.
Emeritus Foundation, DC, $35,000. For matching grant for Emeritus Scientists, Mathematics and Engineers Program. 95.
Family Friends of the National Capital Area, DC, $12,500. For expansion and training services for new volunteers. 95.
Iona Senior Services, Iona House, DC, $17,500. For Community Education Program. 95.
Jewish Social Service Agency, Rockville, MD, $35,000. For Frail Elders Program. 95.
Marys Center for Maternal and Child Care, DC, $15,000. For home visit program. 95.
Pediatric AIDS/HIV Care, DC, $12,500. For general support for Family Respite Care Center. 95.
Sarahs Circle, DC, $12,500. For general support. 95.
United Seniors Health Cooperative, DC, $20,000. To develop Personal Advocates Services Program. 95.

178
The Charles Delmar Foundation
918 16th St., N.W., No. 203
Washington 20006 (202) 293-2494
Contact: Mareen D. Hughes, Pres.

Trust established in 1957 in DC.
Donor(s): Charles Delmar.‡
Financial data (yr. ended 12/31/95): Assets, $5,750,182 (M); expenditures, $210,640; qualifying distributions, $192,934, including $186,624 for 127 grants (high: $8,000; low: $200).
Purpose and activities: Special interests include inter-American studies, higher, secondary, elementary, and other education, underprivileged youth, the disadvantaged, the aged, the homeless and housing issues, general welfare organizations, and fine and performing arts.
Fields of interest: Visual arts; Museums; Performing arts; Theater; Music; Historic preservation/historical societies; Elementary school/education; Secondary school/education; Higher education; Adult education—literacy & basic skills; Reading; Natural resource conservation & protection; Hospitals (general); Family planning; Substance abuse, services; Health associations; Cancer; Cancer research; Housing/shelter, development; Human services; Children & youth, services; Family services; Hospices; Aging, centers & services; Homeless, human services; International affairs, goodwill promotion; International affairs; Race/intergroup relations; Native Americans; Disabled; Aging; Economically disadvantaged; Homeless; Haiti; Latin America.
Types of support: Continuing support, annual campaigns, conferences/seminars, seed money, scholarship funds.
Limitations: Giving primarily in Washington, DC, and Latin America. No grants to individuals, or for building or endowment funds, or matching gifts; no loans.
Application information: Application form not required.
Initial approach: Letter
Copies of proposal: 1
Deadline(s): None
Board meeting date(s): As required
Officers and Trustees:* Mareen D. Hughes,* Pres.; R. Bruce Hughes,* Secy.-Treas.
Number of staff: None.
EIN: 526035345

179
John Edward Fowler Memorial Foundation
1725 K St., N.W., Suite 1201
Washington 20006 (202) 728-9080
Contact: Richard H. Lee, Pres.

Incorporated in 1964 in DE.
Donor(s): Pearl Gunn Fowler.‡
Financial data (yr. ended 12/31/95): Assets, $18,939,783 (M); expenditures, $1,034,992; qualifying distributions, $912,046, including $816,460 for 69 grants (high: $70,000; low: $5,000; average: $5,000-$10,000).
Purpose and activities: Primary areas of interest include the disadvantaged, with emphasis on the homeless and housing. Giving primarily to small community service organizations without public funding, especially for programs that benefit children and youth; support also for social service agencies, literacy programs, and programs that help the elderly maintain their independence.
Fields of interest: Child development, education; Adult education—literacy & basic skills; Reading; Food services; Housing/shelter, development; Human services; Children & youth, services; Child development, services; Aging, centers & services; Homeless, human services; African Americans; Latinos; Aging; Immigrants/refugees; Economically disadvantaged; Homeless.

Types of support: General/operating support, building/renovation, equipment, program development, matching funds.
Limitations: Giving limited to the metropolitan Washington, DC, area. No support for agencies principally funded by local, state, or federal government sources. No grants to individuals, or for medical research programs; no loans.
Publications: Application guidelines, grants list.
Application information: WRAG Common Grant Application Form required for requests over $5,000. Application form required.
Initial approach: Letter requesting application form and guidelines
Copies of proposal: 1
Deadline(s): None
Board meeting date(s): Periodically
Final notification: Approximately 6 months
Officers and Trustees:* Richard H. Lee,* Pres.; Michael P. Bentzen,* Secy.; Jeffery P. Capron,* Treas.
Number of staff: 1 part-time professional.
EIN: 516019469
Grants for Aging:
Christian Communities Group Homes, DC, $10,000. 95.
Downtown Clusters Geriatric Day Care Center, DC, $10,000. 95.
Emmaus Services for the Aging, DC, $20,000. 95.

180
Giant Food Corporate Contributions Program

P.O. Box 1804 D-599
Washington 20013 (301) 341-4710
Contact: Barry F. Scher, V.P., Public Affairs

Established in 1936.
Financial data (yr. ended 02/24/96): Total giving, $565,000, including $490,000 for grants (high: $10,000; low: $50; average: $10-$250) and $75,000 for in-kind gifts.
Purpose and activities: For the past 60 years, Giant Food has operated under the philisophy that it is a privilege to be a corporate citizen of the communities it serves. As such, the company feels it has a responsibility to give back to the citizens and organizations whose patronage has made the company strong. Giant Food and its associates take great pride in the realization that its efforts are making a positive difference in communities where emplyees live and work.
Fields of interest: Youth development; Aging; Homeless.
Types of support: General/operating support, annual campaigns, equipment, emergency funds, program development, scholarship funds, cause-related marketing, loaned talent, public relations services, donated equipment, donated products, in-kind gifts.
Limitations: Giving primarily in DC, DE, MD, NJ, PA, and VA.
Application information: The Public Affairs Dept. handles contributions.
Initial approach: Letter of request to headquarters or nearest company location with appropriate documentation attached
Copies of proposal: 1
Number of staff: 1 part-time professional; 1 full-time support.

181
Jacob and Charlotte Lehrman Foundation, Inc.

1027 33rd St., N.W., 2nd Fl.
Washington 20007
Contact: Robert Lehrman, V.P.

Incorporated in 1953 in DC.
Donor(s): Jacob J. Lehrman,‡ Charlotte F. Lehrman.‡
Financial data (yr. ended 10/31/94): Assets, $8,682,187 (M); expenditures, $471,282; qualifying distributions, $428,750, including $428,750 for 51 grants (high: $175,000; low: $100; average: $500-$10,000).
Purpose and activities: Giving to establish scholarships and fellowships at institutions of learning, and to foster research in medicine and science; grants also for Jewish welfare funds, care of the aged and sick, cancer research, the establishment of trade schools, the fostering of religious observance, museums, and aid to refugees.
Fields of interest: Museums; Vocational education; Education; Health care; Cancer; Health organizations; Medical research; Cancer research; Human services; Aging, centers & services; Community development; Jewish federated giving programs; Jewish agencies & temples; Aging.
Types of support: General/operating support, fellowships, scholarship funds, research, matching funds.
Limitations: Giving primarily in metropolitan Washington, DC. No grants to individuals; no loans.
Application information: Application form not required.
Initial approach: Proposal
Copies of proposal: 1
Deadline(s): Submit proposal preferably in May, or by Sept.; deadline Oct. 15
Board meeting date(s): May and Sept. or Oct.
Officers: Fredrica Carmichael, Pres.; Heidi Berry, V.P.; Robert Lehrman, V.P.; Samuel Lehrman, V.P.; Leslie Handler, Secy.; Robert Barry Wertlieb, Treas.
Number of staff: None.
EIN: 526035666

182
Eugene and Agnes E. Meyer Foundation

1400 16th St., N.W., Suite 360
Washington 20036 (202) 483-8294
Contact: Julie L. Rogers, Pres.

Incorporated in 1944 in NY.
Donor(s): Eugene Meyer,‡ Agnes E. Meyer.‡
Financial data (yr. ended 12/31/95): Assets, $102,894,883 (M); expenditures, $4,252,483; qualifying distributions, $3,616,517, including $3,444,017 for 170 grants (high: $500,000; low: $500; average: $10,000-$40,000) and $172,500 for 8 program-related investments.
Purpose and activities: Grants principally for neighborhood development/housing, education, health and mental health, the arts and humanities, law and justice, and community service.
Fields of interest: Theater; Humanities; Arts/cultural programs; Early childhood education; Child development, education; Elementary school/education; Secondary school/education; Vocational education; Adult education—literacy & basic skills; Reading; Education; Family planning; Medical care, rehabilitation; Health care; Substance abuse, services; Mental health/crisis services; Health organizations; Legal services; Crime/law enforcement; Employment; Housing/shelter, development; Youth development, services; Human services; Children & youth, services; Youth, services; Child development, services; Family services; Aging, centers & services; Women, centers & services; Minorities/immigrants, centers & services; Homeless, human services; Race/intergroup relations; Civil rights; Urban/community development; Community development; Voluntarism promotion; Leadership development; Minorities; Aging; Women; Immigrants/refugees; Economically disadvantaged; Homeless; General charitable giving.
Types of support: General/operating support, capital campaigns, program development, seed money, technical assistance, program-related investments/loans, matching funds.
Limitations: Giving limited to the metropolitan Washington, DC, area, including VA and MD. No support for sectarian purposes, or for programs that are national or international in scope. No grants to individuals, or for annual campaigns, deficit financing, endowment funds, equipment, scholarships, fellowships, scientific or medical research, publications, special events or conferences.
Publications: Annual report (including application guidelines), grants list.
Application information: For a thorough understanding of application procedures, interested parties are strongly urged to read the foundation's annual report and guidelines. Accepts WRAG Common Grant Application Form. Application form not required.
Initial approach: 2-page letter of inquiry
Copies of proposal: 4
Deadline(s): Mar. 15, July 15, and Nov. 15
Board meeting date(s): Applications considered only at Feb., June, and Oct. meetings; board meets also in Apr. and Dec.
Final notification: 1 month after board meetings
Officers and Directors:* David W. Rutstein,* Chair.; Carrie Thornhill,* Vice-Chair.; Julie L. Rogers, Pres.; Maureen E. Dwyer,* Secy.-Treas.; Maureen Bunyan, Newman T. Halvorson, Jr., Boisfeuillet Jones, Jr., James Jones, Patricia McGuire, Robert L. Moore, James T. Speight, Jr., Ricardo M. Urbina.
Staff: Irene S. Lee, Sr. Prog. Officer; Katherine T. Freshley, Prog. Officer; Benita Kornegay-Henry, Prog. Officer; Katherina Pfeil, Grants Asst.
Number of staff: 4 full-time professional; 1 part-time professional; 1 full-time support; 1 part-time support.
EIN: 530241716
Grants for Aging:
Christian Communities Group Homes, DC, $15,000. For general support and to expand age-in-place outreach program to seniors. 95.
Iona Senior Services, DC, $10,000. For efforts of long-term care coalition. 95.

Marys Center for Maternal and Child Care, DC, $30,000. For prenatal, pediatric, adolescent and home visiting programs. 95.

183
Public Welfare Foundation, Inc.

2600 Virginia Ave., N.W., Rm. 505
Washington 20037-1977 (202) 965-1800
Contact: Review Comm.

Incorporated in 1947 in TX; reincorporated in 1951 in DE.
Donor(s): Charles Edward Marsh.‡
Financial data (yr. ended 10/31/95): Assets, $322,962,654 (M); expenditures, $23,552,242; qualifying distributions, $20,296,400, including $20,296,400 for 505 grants (high: $250,000; low: $1,000; average: $25,000-$50,000).
Purpose and activities: Grants primarily to grassroots organizations in the U.S. and abroad, with emphasis on the environment, population and reproductive health, health, the disadvantaged elderly, disadvantaged youth, and criminal justice; support also for select community services. Programs must serve low-income populations, with preference to short-term needs.
Fields of interest: Environment; Health care, reproductive health; Family planning; Health care; AIDS; Health organizations; Crime/violence prevention; Gun control; Offenders/ex-offenders, rehabilitation; Offenders/ex-offenders, prison alternatives; Domestic violence prevention; Legal services; Nutrition; Housing/shelter, development; Children & youth, services; Youth, services; Minorities/immigrants, centers & services; Homeless, human services; Arms control; Human rights (international); Race/intergroup relations; Civil rights; Community development; Minorities; Aging; Immigrants/refugees; Economically disadvantaged; Homeless.
Types of support: General/operating support, continuing support, program development, seed money, matching funds.
Limitations: Giving is generally limited to the U.S. (more than 90 percent). No support for religious purposes. No grants to individuals, or for building funds, capital improvements, endowments, scholarships, graduate work, foreign study, conferences, seminars, publications, research, workshops, or annual campaigns; no loans.
Publications: Annual report (including application guidelines), grants list, informational brochure (including application guidelines).
Application information: WRAG and NNG Common Grant Application forms accepted. Application form not required.
Initial approach: 2-page letter of inquiry. Call for guidelines
Copies of proposal: 1
Deadline(s): None
Board meeting date(s): Board (or a committee of the board) meets 8 times annually
Final notification: 3 to 4 months
Officers and Directors:* Thomas J. Scanlon,* Chair.; Robert H. Haskell,* Vice-Chair.; Linda J. Campbell, Secy.; Antoinette M. Haskell,* Treas.; Larry Kressley, Exec. Dir.; Thomas Ehrlich, Brent L. Henry, Robert R. Nathan, Myrtis H. Powell, Thomas W. Scoville, Jerome W.D. Stokes, C. Elizabeth Warner.
Staff: Anne Townsend, Deputy Dir.; Rebecca A. Davis, Sr. Prog. Officer; Dana A. Alston, Prog. Officer, Environment; Leonard Berman, Prog. Officer, Criminal Justice, Disadvan. Youth; Adisa Douglas, Prog. Officer, Population; Teresa Langston, Prog. Officer, Health, Disadvantaged Elderly; Jodi Williams, Grants Mgr.; Millie Brobston, Prog. Assoc.; Jason Walker, Prog. Assoc.
Number of staff: 12 full-time professional; 5 full-time support; 1 part-time support.
EIN: 540597601
Grants for Aging:
Bayview-Hunters Point Network for Elders, San Francisco, CA, $30,000. For general support to prevent premature institutionalization and elder abuse among predominately African-American poor in district. 95.
Catholic Community Services of Juneau, Juneau, AK, $25,000. For Care Coordination Program, which helps older persons remain at home and live as independently as possible. 95.
Coalition for Elders Independence, Berkeley, CA, $100,000. For start-up support for PACE (Program of All-Inclusive Care for the Elderly) Site in Oakland. 95.
Downtown Clusters Geriatric Day Care Center, DC, $25,000. For general support. 95.
Emmaus Services for the Aging, DC, $25,000. For general support. 95.
Legal Services for Prisoners with Children, San Francisco, CA, $50,000. For Grandparent Caregiver Advocacy Project, with emphasis on working with local child advocates to prepare and disseminate manuals detailing how grandparents and caregivers of children with incarcerated parents can access public benefits for support of children. 95.
Local Enterprise Assistance Fund, Boston, MA, $25,000. For Health Care Lending Initiative, which develops worker-owned home health care companies. 95.
Medicare Beneficiaries Defense Fund, NYC, NY, $45,000. For general support for work to ensure rights of seniors and people with disabilities to quality, affordable health care through direct services, public education and advocacy. 95.
Minnesota Senior Federation, Saint Paul, MN, $48,000. To organize seniors around health care issues and to expand Senior Partners Care, especially in rural areas of Minnesota. 95.
National Council on the Aging, DC, $100,000. For start-up support for National Council of Consumer Organizations in Aging, which will represent grassroots consumer groups of low-income seniors throughout the nation. 95.
Older Womens League (OWL), DC, $50,000. For Health Care - Don't Break the Promise, in defense of Medicaid and Medicare. 95.
Osceola County Council on Aging, Kissimmee, FL, $40,000. For Coming Home, consortium of community agencies to provide continuim of care and services to indigent elderly. 95.
Senior Citizens of Savannah-Chatham County, Savannah, GA, $46,300. To institute Benefits Outreach and Screening Service to assess eligibility and obtain benefits for elderly people. 95.
Seniors with Power United for Rights (SPUR), New Orleans, LA, $25,000. For general support. 95.
Tempe Community Action Agency, Tempe, AZ, $30,000. For Healthy Way, community-based wellness program for disadvantaged elderly. 95.
Time Dollar of Greater Miami, DC, $30,000. For Intergenerational Project for seniors in need of services that can help them continue to live independently. 95.
University of California, San Francisco, CA, $25,000. For start-up support for project to document and disseminate best practices and strategies that promote comprehensive, community-based long-term care for the elderly and disabled. 95.

184
Henry S. and Anne S. Reich Family Foundation

1156 15th St., N.W., Suite 329
Washington 20005 (202) 785-8887
Contact: Stephen A. Bodzin, Esq., V.P.

Established in 1983 in DC.
Donor(s): Anne S. Reich 1983 Charitable Lead Trust No. 1, Anne S. Reich 1983 Charitable Lead Trust No. 2.
Financial data (yr. ended 05/31/95): Assets, $671,560 (M); gifts received, $176,000; expenditures, $200,594; qualifying distributions, $172,165, including $166,280 for 69 grants (high: $37,500; low: $26).
Purpose and activities: Giving for Jewish welfare, temple support, and yeshivas; support also for the performing arts and education.
Fields of interest: Performing arts; Elementary/secondary education; Education; Human services; Jewish federated giving programs; Jewish agencies & temples; Religion; Aging; Women; Israel.
Types of support: General/operating support, continuing support, capital campaigns, emergency funds, program development, seed money, curriculum development, research, program-related investments/loans.
Limitations: Giving primarily in Washington, DC, MD, and VA. No grants to individuals.
Application information: Application form not required.
Initial approach: Letter
Deadline(s): None
Board meeting date(s): May 31
Officers and Directors:* Steven M. Reich,* Pres. and Treas.; Stephen A. Bodzin,* V.P. and Secy.; Albert Abramson.
Number of staff: None.
EIN: 521308578
Grants for Aging:
Hebrew Home of Greater Washington, Rockville, MD, $7,000. 95.
Hebrew Home of Greater Washington, Rockville, MD, $2,500. 95.
Jewish Council for the Aging of Greater Washington, Rockville, MD, $5,000. 94.
Jewish Council for the Aging of Greater Washington, Rockville, MD, $2,500. 95.

185
Walter G. Ross Foundation
c/o ASB Capital Mgmt., Inc.
1101 Pennsylvania Ave., N.W., 3rd Fl.
Washington 20004
Contact: Scott Amling

Trust established about 1964 in DC.
Financial data (yr. ended 12/31/95): Assets, $4,842,841 (M); expenditures, $1,044,002; qualifying distributions, $990,000, including $990,000 for 9 grants (high: $500,000; low: $20,000).
Purpose and activities: Giving primarily for medical research and programs for the elderly, mentally or physically handicapped; support also for higher education and the disadvantaged, including family services and child welfare and development.
Fields of interest: Higher education; Hospitals (general); Health care; Health associations; Heart/circulatory disease; Medical research; Heart/circulatory research; Human services; Children & youth, services; Child development, services; Family services; Hospices; Disabled; Aging; Economically disadvantaged.
Types of support: General/operating support, endowment funds, research, matching funds.
Limitations: Giving limited to the Washington, DC, area, and FL. No grants to individuals, or for scholarships or fellowships; no loans.
Publications: Application guidelines.
Application information: Application form not required.
Initial approach: Letter
Copies of proposal: 1
Deadline(s): Submit proposal preferably in Aug.; deadline Sept. 15
Board meeting date(s): Oct.
Final notification: 1 month after annual meeting
Trustees: Lloyd H. Elliott, Chair.; Eugene L. Bernard, J. Hillman Zahn.
EIN: 526057560

186
George Wasserman Foundation, Inc.
3134 Ellicott St., N.W.
Washington 20008-2025 (202) 966-3355
Contact: Janice W. Goldsten, Pres.

Established in 1948.
Donor(s): George Wasserman.‡
Financial data (yr. ended 12/31/95): Assets, $5,495,433 (M); expenditures, $196,226; qualifying distributions, $177,500, including $177,500 for 7 grants (high: $75,000; low: $10,000).
Purpose and activities: Grants primarily for Jewish welfare funds, theological studies, and temple support; giving also for social services and health.
Fields of interest: Nursing home/convalescent facility; Human services; Jewish federated giving programs; Science; Jewish agencies & temples.
Types of support: General/operating support, continuing support, annual campaigns, building/renovation, endowment funds, program development, seed money, scholarship funds, research, technical assistance, exchange programs.
Limitations: Giving primarily in Washington, DC. No grants to individuals.
Application information:
Initial approach: Letter
Deadline(s): None
Officers and Directors:* Janice W. Goldsten,* Pres. and Treas.; Carolyn Stopak,* V.P. and Secy.; Lisa Gill,* V.P.
EIN: 526035888
Grants for Aging:
Hebrew Home of Greater Washington, Rockville, MD, $75,000. 95.

FLORIDA

187
John E. and Nellie J. Bastien Memorial Foundation
440 East Sample Rd., Suite 209
Pompano Beach 33064 (954) 942-3203
Contact: The Trustees

Trust established in 1965 in FL.
Donor(s): Nellie J. Bastien.‡
Financial data (yr. ended 12/31/93): Assets, $10,195,090 (M); expenditures, $517,455; qualifying distributions, $421,092, including $349,430 for 116 grants (high: $13,750; low: $100).
Fields of interest: Performing arts; Child development, education; Higher education; Environment; Animal welfare; Hospitals (general); Health care; Substance abuse, services; Cancer; Heart/circulatory disease; AIDS; Alcoholism; Biomedicine; Health organizations; Medical research; Cancer research; Heart/circulatory research; AIDS research; Human services; Youth, services; Child development, services; Family services; Hospices; Aging, centers & services; Roman Catholic federated giving programs; Marine science; Religion; Aging; Economically disadvantaged.
Types of support: General/operating support, scholarship funds.
Limitations: Giving primarily in FL.
Application information: Application form not required.
Deadline(s): None
Trustees: Carol R. Kearns, Gene F. Schneider, J. Wallace Wrightson.
EIN: 596160694

188
BCR Foundation, Inc.
P.O. Box 13307
Pensacola 32591-3307 (904) 438-2509
Contact: Betty G. Rainwater, Chair.

Established in 1986.
Financial data (yr. ended 08/31/95): Assets, $3,103,672 (M); expenditures, $84,332; qualifying distributions, $62,950, including $62,950 for 24 grants (high: $9,350; low: $500).
Purpose and activities: Giving primarily for social services, including programs for children; support also for higher education and conservation.
Fields of interest: Education, fund raising; Higher education; Libraries/library science; Education; Natural resource conservation & protection; Environment; Animal welfare; Wildlife preservation & protection; Family planning; Medical care, rehabilitation; Health associations; Cancer; AIDS; Cancer research; AIDS research; Crime/law enforcement; Food services; Housing/shelter, development; Human services; Children & youth, services; Youth, services; Family services; Aging, centers & services; Homeless, human services; Disabled; Aging; Economically disadvantaged; Homeless.
Types of support: Capital campaigns, emergency funds, matching funds.
Limitations: Applications not accepted. Giving primarily in FL. No grants to individuals.
Application information: Contributes only to pre-selected organizations.
Officers and Trustees:* Betty Gregg Rainwater,* Chair. and Pres.; Betty Nickinson,* V.P.; Miriam Flannagan,* Secy.
Number of staff: 1
EIN: 592728836

189
The Frank Stanley Beveridge Foundation, Inc.
301 N.E. 51st St., Suite 1130
Boca Raton 33431-4929 (561) 241-8388
Contact: Philip Caswell, Pres.
Additional tel.: (800) 600-3723; FAX: (407) 241-8332

Trust established in 1947 in MA; incorporated in 1956.
Donor(s): Frank Stanley Beveridge.‡
Financial data (yr. ended 12/31/95): Assets, $44,724,904 (M); expenditures, $2,806,751; qualifying distributions, $2,631,841, including $2,396,328 for 107 grants (high: $1,302,000; low: $100; average: $1,000-$25,000) and $4,000 for 1 in-kind gift.
Purpose and activities: A portion of the income designated for maintenance of a local park established by the donor in Westfield, MA; the balance for general giving, including higher and secondary education institutions attended by the Beveridge Family, social service and youth agencies, community development, culture, health, minorities, ecological programs, and religious organizations attended by the Beveridge Family.
Fields of interest: Historic preservation/historical societies; Education, fund raising; Early childhood education; Child development, education; Elementary school/education; Secondary school/education; Higher education; Adult/continuing education; Education; Animal welfare; Hospitals (general); Health care; Mental health/crisis services; Health organizations; Nutrition; Housing/shelter, development; Human services; Youth, services; Child development, services; Family services; Hospices; Aging, centers & services; Minorities/immigrants, centers & services; Voluntarism promotion; Christian agencies & churches; Protestant agencies & churches; Religion; Minorities; Disabled; Aging.
Types of support: Capital campaigns, building/renovation, equipment, land acquisition, seed money, technical assistance, in-kind gifts, matching funds.

Limitations: Giving primarily in Hampden and Hampshire counties, MA, and Hillsborough and Palm Beach counties, FL. No support for tax-supported organizations. No grants to individuals, or for endowment or operating funds, scholarships, or fellowships; no loans.
Publications: Informational brochure (including application guidelines).
Application information: Application form required.
Initial approach: Letter
Copies of proposal: 1
Deadline(s): Feb. 1 and Aug. 1
Board meeting date(s): Apr. and Oct.
Final notification: 1 month after meeting date
Officers and Directors:* Philip Caswell,* Pres.; Carole S. Lenhart, Treas.; David F. Woods,* Clerk; Sarah Caswell Bartelt, John Beveridge Caswell, Ward S. Caswell, Latimer B. Eddy, Alfred L. Griggs, Joseph Beveridge Palmer, Patsy Palmer Stecher, J. Thomas Touchton.
Number of staff: 1 full-time professional; 1 part-time professional.
EIN: 046032164

190
Blank Family Foundation, Inc.
9350 South Dixie Hwy., Suite 900
Miami 33156
Contact: Robert J. Puck, Secy.-Treas.

Established in 1987 in FL.
Donor(s): Rose Kramer.
Financial data (yr. ended 12/31/93): Assets, $13,580,265 (M); expenditures, $706,747; qualifying distributions, $611,465, including $611,465 for 70 grants (high: $125,000; low: $50).
Fields of interest: Arts/cultural programs; Higher education; Natural resource conservation & protection; Animals/wildlife; Hospitals (general); Human services; Jewish federated giving programs; Jewish agencies & temples; Aging.
Limitations: Applications not accepted. Giving primarily in the Miami, FL, area. No grants to individuals.
Officers and Directors:* Jerome Blank,* Pres.; Andrew Blank,* V.P.; Mark Blank,* V.P.; Robert J. Puck, Secy.-Treas.
EIN: 650060771

191
Edyth Bush Charitable Foundation, Inc.
199 East Welbourne Ave.
P.O. Box 1967
Winter Park 32790-1967 (407) 647-4322
Contact: David A. Odahowski, Pres.
FAX: (407) 647-7716

Originally incorporated in 1966 in MN; reincorporated in 1973 in FL.
Donor(s): Edyth Bassler Bush.‡
Financial data (yr. ended 08/31/95): Assets, $57,718,383 (M); expenditures, $2,959,096; qualifying distributions, $2,989,440, including $2,012,230 for grants (high: $130,000; low: $2,000; average: $20,000-$75,000), $35,240 for foundation-administered programs and $25,000 for program-related investments.
Purpose and activities: Support for charitable, educational, and health service organizations, with emphasis on human services and health, higher education, the elderly, youth services, the handicapped, and demonstrated nationally-recognized quality arts or cultural programs. Provides limited number of program-related investment loans for construction, land purchase, emergency or similar purposes to organizations otherwise qualified to receive grants. Active programs directly managed and/or financed for management/volunteer development of nonprofits.
Fields of interest: Arts/cultural programs; Higher education; Education; Hospitals (general); Health care; Domestic violence prevention; Human services; Youth, services; Aging, centers & services; Nonprofit management; Philanthropy/voluntarism, association; African Americans; Latinos; Native Americans; Disabled; Aging; Women; Economically disadvantaged; Homeless.
Types of support: Continuing support, capital campaigns, building/renovation, equipment, land acquisition, emergency funds, program development, conferences/seminars, seed money, technical assistance, consulting services, program-related investments/loans, matching funds.
Limitations: Giving primarily within a 100-mile radius of Winter Park, FL, with special emphasis on Orange, Seminole, Osceola and Lake counties. No support for alcohol or drug abuse projects or organizations, church, denominational, sacramental, or religious facilities or functions; primarily (50 percent or more) tax-supported institutions; advocacy organizations; foreign organizations; or generally for cultural programs. No grants to individuals, or for scholarships or individual research projects, endowments, fellowships, travel, routine operating expenses, annual campaigns, or deficit financing.
Publications: 990-PF, program policy statement, application guidelines, financial statement.
Application information: Outline required for applications; see Policy Statement before applying. Application guidelines available upon request. Application form not required.
Initial approach: Telephone
Copies of proposal: 2
Deadline(s): Sept. 1 or Jan. 31
Board meeting date(s): Usually in Nov., Apr., and as required
Final notification: 2 weeks after board meetings
Officers and Directors:* H. Clifford Lee,* Chair.; Mary Gretchen Belloff, Vice-Chair.; David A. Odahowski,* Pres. and C.E.O.; Michael R. Cross, V.P., Finance, and Treas.; Edith M. Walsh, Corp. Secy.; Guy D. Colado, Charlotte H. Forward, Gerald F. Hilbrich, Herbert W. Holm, David R. Roberts, Vernon Swartsel, Robert E. Waggoner.
Number of staff: 2 full-time professional; 4 full-time support.
EIN: 237318041

192
Kathleen K. Catlin Charitable Trust
c/o Barnett Banks Trust Co., N.A.
P.O. Box 676
Venice 34284-0676 (941) 951-4441
Contact: Stephen D. Edwards, Trust Officer, Barnett Banks Trust Co., N.A.

Established in 1987 in FL.
Financial data (yr. ended 02/28/95): Assets, $5,854,913 (M); expenditures, $312,970; qualifying distributions, $284,534, including $271,250 for grants.
Fields of interest: Secondary school/education; Hospitals (general); Health care; Health associations; Human services; Aging, centers & services; Aging; Economically disadvantaged.
Types of support: General/operating support, building/renovation, equipment, program development.
Limitations: Giving primarily in Venice and Sarasota, FL. No grants to individuals.
Application information: Application form required.
Deadline(s): None
Trustee: Barnett Banks Trust Co., N.A.
EIN: 596877094

193
George M. Cohen Foundation, Inc.
c/o Shorstein & Shorstein
8265 Bayberry Rd.
Jacksonville 32256

Established in 1984 in FL.
Donor(s): George M. Cohen, Lawrence J. DuBow.
Financial data (yr. ended 11/30/94): Assets, $4,089,952 (M); expenditures, $204,191; qualifying distributions, $198,981, including $198,415 for grants.
Purpose and activities: Giving primarily for Jewish welfare and a home for the aged.
Fields of interest: Human services; Aging, centers & services; Jewish federated giving programs; Jewish agencies & temples; Aging.
Limitations: Applications not accepted. Giving primarily in Jacksonville, FL. No grants to individuals.
Application information: Contributes only to pre-selected organizations.
Officers and Trustees:* George M. Cohen,* Pres. and Mgr.; Lawrence J. DuBow,* Secy.; Samuel R. Shorstein,* Treas.; Carolyn Cohen.
EIN: 592469069

194
The Colen Foundation, Inc.
(Formerly The On Top of the World Foundation, Inc.)
8700 S.W. 99th St.
Ocala 32676 (352) 854-0805
Contact: Kenneth D. Colen, Dir.

Established in 1984.
Donor(s): Kenneth D. Colen, Sidney Colen.
Financial data (yr. ended 11/30/94): Assets, $5,021,042 (M); gifts received, $3,550,000; expenditures, $88,887; qualifying distributions, $70,736, including $66,902 for grants.

Fields of interest: Performing arts; Aging, centers & services; Jewish agencies & temples; Aging.
Limitations: Giving limited to FL.
Application information: Application form not required.
Deadline(s): None
Officer: William J. Hussar, Secy.
Directors: Ina A. Colen, Kenneth D. Colen, Sidney Colen, Raymond J. Funk.
EIN: 592474711

195
Community Foundation of Brevard County, Inc.

P.O. Box 361284
Melbourne 32936-1284 (407) 724-6133
Contact: Walt Robinson, Exec. Dir.

Community foundation established in 1981 in FL.
Foundation type: Community
Financial data (yr. ended 12/31/94): Assets, $419,137 (M); gifts received, $29,878; expenditures, $57,760, including $30,292 for grants.
Fields of interest: Museums; Historic preservation/historical societies; Arts/cultural programs; Education; Natural resource conservation & protection; Environment; Animal welfare; Substance abuse, services; Recreation; Children & youth, services; Aging, centers & services; Community development; Aging.
Types of support: Building/renovation, equipment, program development, seed money, scholarship funds, technical assistance.
Limitations: Giving limited to Brevard County, FL.
Publications: Application guidelines, grants list, informational brochure.
Application information: Application form required.
Copies of proposal: 1
Deadline(s): June 1 and Dec. 1
Board meeting date(s): Bimonthly
Final notification: 90 days after deadline
Officers and Directors:* Yvonne Bixby,* Pres.; Abe Collinsworth,* V.P.; Karen Dee,* Secy.; Walt Secrest,* Treas.; Walt Robinson, Exec. Dir.; Gene Bjerning, Ernie Briel, Ron Heimann, Daria Jones-Francey, Roger Manley, Don Molitor, Patti Patch, James W. Peeples III, Steve Ridder, Thurman Stephens, Don Welk.
Number of staff: 1 part-time professional; 1 part-time support.
EIN: 592114988

196
The Community Foundation of Greater Tampa, Inc.

315 East Madison St., Suite 600
Tampa 33602-4818 (813) 221-1776
Contact: George J. Baxter, Pres.

Established in 1990 in FL.
Foundation type: Community
Financial data (yr. ended 06/30/95): Assets, $9,205,623 (M); gifts received, $3,051,484; expenditures, $1,477,253, including $1,260,688 for 345 grants (high: $250,000; low: $60; average: $500-$5,000) and $16,500 for in-kind gifts.
Purpose and activities: Primary areas of interest include the arts, child welfare, elementary and higher education, and homelessness.
Fields of interest: Visual arts; Performing arts; Historic preservation/historical societies; Arts/cultural programs; Elementary school/education; Higher education; Education; Environment; Health care; Medical research; Housing/shelter, development; Human services; Children & youth, services; Youth, services; Aging, centers & services; Homeless, human services; Community development; Government/public administration; Public affairs; Religion; Aging; Homeless.
Types of support: Building/renovation, equipment, emergency funds, program development, seed money, curriculum development, scholarship funds, technical assistance, consulting services.
Limitations: Giving primarily in the Hillsborough County, FL, area. No grants to individuals, or for operating costs of established programs, advertising or tickets to sponsor events.
Publications: Annual report, informational brochure, newsletter.
Application information: Application form not required.
Initial approach: Letter
Copies of proposal: 1
Board meeting date(s): Jan., May, and Oct.
Officers and Trustees:* James H. Shimberg,* Chair.; Jerry L. Williams,* Vice-Chair.; George J. Baxter,* Pres.; Harold W. Mullis, Jr.,* Secy.; Arthur L. Stuckey,* Treas.; E. Jackson Boggs, Advisory Comm. Chair.; Elizabeth W. Kennedy, Grants Comm. Chair.; John M. Tapley, Fund Acceptance Comm. Chair.; Joyce Wellman, Public Information Comm. Chair.; and 32 additional trustees.
Number of staff: 2 full-time professional; 1 full-time support; 1 part-time support.
EIN: 593001853

197
The Coyne Family Foundation, Inc.

(Formerly The Martin L. & Wileen T. Coyne Foundation, Inc.)
8812 Twin Lake Dr.
Boca Raton 33496 (561) 487-0440
Contact: Martin L. Coyne, Pres., or Deborah P. Coyne, Exec. Dir.

Established in 1985 in FL.
Donor(s): Martin L. Coyne, Melissa Ann Coyne, Russell Coyne.
Financial data (yr. ended 12/31/94): Assets, $911,874 (M); expenditures, $131,957; qualifying distributions, $122,105, including $122,105 for 21 grants (high: $67,000; low: $250).
Fields of interest: Arts/cultural programs; Hospitals (general); Health care; Cancer; AIDS; Health organizations; Medical research; Cancer research; AIDS research; Human services; Children & youth, services; Aging, centers & services; Disabled; Aging; Economically disadvantaged; General charitable giving.
Types of support: General/operating support, continuing support, annual campaigns, program development, seed money, scholarship funds, research.
Limitations: Giving limited to Palm Beach County, FL. No grants to individuals.
Application information: Application form not required.
Initial approach: Proposal
Copies of proposal: 1
Deadline(s): Oct. 15
Board meeting date(s): Nov.
Final notification: Before year end
Officers: Martin L. Coyne, Pres.; Melissa Ann Coyne, Secy.; Russell Coyne, Treas.; Deborah P. Coyne, Exec. Dir.
Director: William Livingston.
Number of staff: None.
EIN: 592473967

198
Crossroads Foundation, Inc.

P.O. Box 1927
Winter Park 32790-1927
Contact: Philip B. Crosby, Founder

Established in 1986 in FL.
Donor(s): Nicholas Wright, Phylis Crosby-Wright.
Financial data (yr. ended 12/31/94): Assets, $9,318 (M); gifts received, $74,955; expenditures, $74,727; qualifying distributions, $73,475, including $73,475 for 16 grants (high: $15,000; low: $250).
Fields of interest: Visual arts; Museums; Performing arts; Arts/cultural programs; Child development, education; Elementary school/education; Higher education; Hospitals (general); Health care; Substance abuse, services; Cancer; Health organizations; Cancer research; Human services; Children & youth, services; Youth, services; Child development, services; Aging, centers & services; Homeless, human services; Christian agencies & churches; Disabled; Aging; Economically disadvantaged; Homeless.
Types of support: General/operating support, continuing support, capital campaigns, building/renovation, equipment, program development.
Limitations: Applications not accepted. Giving primarily in central FL. No grants to individuals.
Publications: Program policy statement.
Application information: Contributes only to pre-selected organizations.
Board meeting date(s): Annually
Officers: Peggy D. Crosby, Founder; Philip B. Crosby, Founder; Mindy Raymond, Administrator.
Number of staff: None.
EIN: 592714846

199
Dade Community Foundation, Inc.

(Formerly Dade Foundation)
200 South Biscayne Blvd., Suite 2780
Miami 33131-2343 (305) 371-2711
Contact: Ruth Shack, Pres.

Established in 1967 in FL.
Foundation type: Community
Financial data (yr. ended 12/31/95): Assets, $38,976,770 (M); gifts received, $4,436,059;

expenditures, $5,112,507, including $3,078,423 for 586 grants (high: $200,000; low: $100; average: $100-$200,000), $21,000 for 18 grants to individuals (high: $2,000; low: $500; average: $500-$10,000) and $23,000 for 5 loans.
Purpose and activities: Support for projects which: provide an innovative response to a recognized community need but which do not duplicate other efforts; help an organization build internal stability; promise to affect a broad segment of the residents of Dade County; and exert a leverage or multiplier effect in addressing community problems to be solved. Primary areas of support are AIDS, community development, the disadvantaged, leadership development, and housing; other areas of support include health, social services, the homeless and housing, civic affairs, education, arts and culture, and religious organizations.
Fields of interest: Arts/cultural programs; Law school/education; Adult education—literacy & basic skills; Reading; Education; Animal welfare; Family planning; Health care; AIDS; AIDS research; Housing/shelter, development; Youth development, services; Youth development, citizenship; Human services; Children & youth, services; Aging, centers & services; Women, centers & services; Homeless, human services; Community development; Government/public administration; Public affairs, citizen participation; Leadership development; Aging; Women; Economically disadvantaged.
Types of support: General/operating support, continuing support, building/renovation, equipment, land acquisition, endowment funds, emergency funds, program development, publication, seed money, internships, scholarship funds, research, technical assistance, consulting services, program-related investments/loans, grants to individuals, scholarships—to individuals, matching funds.
Limitations: Giving limited to Dade County, FL. No grants for deficit financing or conferences.
Publications: Annual report, application guidelines, newsletter, occasional report.
Application information: Application form not required.
Initial approach: Letter
Copies of proposal: 1
Deadline(s): Submit proposal preferably in Nov.; deadline Nov. 30
Board meeting date(s): Feb., May, Sept., and Nov.
Final notification: 1st quarter of the year
Officers and Governors:* Maria Elena Prio,* Chair.; David Lawrence,* Vice-Chair.; Ruth Shack, Pres.; Ghislain Gouraige, Jr., Secy.; Christopher Economides, Treas.; and 17 additional governors.
Investment Managers: Barnett Banks Trust Co., N.A., Fiduciary Trust International of the South, First Union National Bank of Florida, Fox Asset Management, GSB, Nicholas Applegate, Northern Trust Bank of Florida, N.A., SunTrust Bank, Miami, N.A., TIFF.
Number of staff: 4 full-time professional; 1 part-time professional; 3 part-time support.
EIN: 650350357
Grants for Aging:
North Miami Foundation for Senior Citizens, Miami, FL, $10,000. For Loving Touch, human and animal interaction and animal care program. 94.

200
The Leonard and Sophie Davis Foundation, Inc.
601 Clearwater Park Rd.
West Palm Beach 33401-6233 (561) 832-6466
Contact: Marilyn Hoadley, Pres.

Incorporated in 1961 in NY.
Donor(s): Leonard Davis, Sophie Davis.
Financial data (yr. ended 12/31/93): Assets, $20,206,244 (M); gifts received, $1,632,406; expenditures, $2,452,544; qualifying distributions, $2,425,818, including $2,404,325 for grants.
Purpose and activities: Grants primarily for Jewish charitable, religious, and educational organizations, and for higher education; support also for the arts, community services, and health agencies and hospitals; limited giving to public interest groups.
Fields of interest: Museums; Dance; Music; Arts/cultural programs; Higher education; Hospitals (general); Health care; AIDS; AIDS research; Human services; Hospices; Aging, centers & services; Federated giving programs; Jewish federated giving programs; Public policy, research; Jewish agencies & temples; Aging.
Types of support: Continuing support, annual campaigns, building/renovation, conferences/seminars.
Limitations: Applications not accepted. Giving primarily in Palm Beach County, FL, and New York, NY. No grants to individuals.
Application information:
Board meeting date(s): As required
Officers: Marilyn Hoadley, Pres.; Leonard Davis, V.P.; Sophie Davis, V.P.
Directors: Alan Davis, Michael Davis.
Number of staff: None.
EIN: 136062579
Grants for Aging:
University of Southern California, Leonard Davis School of Gerontology, Los Angeles, CA, $76,000. 95.

201
Elsie & Marvin Dekelboum Foundation, Inc.
(Formerly Elmar Foundation, Inc.)
c/o Thaler & Thaler
700 North Olive Ave.
West Palm Beach 33401 (561) 659-1183
Contact: Marvin Dekelboum, Pres.

Established in 1989 in FL.
Donor(s): Marvin Dekelboum, Elsie Dekelboum.
Financial data (yr. ended 12/31/94): Assets, $694,340 (M); gifts received, $192,000; expenditures, $40,106; qualifying distributions, $40,106, including $32,000 for 1 grant.
Fields of interest: Performing arts; Youth, services; Aging.
Application information:
Initial approach: Letter
Deadline(s): None
Officers: Marvin Dekelboum, Pres.; Elsie Dekelboum, V.P.; Manley Thaler, Secy.
EIN: 650121068

202
Doctors Hospital Inc. of Plantation
P.O. Box 15066
Plantation 33318-5066 (954) 475-2455
Contact: Ruth Weis, Grants Consultant

Established as private foundation in 1987 in FL.
Financial data (yr. ended 12/31/93): Assets, $11,527,550 (M); expenditures, $1,004,873; qualifying distributions, $752,520, including $722,420 for 38 grants (high: $620,000; low: $1,000; average: $1,000-$5,000).
Purpose and activities: Primary areas of interest include health issues and community funds.
Fields of interest: Higher education; Health care; Health organizations; Family services; Aging, centers & services; Federated giving programs; Aging.
Types of support: General/operating support, continuing support, professorships, research.
Limitations: Giving limited to Broward, Dade, and West Palm Beach counties, FL. No grants to individuals.
Application information: Application form not required.
Initial approach: Letter of intent
Copies of proposal: 1
Deadline(s): Aug. 15 for letter of intent; Nov. 30 for complete proposal
Final notification: Jan. 30
Officers and Trustees:* Donald L. Gross,* Pres.; Robert L. Perraud,* Secy.; Howard L. Neer,* Treas.
Number of staff: None.
EIN: 590906961

203
Dodson Family Foundation, Inc.
c/o Howard Weiss
7383 Orangewood Ln., Suite 303
Boca Raton 33433

Established in 1992 in FL and DE.
Donor(s): Elizabeth K. Dodson.
Financial data (yr. ended 12/31/93): Assets, $1,684,769 (M); gifts received, $817,250; expenditures, $101,870; qualifying distributions, $100,172, including $63,165 for 16 grants (high: $22,475; low: $20).
Fields of interest: Theater; Elementary/secondary education; Hospitals (general); Alzheimer's disease; American Red Cross.
Limitations: Applications not accepted. Giving primarily in Boca Raton, FL. No grants to individuals.
Application information: Contributes only to pre-selected organizations.
Officers and Director:* Elizabeth K. Dodson,* Pres.; Howard Weiss,* V.P. and Secy.-Treas.; Michael J. Kara,* V.P.; Isabel Vincent,* V.P.
EIN: 510342321

204
Alfred I. duPont Foundation
P.O. Box 1380
Jacksonville 32201 (904) 396-6600

Contact: Rosemary C. Wills, Asst. Secy.

Incorporated in 1936 in FL.
Donor(s): Jessie Ball duPont.‡
Financial data (yr. ended 12/31/93): Assets, $26,890,000 (M); expenditures, $947,000; qualifying distributions, $922,000, including $517,400 for 94 grants (high: $60,000; low: $25) and $394,600 for 200 grants to individuals (high: $12,000; low: $150).
Purpose and activities: Giving primarily to the elderly in distressed situations requiring health, economic, or educational assistance; support also for higher education and medical research.
Fields of interest: Higher education; Medical research; Aging, centers & services; Aging; Economically disadvantaged.
Types of support: General/operating support, grants to individuals.
Limitations: Giving primarily in the Southeast.
Application information: Application form required.
Initial approach: Proposal
Copies of proposal: 1
Deadline(s): None
Officers and Directors:* Braden Ball,* Pres.; J.C. Belin,* V.P. and Treas.; Lillie S. Land,* Secy.; R.E. Nedley.
EIN: 591297267

205
Eagles Memorial Foundation, Inc.
4710 14th St. West
Bradenton 34207 (941) 758-5456
Contact: Thomas J. McGriff, Exec. Secy.
Application address: c/o Richard J. Steinberg, Golden Eagle Fund, P.O. Box 25916, Milwaukee, WI 53225-0916

Established in 1944.
Financial data (yr. ended 05/31/96): Assets, $13,494,887 (M); gifts received, $337,881; expenditures, $805,074; qualifying distributions, $819,457, including $463,217 for grants and $60,461 for grants to individuals.
Purpose and activities: Grants to organizations made through the Golden Eagle Fund, which supports the aged, nutrition, public libraries, and Eagle Village, Inc. The foundation supports scientific research to discover the cause, treatment, and possible cure for Alzheimer's disease. The foundation also gives for educational and medical purposes to children of deceased Eagle servicemen and women, law officers, firefighters, and EMS workers.
Fields of interest: Libraries/library science; Nutrition; Aging, centers & services; Aging; Economically disadvantaged.
Types of support: Program development, research, grants to individuals, scholarships—to individuals.
Limitations: No grants to individuals (except for scholarships and medical expense assistance to Eagle members and families), hospices, private nursing homes, or Aerie clubs.
Application information: Alzheimer grant requests must include research project description sheet written on the letterhead of the applying medical institution. Application form required.
Copies of proposal: 1
Deadline(s): None
Officers and Directors:* Dale E. Webster,* Chair.; Laverne P. Weber,* Vice-Chair.; Vincent Cherry,* Secy.; Thomas J. McGriff,* Exec. Secy.; Ed Bollenbacher, W.E. "Bill" Mason.
EIN: 396126176

206
The Eppler Family Foundation
150 North Ocean Blvd.
Palm Beach 33480

Donor(s): Heinz Eppler.
Financial data (yr. ended 12/31/94): Assets, $235,473 (M); gifts received, $484,204; expenditures, $238,706; qualifying distributions, $235,290, including $235,290 for grants.
Fields of interest: Arts/cultural programs; Human services; Aging, centers & services; Community development; Jewish federated giving programs; Aging.
Limitations: Applications not accepted. Giving primarily in FL and CO. No grants to individuals.
Application information: Contributes only to pre-selected organizations.
Officers: Heinz Eppler, Pres.; Ruthe Eppler, V.P.
Directors: Marcia Colvin, David Michael Eppler, Nancy Eppler Wolff.
EIN: 591949552

207
Claudia S. Morse Evans Private Foundation, Inc.
c/o Coopers & Lybrand
515 North Flagler Dr., No. 400
West Palm Beach 33401-4382

Established in 1987 in FL.
Donor(s): Jeanne and Irwin Levy Foundation, Inc., Claudia S. Morse Evans.
Financial data (yr. ended 09/30/92): Assets, $436,935 (M); expenditures, $72,033; qualifying distributions, $72,033, including $70,000 for 1 grant.
Purpose and activities: Support primarily for a geriatric center.
Fields of interest: Aging, centers & services; Aging.
Limitations: Applications not accepted. Giving primarily in West Palm Beach, FL. No grants to individuals.
Application information: Contributes only to pre-selected organizations.
Officers: Claudia S. Morse Evans, Pres.; Alan Evans, V.P.; Stanley B. Brenner, Secy.; H. Irwin Levy, Treas.
EIN: 592797822

208
The David Falk Foundation, Inc.
c/o SunTrust Bank, Tampa Bay
P.O. Box 1498
Tampa 33601 (813) 224-2626
Contact: John J. Howley, Pres.
FAX: (813) 224-2461

Incorporated in 1945 in FL.
Donor(s): David A. Falk.‡
Financial data (yr. ended 12/31/95): Assets, $2,594,316 (M); expenditures, $157,058; qualifying distributions, $124,557, including $115,111 for 26 grants (high: $12,500; low: $200; average: $100-$10,000).
Fields of interest: Media/communications; Museums; Performing arts; Humanities; Arts/cultural programs; Higher education; Business school/education; Education; Hospitals (general); Medical care, rehabilitation; Health care; Substance abuse, services; Mental health/crisis services; Heart/circulatory disease; Biomedicine; Health organizations; Medical research; Heart/circulatory research; Delinquency prevention/services; Crime/law enforcement; Human services; Children & youth, services; Youth, services; Family services; Hospices; Aging, centers & services; Minorities/immigrants, centers & services; Homeless, human services; Community development; Voluntarism promotion; Minorities; Disabled; Aging; Economically disadvantaged; Homeless; General charitable giving.
Types of support: General/operating support, capital campaigns, building/renovation, equipment, land acquisition, endowment funds, emergency funds, program development, publication, seed money, scholarship funds, research, matching funds.
Limitations: Giving limited to the Tampa Bay, FL, area. No support for community funds or electoral or political projects. No grants to individuals, or for continuing support, annual campaigns, deficit financing, conferences, scholarships, or fellowships; no loans.
Publications: Program policy statement, application guidelines.
Application information: Application form required.
Initial approach: Proposal
Copies of proposal: 1
Deadline(s): None
Board meeting date(s): Mar., June, Sept., and Dec.
Final notification: 90 days after board meeting
Officers and Directors:* Herbert G. McKay,* Chair.; John J. Howley,* Pres.; John C. Peters,* V.P.; H.D. Carrington, Jr., Secy.-Treas.; David C.G. Kerr.
Number of staff: None.
EIN: 591055570

209
Florida Rock Industries Foundation, Inc.
155 East 21st St.
Jacksonville 32206-2104
Contact: H.B. Horner, Secy.
Application address: P.O. Box 4667, Jacksonville, FL 32201

Established in 1981 in FL.
Donor(s): Florida Rock Industries, Inc.
Foundation type: Company-sponsored
Financial data (yr. ended 09/30/94): Assets, $1,673,399 (M); expenditures, $149,680; qualifying distributions, $138,779, including $138,779 for 51 grants (high: $20,000; low: $100).
Fields of interest: Museums; Higher education; Alzheimer's disease; Alzheimer's disease research; Human services; Youth, services.
Types of support: Scholarship funds.

Limitations: No grants to individuals.
Application information:
Initial approach: Proposal
Officers: Edward L. Baker, Pres.; John D. Baker II, V.P.; H.B. Horner, Secy.; Ruggles B. Carlson, Treas.
EIN: 592143326
Grants for Aging:
Alzheimers Care and Research Center at Cypress Village, Jacksonville, FL, $20,000. 94.

210
FPL Group Foundation, Inc.
(Formerly FPL Foundation, Inc.)
700 Universe Blvd.
Juno Beach 33102
Contact: John L. Kitchens, Corp. Contribs. Administrator
Application address: P.O. Box 029100, Miami, FL 33102

Established in 1987 in FL.
Donor(s): Florida Power & Light Co.
Foundation type: Company-sponsored
Financial data (yr. ended 12/31/95): Assets, $3,890,000 (M); gifts received, $1,425,000; expenditures, $1,433,020; qualifying distributions, $1,427,329, including $1,211,329 for 330 grants (high: $30,000; low: $50; average: $500-$10,000) and $216,000 for 200 employee matching gifts.
Purpose and activities: Giving primarily for the environment; support also for health, the arts, education, social services, workforce readiness, and community development.
Fields of interest: Visual arts; Performing arts; Arts/cultural programs; Higher education; Education; Energy; Environment; Health care; Health organizations; Human services; Aging, centers & services; Minorities/immigrants, centers & services; Race/intergroup relations; Community development; Voluntarism promotion; Minorities; African Americans; Latinos; Disabled; Aging; Economically disadvantaged; Homeless.
Types of support: Capital campaigns, endowment funds, employee matching gifts.
Limitations: Giving primarily in areas of company operations which includes most of the east coast of FL and the coast from Bradenton to Naples. No support for religious or political groups or United Way-affiliated agencies. No grants to individuals.
Publications: Application guidelines, 990-PF.
Application information: Application form not required.
Initial approach: Proposal
Copies of proposal: 1
Deadline(s): Aug.
Board meeting date(s): Undesignated
Officers and Directors:* J.L. Broadhead,* Chair.; Paul J. Evanson,* Pres.; L.J. Kelleher III, V.P.; D.P. Coyle,* Secy.
Number of staff: 125 part-time support.
EIN: 650031452

211
FPL Group, Inc. Contributions Program
11770 U.S. Hwy. One, Box 088801
North Palm Beach 33408-3029 (305) 552-4090
Contact: John L. Kitchens, Corp. Contribs. Administrator
Application address: P.O. Box 029100, Miami, FL 33102-9100

Financial data (yr. ended 12/31/94): Total giving, $861,000, including $858,500 for 1,000 grants (high: $10,000; low: $50; average: $50-$10,000) and $2,500 for 1 in-kind gift.
Purpose and activities: The company supports organizations that focus on one of four areas: the environment; social services for those living on low income, the elderly, and minorities; community development; and workforce readiness and organizational effectiveness.
Fields of interest: Performing arts; Arts/cultural programs; Higher education; Engineering school/education; Education; Natural resource conservation & protection; Energy; Environment; Health care; Human services; Aging, centers & services; Minorities/immigrants, centers & services; Community development; Engineering & technology; Engineering; Science; Government/public administration; Minorities; Aging.
Types of support: Annual campaigns, capital campaigns, building/renovation, program development, scholarship funds, employee volunteer services, sponsorships, employee matching gifts, matching funds.
Limitations: Giving limited to service area in FL. No support for religious or political groups. No grants to individuals, or for United Way affiliated agencies.
Publications: Application guidelines.
Application information:
Initial approach: Letter of proposal; send requests to nearest company facility; External Affairs handles all contributions
Copies of proposal: 1
Deadline(s): Applications accepted throughout the year. The budget is completed in Aug. for the upcoming year
Administrator: John L. Kitchens, Corp. Contribs., Administrator.
Number of staff: 2 part-time professional; 1 full-time support.

212
The Greenburg-May Foundation, Inc.
P.O. Box 54-5816
Miami Beach 33154 (305) 864-8639
Contact: Samuel D. May, Pres.

Incorporated in 1947 in DE.
Donor(s): Harry Greenburg.‡
Financial data (yr. ended 12/31/93): Assets, $4,363,259 (M); expenditures, $224,192; qualifying distributions, $198,875, including $191,361 for 50 grants (high: $62,750; low: $25).
Purpose and activities: Grants almost entirely for medical research, primarily in cancer and heart disease; some support also for aging, hospitals, Jewish welfare funds, and temples.
Fields of interest: Hospitals (general); Cancer; Heart/circulatory disease; Medical research; Cancer research; Heart/circulatory research; Human services; Aging, centers & services; Jewish federated giving programs; Jewish agencies & temples; Aging.
Types of support: General/operating support, continuing support, building/renovation, endowment funds, scholarship funds, research.
Limitations: Giving primarily in southern FL, IL, and NY. No grants to individuals, or for conferences; generally no grants for scholarships or fellowships; no loans.
Application information: Application form not required.
Initial approach: Letter
Copies of proposal: 1
Deadline(s): None
Board meeting date(s): Jan., Apr., July, and Oct.
Final notification: 1 to 2 months
Officers and Directors:* Samuel D. May,* Pres. and Treas.; Peter May,* V.P.; Linda Sklar,* V.P.; Isabel May,* Secy.
Number of staff: 2 part-time support.
EIN: 136162935

213
The GTR Foundation, Inc.
1704 Thomasville Rd., No. 194
Tallahassee 32303

Established in 1987 in FL.
Donor(s): William O'Neil III.
Financial data (yr. ended 12/31/94): Assets, $667,333 (M); expenditures, $49,300; qualifying distributions, $48,237, including $42,000 for 8 grants (high: $5,000; low: $3,000) and $5,358 for 1 grant to an individual.
Fields of interest: Food services; Aging, centers & services; Homeless, human services; Disabled; Aging; Economically disadvantaged; Homeless.
Types of support: Grants to individuals.
Limitations: Applications not accepted. Giving limited to FL.
Officers and Directors:* William O'Neil III,* Chair. and Pres.; Nikki Hubbard, Secy.-Treas.
EIN: 592798067

214
Haywood Foundation, Inc.
5585 Las Brisa Dr.
Vero Beach 32967
Contact: Oliver G. Haywood, Pres.

Donor(s): Oliver G. Haywood.
Financial data (yr. ended 12/31/93): Assets, $110,451 (M); expenditures, $11,436; qualifying distributions, $11,436, including $11,217 for grants.
Fields of interest: Higher education; Medical research; Human services; Aging, centers & services; Military/veterans' organizations; Disabled; Aging.
Limitations: Giving on a national basis. No grants to individuals.
Application information: Application form not required.
Deadline(s): None

Officers: Oliver G. Haywood, Pres. and Treas.; Robert G. Haywood, V.P.; Barbara A. Haywood, Secy.
EIN: 237028521

215
Jacarlene Foundation, Inc.
c/o SunBank of Tampa Bay
P.O. Box 1498
Tampa 33601

Established in 1987 in FL.
Donor(s): Jacqueline Preis.
Financial data (yr. ended 12/31/93): Assets, $966,745 (M); gifts received, $340,000; expenditures, $45,510; qualifying distributions, $40,177.
Fields of interest: Museums (science & technology); Health associations; Aging.
Limitations: Applications not accepted. Giving primarily in FL. No grants to individuals.
Officers: Jacqueline Preis, Pres.; John J. Howley, Secy.-Treas.
Director: Allen Steinberg.
EIN: 581762618

216
The Jewish Charity & Elderly Housing Fund, Inc.
999 Washington Ave.
Miami Beach 33139

Financial data (yr. ended 12/31/92): Assets, $11,336 (M); gifts received, $12,500; expenditures, $2,772; qualifying distributions, $2,500, including $2,500 for grants.
Fields of interest: Aging, centers & services; Jewish agencies & temples; Aging.
Limitations: Applications not accepted.
Officers: Hyman P. Galbut, Pres.; Robert N. Galbut, Secy.; David L. Galbut, Treas.
Directors: Abraham A. Galbut, Russell W. Galbut.
EIN: 650076270

217
Lost Tree Charitable Foundation, Inc.
11555 Lost Tree Way
North Palm Beach 33408 (561) 622-3780
Contact: James Gillin, Pres., or Pamela M. Rue, Prog. Dir.

Incorporated in 1982 in FL.
Foundation type: Community
Financial data (yr. ended 12/31/94): Assets, $2,249,124 (M); gifts received, $560,456; expenditures, $667,061, including $581,970 for 37 grants (high: $50,000; low: $1,000).
Purpose and activities: Giving primarily for family and social services, including programs for rehabilitation, alcohol and drug abuse, and the disabled; support also for higher, medical, early childhood and other education, and health services.
Fields of interest: Early childhood education; Child development, education; Higher education; Education; Hospitals (general); Medical care, rehabilitation; Health care; Substance abuse, services; Mental health/crisis services; Alcoholism; Health organizations; Food services; Youth development, services; Human services; Youth, services; Child development, services; Family services; Hospices; Aging, centers & services; Homeless, human services; Roman Catholic federated giving programs; Leadership development; Disabled; Aging; Economically disadvantaged; Homeless.
Types of support: General/operating support, continuing support, capital campaigns, building/renovation, equipment, program development, seed money, scholarship funds, matching funds.
Limitations: Giving limited to Palm Beach and Martin counties, FL. No grants to individuals.
Publications: Annual report, newsletter, occasional report, informational brochure.
Application information:
Initial approach: Letter
Copies of proposal: 1
Deadline(s): Sept. 30 for consideration in fall and spring of following year
Officers and Trustees:* James Gillin,* Pres.; John W. Fauver,* Exec. V.P.; David R. Clare,* V.P.; Joseph D. Harnett,* V.P.; Mrs. Frank R. Milnor,* V.P.; Robert A. Waidner,* V.P.; William N. Poundstone,* Secy.; Joseph M. Hickey, Jr.,* Treas.
Staff: Pamela M. Rue, Prog. Dir.
Number of staff: 1 full-time professional; 1 part-time support.
EIN: 592104920

218
The Milton and Tamar Maltz Family Foundation, Inc.
4300 South U.S. Hwy. No. 1, 203-328
Jupiter 33477-1125

Established in 1989 in FL.
Donor(s): Milton S. Maltz, Thelma Maltz.
Financial data (yr. ended 06/30/95): Assets, $1,132,331 (M); expenditures, $75,053; qualifying distributions, $138,869, including $47,000 for 2 grants (high: $45,000; low: $2,000) and $91,869 for 2 foundation-administered programs.
Fields of interest: Human services; Aging, centers & services; Jewish federated giving programs; Aging.
Limitations: Applications not accepted. No grants to individuals.
Application information: Contributes only to pre-selected organizations.
Officers: Milton S. Maltz, Pres.; Julie E. Konigsberg, V.P.; Daniel Maltz, V.P.; Thelma Maltz, Secy.; David Maltz, Treas.
EIN: 650164300

219
The Baron de Hirsch Meyer Foundation
407 Lincoln Rd., Suite 6J
Miami Beach 33139

Incorporated in 1940 in FL.
Donor(s): Baron de Hirsch Meyer.‡
Financial data (yr. ended 12/31/93): Assets, $3,443,388 (M); gifts received, $200; expenditures, $177,451; qualifying distributions, $96,776, including $82,497 for 22 grants (high: $26,176; low: $20).
Fields of interest: Performing arts; Animal welfare; Hospitals (general); Health care; Cancer; Cancer research; Human services; Children & youth, services; Aging, centers & services; Jewish federated giving programs; Religious federated giving programs; Roman Catholic agencies & churches; Aging; General charitable giving.
Types of support: Building/renovation.
Limitations: Giving primarily in southern FL. No grants to individuals.
Publications: Informational brochure (including application guidelines).
Application information: Application form not required.
Initial approach: Proposal or letter
Copies of proposal: 1
Board meeting date(s): Feb.
Officers and Directors:* Polly de Hirsch Meyer,* Pres. and Treas.; Marie Williams,* V.P.; Martin Steedman,* Secy.
Number of staff: 2
EIN: 596129646

220
Mote Scientific Foundation, Inc.
603 Longboat Club Way, 1101N
Longboat Key 34228
Contact: William R. Mote, Pres.

Incorporated in 1950 in NY.
Donor(s): William R. Mote, T.R. Bartels, Theodore R. Bartels.
Financial data (yr. ended 11/30/94): Assets, $7,794,668 (M); gifts received, $5,183,882; expenditures, $269,978; qualifying distributions, $238,966, including $235,600 for grants.
Purpose and activities: Giving mainly for oceanography; support primarily for the Mote Marine Laboratory; support also for social services.
Fields of interest: Environment; Human services; Marine science; Aging.
Types of support: General/operating support, research.
Limitations: Applications not accepted. Giving primarily in FL. No grants to individuals.
Publications: Annual report.
Application information: Contributes only to pre-selected organizations.
Officers: William R. Mote, Pres.; Jaqulin Prindle, Secy.
Number of staff: 1 part-time support.
EIN: 136117615

221
NationsBank Community Foundation
(Formerly NCNB Community Foundation)
c/o NationsBank of Florida, N.A.
2470 Ringling Blvd.
Sarasota 34237-7243
Contact: Stephen J. Smith, V.P. and Trust Officer, NationsBank of Florida, N.A.

Established in 1961 in FL as the Sarasota Bank and Trust Company Community Foundation.
Donor(s): Eileen Kroeger, Julius Brandenburg.‡

Financial data (yr. ended 12/31/94): Assets, $4,359,124 (M); expenditures, $456,410; qualifying distributions, $394,506, including $394,506 for 37 grants (high: $50,000; low: $100; average: $100-$30,000) and $117,165 for 4 program-related investments.
Fields of interest: Film/video; Visual arts; Museums; Performing arts; Dance; Theater; Humanities; Historic preservation/historical societies; Arts/cultural programs; Education, fund raising; Early childhood education; Child development, education; Elementary school/education; Secondary school/education; Vocational education; Higher education; Adult education—literacy & basic skills; Reading; Education; Natural resource conservation & protection; Environment; Family planning; Health care; Mental health/crisis services; Health associations; AIDS; Biomedicine; Medical research; AIDS research; Delinquency prevention/services; Recreation; Human services; Children & youth, services; Child development, services; Family services; Hospices; Aging, centers & services; Women, centers & services; Minorities/immigrants, centers & services; Homeless, human services; Urban/community development; Community development; Marine science; Chemistry; Computer science; Biological sciences; Government/public administration; Religion; Minorities; Disabled; Aging; Women; Economically disadvantaged; Homeless.
Types of support: Capital campaigns, building/renovation, equipment, program development, publication, seed money, matching funds.
Limitations: Giving limited to Sarasota County, FL, and surrounding counties. No grants to individuals, or for endowments or general operating support.
Publications: Application guidelines.
Application information: Application form required.
Initial approach: Proposal
Copies of proposal: 10
Deadline(s): May 1 and Nov. 1
Board meeting date(s): End of June and Nov.
Final notification: July 1 and Jan. 1
Trustee: NationsBank of Florida, N.A.
Number of staff: None.
EIN: 596142753
Grants for Aging:
Pines of Sarasota, Saraso'a, FL, $15,000. 94.

222
Samuel E. & Julienne M. Newey Family Foundation, Inc.
720 Oaks Field Rd.
Jacksonville 32211

Established in 1985 in FL.
Donor(s): Samuel E. Newey.
Financial data (yr. ended 08/31/94): Assets, $29,516 (M); expenditures, $4,871; qualifying distributions, $4,325, including $4,000 for grants.
Fields of interest: Aging, centers & services; Religion; Aging.
Limitations: Applications not accepted. Giving primarily in Jacksonville, FL, and Englewood, NJ. No grants to individuals.
Application information: Contributes only to pre-selected organizations.
Officers and Trustees:* Samuel E. Newey,* Pres.; Julienne M. Newey,* Secy.-Treas.; Pamela J. Newey.
EIN: 592612332

223
The Dr. P. Phillips Foundation
60 West Robinson St.
P.O. Box 3753
Orlando 32802 (407) 422-6105
Contact: J.A. Hinson, Pres. or Ann F. Manley, Ed.D., Exec. Dir.

Incorporated in 1953 in FL.
Donor(s): Della Phillips,‡ Howard Phillips,‡ Dr. Phillips, Inc.
Financial data (yr. ended 05/31/95): Assets, $28,694,763 (M); gifts received, $3,193; expenditures, $1,227,642; qualifying distributions, $1,266,989, including $1,129,266 for 69 grants (high: $500,900; low: $250), $56,784 for 1 foundation-administered program and $55,547 for 3 program-related investments.
Purpose and activities: Emphasis on education, child development and welfare, youth, the elderly, and community development, including arts and culture, museums, recreation, and social and family services.
Fields of interest: Arts/cultural programs; Child development, education; Education; Human services; Children & youth, services; Youth, services; Child development, services; Family services; Aging, centers & services; Community development; Aging.
Types of support: Capital campaigns, building/renovation, equipment, program development, program-related investments/loans, matching funds.
Limitations: Giving generally limited to Orange County, FL. No grants to individuals, or for endowment funds.
Publications: Application guidelines.
Application information: Application form not required.
Initial approach: Letter (no more than 3 pages)
Copies of proposal: 1
Deadline(s): None
Board meeting date(s): Semiannually
Final notification: Varies
Officers and Directors:* J.A. Hinson,* Chair. and Pres.; R.A. Simon,* V.P.; E.F. Furey, Secy.-Treas.; Ann F. Manley, Ed.D., Exec. Dir.
Number of staff: 1 full-time professional.
EIN: 596135403

224
The Purcell Family Foundation, Inc.
c/o Grenadier Assocs., Ltd.
1155 U.S. 1, Rm. 310
Juno Beach 33408

Established in 1992 in FL and DE.
Donor(s): John R. Purcell, Sr., Sheryl I. Purcell.
Financial data (yr. ended 12/31/93): Assets, $2,383,993 (M); gifts received, $182,500; expenditures, $45,318; qualifying distributions, $14,083, including $10,000 for 2 grants of $5,000 each.
Fields of interest: Medical research; Aging.
Limitations: Applications not accepted. No grants to individuals.
Application information: Contributes only to pre-selected organizations.
Officers: John R. Purcell, Sr., Chair.; Sheryl I. Purcell, Secy.
EIN: 161425579

225
William G. Selby and Marie Selby Foundation
1800 Second St., Suite 905
Sarasota 34236 (941) 957-0442
Contact: Robert E. Perkins, Exec. Dir.

Trust established in 1955 in FL.
Donor(s): William G. Selby,‡ Marie Selby.‡
Financial data (yr. ended 05/31/95): Assets, $59,026,157 (M); expenditures, $3,190,039; qualifying distributions, $2,957,483, including $2,754,059 for 79 grants (high: $365,500; low: $800).
Purpose and activities: Emphasis on scholarships and capital grants for giving directly to Florida colleges and universities; local giving also for the aged, hospitals, social service and youth agencies, and cultural programs.
Fields of interest: Visual arts; Performing arts; Arts/cultural programs; Child development, education; Elementary school/education; Secondary school/education; Higher education; Education; Housing/shelter, development; Human services; Youth, services; Child development, services; Aging, centers & services; Community development; Aging; General charitable giving.
Types of support: Capital campaigns, building/renovation, equipment, land acquisition, scholarship funds, scholarships—to individuals, matching funds.
Limitations: Giving limited to Sarasota, Manatee, Charlotte, and DeSoto counties, FL. No support for grantmaking foundations or for non 501(c)(3) organizations. No grants to individuals (except for the Direct Scholarship Program), or for general purposes, continuing support, annual campaigns, deficit financing, seed money, emergency funds, operating budgets, endowment funds, special projects, surveys, program advertising, research, graduate study, publications, seminars, workshops, or conferences; no loans.
Publications: Informational brochure, program policy statement, application guidelines.
Application information: Application form required.
Initial approach: Letter
Copies of proposal: 3
Deadline(s): Aug. 1 and Feb. 1
Board meeting date(s): Apr. and Oct.
Final notification: 2 to 6 months
Trustee: First Union National Bank of Florida.
Administrative Committee: Charles E. Stottlemyer, Chair.; Robert E. Perkins, Exec. Dir.; John B. Davidson, Wendel Kent, Sid Schwalbe, Neil Scott, Susan Scott.
Number of staff: 1 full-time professional; 2 full-time support.
EIN: 596121242
Grants for Aging:
Jefferson Center, Sarasota, FL, $19,600. 95.

226
Ida M. Stevens Foundation, Inc.

4595 Lexington Ave., No. 100
Jacksonville 32210-2058 (904) 396-5831
Contact: Ben W. Hightower, Trustee

Established in 1967 in FL.
Donor(s): Virgil A. Stevens.‡
Foundation type: Operating
Financial data (yr. ended 12/31/94): Assets, $14,811,846 (M); expenditures, $1,097,318; qualifying distributions, $819,392, including $507,764 for 37 grants (high: $76,471; low: $300) and $244,755 for 3 foundation-administered programs.
Purpose and activities: A private operating foundation; giving for social services, rent subsidy, and health programs benefiting the elderly.
Fields of interest: Health care; Health organizations; Housing/shelter, development; Aging, centers & services; Aging.
Types of support: General/operating support, land acquisition, conferences/seminars, technical assistance, program-related investments/loans.
Limitations: Giving limited to Jacksonville, FL.
Publications: 990-PF, financial statement.
Application information: Application form required.
Initial approach: Proposal
Copies of proposal: 1
Deadline(s): None
Trustees: G.L. Garnett Ashby, Ben W. Hightower, David Lemmel, Douglas J. Milne.
Number of staff: 2 full-time support; 2 part-time support.
EIN: 591746148

227
Carl S. Swisher Foundation, Inc.

P.O. Box 14790
Jacksonville 32238-1790
Contact: E.A. Middlebrooks, Jr., Secy.-Treas.

Incorporated in 1949 in FL.
Donor(s): Carl S. Swisher.‡
Financial data (yr. ended 12/31/94): Assets, $6,687,015 (M); expenditures, $293,708; qualifying distributions, $270,876, including $258,500 for 46 grants (high: $50,000; low: $500; average: $300-$50,000).
Purpose and activities: Support for higher education; grants also for youth agencies, hospitals, and social services.
Fields of interest: Arts/cultural programs; Higher education; Adult/continuing education; Education; Hospitals (general); Human services; Children & youth, services; Aging, centers & services; Federated giving programs; Minorities; Aging.
Types of support: General/operating support, scholarship funds, matching funds.
Limitations: Giving primarily in the Jacksonville, FL, area. No grants to individuals; no loans.
Application information: Application form not required.
Initial approach: Letter
Copies of proposal: 1
Deadline(s): None
Board meeting date(s): Usually quarterly
Officers and Trustees:* George S. Coulter,* Pres.; Kenneth G. Anderson,* V.P.; Harold W. Smith,* V.P.; E.A. Middlebrooks, Jr.,* Secy.-Treas.
Number of staff: 1 part-time professional.
EIN: 590998262

228
The Thoresen Foundation

2300 West Bay Dr.
Largo 34640
Contact: George V. Berger, Trustee

Established in 1952 in IL.
Donor(s): William E. Thoresen,‡ Catherine E. Thoresen.‡
Financial data (yr. ended 02/28/94): Assets, $28,151,457 (M); gifts received, $1,816; expenditures, $2,356,471; qualifying distributions, $2,000,160, including $2,000,000 for grants.
Purpose and activities: Giving primarily to a women's college; support also for the opera and fine arts.
Fields of interest: Visual arts; Museums; Performing arts; Music; Higher education; Dental school/education; Medical school/education; Nursing school/education; Education; Domestic violence prevention; Civil rights, immigrants; Civil rights, minorities; Civil rights, disabled; Civil rights, women; Civil rights, aging; Civil rights, gays/lesbians; Asians/Pacific Islanders; African Americans; Latinos; Native Americans; Disabled; Aging; People with AIDS (PWAs); Gays/lesbians; Immigrants/refugees; Economically disadvantaged; Homeless.
Limitations: Giving primarily in VA, FL, and IL. No grants to individuals, or for scholarships.
Application information:
Initial approach: Letter
Deadline(s): None
Board meeting date(s): As required
Trustees: George V. Berger, Katherine Culver, Paul V. O'Connell, Michael Thoresen.
Number of staff: None.
EIN: 366102493

229
Vero Beach Foundation for the Elderly

c/o First Union National Bank of Florida
500 Beach Land Blvd.
Vero Beach 32963 (561) 770-0044
Contact: Richard L. Mead, Chair.
Application address: 2800 Indian River Blvd., Apt. U-2, Vero Beach, FL 32960

Established in 1967 in FL.
Donor(s): Myrtle Peebles.‡
Financial data (yr. ended 12/31/93): Assets, $1,236,823 (M); expenditures, $130,312; qualifying distributions, $98,421, including $96,944 for grants to individuals.
Purpose and activities: Provides relief assistance to indigent individuals for medical and convalescent care, as well as for food and general assistance. Recipients must be 65 or older and residents of the Vero Beach, FL, area.
Fields of interest: Aging, centers & services; Aging; Economically disadvantaged.
Types of support: Grants to individuals.
Limitations: Giving limited to residents of Vero Beach, FL.
Application information: Applicants must be at least 65 years of age; assistance payments may be made directly to recipient or to physicians and medical facilities. Application form required.
Initial approach: All applications must come through Indian River County Council on Aging
Deadline(s): None
Board meeting date(s): 1st Monday of each month
Officers and Directors:* Richard L. Mead, Chair.; Pat Tibbetts,* Secy.; Paul Johnson,* Treas.
Trustee: First Union National Bank of Florida.
Number of staff: None.
EIN: 596214870

230
Benjamin Volen Charitable Trust

c/o Northern Trust Bank of Florida, N.A.
700 Brickell Ave.
Miami 33131-2804

Established in 1988 in FL.
Donor(s): Benjamin Volen.
Financial data (yr. ended 12/31/94): Assets, $10,259,151 (M); expenditures, $598,570; qualifying distributions, $540,336, including $531,074 for 1 grant.
Purpose and activities: Giving primarily for the May Volen Senior Center.
Fields of interest: Aging, centers & services; Aging.
Types of support: General/operating support.
Limitations: Applications not accepted. Giving primarily in Boca Raton, FL. No grants to individuals.
Application information: Contributes only to pre-selected organizations.
Trustee: Northern Trust Bank of Florida, N.A.
Number of staff: None.
EIN: 656018806
Grants for Aging:
Mae Volen Senior Center, Boca Raton, FL, $531,074. 94.

231
The I. Waldbaum Family Foundation, Inc.

16519 Ironwood Dr.
Delray Beach 33445
Contact: Nancy Waldbaum
Application address: 225 West 83rd St., Suite 232, New York, NY 10024, Tel.: (212) 724-4148

Incorporated in 1961 in NY.
Donor(s): Bernice Waldbaum, Ira Waldbaum, Waldbaum, Inc.
Financial data (yr. ended 12/31/93): Assets, $10,362,336 (M); expenditures, $557,983; qualifying distributions, $419,318, including $411,475 for 78 grants (high: $175,000; low: $25).
Purpose and activities: Giving primarily to Jewish organizations, including welfare funds, religious schools, and temple support, and to cultural programs and hospitals.
Fields of interest: Arts/cultural programs; Elementary/secondary education; Child development, education; Education; Hospitals (general); Human services; Child development,

services; Aging, centers & services; Community development; Jewish federated giving programs; Jewish agencies & temples; Religion; Aging.
Types of support: Building/renovation, seed money.
Limitations: Giving primarily in the metropolitan New York, NY, area.
Application information:
Initial approach: Proposal
Officers: Ira Waldbaum, Pres.; Bernice Waldbaum, Treas.
Directors: Randie Malinsky, Julia Waldbaum.
Number of staff: 1 full-time professional.
EIN: 136145916

232
Wilson-Wood Foundation, Inc.
(Formerly Hugh & Mary Wilson Foundation, Inc.)
7188 Beneva Rd.
Sarasota 34238 (941) 921-2856
Contact: John R. Wood II, Dir., or Susan Wood, Treas. and Assoc. Dir.

Established in 1983 in FL.
Donor(s): Hugh H. Wilson,‡ Mary P. Wilson.‡
Financial data (yr. ended 12/31/95): Assets, $6,625,652 (M); expenditures, $357,912; qualifying distributions, $290,776, including $244,899 for 20 grants (high: $30,000; low: $1,400; average: $28,600).
Fields of interest: Adult education—literacy & basic skills; Reading; Education; Health care; Nutrition; Housing/shelter, development; Human services; Children & youth, services; Youth, services; Aging, centers & services; Women, centers & services; Minorities/immigrants, centers & services; Disabled; Aging; Women; Economically disadvantaged; General charitable giving.
Types of support: General/operating support, capital campaigns, building/renovation, equipment.
Limitations: Giving limited to the Manatee-Sarasota, FL, area. No support for foreign organizations or private foundations. No grants to individuals, or for endowment funds, deficit financing, travel projects, research, fundraising costs, or multi-year projects.
Publications: Annual report (including application guidelines).
Application information: The foundation no longer funds awards or prizes to individuals. Application form not required.
Initial approach: Letter of inquiry
Copies of proposal: 1
Deadline(s): Sept. 1; initial letter of inquiry must be received by June 1
Board meeting date(s): Mar., June, and Oct.
Final notification: Oct.
Officers and Directors:* John R. Wood,* Pres.; George Fraley,* V.P.; Harry Klinger,* V.P.; Sadie L. Wood,* Secy.; Susan Wood,* Treas.; John R. Wood II.
Number of staff: 2 part-time professional.
EIN: 592243926

GEORGIA

233
Asbury-Warren Foundation
c/o SunTrust Bank, Atlanta
P.O. Box 4655
Atlanta 30302-4655 (404) 588-8449
Contact: Dale Welch, Advisory Committee Member

Donor(s): Josephine W. Asbury.
Financial data (yr. ended 09/30/94): Assets, $555,046 (M); expenditures, $33,445; qualifying distributions, $29,495, including $26,600 for grants.
Fields of interest: Higher education; Aging, centers & services; Protestant agencies & churches; Aging.
Types of support: General/operating support.
Limitations: Giving primarily in KY.
Application information:
Initial approach: Letter or proposal
Deadline(s): None
Trustee: SunTrust Bank, Atlanta.
Advisory Committee: Edward P. Gould, Jesse C. Hall, Dale Welch.
EIN: 581378820

234
Beloco Foundation, Inc.
P.O. Box 140
Columbus 31902 (706) 571-6040
Contact: Lovick P. Corn, Pres.

Established in 1967 in GA.
Donor(s): Lovick P. Corn, Elizabeth T. Corn.
Financial data (yr. ended 06/30/94): Assets, $3,791,261 (M); gifts received, $545,030; expenditures, $157,833; qualifying distributions, $149,883, including $149,500 for 15 grants (high: $50,000; low: $500).
Fields of interest: Arts/cultural programs; Higher education; Education; Nursing home/convalescent facility.
Types of support: General/operating support, continuing support, capital campaigns.
Limitations: Giving primarily in GA.
Application information:
Initial approach: Letter
Deadline(s): None
Officers and Trustees:* Lovick P. Corn,* Pres.; Elizabeth C. Ogie,* V.P.; Elizabeth T. Corn, Secy.; Polly C. Miller, Treas.
EIN: 586065378
Grants for Aging:
Methodist Home for the Aging of South Georgia, Americus, GA, $25,000. 94.

235
Callaway Foundation, Inc.
209 Broome St.
P.O. Box 790
La Grange 30241 (706) 884-7348
Contact: J.T. Gresham, Pres.

Incorporated in 1943 in GA.
Donor(s): Textile Benefit Assn., Callaway Mills, Callaway Institute, Inc.
Financial data (yr. ended 09/30/95): Assets, $167,871,297 (M); expenditures, $7,711,571; qualifying distributions, $7,197,834, including $5,809,668 for 70 grants (high: $1,135,249; low: $175; average: $1,000-$100,000) and $1,092,062 for 5 in-kind gifts.
Purpose and activities: Giving for elementary, higher, and secondary education, including libraries and buildings, and equipment; health and hospitals; community funds; care for the aged; community development; historic preservation; and church support.
Fields of interest: Historic preservation/historical societies; Elementary school/education; Secondary school/education; Higher education; Libraries/library science; Education; Hospitals (general); Health care; Health organizations; Aging, centers & services; Community development; Christian agencies & churches; Aging; General charitable giving.
Types of support: General/operating support, continuing support, annual campaigns, capital campaigns, building/renovation, equipment, land acquisition, matching funds.
Limitations: Giving primarily in GA, with emphasis on the City of LaGrange and Troup County. No grants to individuals, or for endowment funds, deficit financing, scholarships, or fellowships; no loans.
Publications: Annual report (including application guidelines).
Application information: Application form not required.
Initial approach: Letter
Copies of proposal: 1
Deadline(s): End of month preceding board meetings
Board meeting date(s): Jan., Apr., July, and Oct.
Final notification: 2 months
Officers and Trustees:* J.T. Gresham, Pres., Treas., and General Mgr.; Charles D. Hudson,* V.P.; C.L. Pitts, Secy.; Mark Clayton Callaway, Charles D. Hudson, Jr., James R. Lewis, Fred L. Turner.
Number of staff: None.
EIN: 580566147

236
The Conboy Foundation
1100 Peachtree St. N.E., Suite 2050
Atlanta 30309-4520

Established in 1987 in GA.
Donor(s): James J. Conboy, Lynne D. Conboy.
Financial data (yr. ended 12/31/94): Assets, $1,345,340 (M); expenditures, $90,996; qualifying distributions, $80,000, including $80,000 for 12 grants (high: $13,000; low: $1,000).
Fields of interest: Performing arts; Housing/shelter, development; Human services; Aging, centers & services; Public affairs; Christian agencies & churches.
Limitations: Applications not accepted. Giving primarily in GA. No grants to individuals.
Application information: Contributes only to pre-selected organizations.
Trustees: Opal Duke Abbink, James J. Conboy, Lynne D. Conboy.
EIN: 581742620
Grants for Aging:

Senior Citizens Services of Metropolitan Atlanta, Atlanta, GA, $10,000. For Meals on Wheels program. 94.

237
The Florence C. and Harry L. English Memorial Fund

c/o SunTrust Bank, Atlanta
P.O. Box 4418, MC 041
Atlanta 30302-4418 (404) 588-8246
Contact: William R. Bowdoin, Jr., 1st. V.P.
FAX: (404) 230-5550

Established in 1964 in GA.
Donor(s): Florence Cruft English.‡
Financial data (yr. ended 12/31/94): Assets, $10,809,874 (M); expenditures, $551,195; qualifying distributions, $513,945, including $513,945 for grants (average: $3,000-$5,000).
Purpose and activities: Grants only for education, health, general welfare, and culture, with emphasis on assisting the aged and chronically ill, the blind, and those persons generally designated as the "underprivileged."
Fields of interest: Arts/cultural programs; Higher education; Education; Health care; Health associations; Human services; Aging, centers & services; Homeless, human services; Community development; Disabled; Aging; Economically disadvantaged.
Types of support: Capital campaigns, building/renovation, equipment, program development.
Limitations: Giving limited to the metropolitan Atlanta, GA, area. No support for veterans' organizations or organizations which have not been operating without a deficit for at least a year. No grants to individuals; no loans.
Publications: Program policy statement, application guidelines.
Application information: Application form required.
Initial approach: Letter
Copies of proposal: 1
Deadline(s): Mar. 1, June 1, Sept. 1, and Dec. 1
Board meeting date(s): Jan., Apr., July, and Oct.
Distribution Committee: Robert R. Long, Chair.; William R. Bowdoin, Jr., 1st. V.P.; L.P. Humann, John W. Spiegel, James B. Williams, E. Jenner Wood III.
Trustee: SunTrust Bank, Atlanta.
Number of staff: 1 full-time professional; 1 full-time support.
EIN: 586045781

238
S. W. Frankenthal Memorial Foundation, Inc.

(Formerly Frankenthal Family Foundation, Inc.)
120 Blenheim Place
Dunwoody 30350

Incorporated in 1967 in WI.
Donor(s): Members of the Frankenthal family.
Financial data (yr. ended 08/31/92): Assets, $853,331 (M); expenditures, $50,200; qualifying distributions, $27,310, including $27,310 for 6 grants (high: $26,000; low: $50).
Purpose and activities: Giving for hospitals, higher education, and Jewish welfare funds; some support for the aged, community funds, and youth agencies.
Fields of interest: Higher education; Hospitals (general); Human services; Youth, services; Aging, centers & services; Federated giving programs; Jewish federated giving programs; Aging.
Types of support: General/operating support, building/renovation, equipment, land acquisition, endowment funds, professorships, scholarship funds, matching funds.
Limitations: Applications not accepted. Giving primarily in WI and KY. No grants to individuals; no loans.
Application information: Contributes only to pre-selected organizations.
Board meeting date(s): Aug.
Officers and Directors:* Betty F. Behr,* Pres.; Kenneth B. Behr,* V.P.; Isle L. Meyer,* Secy.
Number of staff: 2
EIN: 396106541

239
Georgia Power Company Corporate Giving Program

333 Piedmont Ave., 20th Fl.
Atlanta 30302 (404) 526-6784
Contact: Judy M. Anderson, V.P. and Corp. Secy.

Established in 1930 in GA.
Financial data (yr. ended 12/31/92): Total giving, $2,402,000, including $2,300,000 for 1,052 grants (high: $1,200,000; low: $25) and $102,000 for 663 employee matching gifts.
Fields of interest: Journalism & publishing; Visual arts; Performing arts; Humanities; Historic preservation/historical societies; Arts/cultural programs; Education, association; Education, research; Education, fund raising; Early childhood education; Elementary school/education; Higher education; Business school/education; Education; Natural resource conservation & protection; Hospitals (general); Medical care, rehabilitation; Health care; Substance abuse, services; Health associations; Heart/circulatory disease; AIDS; Heart/circulatory research; AIDS research; Food services; Housing/shelter, development; Human services; Children & youth, services; Family services; Hospices; Aging, centers & services; Homeless, human services; International affairs, goodwill promotion; International relief; Human rights (international); Race/intergroup relations; Civil rights; Federated giving programs; Government/public administration; Minorities; Disabled; Aging; Economically disadvantaged; Homeless; Latin America.
Types of support: General/operating support, continuing support, annual campaigns, capital campaigns, building/renovation, endowment funds, debt reduction, emergency funds, program development, conferences/seminars, professorships, seed money, scholarship funds, research, technical assistance, employee volunteer services, loaned talent, use of facilities, employee matching gifts, employee-related scholarships, donated equipment, donated products.
Limitations: Giving primarily in GA.
Publications: Corporate report.
Application information: Corporate Secretary's office handles giving; grants are only for 501(c)(3) organizations. Application form not required.
Initial approach: Letter to headquarters
Copies of proposal: 1
Deadline(s): None
Board meeting date(s): 1st week of each month
Final notification: After board review
Administrator: Michael E. Gregory, Coord., Philanthropy.
Number of staff: 2 part-time professional; 1 part-time support.

240
Georgia Power Foundation, Inc.

333 Piedmont Ave., Bin 10200
Atlanta 30308-3374 (404) 526-6784
Contact: Ms. Judy M. Anderson, Exec. Dir.
FAX: (404) 526-2945

Established in 1986 in GA.
Donor(s): Georgia Power Co.
Foundation type: Company-sponsored
Financial data (yr. ended 12/31/95): Assets, $71,598,886 (M); expenditures, $3,475,872; qualifying distributions, $3,475,872, including $3,467,331 for 324 grants (high: $338,334; low: $250).
Purpose and activities: Primary areas of interest include social and family services, youth, civic affairs and community development, the arts, health, and education. Support also for the aged, AIDS, cancer, race relations, the homeless, rehabilitation, human rights, leadership development, legal services, libraries, medical research, museums, performing arts, theater, historic preservation, fine arts, and environmental conservation.
Fields of interest: Journalism & publishing; Museums; Theater; Music; History & archaeology; Arts/cultural programs; Education, research; Early childhood education; Elementary school/education; Higher education; Business school/education; Law school/education; Medical school/education; Engineering school/education; Libraries/library science; Education; Natural resource conservation & protection; Environment; Wildlife preservation & protection; Hospitals (general); Medical care, rehabilitation; Health care; Substance abuse, services; Cancer; Heart/circulatory disease; Health organizations; Medical research; Cancer research; Heart/circulatory research; Legal services; Crime/law enforcement; Housing/shelter, development; Youth development, services; Human services; Children & youth, services; Youth, services; Family services; Aging, centers & services; Women, centers & services; Minorities/immigrants, centers & services; Homeless, human services; Human rights (international); Civil rights; Community development; Engineering & technology; Engineering; Science; Government/public administration; Leadership development; Jewish agencies & temples; Minorities; African Americans; Latinos; Disabled; Aging; Women; People with AIDS (PWAs); Economically disadvantaged; Homeless.
Types of support: General/operating support, annual campaigns, capital campaigns, building/renovation, equipment, endowment funds, debt reduction, program development,

conferences/seminars, seed money, scholarship funds, research.
Limitations: Giving primarily in GA. No support for private foundations. No grants to individuals.
Publications: Informational brochure (including application guidelines), 990-PF.
Application information: Application form not required.
Initial approach: Letter with proposal
Copies of proposal: 1
Deadline(s): None
Board meeting date(s): Quarterly
Final notification: After board review
Officers and Directors:* Warren Y. Jobe,* Pres.; Judy M. Anderson,* Secy. and Exec. Dir.; Charles O. Rawlins,* Treas.; William C. Archer III, R.L. Boyer, Wayne T. Dahlke, James K. Davis, Robert H. Haubein, Gene R. Hodges, Jeffrey L. Wallace.
Number of staff: None.
EIN: 581709417

241
Gwinnett Foundation, Inc.
1770 Indian Trail Rd., Suite 160
Norcross 30093 (770) 564-3451
Contact: Joseph J. Estafen, Exec. Dir.

Incorporated in 1985 in GA.
Foundation type: Community
Financial data (yr. ended 12/31/95): Assets, $5,137,519 (M); gifts received, $762,721; expenditures, $547,508, including $366,100 for 59 grants (high: $100,000; low: $250; average: $2,500-$5,000) and $20,000 for 2 in-kind gifts.
Fields of interest: Performing arts; Arts/cultural programs; Early childhood education; Child development, education; Elementary school/education; Adult/continuing education; Adult education—literacy & basic skills; Reading; Education; Health care; Health organizations; Food services; Housing/shelter, development; Youth development, services; Human services; Children & youth, services; Youth, services; Child development, services; Family services; Hospices; Aging, centers & services; Homeless, human services; Community development; Government/public administration; Leadership development; Minorities; Disabled; Aging; Economically disadvantaged; Homeless; General charitable giving.
Types of support: Building/renovation, program development, seed money, matching funds.
Limitations: Giving primarily in Gwinnett County, GA. No support for religious organizations for religious purposes, or commonly accepted community services. No grants to individuals, or for endowment support, debt reduction, fundraising or annual campaigns, membership contributions, research, or travel for individuals or groups, or ongoing operating support.
Publications: Annual report (including application guidelines), 990-PF, grants list, newsletter.
Application information:
Initial approach: Telephone
Copies of proposal: 10
Deadline(s): Apr. 15 and Sept. 15
Board meeting date(s): 5 times annually
Final notification: July and Dec.
Officers and Directors:* Thomas D. Jones,* Pres.; Forrest Robinson,* V.P.; Carole E. Kendall, Secy.; Jack Sawyer,* Treas.; Beauty Baldwin, Kenneth Brown, Patricia M. Brown, J.D. Caswell, James H. Cowart, Paul A. Duke, Judy Fowler, Julie Keeton, Jeffry Manry, Wayne H. Mason, William E. McLendon, James F. Pack, Louise Radloff, William R. Short, T. Michael Tennant, Jones Webb, Thomas W. Wheeler, Jr., Glenn White.
Trustees: NationsBank of Georgia, N.A., SunTrust Bank, Atlanta.
Number of staff: 1 full-time professional; 1 full-time support.
EIN: 581557995

242
The Irving Foundation, Inc.
1330 Spartan Ln.
Athens 30606-5324
Contact: Joe Irving, Pres.

Established in 1991 in GA.
Donor(s): Joe D. Irving.
Financial data (yr. ended 12/31/94): Assets, $15,497 (M); gifts received, $47,400; expenditures, $74,888; qualifying distributions, $74,888, including $74,200 for 16 grants (high: $43,000; low: $200).
Fields of interest: Health associations; Aging, centers & services; Aging.
Limitations: Applications not accepted. Giving primarily in GA. No grants to individuals.
Application information: Contributes only to pre-selected organizations.
Officers and Directors:* Joe D. Irving,* Pres. and Treas.; Tony G. Mills,* Secy.; James L. Newland.
EIN: 581943208
Grants for Aging:
Athens Community Council on Aging, Athens, GA, $43,000. 94.

243
Jack M. Jones Foundation
P.O. Box 1955
Thomasville 31799-1955 (912) 226-8354
Contact: Jack M. Jones, Pres.

Financial data (yr. ended 06/30/93): Assets, $671,382 (M); gifts received, $126,470; expenditures, $39,507; qualifying distributions, $39,507, including $34,150 for grants.
Fields of interest: Theological school/education; Nursing home/convalescent facility.
Types of support: Scholarship funds.
Limitations: No grants to individuals.
Application information:
Deadline(s): None
Officers: Jack M. Jones, Pres.; Phyllis J. Jones, Secy.-Treas.
Director: Patricia J. Jackson.
EIN: 581769636

244
The James R. Kuse Foundation
P.O. Box 7172
Atlanta 30357-0172
Contact: Carolyn KoKenge, Dir.

Established in 1989 in GA.
Donor(s): James R. Kuse.
Financial data (yr. ended 12/31/95): Assets, $6,138,236 (M); expenditures, $341,563; qualifying distributions, $306,500, including $306,500 for 35 grants (high: $25,000; low: $1,000; average: $1,000-$5,000).
Purpose and activities: Support for charities primarily in the metropolitan Atlanta, GA, area with special emphasis on programs for children and the elderly.
Fields of interest: Children & youth, services; Aging.
Types of support: General/operating support, building/renovation, annual campaigns, capital campaigns, equipment, endowment funds.
Limitations: Giving primarily in the metropolitan Atlanta, GA, area. No support for private foundations. No grants to individuals.
Publications: Application guidelines.
Application information: Application form not required.
Initial approach: Letter or personal contact
Copies of proposal: 1
Deadline(s): None
Board meeting date(s): Quarterly
Officers and Trustees:* James R. Kuse,* Pres.; Shirley R. Kuse,* Secy.; Carol Ehlen, Lynn Ehret, Michael Kuse.
Number of staff: 1 part-time professional.
EIN: 581845413

245
Mattie H. Marshall Foundation
c/o SunTrust Bank, Atlanta
P.O. Box 4655
Atlanta 30302 (404) 588-8197
Contact: Mr. Kelly McCutchen, Trust Officer, SunTrust Bank, Atlanta

Established in 1963 in GA.
Financial data (yr. ended 12/31/93): Assets, $4,017,148 (M); expenditures, $158,747; qualifying distributions, $133,878, including $120,000 for 20 grants (high: $42,000; low: $1,000).
Purpose and activities: Giving primarily for higher education; support also for churches, hospitals, a clinic, a humane society, and a home for the aged.
Fields of interest: Higher education; Animal welfare; Hospitals (general); Health associations; Aging, centers & services; Christian agencies & churches; Aging.
Types of support: General/operating support, annual campaigns, capital campaigns, building/renovation, endowment funds, program development.
Limitations: Giving limited to GA, with emphasis on Americus and southern GA.
Publications: Application guidelines.
Application information: Application form not required.
Initial approach: Letter
Copies of proposal: 1
Deadline(s): None

Board meeting date(s): Dec.
Officer: Thomas O. Marshall, Chair. and Secy.
Director: Martha M. Dykes.
Number of staff: None.
EIN: 586042019

246
Harriet McDaniel Marshall Trust in Memory of Sanders McDaniel

c/o SunTrust Bank, Atlanta,
Community Affairs Fdn. Prog.
P.O. Box 4418, MC 041
Atlanta 30302 (404) 588-8246
Contact: William R. Bowdoin, Jr., 1st V.P., SunTrust Bank, Atlanta

Trust established in 1962 in GA.
Donor(s): Harriet McDaniel Marshall.‡
Financial data (yr. ended 11/30/94): Assets, \$5,457,342 (M); expenditures, \$296,913; qualifying distributions, \$278,711, including \$278,711 for grants (average: \$3,000-\$5,000).
Purpose and activities: Giving primarily for higher education and building funds for educational institutions, health, and the handicapped; support also for welfare, including organizations assisting the disadvantaged, the homeless, and the elderly, community funds and development, and arts and culture.
Fields of interest: Arts/cultural programs; Higher education; Health care; Health associations; Human services; Aging, centers & services; Homeless, human services; Community development; Federated giving programs; Disabled; Aging; Economically disadvantaged.
Types of support: Capital campaigns, building/renovation, equipment, program development.
Limitations: Giving primarily in the metropolitan Atlanta, GA, area. No grants to individuals, or for scholarships or fellowships; no loans.
Publications: Application guidelines, program policy statement.
Application information: Application form required.
Initial approach: Letter
Copies of proposal: 1
Deadline(s): Mar. 1, June 1, Sept. 1, and Dec. 1
Board meeting date(s): Jan., Apr., July, and Oct.
Distribution Committee: Robert R. Long, Chair.; William R. Bowdoin, Jr., Secy.; L.P. Hamann, John W. Spiegel, James B. Williams, E. Jenner Wood III.
Trustee: SunTrust Bank, Atlanta.
Number of staff: 1 full-time professional; 1 full-time support.
EIN: 586089937

247
Moultrie Manufacturing Company Foundation

P.O. Box 1179
Moultrie 31776

Donor(s): Moultrie Manufacturing Co.
Foundation type: Company-sponsored
Financial data (yr. ended 05/31/92): Assets, \$51,802 (M); expenditures, \$4,305; qualifying distributions, \$3,581, including \$3,360 for 5 grants (high: \$2,100; low: \$100).
Fields of interest: Youth, services; Aging, centers & services; Government/public administration; Aging; General charitable giving.
Limitations: Applications not accepted. Giving limited to the Moultrie, GA, area. No grants to individuals.
Trustees: Anne F. Smith, Anne G. Smith, W.E. Smith, Sr., W.E. Smith, Jr., Moultrie National Bank.
EIN: 580057107

248
Oxford Industries Foundation, Inc.

222 Piedmont Ave., N.E.
Atlanta 30308-3391 (404) 659-2424
Contact: R. William Lee, Jr., Trustee

Established in 1975 in GA.
Foundation type: Company-sponsored
Financial data (yr. ended 12/31/93): Assets, \$901,274 (M); expenditures, \$120,439; qualifying distributions, \$119,921, including \$119,906 for 85 grants (high: \$12,750; low: \$15).
Fields of interest: Visual arts; Museums; Performing arts; Humanities; Arts/cultural programs; Child development, education; Higher education; Business school/education; Adult education—literacy & basic skills; Reading; Education; Animal welfare; Hospitals (general); Health care; Mental health/crisis services; Cancer; AIDS; Health organizations; Cancer research; AIDS research; Food services; Human services; Children & youth, services; Youth, services; Child development, services; Family services; Aging, centers & services; Women, centers & services; Homeless, human services; Human rights (international); Federated giving programs; Aging; Women; Economically disadvantaged; Homeless.
Types of support: General/operating support, continuing support, annual campaigns, capital campaigns, emergency funds, program development, employee matching gifts.
Limitations: No grants to individuals, or for advertising.
Publications: Program policy statement.
Application information: Application form not required.
Initial approach: Proposal
Copies of proposal: 2
Officers and Trustees:* J. Hicks Lanier,* Chair. and Pres.; David Ginn, Counsel; R. William Lee, Jr.
Number of staff: None.
EIN: 581209452

249
Patterson-Barclay Memorial Foundation, Inc.

6487 Peachtree Industrial Blvd., Suite A
Doraville 30360 (770) 396-8400
Contact: Mrs. Lee Barclay Patterson Allen, Pres.

Incorporated in 1953 in GA.
Donor(s): Frederick W. Patterson.‡
Financial data (yr. ended 12/31/95): Assets, \$9,115,409 (M); expenditures, \$450,887; qualifying distributions, \$427,500, including \$427,500 for 107 grants (high: \$15,000; low: \$1,000; average: \$1,000-\$5,000).
Purpose and activities: Giving for Christian organizations, hospitals, and higher, secondary, and other education; grants also for health, social service and youth agencies, arts and culture, and the environment.
Fields of interest: Museums; Performing arts; Theater; Arts/cultural programs; Education, association; Child development, education; Secondary school/education; Higher education; Natural resource conservation & protection; Environment; Wildlife preservation & protection; Hospitals (general); Medical care, rehabilitation; Health care; Substance abuse, services; Human services; Children & youth, services; Child development, services; Hospices; Aging, centers & services; Women, centers & services; Homeless, human services; Community development; Roman Catholic federated giving programs; Government/public administration; Christian agencies & churches; Religion; Aging; Women; Economically disadvantaged; Homeless.
Types of support: General/operating support, continuing support, annual campaigns, capital campaigns, building/renovation, endowment funds, scholarship funds, program-related investments/loans.
Limitations: Giving limited to the metropolitan Atlanta, GA, area. No grants to individuals.
Application information:
Board meeting date(s): 3rd Wednesday in May and Oct.
Officers and Trustees:* Mrs. Lee Barclay Patterson Allen,* Pres. and Treas.; Jack W. Allen,* V.P.; Hugh R. Powell, Jr., Secy.; Ross Arnold, Laurell Allen Rusow.
Number of staff: None.
EIN: 580904580

250
William I. H. and Lula E. Pitts Foundation

c/o SunTrust Bank, Atlanta
P.O. Box 4655
Atlanta 30302 (404) 588-8449
Contact: Clare Ranney, Secy.

Trust established in 1941 in GA.
Donor(s): William I.H. Pitts,‡ Margaret A. Pitts.
Financial data (yr. ended 12/31/94): Assets, \$39,877,070 (M); gifts received, \$30,000; expenditures, \$1,241,583; qualifying distributions, \$1,787,701, including \$1,139,392 for grants (average: \$5,000-\$47,000).
Purpose and activities: Giving exclusively to Methodist church-related institutions in GA; emphasis on higher education and care of the aged.
Fields of interest: Higher education; Human services; Aging, centers & services; Protestant federated giving programs; Protestant agencies & churches; Aging.
Types of support: General/operating support, continuing support, building/renovation.
Limitations: Giving limited to GA. No grants to individuals, or for endowment funds, research, scholarships, fellowships, or matching gifts; no loans.
Application information: Application form not required.

Initial approach: Letter
Copies of proposal: 1
Deadline(s): None
Board meeting date(s): Apr. and Nov.
Officers: Bishop William R. Cannon, Chair.; Clare Ranney, Secy.; John H. Boman, Jr., Mgr.; Carroll Payne Jones, Mgr.; Thomas O. Marshall, Mgr.; Walter Y. Murphy, Mgr.; Margaret A. Pitts, Mgr.; Robert M. Strickland, Mgr.; Kirk Treible, Mgr.
Trustee: SunTrust Bank, Atlanta.
Number of staff: None.
EIN: 586026047

251
The Rich Foundation, Inc.

10 Piedmont Ctr., Suite 802
Atlanta 30305 (404) 262-2266
Contact: Anne Poland Berg, Grant Consultant

Incorporated in 1942 in GA.
Donor(s): Rich's, Inc., and members of the Rich family.
Financial data (yr. ended 01/31/95): Assets, $27,698,768 (M); expenditures, $1,527,654; qualifying distributions, $1,430,528, including $1,369,500 for grants.
Purpose and activities: Giving primarily for the performing arts and other cultural programs, higher education, social services, including programs for the homeless and people with AIDS, youth agencies, and hospitals, including research in heart disease.
Fields of interest: Theater; Arts/cultural programs; Higher education; Education; Hospitals (general); Health care; Heart/circulatory research; Human services; Youth, services; Homeless, human services; Disabled; Aging; People with AIDS (PWAs); Economically disadvantaged; Homeless.
Types of support: General/operating support, continuing support, annual campaigns, capital campaigns, building/renovation, equipment, endowment funds, research, technical assistance.
Limitations: Giving limited to the Atlanta, GA, area. No grants to individuals, or for matching gifts; no loans.
Publications: Application guidelines.
Application information: Application form required.
Initial approach: Letter
Copies of proposal: 6
Deadline(s): Mar. 15, June 15, Sept. 15, and Dec. 15
Board meeting date(s): Feb., May, Aug., and Nov.
Final notification: 2 weeks
Officers and Trustees:* Joel Goldberg,* Pres.; Thomas J. Asher,* V.P.; David S. Baker, Joseph K. Heyman, Margaret S. Weiller.
Number of staff: None.
EIN: 586038037

252
Russell Charitable Trust

P.O. Box 1064
Decatur 30031 (404) 636-0367
Contact: Ernest J. Arnold, Trustee

Established in 1960 in ME.
Donor(s): H.M. Russell.
Financial data (yr. ended 07/31/94): Assets, $720,551 (M); expenditures, $143,741; qualifying distributions, $118,480, including $110,500 for 12 grants (high: $75,000; low: $500).
Fields of interest: Media/communications; Elementary/secondary education; Higher education; Health care; Health organizations; Youth, services; Aging, centers & services; Protestant agencies & churches; Religion; Aging.
Types of support: General/operating support, capital campaigns, endowment funds, seed money.
Limitations: Giving primarily in GA.
Application information:
Initial approach: Proposal
Deadline(s): None
Board meeting date(s): Quarterly
Final notification: Grants are made at the beginning of each calendar quarter
Trustees: Ernest J. Arnold, Frances P. Arnold, Judy A. Moore.
EIN: 016009882

253
Savannah Widows' Society

P.O. Box 30156
Savannah 31410 (912) 232-6312
Contact: Barbara Wall, Pres.

Foundation type: Operating
Financial data (yr. ended 08/31/92): Assets, $1,419,230 (M); expenditures, $96,966; qualifying distributions, $89,984, including $840 for 2 grants of $420 each and $63,974 for 80 grants to individuals (high: $7,350; low: $55).
Purpose and activities: A private operating foundation; giving primarily to single women, 55 or older; also provides aid to seriously disabled or handicapped persons, whose income from other sources is insufficient to provide their care in a reasonably comfortable manner.
Fields of interest: Aging, centers & services; Women, centers & services; Disabled; Aging; Women.
Types of support: Grants to individuals.
Limitations: Giving primarily in the Chatham County, GA, area.
Application information: Application form required.
Deadline(s): None
Officers and Board Members:* Barbara Wall,* Pres.; Ann Stubbs,* 1st V.P.; Marion Levy,* 2nd V.P.; Martha Peeples,* Treas.; Ellen R. Byck, Margaret Callaway, Frances Olsen, Peg Sterling, Becky Traxler, and 13 additional members.
EIN: 580603157

254
William F. Shallenberger Trust Fund

c/o Alston & Bird, One Atlantic Ctr.
1201 West Peachtree St., N.W., Suite 4200
Atlanta 30309-3424 (404) 881-7000
Contact: Benjamin T. White, Mgr.

Established in 1980 in GA.
Financial data (yr. ended 12/31/94): Assets, $5,392,192 (M); expenditures, $251,676; qualifying distributions, $244,523, including $240,000 for 18 grants (high: $35,000; low: $5,000; average: $1,000-$10,000).
Fields of interest: Hospitals (general); Health care; Health organizations; Human services; Aging, centers & services; Aging.
Limitations: Giving primarily in Atlanta, GA. No grants to individuals.
Application information:
Initial approach: Letter
Deadline(s): None
Officer: Benjamin T. White, Mgr.
Trustees: Mark P. Pentecost, Jr., M.D., Frank Wilson, M.D., Charles K. Wright, M.D.
Number of staff: None.
EIN: 581403009
Grants for Aging:
Senior Citizens Services of Metropolitan Atlanta, Atlanta, GA, $15,000. For Foster Grandparent program. 94.

255
Paul and Ferne Sticht Foundation

c/o Wachovia Bank of Georgia, N.A.
191 Peachtree St., N.E., MC GA705
Atlanta 30303
Contact: Kay McMaster

Established in 1986 in GA.
Donor(s): Ferne C. Sticht, J. Paul Sticht.
Financial data (yr. ended 12/31/95): Assets, $1,316,060 (M); expenditures, $75,763; qualifying distributions, $66,750, including $66,750 for 26 grants (high: $20,000; low: $150).
Fields of interest: Higher education; Natural resource conservation & protection; Aging, centers & services; Federated giving programs; Aging.
Limitations: Applications not accepted. Giving primarily in the eastern states. No grants to individuals.
Application information: Contributes only to pre-selected organizations. Unsolicited requests for funds not considered.
Trustees: David S. Sticht, Ferne C. Sticht, J. Paul Sticht, Mark D. Sticht.
Agent: Wachovia Bank of Georgia, N.A.
Number of staff: None.
EIN: 581704090

256
SunTrust Bank Atlanta Foundation

(Formerly Trust Company of Georgia Foundation)
c/o SunTrust Bank, Atlanta
P.O. Box 4418, MC 041
Atlanta 30302-4418 (404) 588-8246
Contact: William R. Bowdoin, Jr., 1st. V.P.
FAX: (404) 230-5550

Trust established in 1959 in GA.
Donor(s): SunTrust Bank, Atlanta.
Foundation type: Company-sponsored
Financial data (yr. ended 12/31/94): Assets, $15,307,985 (M); gifts received, $2,720,000; expenditures, $2,392,499; qualifying distributions, $2,293,351, including $2,224,156 for grants.
Purpose and activities: Emphasis on the fine arts and other cultural programs; health services, including mental health and programs for the handicapped; and education, including

secondary and higher educational institutions; support also for youth agencies, local community development and welfare programs, including a community fund.
Fields of interest: Visual arts; Performing arts; Arts/cultural programs; Education, fund raising; Higher education; Education; Health care; Mental health/crisis services; Human services; Youth, services; Aging, centers & services; Community development; Disabled; Aging; Economically disadvantaged; General charitable giving.
Types of support: Capital campaigns, building/renovation, equipment, program development, employee matching gifts.
Limitations: Giving primarily in metropolitan Atlanta, GA. No support for churches or political organizations. No grants to individuals, or for scholarships, fellowships, maintenance, or debt service; no loans.
Publications: Application guidelines, program policy statement.
Application information: Application form required.
Initial approach: Letter or telephone
Copies of proposal: 1
Deadline(s): 1st of month preceding month of board meeting (Mar. 1, June 1, Sept. 1, and Dec. 1)
Board meeting date(s): Jan., Apr., July, and Oct.
Final notification: By letter
Distribution Committee: Robert R. Long, Chair.; William R. Bowdoin, Jr., 1st V.P.; L. Phillip Humann, John W. Spiegel, James B. Williams.
Trustee: SunTrust Bank, Atlanta.
Number of staff: 1 full-time professional; 1 full-time support.
EIN: 586026063

257
The UPS Foundation

55 Glenlake Pkwy., N.E.
Atlanta 30328 (770) 828-6451
Contact: Gary Lee, Jr., Exec. Dir.
Additional tel.: (404) 828-6374; FAX: (404) 828-6451

Incorporated in 1951 in DE.
Donor(s): UPS, Inc.
Foundation type: Company-sponsored
Financial data (yr. ended 12/31/94): Assets, $69,333,180 (M); gifts received, $14,130,137; expenditures, $12,482,200; qualifying distributions, $13,359,754, including $12,319,906 for grants.
Purpose and activities: Support for philanthropic human welfare or education projects or organizations that are tax-exempt under 501(c)(3) and meet the guidelines of the foundation. Emphasis on programs for families and children in crisis, adult literacy, the distribution of food to hungry Americans, economic opportunity for minorities, programs for the handicapped, and support for higher education, including academic, public policy, and transportation/logistics research.
Fields of interest: Higher education; Adult/continuing education; Adult education—literacy & basic skills; Reading; AIDS; AIDS research; Food services; Human services; Children & youth, services; Youth, services; Aging, centers & services; Public policy, research; Government/public administration; Transportation; Minorities; Aging; Economically disadvantaged.
Types of support: Continuing support, equipment, program development, professorships, seed money, fellowships, internships, scholarship funds, research, employee matching gifts, employee-related scholarships, matching funds.
Limitations: Giving limited to the U.S. and Canada. No support for religious organizations or theological functions, or church-sponsored programs limited to church members. No grants to individuals (except for employee-related scholarships), or for building or endowment funds, operating funds, annual campaigns, emergency funds, deficit financing, land acquisition, or publications; no loans.
Publications: Informational brochure (including application guidelines).
Application information: Application form not required.
Initial approach: Letter (preferably no more than 2 pages), addressing programs, objectives, and cost
Copies of proposal: 1
Deadline(s): Submit proposal Jan. through Aug.
Board meeting date(s): Oct. and Nov.
Final notification: For local programs, Nov. 1; for national programs, Dec. 1
Officers and Trustees:* Kent C. Nelson,* Chair.; Calvin E. Tyler, Jr.,* Secy.; Robert Clanin, Treas.; Gary Lee, Jr., Exec. Dir.; Don Fisher, John J. Kelly, Bud Yard.
Number of staff: 5 full-time professional; 4 full-time support.
EIN: 136099176

258
Joseph B. Whitehead Foundation

50 Hurt Plaza, Suite 1200
Atlanta 30303 (404) 522-6755
Contact: Charles H. McTier, Pres.
FAX: (404) 522-7026

Incorporated in 1937 in GA.
Donor(s): Joseph B. Whitehead, Jr.‡
Financial data (yr. ended 12/31/95): Assets, $790,402,293 (M); expenditures, $26,815,169; qualifying distributions, $26,098,163, including $25,890,000 for 84 grants (high: $2,000,000; low: $15,000; average: $25,000-$750,000).
Purpose and activities: Principal giving interests are focused on the following program areas: human services, particularly for children and youth; elementary and secondary education; health care and education; economic development and civic affairs; literacy and vocational training; art and cultural activities; and conservation of natural resources and environmental protection. Preference is given to one-time capital projects of established private charitable organizations.
Fields of interest: Arts/cultural programs; Elementary/secondary education; Child development, education; Education; Environment; Health care; Health organizations; Children & youth, services; Youth, services; Child development, services; Aging, centers & services; Economic development; Government/public administration; Aging.
Types of support: Capital campaigns, building/renovation, equipment, land acquisition, program development, seed money.
Limitations: Giving limited to metropolitan Atlanta, GA. No grants to individuals, or for endowment funds, research, scholarships, fellowships, or matching gifts; generally no support for operating expenses; no loans.
Publications: Application guidelines, informational brochure (including application guidelines), program policy statement.
Application information: Application form not required.
Initial approach: Letter
Copies of proposal: 1
Deadline(s): 1st of Feb. and Sept.
Board meeting date(s): Apr. and Nov.
Final notification: Within 30 days of trustees meeting
Officers and Trustees:* Joseph W. Jones,* Chair.; James M. Sibley,* Vice-Chair.; Charles H. McTier, Pres.; P. Russell Hardin, V.P. and Secy.; J. Lee Tribble, Treas.; Roberto C. Goizueta.
Number of staff: 10 shared staff
EIN: 586001954
Grants for Aging:
Center for the Visually Impaired, Atlanta, GA, $140,000. For addition of staff members to serve visually-impaired senior citizens. 94.
Downtown Atlanta Senior Services, Atlanta, GA, $15,000. For second payment to provide expertise in board development and fundraising. 94.
Visiting Nurse Health System, Atlanta, GA, $1,500,000. Toward purchase of land at Lenox Park on which to build hospice facility. 94.
Visiting Nurse Health System, Atlanta, GA, $500,000. For challenge grant for construction of hospice facility. 94.

259
Lettie Pate Whitehead Foundation, Inc.

50 Hurt Plaza, Suite 1200
Atlanta 30303 (404) 522-6755
Contact: Charles H. McTier, Pres.
FAX: (404) 522-7026

Incorporated in 1946 in GA.
Donor(s): Conkey Pate Whitehead.‡
Financial data (yr. ended 12/31/95): Assets, $611,485,764 (M); expenditures, $11,943,636, including $11,527,667 for 206 grants (high: $500,000; low: $10,000).
Purpose and activities: Grants to institutions for scholarships for the education of poor Christian girls. While most scholarships go toward undergraduate higher education, the foundation maintains a special interest in health education. A significant number of its scholarship grants support education in the medical, nursing, and allied health care fields. Institutional grants are also awarded to assist poor and aged Christian women residing in a few selected nursing homes and retirement communities in GA, NC, and VA.
Fields of interest: Higher education; Medical school/education; Nursing school/education; Health sciences school/education; Nursing care; Nursing home/convalescent facility; Aging,

centers & services; Women, centers & services; Christian agencies & churches; Aging; Women.
Types of support: Scholarship funds.
Limitations: Giving limited to AL, FL, GA, LA, MS, NC, SC, TN, and VA. No grants to individuals, or for building or endowment funds, or matching gifts; no loans.
Publications: Application guidelines, informational brochure.
Application information: Application form not required.
Initial approach: Letter
Copies of proposal: 1
Deadline(s): Sept. 1
Board meeting date(s): Apr. and Nov.
Final notification: Mar. 1
Officers: Charles H. McTier, Pres.; P. Russell Hardin, V.P. and Secy.; J. Lee Tribble, Treas.
Trustees: Hughes Spalding, Jr., Chair.; Herbert A. Claiborne, Jr., M.D., Vice-Chair.; Lyons Gray.
Number of staff: 9 shared staff
EIN: 586012629

260
Robert W. Woodruff Foundation, Inc.
(Formerly Trebor Foundation, Inc.)
50 Hurt Plaza, Suite 1200
Atlanta 30303 (404) 522-6755
Contact: Charles H. McTier, Pres.
FAX: (404) 522-7026; E-mail: fdns@woodruff.org

Incorporated in 1937 in DE.
Donor(s): Robert W. Woodruff,‡ The Acmaro Securities Corp., and others.
Financial data (yr. ended 12/31/95): Assets, $2,349,578,813 (M); expenditures, $74,747,500; qualifying distributions, $73,303,278, including $72,519,703 for 54 grants (high: $5,000,000; low: $15,000; average: $50,000-$750,000).
Purpose and activities: Principal giving interests are focused on the following program areas: elementary, secondary, and higher education; health care and education; human services, particularly for children and youth; economic development and civic affairs; art and cultural activities; and conservation of natural resources and environmental protection. Preference is given to one-time capital projects of established private charitable organizations.
Fields of interest: Arts/cultural programs; Elementary/secondary education; Higher education; Education; Natural resource conservation & protection; Environment; Health care; Health organizations; Human services; Children & youth, services; Youth, services; Aging, centers & services; Economic development; Government/public administration; Public affairs; Aging.
Types of support: Capital campaigns, building/renovation, equipment, land acquisition, program development.
Limitations: Giving primarily in Atlanta, GA. No grants to individuals, or for endowment funds, research, publications, conferences and seminars, or operating budgets; no loans.
Publications: Application guidelines, informational brochure.
Application information: Application form not required.
Initial approach: Letter
Copies of proposal: 1
Deadline(s): 1st of Feb. and Sept.
Board meeting date(s): Apr. and Nov.
Final notification: Within 30 days of trustee meeting
Officers and Trustees:* Joseph W. Jones,* Chair.; James M. Sibley,* Vice-Chair.; Charles H. McTier, Pres.; P. Russell Hardin, V.P. and Secy.; J. Lee Tribble, Treas.; Ivan Allen, Jr., Wilton Looney, James B. Williams.
Number of staff: 10 shared staff
EIN: 581695425
Grants for Aging:
Emory University, Atlanta, GA, $2,000,000. For capital and endowment campaign to include construction of geriatric primary care outpatient clinic at Wesley Woods. 95.

HAWAII

261
Clarence T. C. Ching Foundation
1001 Bishop St., Suite 2200
Honolulu 96813 (808) 524-4900
Contact: Lawrence S.L. Ching, Chair. (by mail), and Carol L. Hong, Secy. (by telephone)

Established in 1967.
Donor(s): Clarence T.C. Ching,‡ Loyalty Development Co., Ltd.
Financial data (yr. ended 12/31/94): Assets, $3,849,897 (M); gifts received, $1,261,182; expenditures, $32,193; qualifying distributions, $18,047, including $7,500 for 2 grants (high: $5,000; low: $2,500; average: $5,000-$20,000).
Purpose and activities: Giving primarily to the Marinist Center of Hawaii and the Saint Francis Hospital.
Fields of interest: Higher education; Hospitals (general); Christian agencies & churches; Asians/Pacific Islanders; Disabled; Aging; Immigrants/refugees; Economically disadvantaged; Homeless.
Types of support: General/operating support, building/renovation, matching funds.
Limitations: Giving primarily in Honolulu, HI. No grants to individuals.
Application information: Application form not required.
Initial approach: Letter
Copies of proposal: 5
Deadline(s): None
Board meeting date(s): Varies
Officers and Trustees:* Lawrence S.L. Ching,* Chair.; Carol L. Hong,* Secy.; George Chaplin, Wallace S.J. Ching, Paul C.T. Loo.
Number of staff: None.
EIN: 996014634

262
Cooke Foundation, Ltd.
c/o Hawaiian Trust Co., Ltd.
P.O. Box 3170
Honolulu 96802
Contact: Prog. Officer
Application address: Grants Administrator, c/o Hawaii Community Foundation, 900 Fort Street Mall, Suite 1300, Honolulu, HI 96813; Tel.: (808) 537-6333; FAX: (808) 521-6286

Trust established in 1920 in HI; incorporated in 1971.
Donor(s): Anna C. Cooke.‡
Financial data (yr. ended 06/30/95): Assets, $19,877,041 (M); expenditures, $863,380; qualifying distributions, $754,024, including $673,500 for 62 grants (high: $25,000; low: $1,000; average: $1,000-$100,000).
Fields of interest: Humanities; Arts/cultural programs; Education; Environment; Health care; Health associations; Human services; Youth, services; Aging, centers & services; Aging.
Types of support: General/operating support, capital campaigns, building/renovation, program development, seed money, matching funds.
Limitations: Giving limited to HI and organizations serving the people of HI. No support for churches or religious organizations, unless the trustees' "missionary forebears" were involved with them. No grants to individuals, or for scholarships, fellowships, or endowment funds; no loans.
Publications: Annual report (including application guidelines).
Application information: Application form not required.
Initial approach: Telephone or proposal
Copies of proposal: 7
Deadline(s): 2 months before each board meeting
Board meeting date(s): 4th Wednesday in May, Sept., and Jan.
Final notification: 2 weeks after board meeting
Officers and Trustees:* Samuel A. Cooke,* Pres.; Anna D. Blackwell,* V.P. and Secy.; Betty P. Dunford,* V.P. and Treas.; Dale S. Bachman, V.P.; Richard A. Cooke, Jr.,* V.P.; Charles C. Spalding, Jr.,* V.P.
Number of staff: None.
EIN: 237120804

263
Hawaii Community Foundation
(Formerly The Hawaiian Foundation)
900 Fort Street Mall, Suite 1300
Honolulu 96813 (808) 537-6333
Contact: Jane Renfro Smith, C.E.O and Pres.
FAX: (808) 521-6286

Established in 1916 in HI by trust resolution; incorporated in 1987; reorganized in 1988.
Foundation type: Community
Financial data (yr. ended 12/31/95): Assets, $216,707,232 (M); gifts received, $9,189,389; expenditures, $13,831,804, including $8,552,514 for 1,217 grants (high: $150,000; low: $28; average: $500-$50,000) and $354,437 for 831 grants to individuals (high: $3,800; low: $8; average: $50-$1,000).

Purpose and activities: To assist charitable, religious, and educational institutions by the distribution of funds, many of which have been restricted for specific purposes and in some instances for specific institutions. Major discretionary grantmaking areas are: culture, education, health, mental health, elderly, medical research and residential treatment. The foundation also provides scholarships (to Hawaiian residents only).
Fields of interest: Historic preservation/historical societies; Arts/cultural programs; Adult/continuing education; Education; Health care; Mental health, treatment; Medical research; Human services; Residential/custodial care; Aging, centers & services; Aging; Economically disadvantaged.
Types of support: Equipment, program development, conferences/seminars, seed money, scholarship funds, research, technical assistance, consulting services, scholarships—to individuals.
Limitations: Giving limited to HI. No grants for annual campaigns; no loans.
Publications: Program policy statement, application guidelines, informational brochure, annual report, newsletter.
Application information: Application procedures vary with foundation's different grantmaking programs. Application form not required.
Initial approach: Letter requesting application guidelines
Copies of proposal: 1
Deadline(s): 2 months prior to committee meetings
Board meeting date(s): Varies
Final notification: 3 weeks after meeting
Officers and Board Members:* Julia Ann Frohlich,* Chair.; David Iha,* Vice-Chair.; Walter Laskey,* Vice-Chair.; Jane Renfro Smith, C.E.O and Pres.; Janis Reischmann, V.P.; Amy Agbayani,* Secy.; Donald G. Horner,* Treas.; Robert Alm, Zadoc Brown, Jr., Gary L. Gifford, Louise K.Y. Ing, Lawrence M. Johnson, Barbara Kalipi, Gerry Keir, Paul Kosasa, Anton Krucky, Elia A. Long, Dee Jay Mailer, Margaret K. Masunaga, Tom Mitrano, Pepi Nieva, Michael O'Brien, Russell K. Okata, Sada Okumura, Gwen Pacarro, Jan Rudinoff, Thanh-Lo Sananikone, R. Dwayne Steele, Margaret S. Ushijima, Lynne Waihee, Jenai Wall, Ronald Wo.
Trustees: Hawaiian Trust Co., Ltd., First Hawaiian Bank.
Staff: Daniel deCastro, Communications Officer; Janet Oshiro, Funds Admin. Officer; Cynthia Schnack, Dir. of Development; Lynn Haff, Prog. Officer, Scholarships; Susan Jones, Prog. Officer, Education; Steven Kaneshiro, Prog. Officer, Human Svcs.; Robyn Kaufman, Prog. Officer, Health; Karen Masaki, Prog. Officer, Culture and Arts; David Murata, Prog. Officer, Maui; Maralyn Kurshals, Prog. Assoc., Neighborhood/Community Development; Nani Larsen, Prog. Assoc., Kauai; Nan Madsen, Prog. Assoc., West Hawaii; Joanne Yamada, Prog. Assoc., Film, Counseling, the Disabled.
Number of staff: 19 full-time professional; 6 part-time professional; 13 full-time support; 3 part-time support.
EIN: 990261283
Grants for Aging:
Aged to Perfection Club, Honolulu, HI, $23,760. For assistance to elderly, needy clients. 94.
Alzheimers Disease and Related Disorders Association, Honolulu, HI, $15,000. For start-up costs for Hale Kako'o respite center. 94.
Catholic Charities of Honolulu, Honolulu, HI, $15,000. For money management program for elderly individuals. 94.
Hawaii Island Adult Care, Hilo, HI, $38,880. For assistance to elderly, needy clients. 94.
Honolulu Gerontology Program, Honolulu, HI, $10,000. For assistance for older adults. 94.
Kona Adult Day Care Center, Kelakekua, HI, $12,960. For assistance for elderly, needy clients. 94.
Kuakini Adult Day Care Center, Honolulu, HI, $19,008. For assistance for elderly, needy clients. 94.
Malama Makua Adult Day Care Center, Honolulu, HI, $39,960. For assistance for elderly, needy clients for adult day care. 94.
Maui Economic Opportunity, Kahului, HI, $12,000. For elderly individuals in need. 94.
Sacred Heart Parish Outreach, Honolulu, HI, $13,000. For older adults and mentally ill individuals. 94.
Waianae District Comprehensive Health and Hospital Board, Waianae, HI, $51,840. For assistance for elderly, needy clients for adult day care. 94.
Wilcox Hospital Foundation, Lihue, HI, $25,920. For elderly, needy clients for adult day care. 94.
Windward Seniors Day Care Center, Kailua, HI, $16,200. For assistance for elderly, needy clients for adult day care. 94.

264
Teresa F. Hughes Trust

c/o Hawaiian Trust Co., Ltd.
P.O. Box 3170
Honolulu 96802
Application address: c/o Hawaii Community Foundation, 900 Fort Street Mall, Suite 1300, Honolulu, HI 96813; Tel: (808) 566-5570

Established in 1991 in HI.
Donor(s): Teresa F. Hughes.‡
Financial data (yr. ended 03/31/95): Assets, $7,408,418 (M); expenditures, $243,074; qualifying distributions, $213,782, including $15,150 for 2 grants (high: $15,000; low: $150) and $158,378 for 130 grants to individuals (high: $5,900; low: $20).
Purpose and activities: Grants restricted to orphans, half-orphans, social orphans (neglected or abused), children born out-of-wedlock to teen mothers, and indigent and infirmed adults over age 50.
Fields of interest: Human services; Children & youth, services; Family services; Aging, centers & services; Aging; Economically disadvantaged.
Types of support: General/operating support, grants to individuals.
Limitations: Giving limited to HI.
Application information: Social summary must accompany application. Application form required.
Board meeting date(s): Every other month
Trustees: Karen K. White, Hawaiian Trust Co., Ltd.
Number of staff: None.
EIN: 990042494
Grants for Aging:
Adult Day Centers of Hawaii, HI, $20,000. For start-up cost. 94.
Adult Day Centers of Hawaii, HI, $15,000. For study to identify financing options for adult care. 94.
Adult Day Centers of Hawaii, HI, $15,000. For study to identify financing options for adult care. 94.

265
The People's Fund

1325 Nu'uanu Ave., Suite 207
Honolulu 96817 (808) 526-2441
Contact: Richard Rothschiller, Exec. Dir.

Established in 1972 in HI.
Financial data (yr. ended 06/30/94): Assets, $25,875 (L); gifts received, $51,876; expenditures, $75,303; qualifying distributions, $46,552, including $27,000 for 32 grants (high: $2,000; low: $100).
Purpose and activities: The fund provides financial support and technical assistance to progressive grassroots social change organizations, especially those considered too small, too new, or too radical by traditional funders. The fund invites applications from organizations and individuals working against discrimination based on race, sex, age, religion, economic status, sexual orientation, ethnic background, illness/disease or physical or mental disabilities; struggling for the rights of workers; promoting self-determination in low-income and disenfranchised communities; creating alternative arts and media; and promoting peace and responsible U.S. foreign policy. Emergency grants of up to $300 are available for response to issues that arise unexpectedly. Does not affect eligibility for a grant during regularly scheduled funding cycle.
Fields of interest: Environment; Employment, equal rights; Aging, centers & services; Peace; Civil rights, gays/lesbians; Race/intergroup relations; Civil rights; Aging; Asia.
Types of support: General/operating support, emergency funds, seed money.
Limitations: Giving limited to HI and the Pacific Basin. No support for groups with annual budgets exceeding $100,000 or organizations that have received a grant from the fund in past 12-month period.
Publications: Annual report, informational brochure, newsletter, financial statement, application guidelines, grants list, 990-PF.
Application information: Application form required.
Initial approach: Letter or telephone requesting application guidelines
Copies of proposal: 10
Deadline(s): Mar. 1 and Sept. 1; none for emergency grants
Board meeting date(s): Monthly
Final notification: Late Apr. and late Oct.
Officers and Directors:* Lynette Cruz,* Pres.; Gail Hovey,* V.P.; Charlene Sato,* Co-Secy.; Lucy Witeck,* Co-Secy.; Jawea Mockabee,* Treas.; Richard Rothschiller, Exec. Dir.; Ibrahim Aoude, Norma Carr, Gary Gill, Ku'umeaaloha Gomes, Marsha Joyner, Danny Li, Neal Mazer,

Steve Nakano, Setsu Okubo, Rachel Saiki, Judy Sobin, Pete Wilcox.
Number of staff: 1 full-time professional.
EIN: 237250803

266
Theodore A. Vierra Foundation
c/o Hawaiian Trust Co., Ltd.
P.O. Box 3170
Honolulu 96802 (808) 525-8548
Application address: c/o Hawaii Community Foundation, 900 Fort Street Mall, Suite 1300, Honolulu, HI 96813

Financial data (yr. ended 12/31/94): Assets, $375,250 (M); expenditures, $29,717; qualifying distributions, $24,032, including $21,616 for 22 grants to individuals (high: $3,960; low: $180).
Fields of interest: Aging, centers & services; Aging; Economically disadvantaged.
Types of support: Grants to individuals.
Limitations: Giving limited to residents of HI.
Application information: Application form required.
Deadline(s): None
Officers: Theodore A. Vierra, Jr., Pres.; Charles E. Nelson, V.P.; Jeanne Nelson, V.P.; Earlynne Oshiro, Secy.-Treas.
Trustee: Hawaiian Trust Co., Ltd.
EIN: 990241429

267
G. N. Wilcox Trust
c/o Hawaiian Trust Co., Ltd.
130 Merchant St.
Honolulu 96813 (808) 538-4944
Contact: Mrs. Lois C. Loomis, V.P., Hawaiian Trust Co., Ltd.
Mailing address: P.O. Box 3170, Honolulu, HI 96802-3170

Trust established in 1916 in HI.
Donor(s): George N. Wilcox.‡
Financial data (yr. ended 12/31/94): Assets, $14,771,936 (M); expenditures, $784,167; qualifying distributions, $697,621, including $669,400 for 122 grants (high: $28,400; low: $750; average: $1,000-$10,000).
Purpose and activities: Primary areas of interest include social services, child welfare, family services, education, and health. Support also for literacy programs, the elderly, arts and culture, hospices, AIDS services and education, community funds, delinquency and crime prevention, and Protestant church support.
Fields of interest: Arts/cultural programs; Adult education—literacy & basic skills; Reading; Education; Health care; AIDS; Health organizations; Delinquency prevention/services; Crime/law enforcement; Human services; Children & youth, services; Family services; Hospices; Aging, centers & services; Protestant agencies & churches; Religion.
Types of support: General/operating support, capital campaigns, building/renovation, equipment, program development, seed money, scholarship funds, matching funds.
Limitations: Giving limited to HI, particularly the Island of Kauai. No support for government agencies or organizations substantially supported by government funds. No grants to individuals, or for endowment funds, reserve funds, research, or deficit financing; no direct student aid or scholarships; no loans.
Publications: Annual report (including application guidelines).
Application information: Schools' scholarship requests considered at Mar. meeting; capital campaign requests considered at Dec. meeting. Application form not required.
Initial approach: Telephone or proposal
Copies of proposal: 5
Deadline(s): Jan. 15, Apr. 15, July 15, and Oct. 15
Board meeting date(s): Mar., June, Sept., and Dec.
Final notification: 2 to 3 months
Committee on Beneficiaries: Michael A. O'Brien, Chair.; Gale Fisher Carswell, Aletha Kaohi.
Trustee: Hawaiian Trust Co., Ltd.
Number of staff: None.
EIN: 996002445
Grants for Aging:
Alzheimers Disease and Related Disorders Association, Honolulu, HI, $5,000. For respite center start-up fund. 94.
Kauai Senior Centers, Kapaa, HI, $5,000. For Senior Activity Outreach program. 94.

IDAHO

268
Roger and Sybil Ferguson Charitable Foundation
P.O. Box 519
Rexburg 83440-2108 (208) 356-3716
Contact: Diane Clements

Established in 1988 in ID.
Donor(s): Roger N. Ferguson, Sybil Ferguson.
Financial data (yr. ended 12/31/95): Assets, $682,886 (M); expenditures, $38,281; qualifying distributions, $37,135, including $37,135 for 21 grants (high: $20,000; low: $25).
Fields of interest: Secondary school/education; Education; Medicine/medical care, fund raising; Aging, centers & services; Community development.
Types of support: General/operating support.
Limitations: Giving primarily in ID.
Application information: Application form required.
Deadline(s): None
Trustees: Roger N. Ferguson, Sybil Ferguson.
EIN: 820423853

ILLINOIS

269
The Clara Abbott Foundation
200 Abbott Park Rd., D579, Bldg. AP-51
Abbott Park 60064-3537
Contact: Barry R. Wojtak, Exec. Dir.

Established in 1940 in IL. Funds donated by Clara Abbott(deceased).
Donor(s): Clara Abbott.‡
Financial data (yr. ended 12/31/94): Assets, $148,330,446 (M); gifts received, $134,934; expenditures, $9,194,664; qualifying distributions, $8,939,730, including $7,250,970 for 3,198 grants to individuals, $522,756 for 1 foundation-administered program and $1,166,004 for 559 loans to individuals.
Purpose and activities: Grants and loans are made to Abbott Laboratories employees and retirees for financial aid due to financial hardships. Educational grants are made only to dependents of Abbott Laboratories employees and retirees based on a need criteria.
Fields of interest: Education; Human services; Aging; Economically disadvantaged.
Types of support: Continuing support, emergency funds, consulting services, program-related investments/loans, employee-related scholarships, grants to individuals.
Limitations: Giving primarily to Abbott Laboratories employees and retirees worldwide.
Publications: 990-PF, financial statement, informational brochure, annual report.
Application information: Application form required.
Initial approach: Contact consultant contracted with foundation or complete application
Deadline(s): Scholarship application deadline, Mar. 15 (domestic) and Aug. 15 (international); for other financial aid, no deadline
Board meeting date(s): Apr. and Oct.
Final notification: Varies
Officers and Directors:* Eugene L. Woroch,* Pres.; Laurence R. Lee,* V.P.; Dale E. Stavlo,* V.P.; Brian Smith, Secy.; Carol A. Stasiek, Treas.; Barry R. Wojtak, Exec. Dir; Catherine Babington, Joseph M. Bernik, Patricia Coles, John E. Condon, Kenneth W. Farmer, Lester E. Hammar, James A. Hanley, Lucille Heine, Joseph G. Miller, James W. Milne, Paul E. Roge, Marcia A. Thomas, Ellen Walvoord.
Number of staff: 5 full-time professional; 6 full-time support.
EIN: 366069632

270
Allen-Heath Memorial Foundation
222 North LaSalle St., Suite 300
Chicago 60601-1005

Incorporated in 1947 in CA.
Donor(s): Harriet A. Heath,‡ John E.S. Heath.‡
Financial data (yr. ended 12/31/94): Assets, $3,511,137 (M); expenditures, $218,519; qualifying distributions, $186,712, including $185,000 for 25 grants (high: $18,000; low: $1,000; average: $1,000-$30,000).
Purpose and activities: Grants to a limited number of educational institutions, hospitals, museums, air safety organizations, and other charitable institutions.
Fields of interest: Museums; Higher education; Hospitals (general); Safety/disasters; Children & youth, services; Hospices; Aging, centers & services; Women, centers & services; Community development; Federated giving programs; Aging; Women.

Types of support: General/operating support, program development.
Limitations: Applications not accepted. No support for religious or foreign organizations, private foundations, or conduit organizations. No grants to individuals; no loans.
Publications: Annual report.
Application information: Contributes only to pre-selected organizations; unsolicited applications for funds not considered.
Board meeting date(s): Nov.
Officers and Directors:* Charles K. Heath,* Pres.; Ruth R. Hooper,* V.P.; James Harbert, Secy.-Treas.
Number of staff: None.
EIN: 363056910

271
Alton Woman's Home Association
P.O. Box 552
Alton 62002

Established in 1897 in IL.
Foundation type: Operating
Financial data (yr. ended 12/31/94): Assets, $2,058,484 (M); gifts received, $5,901; expenditures, $102,612; qualifying distributions, $100,849, including $97,750 for 14 grants (high: $17,000; low: $1,250).
Purpose and activities: A private operating foundation established to serve local area needy women and children; grants to services for the aged, welfare agencies, and a hospital.
Fields of interest: Human services; Children & youth, services; Aging, centers & services; Women, centers & services; Aging; Women.
Types of support: Continuing support.
Limitations: Giving limited to Madison County, IL. No support for profit-making organizations. No grants to individuals.
Publications: Financial statement.
Application information: Application form required.
Initial approach: Letter
Copies of proposal: 1
Deadline(s): Sept. 1
Board meeting date(s): Mar., June, Sept., Nov., and Dec.
Final notification: Dec. 15
Officers and Directors:* Judith Mottaz,* Pres.; Carol Neudecker,* V.P.; Trudi Weber Allen, Corresponding Secy.; Jacqueline L. Williams,* Recording Secy.; Kathryn Kamp,* Treas.; and 15 additional directors.
Number of staff: None.
EIN: 370799839
Grants for Aging:
Meals on Wheels, IL, $3,200. 94.
Senior Services Plus, Alton, IL, $7,000. 94.

272
Alzheimer's Association
(also known as Alzheimer's Disease and Related Disorders Association)
c/o Medical and Scientific Affairs
919 North Michigan Ave., Suite 1000
Chicago 60611-1676 (800) 272-3900
Contact: Timothy J. Morgan, Dir. of Financial Opers.
Research Grant Office tel.: (312) 335-5779; FAX: (312) 335-1110; URL: http://www.alz.org; E-mail: Develop@alz.org

Established in 1980 in DE.
Financial data (yr. ended 06/30/95): Assets, $44,475,785 (M); gifts received, $25,852,133; expenditures, $25,775,445; qualifying distributions, $19,037,101, including $8,035,727 for grants.
Purpose and activities: The association is a national voluntary health organization dedicated to researching the prevention, cure, and treatment of Alzheimer's disease and related disorders, and providing support and assistance to afflicted individuals and their families. Grants are made to qualified medical science investigators at nonprofit institutions who are involved in biological, clinical, and social/behavioral research relevant to degenerative brain diseases, such as Alzheimer's disease.
Fields of interest: Alzheimer's disease; Alzheimer's disease research.
Types of support: Research.
Publications: Annual report, informational brochure, newsletter.
Application information: Contact association for current application guidelines. A portion of the association's grantmaking is directed to chapter organizations. Application form required.
Initial approach: Letter or telephone
Deadline(s): Jan. 13 for Investigator-Initiated Research Grants and Faculty Scholar Awards; June 30 for Pilot Research Grants; Aug. 11 for Zenith Awards
Board meeting date(s): Jan., May, and Oct.
Officers and Directors:* Stuart C. Roth,* Chair.; Hon. Griff Steinke, Sr. Vice-Chair.; Mrs. George F. Berlinger,* Vice-Chair.; Mrs. Samuel A. Blank, Vice-Chair.; Princess Yasmin Aga Khan, Vice-Chair.; Nancy Emerson Lombardo, Ph.D., Vice-Chair.; William L. McLennan, Vice-Chair.; Hilda Pridgeon, Vice-Chair.; Irvine D. Flinn,* Secy.; Lonnie E. Wollin,* Treas.; Kitty Allen, and 51 additional directors.
EIN: 133039601

273
Ameritech Corporate Giving Program
30 South Wacker Dr., 34th Fl.
Chicago 60606
Contact: Michael E. Kuhlin, Sr. Dir., Corp. Contribs. and Ameritech Fdn.
Donna Jernigan, Dir., Corp. Contribs. IL, 225 West Randolph 30-A, Chicago, IL 60606; Lesley Livengood, Dir., Corp. Contribs. IN, 240 North Meridian, Rm. 1811, Indianapolis, IN 46204; Lyn Allen, Dir., Corp. Contribs. MI, 444 Michigan Ave., 1550, Detroit, MI 48226; Bill Boag, Dir., Corp. Contribs. OH, 45 Erieview Plaza, Rm. 1457, Cleveland, OH 44114; Peggy Larson, Dir., Corp. Contribs. WI, 722 North Broadway, 13th Fl., Milwaukee, WI 53202; or for Regional/National/Intl. Progs., Michael Kuhlin, Sr. Dir., Corp. Contribs. and Ameritech Fdn., 30 South Wacker Dr., 34th Fl., Chicago, IL 60606. URL: http://www.ameritech.com/news/contributions

Financial data (yr. ended 12/31/95): Total giving, $23,848,000, including $20,558,000 for grants (high: $1,800,000; low: $1,000) and $3,290,000 for employee matching gifts.
Purpose and activities: Ameritech's contributions program complements the company's commitment to improving the quality of life. As a good corporate citizen, Ameritech invests a good portion of its earnings in selected educational, civic, health, and cultural organizations. IL, IN, MI, OH, and WI each have a director of corporate contributions to represent business interests locally on behalf of all Ameritech entities and their people. Grant seekers should direct their requests to the appropriate director.
Fields of interest: Arts/cultural programs; Education; Environment; Health care; Mental health/crisis services; Crime/violence prevention; Offenders/ex-offenders, rehabilitation; Housing/shelter; Youth development, services; Youth development; Aging, centers & services; Human services; Community development, neighborhood development; Economic development; Engineering & technology; Computer science; Science; Telecommunications.
Types of support: Continuing support, capital campaigns, program development, conferences/seminars, professorships, curriculum development, research, cause-related marketing, employee volunteer services, sponsorships, employee matching gifts.
Limitations: Giving primarily in areas of operations in IL, IN, MI, OH, and WI. No support for national health organizations, organizations that discriminate on the basis of race, color, creed, or nationality, denominational or sectarian religious organizations, organizations receiving government support, affiliates of labor organizations, for-profit organizations, nursing or retirement homes, local athletics or sports programs (excluding Special Olympics and U.S. Olympics), organizations only benefitting a few people, United Way supported agencies, service organizations raising money for community purposes, political organizations or candidates, or disease or disorder-specific organizations. No grants to individuals, or for lobbying, medical research, advertising, hospital capital campaigns, travel, or for operating support.
Publications: Application guidelines.
Application information: Application forms are available to employees through the company's employee publication. Application form not required.
Initial approach: Brief letter of inquiry to contributions manager of nearest individual subsidiary
Copies of proposal: 1
Deadline(s): None
Final notification: 6 weeks
Directors: Michael E. Kuhlin, Sr. Dir., Corp. Contribs. and Ameritech Fdn.; Lyn Allen, Dir., Corp. Contribs. for MI; Bill Boag, Dir., Corp. Contribs. for OH; Donna Jernigan, Dir., Corp. Contribs. for IL; Peggy Larson, Dir., Corp. Contribs. for WI; Lesly Livengood, Dir., Corp. Contribs. for IN.
Number of staff: 6 full-time professional; 3 full-time support.

274
Roland G. Balg Charitable Trust
c/o Bank of America Illinois
231 South LaSalle St.
Chicago 60697 (312) 828-1785
Contact: M.C. Ryan

Established in 1977 in IL.
Financial data (yr. ended 08/31/94): Assets, $1,584,929 (M); expenditures, $69,484; qualifying distributions, $53,992, including $52,512 for 5 grants of $10,502 each.
Fields of interest: Higher education; Animal welfare; Hospitals (general); Children & youth, services; Aging, centers & services; Aging.
Limitations: Giving limited to IL and WI. No grants to individuals.
Application information: Application form not required.
Initial approach: Letter
Deadline(s): None
Trustee: Bank of America Illinois.
EIN: 366650606

275
Francis Beidler Charitable Trust
53 West Jackson Blvd., Rm. 530
Chicago 60604 (312) 922-3792
Contact: Rosemarie Smith, Trustee

Trust established in 1924 in IL.
Donor(s): Francis Beidler.‡
Financial data (yr. ended 12/31/94): Assets, $8,632,537 (L); expenditures, $368,806; qualifying distributions, $319,142, including $319,142 for grants.
Purpose and activities: To aid public and operating charitable organizations; giving for social services, including care of the aged or crippled, family planning, youth agencies, child development and welfare, and education; support also for legal services and education, the mental and behavioral sciences, international affairs and foreign policy, arms control, and the environment. No beneficiary may receive more than one-fifth of the net income yearly.
Fields of interest: Child development, education; Law school/education; Education; Environment; Family planning; Mental health, treatment; Mental health/crisis services; Legal services; Crime/law enforcement; Human services; Children & youth, services; Child development, services; Aging, centers & services; Arms control; Foreign policy; International affairs; Community development; Psychology/behavioral science; Disabled; Aging; Economically disadvantaged.
Types of support: General/operating support, continuing support.
Limitations: Giving primarily in IL. No grants to individuals, or for building funds, research, or matching gifts; no loans.
Application information: Application form not required.
Initial approach: Letter
Copies of proposal: 1
Deadline(s): None
Board meeting date(s): May or June
Trustees: Francis Beidler III, Thomas B. Dorris, Rosemarie Smith.
Number of staff: None.
EIN: 362166969

276
Daniel L. & Rosalind Benton Foundation
c/o Michael Silver & Co.
8833 Gross Point Rd., Suite 306
Skokie 60077-1810

Established in 1961.
Financial data (yr. ended 05/31/94): Assets, $101,772 (M); expenditures, $56,066; qualifying distributions, $54,741, including $54,741 for 20 grants (high: $25,250; low: $25).
Fields of interest: Aging, centers & services; Jewish agencies & temples; Aging.
Limitations: Applications not accepted. Giving primarily in Palm Springs, CA.
Application information: Contributes only to pre-selected organizations.
Officers and Directors:* Daniel L. Benton,* Pres.; Bruce K. Benton,* Secy.; Robert Benton, Ellen Gutterman.
EIN: 366116745
Grants for Aging:
Mizell Senior Center, Palm Springs, CA, $25,250. 94.

277
Helen Brach Foundation
55 West Wacker Dr., Suite 701
Chicago 60601 (312) 372-4417
Contact: Raymond F. Simon, Pres.

Established in 1974 in IL.
Donor(s): Helen Brach.‡
Financial data (yr. ended 03/31/95): Assets, $69,152,658 (M); expenditures, $2,955,620; qualifying distributions, $2,696,355, including $2,531,746 for grants (high: $25,000; low: $3,000; average: $5,000-$25,000).
Purpose and activities: Support for the prevention of cruelty to animals; programs that test public safety; social and family services, including programs for the prevention of cruelty to children, youth and child welfare, the homeless and housing, the aged, women, the disabled, and the disadvantaged; conservation of the environment; secondary, higher, and other education; and general health.
Fields of interest: Child development, education; Secondary school/education; Higher education; Education; Natural resource conservation & protection; Environment; Animal welfare; Hospitals (general); Health care; Food services; Housing/shelter, development; Safety/disasters; Youth development, citizenship; Human services; Children & youth, services; Youth, services; Child development, services; Family services; Aging, centers & services; Women, centers & services; Homeless, human services; Disabled; Aging; Women; Economically disadvantaged; Homeless.
Types of support: General/operating support, annual campaigns, building/renovation, equipment, program development, publication, scholarship funds, research.
Limitations: Giving primarily in the Midwest. No grants to individuals, or for organizations with less than one year of budget history.
Publications: Multi-year report (including application guidelines), application guidelines.
Application information: Application form required.
Initial approach: Letter
Copies of proposal: 1
Deadline(s): Dec. 31 (earlier preferred)
Board meeting date(s): Quarterly
Final notification: Mar.
Officers and Directors:* Charles M. Vorhees,* Chair.; Raymond F. Simon,* Pres.; James J. O'Connor,* V.P.; John J. Sheridan,* Secy.-Treas.; R. Matthew Simon, Charles A. Vorhees.
Number of staff: 1 part-time support.
EIN: 237376427
Grants for Aging:
Northwest Home for the Aged, Chicago, IL, $20,000. 95.
Saint Josephs Home for the Elderly of Little Sisters of the Poor, Palatine, IL, $10,000. 95.

278
Harry F. and Elaine Chaddick Foundation, Inc.
123 West Madison St., Suite 200
Chicago 60602-4511 (312) 704-4100
Contact: Elaine M. Chaddick, Pres.

Established in 1986 in IL.
Donor(s): Harry F. Chaddick,‡ Elaine Chaddick.
Financial data (yr. ended 06/30/95): Assets, $3,079,783 (M); gifts received, $1,000,000; expenditures, $158,131; qualifying distributions, $113,900, including $113,900 for 15 grants (high: $50,000; low: $1,000).
Fields of interest: Historic preservation/historical societies; Arts/cultural programs; Education, research; Secondary school/education; Vocational education; Higher education; Education; Medical care, rehabilitation; Health care; Health associations; Cancer; Heart/circulatory disease; Medical research; Cancer research; Heart/circulatory research; Youth development, services; Human services; Youth, services; Aging, centers & services; Urban/community development; Community development; Roman Catholic federated giving programs; Engineering & technology; Science; Leadership development; Public affairs; Disabled; Aging; Economically disadvantaged; General charitable giving.
Types of support: Continuing support, building/renovation, equipment, program development, conferences/seminars, curriculum development, scholarship funds, research.
Limitations: Giving primarily in the metropolitan Chicago, IL, area. No grants to individuals.
Application information: Application form required.
Initial approach: Letter
Copies of proposal: 1
Deadline(s): Apr. 1
Board meeting date(s): Various; annual meeting in June
Officers and Directors:* Elaine M. Chaddick,* Pres.; John P. Murray,* Secy.; Camille Hatzenbuehler,* Treas.; Wayne Moretii.
Number of staff: 1 part-time professional; 1 full-time support.
EIN: 363320988
Grants for Aging:

Housing Opportunities and Maintenance for the Elderly (HOME), Chicago, IL, $5,000. 95.

279
The Chicago Community Trust

222 North LaSalle St., Suite 1400
Chicago 60601-1009 (312) 372-3356
Contact: Ms. Sandy Chears, Grants Mgr. (grants to organizations)

Established in 1915 in IL by bank resolution and declaration of trust.
Donor(s): Albert W. Harris, and members of the Harris family.
Foundation type: Community
Financial data (yr. ended 09/30/95): Assets, $477,758,400 (M); gifts received, $30,551,461; expenditures, $38,170,309, including $30,962,680 for grants (average: $10,000-$50,000).
Purpose and activities: Established "for such charitable purposes as will . . . best make for the mental, moral, intellectual and physical improvement, assistance and relief of the inhabitants of the County of Cook, State of IL." Grants for both general operating support and specific programs and projects in the areas of health and social services, youth agencies, education, cultural and civic affairs; awards fellowships to individuals in leadership positions in local community service organizations.
Fields of interest: Visual arts; Performing arts; Arts/cultural programs; Child development, education; Elementary school/education; Secondary school/education; Higher education; Libraries/library science; Environment; Health care; AIDS; Health organizations; Housing/shelter, development; Youth development, services; Human services; Youth, services; Child development, services; Aging, centers & services; Women, centers & services; Minorities/immigrants, centers & services; Homeless, human services; Economic development; Community development; Public policy, research; Government/public administration; Leadership development; Minorities; Disabled; Aging; Women; Homeless.
Types of support: General/operating support, continuing support, capital campaigns, building/renovation, equipment, land acquisition, emergency funds, program development, seed money, research, technical assistance, program-related investments/loans, matching funds.
Limitations: Giving primarily in Cook County, IL. No support for religious purposes. No grants to individuals, (except for limited fellowship programs) or for annual campaigns, deficit financing, endowment funds, publications, conferences, or scholarships; no support for the purchase of computer hardware; no general operating support for agencies or institutions whose program activities substantially duplicate those already undertaken by others.
Publications: Annual report, informational brochure, financial statement, application guidelines, newsletter.
Application information: Application form required for various special programs.
Initial approach: Proposal
Copies of proposal: 2
Deadline(s): Proposals scheduled for next available board meeting; no set deadline
Board meeting date(s): Jan., May, and Sept.
Final notification: 4 to 6 months after submission
Officers: Carol Crenshaw, C.F.O.; Bruce L. Newman, Exec. Dir.
Executive Committee: Rev. Dr. Kenneth B. Smith, Chair.; Judith S. Block, Milton Davis, Sue Ling Gin, James J. Glasser, Margaret D. Hartigan, Homer J. Livingston, Lewis Manilow, Virginia F. Ojeda, Cordell Reed, Shirley W. Ryan, Eugene A. Tracy, Ormand J. Wade.
Trustees: American National Bank & Trust Co. of Chicago, Bank of America Illinois, Chicago Title and Trust Co., First Bank, First National Bank of Chicago, Harris Trust & Savings Bank, Heritage Pullman Bank, LaSalle National Bank, The Northern Trust Co.
Staff: Marvin R. Cohen, Dir., Children, Youth & Family Initiative; Janice B. Bennett, Sr. Staff Assoc., Civic Affairs & Environment; Margo De Ley, Sr. Staff Assoc., Social Services; Ada Mary Gugenheim, Sr. Staff Assoc., Health; Michael S. Marcus, Sr. Staff Assoc., Social Services & Aging; Sarah Solotaroff, Sr. Staff Assoc., Cultural Arts; Maria Whelan, Sr. Staff Assoc., Social Services & Education; Daryl Woods, Sr. Staff Assoc., Social Services; Sandy Chears, Grants Mgr.
Number of staff: 22 full-time professional; 1 part-time professional; 13 full-time support; 3 part-time support.
EIN: 362167000
Grants for Aging:
Casa Central, Chicago, IL, $200,000. For pre-development support to construct new multi-purpose building. 95.
Chicago Commons Association, Chicago, IL, $35,000. For wheelchair/disabled access van for Comprehensive Senior Care Program. 95.
Chicago Commons Association, Chicago, IL, $34,000. For adult day care health coordinator for Comprehensive Senior Care Program. 95.
Chicago Commons Association, Chicago, IL, $25,000. To develop information system for Comprehensive Senior Care Program. 95.
Coalition of Limited English Speaking Elderly (CLESE), Chicago, IL, $20,000. For general operating support. 95.
Council for Jewish Elderly, Chicago, IL, $72,000. For redesign project for Benefits Eligibility Check-Up System's Living-at-Home Program. 95.
Illinois Alliance for Aging, Chicago, IL, $12,500. For start-up support for Senior Net. 95.
Maple Park United Methodist Church, Chicago, IL, $15,000. To establish Alzheimer's Respite Care Program at Phoebe's Place. 95.
North Shore Senior Center, Northfield, IL, $15,000. For part-time controller, to train staff and for accounting software. 95.
Northwestern University, Center for Health Services and Policy Research, Evanston, IL, $99,754. For study of managed-care programs for elderly and disabled. 95.
South Austin Coalition Community Council, Chicago, IL, $25,000. To establish senior information and advocacy center. 95.
Suburban Area Agency on Aging, Oak Park, IL, $200,000. For Collaborative Seniors Advocate Program. 95.
University of Chicago, Chicago, IL, $151,375. For study on emergency care for Chicago's elderly. 95.
White Crane Wellness Center, Chicago, IL, $46,000. For part-time administrative assistant and part-time nurse practitioner. 95.
White Crane Wellness Center, Chicago, IL, $24,950. For program evaluation project. 95.

280
Community Foundation of Champaign County

c/o BankIllinois
100 West University Ave., P.O. Box 826
Champaign 61824-0826 (217) 351-6607
Contact: Betty J. Zeedyk, Secy.

Incorporated in 1972 in IL.
Foundation type: Community
Financial data (yr. ended 03/31/94): Assets, $2,666,062 (M); gifts received, $450,166; expenditures, $255,341, including $204,029 for grants (average: $200-$12,000).
Fields of interest: Humanities; Arts/cultural programs; Education; Health care; Health organizations; Abuse prevention; Human services; Government/public administration; African Americans; Disabled; Aging; Gays/lesbians; Economically disadvantaged; Homeless.
Types of support: Continuing support, annual campaigns, building/renovation, equipment, publication, consulting services, program-related investments/loans, scholarships—to individuals.
Limitations: Giving primarily in Champaign, IL.
Publications: Annual report.
Application information: Application form required.
Copies of proposal: 1
Deadline(s): Feb. 1
Board meeting date(s): Feb. 15
Final notification: Mar. 1
Officers: Christopher Moyer, Pres.; W. Larry Shelby, V.P.; Betty J. Zeedyk, Secy.; Mary McGrath, Treas.
Number of staff: 1 part-time support.
EIN: 237176723
Grants for Aging:
Peace Meal Senior Nutrition Program, $650. 94.

281
Margaret O'Maller DeSylvester Charitable Foundation

Ten South Wacker Dr., No. 4000
Chicago 60606

Established in 1990 in IL.
Donor(s): Margaret O'Malley DeSylvester.‡
Financial data (yr. ended 08/31/92): Assets, $818,572 (M); expenditures, $92,747; qualifying distributions, $92,070, including $80,000 for grants.
Fields of interest: Higher education; Health associations; Aging, centers & services; Disabled; Aging.
Limitations: Applications not accepted.
Application information: Contributes only to pre-selected organizations.
Trustees: Donald A. Gillies, Richard E. Zscheile.

EIN: 366886118

282
Mary Lou Downs Foundation
c/o Paul F. Gerbosi
200 West Adams St., No. 2500
Chicago 60606

Established in 1991 in IL.
Donor(s): Mary Lou McIlrath.
Financial data (yr. ended 12/31/93): Assets, $31,943 (M); gifts received, $44,500; expenditures, $44,025; qualifying distributions, $44,000, including $44,000 for grants.
Fields of interest: Aging, centers & services; Christian agencies & churches.
Limitations: Applications not accepted. Giving limited to IL. No grants to individuals.
Application information: Contributes only to pre-selected organizations.
Trustees: Paul F. Gerbosi, Mary Lou McIlrath.
EIN: 363797797

283
Evanston Community Foundation
828 Davis St., Suite 300
Evanston 60201 (847) 475-2402
Contact: Thomas K. Jager, Administrator

Established in 1986 in IL.
Foundation type: Community
Financial data (yr. ended 12/31/95): Assets, $1,034,213 (M); gifts received, $83,997; expenditures, $65,080, including $32,580 for 10 grants (high: $5,000; low: $1,500; average: $3,500).
Fields of interest: Arts/cultural programs; Early childhood education; Education; Health care; Mental health/crisis services; Health associations; AIDS; Delinquency prevention/services; Housing/shelter, development; Youth development, services; Human services; Youth, services; Family services; Aging, centers & services; Minorities/immigrants, centers & services; Homeless, human services; Community development; Public affairs, citizen participation; Leadership development; Minorities; Disabled; Aging; Economically disadvantaged; Homeless.
Types of support: General/operating support, continuing support, emergency funds, program development, seed money.
Limitations: Giving limited to Evanston, IL. No grants to individuals.
Publications: Annual report, newsletter, application guidelines, informational brochure.
Application information: Application form required.
Initial approach: Letter
Copies of proposal: 12
Deadline(s): Mar. 25
Board meeting date(s): Monthly
Final notification: June 1
Officers and Directors:* Betty Papangelis,* Chair.; Thomas K. Jager,* Administrator; Joy Creamer, Jay Lytle, Ralph Segall, Larry TerMolen, and 17 additional directors.
Number of staff: 2 part-time professional.
EIN: 363466802

284
The Field Foundation of Illinois, Inc.
200 South Wacker Dr., Suite 2080
Chicago 60606 (312) 831-0910
Contact: Handy L. Lindsey, Jr., Exec. Dir.

Incorporated in 1960 in IL.
Donor(s): Marshall Field IV.‡
Financial data (yr. ended 04/30/94): Assets, $34,302,417 (M); expenditures, $1,830,787; qualifying distributions, $1,485,855, including $1,165,643 for 133 grants (high: $50,000; low: $100; average: $5,000-$25,000).
Purpose and activities: Giving in the fields of health, community welfare, primary and secondary education, cultural activities, conservation, and urban and community affairs.
Fields of interest: Museums; Arts/cultural programs; Early childhood education; Elementary school/education; Secondary school/education; Adult education—literacy & basic skills; Reading; Education; Natural resource conservation & protection; Environment; Medical care, rehabilitation; Health care; Substance abuse, services; Mental health/crisis services; AIDS; Health organizations; Employment; Food services; Human services; Children & youth, services; Youth, services; Aging, centers & services; Homeless, human services; Race/intergroup relations; Community development; Public policy, research; Public affairs; Aging; Economically disadvantaged; Homeless.
Types of support: Capital campaigns, building/renovation, equipment, land acquisition, emergency funds, program development, seed money, curriculum development, technical assistance, employee matching gifts.
Limitations: Giving primarily in the Chicago, IL, area. No support for member agencies of community funds, national health agencies, neighborhood health clinics, small cultural groups, or for religious purposes. No grants to individuals, or for endowment funds, continuing operating support, medical research, conferences, operating support of day care centers, fundraising events, advertising, scholarships, printed materials or video equipment, or fellowships; no loans.
Publications: Biennial report (including application guidelines).
Application information: Application form not required.
Initial approach: Proposal
Copies of proposal: 1
Deadline(s): None
Board meeting date(s): 3 times a year
Officers and Directors:* Arthur F. Quern,* Chair.; Gary H. Kline,* Secy.; Handy L. Lindsey, Jr.,* Treas. and Exec. Dir.; Berlean Miller Burris, Milton Davis, Marshall Field, Philip Wayne Hummer, George A. Ranney, Jr., Christine M. Tchen.
Number of staff: 2 full-time professional; 1 part-time professional; 1 full-time support; 1 part-time support.
EIN: 366059408

285
Mrs. Zollie S. Frank Fund
(Formerly Zollie and Elaine Frank Fund)
666 Garland Place
Des Plaines 60016
Contact: Elaine S. Frank, Pres.

Incorporated in 1953 in IL.
Donor(s): Zollie S. Frank, Elaine S. Frank, Z. Frank, Inc., Four Wheels, Inc., Wheels, Inc.
Financial data (yr. ended 12/31/94): Assets, $2,519,929 (M); gifts received, $535,000; expenditures, $668,692; qualifying distributions, $663,785, including $656,557 for grants.
Purpose and activities: Emphasis on Jewish welfare funds and temple support; grants also for higher education, hospitals, youth clubs, a senior citizens' center, and organized charities.
Fields of interest: Higher education; Hospitals (general); Human services; Youth, services; Aging, centers & services; Jewish federated giving programs; Jewish agencies & temples; Aging.
Types of support: General/operating support.
Limitations: Giving primarily in IL.
Application information:
Initial approach: Letter
Deadline(s): None
Officers: Elaine S. Frank, Pres.; James S. Frank, Secy.
EIN: 366118400

286
Benjamin Benedict Green-Field Foundation
Eight South Michigan, Suite 2900
Chicago 60603
Contact: Harriet Brady, Secy.

Established in 1988 in IL.
Donor(s): Benjamin Benedict Green-Field.‡
Financial data (yr. ended 12/31/94): Assets, $5,005,248 (M); expenditures, $323,003; qualifying distributions, $323,003, including $237,000 for 9 grants (high: $120,000; low: $500).
Purpose and activities: Giving to organizations that promote the interests of the young and/or the elderly; support also for health associations, with emphasis on Alzheimer's disease and its related disorders.
Fields of interest: Health associations; Alzheimer's disease; Children & youth, services; Aging, centers & services; Aging.
Limitations: Giving primarily in the metropolitan Chicago, IL, area. No grants to individuals.
Application information:
Initial approach: Letter
Deadline(s): None
Officers and Directors:* Colin K. Fisher,* Pres.; Daniel Jarke,* V.P.; Harriet Brady,* Secy.; Sheldon Rachman,* Treas.; Hyman Spiegel,* Treas.
EIN: 363559017
Grants for Aging:
Alzheimers Disease and Related Disorders Association, Chicago, IL, $120,000. 94.
Council for Jewish Elderly, Chicago, IL, $20,000. 94.

287
Arthur W. Hill Foundation

c/o Cottle & Cottle, Ltd.
120 South LaSalle St., Suite 640
Chicago 60603

Financial data (yr. ended 10/31/94): Assets, $549,946 (M); expenditures, $24,993; qualifying distributions, $22,003, including $19,250 for grants.
Fields of interest: Higher education; Hospitals (general); Aging, centers & services; Christian agencies & churches; Aging.
Limitations: Applications not accepted. Giving primarily in the midwestern U.S. No grants to individuals.
Application information: Contributes only to pre-selected organizations.
Officers: Doryce Maher, Pres. and Secy.; Nancy Tefft, V.P.; Robert E. Maher, Treas.
EIN: 366050191

288
Household International Corporate Giving Program

2700 Sanders Rd.
Prospect Heights 60070 (847) 564-6010
Contact: Donna M. Funk, Mgr., Philanthropic Services

Established in 1974.
Financial data (yr. ended 12/31/95): Total giving, $3,070,646, including $2,481,681 for grants (high: $20,000; low: $300), $57,600 for grants to individuals, $474,320 for 1,860 employee matching gifts and $57,045 for in-kind gifts.
Purpose and activities: "Household International is committed to good corporate citizenship and to an active involvement in the communities in which it operates. The company invests in the works of numerous nonprofit organizations that advance its philanthropic objectives. Household considers itself in partnership with its employees and the communities in which it does business, working to foster an environment that enhances the quality of life through educational, health and human services, cultural, civic, and community development programs. Household International and its subsidiaries believe in good corporate citizenship. Each business group goes beyond a basic commitment for efficient and responsive consumer financial services through their support of a variety of community-oriented activities including: making cash and in-kind contributions to local nonprofit organizations that serve the communities in which they are located and best respond to the issues and needs of our shareholders, customers, and employees; encouraging employee volunteerism; and initiating or supporting responsive projects and programs to enhance the quality of life in their neighborhoods."
Fields of interest: Arts/cultural programs; Early childhood education; Higher education; Adult/continuing education; Mental health/crisis services; Employment; Housing/shelter; Youth development; Human services; Children & youth, services; Family services; Women, centers & services; Minorities/immigrants, centers & services; Homeless, human services; Human services; Economic development; Urban/community development; Rural development; Community development; Voluntarism promotion; Minorities; Disabled; Aging; Women; Economically disadvantaged.
Types of support: General/operating support, continuing support, annual campaigns, capital campaigns, endowment funds, program development, conferences/seminars, seed money, scholarship funds, research, cause-related marketing, employee volunteer services, employee matching gifts, employee-related scholarships, donated equipment, in-kind gifts, matching funds.
Limitations: Giving primarily in headquarters and operating locations, including Canada and the U.K. No support for political, lobbying, or voter registration programs or those supporting the candidacy of a particular individual; or fraternal, veterans', labor, athletic, or religious organizations serving a limited constituency, or Student Aid or scholarship programs aside from those already establihed by Household International or its business group, or organizations which might in any way pose a conflict with corporate goals, products, customers, or employees; or nonprofit organizations with exemptions other than those covered in section 501(c)(3) of the Internal Revenue Code. No grants to individuals, for fundraising events or benefits, including sponsorship tickets or courtesy advertising.
Publications: Corporate report, program policy statement (including application guidelines), corporate giving report.
Application information: Application form required.
Initial approach: Request guidelines
Copies of proposal: 1
Deadline(s): Ongoing
Board meeting date(s): Ongoing with the exception of Help for Communities and Communities Need You. Contact the appropriate business unit for those procedures and deadlines
Final notification: 2 to 12 weeks in writing
Administrator: Donna M. Funk, Mgr., Philanthropic Serv.
Number of staff: 3 full-time professional; 1 full-time support; 1 part-time support.

289
Inland Steel-Ryerson Foundation, Inc.

30 West Monroe St.
Chicago 60603 (312) 899-3420
Contact: David C. Hawley, Secy.

Incorporated in 1945 in IL as Inland Steel Foundation, Inc.
Donor(s): Inland Steel Co., its subsidiaries and divisions.
Foundation type: Company-sponsored
Financial data (yr. ended 12/31/93): Assets, $11,046 (M); gifts received, $765,000; expenditures, $777,069; qualifying distributions, $777,069, including $762,346 for 125 grants (high: $250,000; low: $250; average: $500-$20,000).
Purpose and activities: The foundation's funding priorities are as follows: 1) support for the United Way in areas where business units are located; 2) programs that encourage student, especially minority, participation in science, math, engineering, and business; 3) programs that provide scholarships to the sons and daughters of company employees; 4) funding of capital projects which will improve the physical and equipment needs of the instruction of science, math, engineering, or business at private post-secondary institutions; 5) funding of local nonprofit agencies which address a need not served by the local United Way.
Fields of interest: Education, association; Education, fund raising; Secondary school/education; Higher education; Business school/education; Engineering school/education; Adult education—literacy & basic skills; Reading; Education; Hospitals (general); Medical care, rehabilitation; Mental health/crisis services; Human services; Youth, services; Hospices; Aging, centers & services; Minorities/immigrants, centers & services; Human rights (international); Civil rights; Urban/community development; Community development; Federated giving programs; Chemistry; Mathematics; Engineering & technology; Engineering; Science; Minorities; Disabled; Aging; Economically disadvantaged.
Types of support: General/operating support, capital campaigns, program development, fellowships, scholarship funds, employee-related scholarships.
Limitations: Giving primarily in areas of company operations, particularly Chicago, IL, and northwest IN. Generally no grants for sectarian or religious organizations (except churches under the category of social welfare). No grants to individuals directly, or for endowment funds, capital programs, matching grants, publications, conferences, seminars, or benefit affairs. Scholarships awarded under the All Inland Scholarship Plan and the National Merit and National Achievement Scholarship programs are restricted to children of company employees. Lawndale Community Scholarships are for area high school seniors.
Publications: Application guidelines.
Application information: Application forms required for scholarships only.
Initial approach: Letter or telephone
Copies of proposal: 1
Deadline(s): Sept. 30
Board meeting date(s): Dec.
Final notification: 3 to 4 months
Officers and Directors:* David B. Anderson,* Pres.; W. Gordon Kay,* V.P.; David C. Hawley,* Secy.; Jay E. Dittus,* Treas.; Judd R. Cool, Robert J. Darnall.
Number of staff: 1 part-time professional; 1 part-time support.
EIN: 366046944

290
George Zoltan Lefton Family Foundation

c/o Geo. Zoltan Lefton Co.
3622 South Morgan St.
Chicago 60609 (773) 254-4344

Financial data (yr. ended 12/31/94): Assets, $835,866 (M); expenditures, $53,240; qualifying distributions, $46,350, including $46,350 for 8 grants (high: $10,000; low: $350).

Fields of interest: Hospitals (general); Nursing home/convalescent facility; Cancer; Alzheimer's disease; Israel.
Limitations: Giving primarily in FL, IL, and Isreal.
Application information: Application form not required.
Deadline(s): None
Final notification: Within 2 months
Officers and Directors:* Margo Lefton,* V.P.; Magda Lefton,* Secy.
EIN: 362851551

291
Marcus and Theresa Levie Educational Fund
c/o Jewish Federation of Metropolitan Chicago
One South Franklin St.
Chicago 60606 (312) 357-4500
Contact: Scholarship Secy.

Trust established in 1959 in IL.
Donor(s): Maude M. Levie,‡ Jerome M. Levie,‡ Charles M. Levie.‡
Financial data (yr. ended 07/31/94): Assets, $2,600,000 (M); expenditures, $220,000; qualifying distributions, $155,500, including $155,500 for 32 grants to individuals (average: $3,000-$6,000).
Purpose and activities: Scholarships awarded to Jewish students who are residents of Cook County and who have demonstrated career promise and have financial need to complete their professional or vocational training in the helping professions.
Fields of interest: Early childhood education; Child development, education; Elementary school/education; Vocational education; Higher education; Medical school/education; Theological school/education; Adult/continuing education; Education; Dental care; Speech & hearing centers; Nursing care; Health care; Mental health, treatment; Mental health/crisis services; Health organizations; Crime/law enforcement; Human services; Children & youth, services; Child development, services; Family services; Aging, centers & services; Psychology/behavioral science; Disabled; Aging.
Types of support: Scholarships—to individuals.
Limitations: Giving limited to Cook County, IL. No grants for general support, or for building or endowment funds, research, or matching gifts; no loans.
Publications: Application guidelines, program policy statement.
Application information: Application form required.
Initial approach: Letter or telephone
Copies of proposal: 2
Deadline(s): Submit scholarship application between Nov. and Feb.; deadline Mar. 1
Board meeting date(s): As required, usually in July
Final notification: July or Aug.
Trustee: Chicago Title and Trust Co.
Number of staff: 14 part-time professional; 1 full-time support; 1 part-time support.
EIN: 366010074

292
LMP Fund
764 Judson Ave.
Highland Park 60035
Contact: Laura Fisher, Dir.

Established in 1976.
Donor(s): Laura Pollak Fisher.
Financial data (yr. ended 12/31/94): Assets, $55,718 (M); gifts received, $84,443; expenditures, $38,220; qualifying distributions, $37,905, including $37,905 for 103 grants (high: $10,250; low: $15; average: $25-$18,000).
Fields of interest: Arts/cultural programs; Human services; Youth, services; Aging, centers & services; International relief; International affairs, U.N.; Civil rights, minorities; Reproductive rights; Jewish agencies & temples; Minorities; African Americans; Aging; Immigrants/refugees; Homeless; General charitable giving.
Types of support: General/operating support, continuing support, capital campaigns, scholarship funds.
Limitations: Applications not accepted. Giving primarily in Chicago, IL.
Application information: Contributes only to pre-selected organizations.
Board meeting date(s): As necessary
Directors: Laura Pollak Fisher, Stephen Pollak, Louise Saltzman.
Number of staff: None.
EIN: 237312903

293
Mattison Foundation, Inc.
545 Blackhawk Park Ave.
Rockford 61104 (815) 962-5521
Contact: R.W. Mattison, Pres.

Established in 1966.
Financial data (yr. ended 06/30/93): Assets, $219,750 (M); expenditures, $78,987; qualifying distributions, $76,835, including $75,291 for 72 grants (high: $5,000; low: $50).
Fields of interest: Performing arts; Secondary school/education; Higher education; Health associations; Human services; Youth, services; Aging, centers & services; Federated giving programs; Aging.
Limitations: Giving primarily in Rockford, IL.
Application information:
Initial approach: Letter
Deadline(s): None
Officers: R.W. Mattison, Pres.; R.L. Mattison, V.P.; Phil L. Mattison, Secy.; A.M. Mattison, Treas.
Number of staff: None.
EIN: 366134793

294
McDonald's Contributions Department
McDonald's Plaza
Oak Brook 60521 (630) 575-3000
Contact: Kenneth L. Barun, Supervisor, Contribs.

Purpose and activities: Support is given in five major focus areas; education, health, arts and culture, civic affairs, and community development.
Fields of interest: Music; Historic preservation/historical societies; Arts/cultural programs; Elementary school/education; Secondary school/education; Vocational education; Higher education; Adult education—literacy & basic skills; Reading; Education; Natural resource conservation & protection; Environment; Hospitals (general); Medical care, rehabilitation; Health care; Substance abuse, services; Alcoholism; Health organizations; Medical research; Employment; Nutrition; Human services; Youth, services; Aging, centers & services; Women, centers & services; Minorities/immigrants, centers & services; Civil rights; Business & industry; Community development; Mathematics; Engineering & technology; Science; Economics; Government/public administration; Minorities; Disabled; Aging; Women; Economically disadvantaged.
Types of support: Program development, seed money, employee matching gifts, in-kind gifts, matching funds.
Limitations: Giving primarily in operating locations, through restaurants, and nationally through the corporation. No support for fraternal, veterans', religious, political, or sectarian programs, intermediary funding organizations, or the United Way outside of the Chicago area. No grants to individuals, or for capital funds, general operating purposes, endowments, investment funds, advertising, unspecified funds for specific elementary or secondary schools, multi-year grants, or research; no loans.
Publications: Corporate giving report, informational brochure.
Application information: Application form not required.
Initial approach: Full proposal (submit only one proposal per year)
Copies of proposal: 1
Deadline(s): None
Board meeting date(s): Review proposals on an on-going basis
Final notification: Within 3 months
Administrators: Kenneth L. Barun, Supervisor, Contribs.; Jackie Meara, Admin. Secy.

295
Molner Foundation
208 South LaSalle St., Suite 1100
Chicago 60604-1101 (312) 759-7246
Contact: Morton John Barnard, Trustee

Established in 1980 in IL.
Financial data (yr. ended 12/31/94): Assets, $859,239 (M); expenditures, $90,039; qualifying distributions, $72,550, including $72,550 for 48 grants (high: $20,000; low: $200).
Fields of interest: Museums; Performing arts; Theater; Music; Historic preservation/historical societies; Arts/cultural programs; Education, association; Education, fund raising; Elementary/secondary education; Secondary school/education; Higher education; Law school/education; Education; Hospitals (general); Speech & hearing centers; Health care; Mental health/crisis services; Health

associations; Cancer; Heart/circulatory disease; Biomedicine; Medical research; Cancer research; Heart/circulatory research; Legal services; Crime/law enforcement; Food services; Housing/shelter, development; Youth development, citizenship; Human services; Youth, services; Family services; Aging, centers & services; Homeless, human services; Human rights (international); Civil rights; Federated giving programs; Jewish federated giving programs; Religious federated giving programs; Government/public administration; Public affairs, citizen participation; Jewish agencies & temples; Religion; Minorities; Disabled; Aging; Homeless; General charitable giving; Middle East; Israel.
Types of support: General/operating support, continuing support, annual campaigns, building/renovation, emergency funds, scholarship funds.
Limitations: Applications not accepted. Giving primarily in IL. No grants to individuals.
Application information: Contributes only to pre-selected organizations.
Trustee: Morton John Barnard.
Number of staff: None.
EIN: 366702256

296
Mark Morton Memorial Fund
100 North Riverside Plaza
Chicago 60606-1596

Established in 1951 in IL.
Financial data (yr. ended 12/31/93): Assets, $14,072,231 (M); expenditures, $897,651; qualifying distributions, $799,903, including $707,307 for grants to individuals.
Purpose and activities: Grants limited to individuals who are verifiable employees of the Morton Salt Co. on or before June 30, 1971, to assist with hospital, medical, and surgical expenses, as well as assistance to the aged, blind, or disabled.
Fields of interest: Disabled; Aging; Economically disadvantaged.
Types of support: Grants to individuals.
Limitations: Giving primarily in TX.
Officers and Directors:* Scott Ellwood,* Pres.; Robert B. Gerrie,* V.P.; Davis Roenisch,* V.P.; Leonard E. Zak,* V.P.; Helen Hines, Secy.-Treas.
Number of staff: 2
EIN: 237181380

297
OMRON Foundation, Inc.
1375 East Woodfield Rd., Suite 520
Schaumburg 60173 (847) 240-5330
Contact: Nicholas Hahn, Dir.
Application address: One East Commerce Dr., Schaumburg, IL 60173; Tel.: (847) 843-7900; FAX: (847) 240-5362

Established in 1989 in IL.
Donor(s): OMRON Electronics, Inc., OMRON Management Center of America, OMRON Systems of America, Inc., OMRON Healthcare, Inc., OMRON Advanced Systems, Inc., OMRON Office Automation Products, Inc.
Foundation type: Company-sponsored
Financial data (yr. ended 03/31/94): Assets, $643,222 (M); gifts received, $331,846; expenditures, $143,951; qualifying distributions, $142,566, including $142,566 for 105 grants (high: $25,000; low: $10).
Purpose and activities: Primary areas of interest include higher and other education, the handicapped, cultural programs, the environment, and the elderly.
Fields of interest: Museums; Performing arts; Music; Humanities; Language & linguistics; Literature; Arts/cultural programs; Education, fund raising; Early childhood education; Child development, education; Secondary school/education; Higher education; Adult/continuing education; Libraries/library science; Education; Natural resource conservation & protection; Energy; Environment; Wildlife preservation & protection; Medical care, rehabilitation; Health care; Substance abuse, services; Mental health/crisis services; Health associations; Cancer; Alcoholism; Biomedicine; Medical research; Cancer research; Employment; Safety/disasters; Youth development, citizenship; Human services; Children & youth, services; Child development, services; Hospices; Aging, centers & services; Women, centers & services; Minorities/immigrants, centers & services; Homeless, human services; International economic development; Peace; Foreign policy; Human rights (international); International affairs; Race/intergroup relations; Civil rights; Community development; Voluntarism promotion; Federated giving programs; Engineering & technology; Science; Population studies; Public policy, research; Public affairs, citizen participation; Public affairs; Minorities; Disabled; Aging; Women; Immigrants/refugees; Homeless; General charitable giving; Asia; Japan.
Types of support: General/operating support, continuing support, building/renovation, scholarship funds, employee matching gifts, employee-related scholarships, in-kind gifts.
Limitations: Giving primarily in Chicago, IL; minor support for non-IL organizations. No grants to individuals.
Publications: Grants list, informational brochure, program policy statement, application guidelines.
Application information: Application form not required.
Initial approach: Letter
Deadline(s): None
Board meeting date(s): Quarterly
Officers: Akitoshi Shirakawa, Secy.; S. Kobayashi, Treas.
Directors: Nicholas G. Hahn, and 5 additional directors.
Number of staff: None.
EIN: 363644055

298
Peoria Area Community Foundation
Bank One Bldg.
124 S.W. Adams St., Mezzanine, Suite 1
Peoria 61602 (309) 674-8730
Contact: George H. Kreiss, Exec. Dir.
FAX: (309) 674-8754

Incorporated in 1987 in IL.
Foundation type: Community
Financial data (yr. ended 06/30/95): Assets, $2,422,502 (M); gifts received, $1,014,459; expenditures, $525,176, including $373,113 for 50 grants (high: $12,500; low: $500).
Purpose and activities: Primary areas of interest include community development, the arts and humanities, education, and health.
Fields of interest: Visual arts; Museums; Performing arts; Dance; Humanities; Historic preservation/historical societies; Arts/cultural programs; Early childhood education; Child development, education; Elementary school/education; Secondary school/education; Higher education; Adult/continuing education; Adult education—literacy & basic skills; Reading; Education; Natural resource conservation & protection; Environment; Animal welfare; Wildlife preservation & protection; Family planning; Medical care, rehabilitation; Health care; Substance abuse, services; Mental health/crisis services; Health associations; Cancer; Heart/circulatory disease; AIDS; Alcoholism; Cancer research; Heart/circulatory research; AIDS research; Delinquency prevention/services; Food services; Nutrition; Recreation; Youth development, services; Human services; Children & youth, services; Child development, services; Family services; Aging, centers & services; Homeless, human services; Civil rights; Urban/community development; Community development; Voluntarism promotion; Federated giving programs; Social sciences; Government/public administration; Leadership development; Minorities; Disabled; Aging; Economically disadvantaged; Homeless; General charitable giving.
Types of support: General/operating support, capital campaigns, equipment, program development, seed money, scholarship funds, in-kind gifts.
Limitations: Giving limited to the central IL area. No support for sectarian religious purposes. No grants to individuals (except designated scholarship funds), or for annual campaigns or endowments; no loans.
Publications: Annual report (including application guidelines), application guidelines, newsletter, informational brochure.
Application information: Application form required.
Initial approach: Letter or telephone
Copies of proposal: 17
Deadline(s): Feb. 1 and July 1 for preliminary application; Mar. 15 and Sept. 1 for final application
Board meeting date(s): Monthly
Final notification: Oct. and Apr.
Officers and Directors:* Ross Canterbury,* Pres.; Vicky Stewart,* V.P.; Pat Barton,* Secy.; Dennis Ewald,* Treas.; Romaine Bayless, David Bielfeldt, Jane Converse, Gerald Flaherty, Taylor French, Lowell Grieves, Michel McCord, Harriet Parkhurst, William Shay, Joseph Solovy, M.D., Harriett Swager, William Tunis, Jay Vonachen, Murray M. Yeomans.
Number of staff: 1 full-time professional; 1 part-time professional; 1 full-time support.
EIN: 371185713
Grants for Aging:

Alzheimers Disease and Related Disorders Association, Chicago, IL, $741. For materials. 94.
Center for the Prevention of Abuse, $1,000. For program for abused senior women. 94.

299
Phillips-Green Foundation, Inc.

5800 Blackstone Ave.
Chicago 60637
Contact: Carol P. Green, Pres.

Established in 1986 in IL.
Donor(s): Lawrence Phillips, Seymour Phillips,‡ Carol P. Green, Madelyn Phillips.
Financial data (yr. ended 08/31/95): Assets, $6,375,255 (M); gifts received, $650,000; expenditures, $862,672; qualifying distributions, $803,442, including $773,819 for 114 grants (high: $501,700; low: $25; average: $500-$1,000).
Fields of interest: Medical school/education; Nursing school/education; Medical research; Cancer research; Gun control; Domestic violence prevention; Human rights (international); Civil rights, women; Reproductive rights; Jewish agencies & temples; African Americans; Native Americans; Aging; Women; People with AIDS (PWAs); Immigrants/refugees; Economically disadvantaged.
Types of support: General/operating support, annual campaigns, capital campaigns, endowment funds, research.
Limitations: Applications not accepted.
Application information: Contributes only to pre-selected organizations.
Officers and Directors:* Carol P. Green,* Pres.; Lawrence Phillips,* V.P.; Cathy J. Green,* Secy.; Janet A. Mikkelsen,* Treas.; Douglas M. Green, David L. Phillips, Laura Phillips.
Number of staff: 1 part-time support.
EIN: 133334090

300
The Retirement Research Foundation

8765 West Higgins Rd., Suite 401
Chicago 60631 (773) 714-8080
Contact: Marilyn Hennessy, Pres.
FAX: (773) 714-8089

Incorporated in 1950 in MI.
Donor(s): John D. MacArthur.‡
Financial data (yr. ended 12/31/95): Assets, $155,120,302 (M); expenditures, $9,089,024; qualifying distributions, $8,229,844, including $6,732,056 for 264 grants (high: $400,000; low: $1,000; average: $5,000-$50,000), $22,000 for 21 grants to individuals (high: $5,000; low: $250; average: $500-$1,000), $139,842 for employee matching gifts and $1,405,946 for 3 program-related investments.
Purpose and activities: Support principally to improve the quality of life of older persons in the U.S. Priority interests are innovative model projects and research designed to: 1) improve the availability and quality of community-based long term care by: increasing the availability and effectiveness of community programs designed to maintain older persons in their own homes, as well as those in residential settings; improving the quality of nursing home care; and integrating the provision of acute and long term care for older persons with chronic conditions by supporting efforts that provide continuity of care, prevention, early intervention and client education; 2) provide new and expanded opportunities for older adults to engage in meaningful roles in society such as employment and volunteerism, that will strengthen the community through activities including, but not limited to, advocacy, community leadership, community services, and intergenerational programs; 3) seek causes and solutions to significant problems of older adults through support of selected basic, applied, and policy research for which federal funding is not available; and 4) increase the number of professionals and para-professionals adequately prepared to serve the elderly population through support of selected education and training initiatives which enhance knowledge and skills of participants.
Fields of interest: Health care; Mental health/crisis services; Health organizations; Medical research; Employment; Human services; Aging, centers & services; Homeless, human services; Social sciences; Public policy, research; Aging; Homeless.
Types of support: Program development, seed money, research, program-related investments/loans, employee matching gifts, matching funds.
Limitations: Giving limited to the Midwest (IL, IN, IA, KY, MI, MO, WI) and FL for service projects not having the potential of national impact. No grants to individuals (except through National Media Awards Program), or for construction, general operating expenses of established organizations, endowment or developmental campaigns, emergency funds, deficit financing, land acquisition, publications, conferences, scholarships, media productions, dissertation research, annual campaigns, or renovation projects.
Publications: Biennial report (including application guidelines), occasional report, program policy statement, grants list, informational brochure.
Application information: All proposals must relate to aged population. Application form not required.
Initial approach: Letter or proposal
Copies of proposal: 3
Deadline(s): Submit proposal preferably in Jan., Apr., or July; deadlines Feb. 1, May 1, and Aug. 1
Board meeting date(s): Feb., May, Aug., and Oct.
Final notification: 4 to 6 months
Officers and Trustees:* Edward J. Kelly,* Chair.; Marilyn Hennessy, Pres.; Brian F. Hofland, Sr. V.P.; Marilyn Stein LeFeber, Assoc. V.P.; Sharon F. Markham, Assoc. V.P.; Robert P. Ewing,* Secy.; William Gentle, Webster Hurley, Nathaniel McParland, M.D., Marvin Meyerson, John F. Santos, Sister Stella Louise, C.S.F.N., Ruth Ann Watkins.
Number of staff: 4 full-time professional; 4 full-time support; 1 part-time support.
EIN: 362429540
Grants for Aging:
AMC Cancer Research Center, Denver, CO, $41,414. For research to measure urinary estrogen metabolites in healthy menopausal women to assess relationship between estrogen metabolism and aging-related diseases in women. 95.
American Association of Retired Persons, DC, $20,000. Toward conferences on images of aging for news media and entertainment industry. 95.
American Longevity Research Institute, Chicago, IL, $30,000. To disseminate information on preventive medicine and advances in aging research. 95.
American Society on Aging, San Francisco, CA, $24,875. For participation of minority aging service providers from Midwest and Florida in New Ventures in Leadership Program. 95.
Apostles Lutheran Church, Melrose Park, IL, $12,500. To develop ministry to seniors. 95.
Asi, Inc., Chicago, IL, $11,270. To update and expand Hispanic Social Services Directory. 95.
Asian Human Services of Chicago, Chicago, IL, $10,000. For Northwest Chicago Senior Care Center. 95.
Association of Community Organizations for Reform Now (ACORN), Chicago, IL, $10,000. For senior leadership skills and community organizing capabilities of community seniors. 95.
Big Brothers/Big Sisters of America, Philadelphia, PA, $45,389. To continue intergenerational initiative connecting older adults to children at risk. 95.
Catholic Charities of the Archdiocese of Chicago, Chicago, IL, $62,805. To develop parish-based social service programs for elderly in Northwest Cook County. 95.
Catholic Charities of the Diocese of Palm Beach, West Palm Beach, FL, $105,000. Toward developing and operating senior housing facility. 95.
Catholic Social Services of the Archdiocese of Milwaukee, Milwaukee, WI, $80,000. For matching grant to work with parishes in southeastern Wisconsin to conduct assessment on aging needs and issues and develop relevant programs. 95.
Center for Information and Crisis Services, Lantana, FL, $118,208. For continued support of Elder Crisis Outreach Program. 95.
Center for New Television, Chicago, IL, $90,182. For National Media Owl Awards. 95.
Chicago Department of Aging, Chicago, IL, $136,452. For Benefit Eligibility Checklist Outreach Program. 95.
Cleveland Works, Cleveland, OH, $26,115. For Nursing Assistant Job Retention Project, which will prepare 120 welfare recipients to be entry-level, state-tested nursing assistants. 95.
Community Renewal Society, Chicago, IL, $50,000. To develop programs to serve seniors in African-American and Hispanic congregations and neighborhoods. 95.
Community Support Services, Brookfield, IL, $11,500. To develop intergenerational program using senior volunteers to work with developmentally disabled young adults to assist them in community orientation and participation. 95.
Congregation Bnai Shalom, Buffalo Grove, IL, $10,000. To develop intergenerational program. 95.
Contact Chicago, Chicago, IL, $10,049. To develop intergenerational volunteer program. 95.

Council for Jewish Elderly, Chicago, IL, $24,869. For three-part planning process to develop evaluation of Managed Community Care Demonstration Project. 95.
Council for Jewish Elderly, Chicago, IL, $10,689. For Peapod Shop-at-Home Program. 95.
District 15 Educational Foundation, Palatine, IL, $25,000. For ENCORE award for Generation Exchange/Senior Exchange Program. 95.
Doctor William M. Scholl College of Podiatric Medicine, Chicago, IL, $22,715. Toward research to describe mechanical characteristics responsible for differences in susceptibility of articular cartilage from different joints to arthritic diseases. 95.
Doctor William M. Scholl College of Podiatric Medicine, Chicago, IL, $22,715. Toward second-year support of research to describe mechanical characteristics responsible for differences in susceptibility of articular cartilage from different joints to arthritic diseases. 95.
Donors Forum of Chicago, Chicago, IL, $12,399. For membership dues. 95.
Duke University Medical Center, Durham, NC, $27,000. To develop measure of religious coping in medically ill elderly. 95.
Dunn County Office on Aging, Menomonie, WI, $69,828. For mental health counseling to older adults in their homes in rural Wisconsin county. 95.
Edgewater Shores Senior Foundation, Chicago, IL, $150,000. For support services to low-income elderly residents of Edgewater Shores for Independent Retirement Living. 95.
El Valor Corporation, Chicago, IL, $30,000. To hire coordinator to develop intergenerational program centered in Pilsen neighborhood. 95.
Episcopal Church Council at University of Chicago, Chicago, IL, $10,000. For intergenerational productions at Shoestring Theater. 95.
Florida Foundation on Active Aging, Tallahassee, FL, $24,850. To continue project designed to develop sense of community among seniors who have retired to Florida. 95.
Foundation for Rural Housing, Madison, WI, $180,400. To begin volunteer home repair program for low-income senior homeowners in rural counties in Wisconsin. 95.
Franciscan Village, Lemont, IL, $11,335. To develop intergenerational volunteer program. 95.
Franciscan Village, Lemont, IL, $11,335. For intergenerational volunteer program. 95.
George Washington University Medical Center, DC, $493,290. For SourceBook on Dying project. 95.
Glenkirk Foundation, Northbrook, IL, $24,000. For continued expansion of Masters program serving developmentally disabled seniors. 95.
Greek-American Community Services, Chicago, IL, $91,000. To expand adult day care program. 95.
Heartland Alliance for Human Needs and Human Rights, Chicago, IL, $45,000. For comprehensive supportive services to low-income elderly residents of Rebecca Walker House. 95.
Hudson Institute, Indianapolis, IN, $15,000. For publication of previously funded project on pensions. 95.
Illinois Association of Chiefs of Police, Springfield, IL, $69,000. Toward project to develop protocols in reporting, investigating and prosecuting of crimes against older adults in Illinois. 95.
Illinois State University, Normal, IL, $24,994. For model program to inform community leaders and service providers in Illinois about rural older adults' needs and to facilitate planning to address those needs. 95.
Indiana University, Bloomington, IN, $46,145. For training for work with family and other survivors of geriatric suicide. 95.
Indochinese Pastoral Center, Chicago, IL, $103,613. To expand services to Vietnamese elderly and to establish drop-in center. 95.
Jane Addams Senior Caucus, Chicago, IL, $35,000. For Ruth Shriman Affordable Housing Campaign. 95.
Korean American Senior Center, Chicago, IL, $75,000. To develop home-based care management program. 95.
Law Enforcement Foundation of Illinois, Springfield, IL, $69,000. Toward project to develop protocols in reporting, investigating and prosecuting of crimes against older adults in Illinois. 95.
Lifelink Housing Corporation, Bensenville, IL, $87,100. To maintain intergenerational program and expand program to all extended care facilities and Illinois senior housing residences. 95.
Little Brothers Friends of the Elderly, Chicago, IL, $10,000. For intergenerational programming between college students and older adults. 95.
Logan Square Neighborhood Association, Chicago, IL, $60,000. For continuation of Senior Citizen Organizing Project. 95.
Lourdes College, Sylvania, OH, $101,640. For model apartment for promoting independence in older adults and training opportunities for students. 95.
Loyola University Medical Center, Maywood, IL, $75,582. For prognostic markers for prostate cancer. 95.
Lutheran Family Mission, Chicago, IL, $12,000. To develop program to identify and train senior leaders. 95.
Mae Volen Senior Center, Boca Raton, FL, $25,000. For passenger van for transportation for elderly adult day care clients. 95.
Marquette University, Milwaukee, WI, $11,506. For marketing and distribution effort for materials produced from Multicultural Focus on Advance Directives Project also funded by Retirement Research Foundation. 95.
Medic Alert Foundation (MAF) International, Turlock, CA, $23,000. For reprinting of Geriatric Emergencies: An EMT Teaching Manual. 95.
National Academy of Social Insurance, DC, $24,500. Toward research internship program in long-term care financing. 95.
National Committee for Responsive Philanthropy, DC, $10,000. Toward advocacy effort on behalf of retention of social justice organizations in workplace giving programs. 95.
Newberry Academy, Friends of, Chicago, IL, $10,000. For intergenerational programming. 95.
Nonprofit Financial Center, Chicago, IL, $30,000. To provide Retirement Research Foundation grantees with intensive financial management technical assistance. 95.
Northwest Neighborhood Federation, Chicago, IL, $10,000. For Senior Project. 95.
Northwestern University, Evanston, IL, $20,539. For project examining mission of nursing homes under health care reform and developing strategies for 21st century. 95.
Northwestern University, Buehler Center on Aging, Evanston, IL, $32,000. For project, Accessing the Media: The Use of Film and Video in Teaching Gerontology. 95.
Norton Gallery and School of Art, West Palm Beach, FL, $10,000. For museum services targeted to senior citizens. 95.
Older Womens League of Illinois, Chicago, IL, $22,810. To develop new chapters and increase awareness of issues. 95.
Palatine Township Senior Citizens Council, Palatine, IL, $15,000. For Senior Centers/Minority Outreach project. 95.
Peoples Reinvestment and Development Effort, Chicago, IL, $10,000. To purchase furniture for SRO units in Rebecca Walker Housing Complex. 95.
Pilsen Coalition for Families, Chicago, IL, $10,000. To develop community-based health care program for seniors. 95.
Polish Welfare Association, Chicago, IL, $21,235. For program for elderly Polish residents of Chicago. 95.
Prairie State Legal Services, Rockford, IL, $25,000. For ENCORE award for Senior Citizens Legal Services. 95.
Provenant Health Foundation/Provenant Health Partners, Denver, CO, $267,298. To implement and study differentiated practice model of nursing care for older adults in long-term care. 95.
Public/Private Ventures, Philadelphia, PA, $200,000. To mobilize time, talent and resources of older Americans on behalf of children in poverty. 95.
Redemptorist Parish Ministry Services to the Aging and Needy, Kansas City, MO, $35,000. For expansion of senior center. 95.
RespiteCare, Evanston, IL, $25,000. For ENCORE award for Respite Care Older Adult Program. 95.
Rush-Presbyterian-Saint Lukes Medical Center, Chicago, IL, $45,000. For research to evaluate whether integrated, multimodality program of health promotion practices can slow or possibly reverse aging processes in elderly. 95.
Sacred Heart Home, Avilla, IN, $25,860. Toward expansion of Alzheimer's special care unit. 95.
Saint Joseph Health Care Foundation, Chicago, IL, $45,000. For research to evaluate whether integrated, multimodality program of health promotion practices can slow or possibly reverse aging processes in elderly. 95.
Saint Josephs Home for the Elderly of Little Sisters of the Poor, Palatine, IL, $100,000. Toward construction of low-income independent living apartments. 95.
Saint Mary of the Assumption Church, Elizabeth, NJ, $10,083. For Senior Program. 95.
Saint Vincent de Paul Center, Chicago, IL, $25,000. For Laboure House, intergenerational assisted-living facility for elderly poor. 95.
Seguin Services, Cicero, IL, $17,541. For project integrating older adults with developmental

disabilities into community senior programs. 95.
Senior Home Sharing, Lombard, IL, $40,000. For outreach campaign to increase awareness of shared housing and to increase referral sources and referrals. 95.
Shepherds Centers of America, Kansas City, MO, $150,000. To expand number of Shepherds Centers nationally and create nationwide information network to serve older adults in communities where there is not a Shepherds Center. 95.
Simon Foundation for Continence, Wilmette, IL, $150,000. To develop national continence cooperative project. 95.
Sisters of the Holy Family of Nazareth, Monroe, CT, $15,000. For access to Elderhostel Program. 95.
South Austin Coalition Community Council, Chicago, IL, $20,000. To continue senior organizing project and to establish senior information and advocacy center. 95.
Southeast Asia Center, Chicago, IL, $10,000. To develop health and wellness program for seniors. 95.
Suburban Area Agency on Aging, Oak Park, IL, $200,000. For Collaborative Senior Advocate Program that trains seniors as advocates to assist other seniors. 95.
Swedish Covenant Hospital, Chicago, IL, $11,152. For psychiatric home visits for older adults. 95.
Temple Judea Mizpah, Skokie, IL, $10,773. For senior program, The Place. 95.
Temple University, Philadelphia, PA, $158,887. For intergenerational program at Elmire Jeffries Nursing Home involving residents, community residents and university students. 95.
Terra Nova Films, Chicago, IL, $10,000. Toward video examining impact of guardianship upon older adults and ethical issues surrounding guardianship decisionmaking process. 95.
Third Baptist Church, San Francisco, CA, $12,500. For senior ministry. 95.
Tufts University, Medford, MA, $210,758. For research on decisionmaking process used by HMOs to utilize medical technology to treat elderly patients and to develop and disseminate practical guidelines on use of technology by range of managed care and other providers. 95.
United Methodist Homes and Services, Chicago, IL, $65,000. Toward renovation of apartment building to provide low-cost independent living for seniors. 95.
University of Alabama, Birmingham, AL, $95,592. For research project to investigate impact of reading group activities on behavior of Alzheimer patients. 95.
University of California, Los Angeles, CA, $32,000. For prototype microphone array system for improved hearing aid preprocessor. 95.
University of Chicago Hospitals, Chicago, IL, $138,761. For study to describe what happens to older patients prior to, during and following presentation at Emergency Department. 95.
University of Louisville, Louisville, KY, $76,144. For research project to investigate role of estrogen in neurodegenerative disorders in women. 95.
University of Minnesota, Minneapolis, MN, $203,378. For study to determine whether hospital discharge planning process featuring professional-patient partnership improves outcomes for elderly patients with congestive heart failure and their caregivers. 95.
University of South Florida, Tampa, FL, $194,917. To establish certification program providing training to nurses aides on effective care and management of confused and memory-impaired older adults. 95.
University of South Florida, Institute on Aging, Tampa, FL, $11,000. For faculty intensives to develop interdisciplinary linkage of core courses for new Ph.D. in Aging studies. 95.
W. W. Outreach, Chicago, IL, $10,000. For intergenerational housing program. 95.
Westside Health Authority, Chicago, IL, $10,000. For intergenerational program linking seniors and students at Austin High School. 95.
White Crane Senior Health Center, Chicago, IL, $36,551. To expand wellness classes and to evaluate all program services. 95.
YMCA of Metropolitan Chicago, Chicago, IL, $300,000. For senior residents to maintain their independence through development of supportive program of case management health services, social and recreational activities and family reunification. 95.

301
Hulda B. & Maurice L. Rothschild Foundation

c/o First National Bank of Chicago
791 Elm St.
Winnetka 60093 (847) 441-3060
Contact: Donald A. Kress, V.P., First National Bank of Chicago
FAX: (847) 441-0718

Established in 1981 in IL.
Donor(s): Hulda B. Rothschild.‡
Financial data (yr. ended 12/31/94): Assets, $8,498,979 (M); expenditures, $346,483; qualifying distributions, $270,954, including $256,230 for 13 grants (high: $59,495; low: $5,000; average: $5,000-$10,000).
Purpose and activities: "To improve the quality of life for older adults in the Chicago metropolitan area; the foundation is interested in innovative projects which develop and/or demonstrate new approaches and creative solutions to the problems of older adults and which have the potential for significant impact, especially programs of cultural outreach."
Fields of interest: Arts/cultural programs; Aging, centers & services; Aging.
Types of support: Program development, publication, seed money, research, matching funds.
Limitations: Giving primarily in the metropolitan Chicago, IL, area. No support for projects outside the U.S. No grants to individuals, or for general purposes, construction, operating budgets, endowment or development campaigns, or scholarships; no loans.
Publications: Application guidelines.
Application information: Priority given to organizations which have clear objectives, well-defined outcomes or impact, and cost effective approaches. Application form not required.
Initial approach: Letter
Copies of proposal: 1
Deadline(s): None
Final notification: 30 to 45 days
Officer and Trustees:* Robert N. Mayer,* Pres.; Beatrice Mayer, First National Bank of Chicago.
Number of staff: None.
EIN: 366752787

302
Elsie O. and Philip D. Sang Foundation

180 East Pearson St., Apt. 5805
Chicago 60611
Contact: Elsie O. Sang, Pres.

Established in 1954.
Financial data (yr. ended 10/31/93): Assets, $2,238,558 (M); expenditures, $154,270; qualifying distributions, $154,270, including $151,650 for 34 grants (high: $75,000; low: $100).
Fields of interest: Arts, multipurpose centers/programs; Education; Hospitals (general); Children & youth, services; Aging, centers & services; Jewish federated giving programs; Jewish agencies & temples.
Limitations: Giving primarily in Chicago, IL. No grants to individuals.
Application information: Application form not required.
Initial approach: Letter
Deadline(s): None
Board meeting date(s): As required
Officers: Elsie O. Sang, Pres.; Bernard G. Sang, Secy.
Number of staff: None.
EIN: 366214200

303
Sara Lee Foundation

Three First National Plaza
Chicago 60602-4260 (312) 558-8448
Contact: Robin S. Tryloff, Exec. Dir.

Incorporated in 1981 in IL.
Donor(s): Sara Lee Corporation.
Foundation type: Company-sponsored
Financial data (yr. ended 07/01/95): Assets, $11,434,550 (M); gifts received, $667,309; expenditures, $7,574,907; qualifying distributions, $5,517,075, including $4,213,589 for 372 grants (high: $400,000; low: $2,500; average: $2,500-$7,500) and $1,303,486 for 5,349 employee matching gifts.
Purpose and activities: Primary focus is on social service organizations assisting women, the homeless, and the disadvantaged, and arts and cultural organizations.
Fields of interest: Visual arts; Museums; Performing arts; Dance; Theater; Music; Arts/cultural programs; Child development, education; Adult/continuing education; Adult education—literacy & basic skills; Libraries/library science; Reading; AIDS; AIDS research; Employment; Food services; Housing/shelter, development; Human services; Children & youth, services; Youth, services; Child development, services; Family services; Aging, centers & services; Women, centers & services; Minorities/immigrants, centers & services; Homeless, human services; Urban/community development; Community development; Minorities; Disabled; Aging;

Women; Economically disadvantaged; Homeless.
Types of support: General/operating support, continuing support, annual campaigns, program development, employee matching gifts, employee-related scholarships.
Limitations: Giving primarily in the Chicago, IL, area. No support for elementary or secondary schools, religious organizations, disease-specific health organizations, fraternal, political, or veterans' organizations, or national or international organizations with limited relationships to local company operations. No grants to individuals, or for fundraising events, goodwill advertising, endowments, or capital campaigns.
Publications: Informational brochure (including application guidelines), application guidelines.
Application information: Application form required.
Initial approach: Letter or telephone
Copies of proposal: 1
Deadline(s): 1st working day of Mar., Sept., or Dec.
Board meeting date(s): 8 to 10 weeks following deadline
Final notification: 1 to 2 weeks after Mgmt. Donations Comm. meetings
Officers and Directors:* Michael E. Murphy,* Pres.; Janet Kelly, V.P. and Secy.; Maureen Culhane, Treas.; Robin S. Tryloff, Exec. Dir.; John H. Bryan, Elynor Williams.
Staff: Valerie Cobb, Grants Coodinator.
Number of staff: 7 full-time professional.
EIN: 363150460

304
Dr. Scholl Foundation
11 South LaSalle St., Suite 2100
Chicago 60603 (312) 782-5210
Contact: Pamela Scholl, Pres.

Incorporated in 1947 in IL.
Donor(s): William M. Scholl, M.D.‡
Financial data (yr. ended 12/31/94): Assets, $127,788,300 (M); expenditures, $9,906,647; qualifying distributions, $9,032,099, including $8,536,800 for 356 grants (high: $500,000; low: $2,000; average: $5,000-$50,000).
Purpose and activities: Support for private education at all levels, including elementary, secondary, and post-secondary schools, colleges and universities, and medical and nursing institutions; general charitable programs, including grants to hospitals, and programs for children, the developmentally disabled, and senior citizens; and civic, cultural, social welfare, economic, and religious activities.
Fields of interest: Film/video; Visual arts; Museums; Performing arts; Dance; Theater; History & archaeology; Arts/cultural programs; Elementary/secondary education; Early childhood education; Child development, education; Elementary school/education; Secondary school/education; Higher education; Business school/education; Law school/education; Medical school/education; Adult education—literacy & basic skills; Libraries/library science; Reading; Education; Natural resource conservation & protection; Animal welfare; Hospitals (general); Nursing care; Health care; Mental health/crisis services; Cancer; Heart/circulatory disease; AIDS; Alcoholism; Health organizations; Medical research; Cancer research; Heart/circulatory research; AIDS research; Delinquency prevention/services; Legal services; Housing/shelter, development; Human services; Children & youth, services; Youth, services; Child development, services; Family services; Hospices; Aging, centers & services; Minorities/immigrants, centers & services; Homeless, human services; Civil rights; Community development; Jewish federated giving programs; Engineering & technology; Computer science; Science; Economics; Government/public administration; Roman Catholic agencies & churches; Religion; Minorities; Disabled; Aging; Economically disadvantaged; Homeless.
Types of support: Building/renovation, equipment, endowment funds, program development, conferences/seminars, fellowships, research.
Limitations: No support for public education. No grants to individuals, or for general support, continuing support, operating budgets, deficit financing, or unrestricted purposes.
Publications: Informational brochure (including application guidelines), application guidelines.
Application information: The scholarship program for the children of company employees has been discontinued. Application form required.
Copies of proposal: 1
Deadline(s): May 15
Board meeting date(s): Feb., May, Aug., and Oct.
Final notification: Nov.
Officers and Trustees:* William H. Scholl, Chair.; Pamela Scholl,* Pres.; Jack E. Scholl,* V.P. and Secy.; Leonard J. Knirko, Treas.; George W. Alexander, Neil Flanagin, Jeanne M. Scholl, Michael W. Scholl, Susan Scholl, Douglas C. Witherspoon.
Number of staff: 3 full-time professional; 2 part-time professional; 3 full-time support.
EIN: 366068724
Grants for Aging:
Alzheimers Disease and Related Disorders Association, Chicago, IL, $15,000. Toward Pilot research grant. 94.
Alzheimers Disease and Related Disorders Association, Skokie, IL, $15,000. For family support programs. 94.
Casa Central, Chicago, IL, $15,000. Toward La Posada program. 94.
Christian Appalachian Project, Lancaster, KY, $15,000. For elderly visitation program. 94.
Illinois Alliance for Aging, Chicago, IL, $10,000. For elderly substance abuse program. 94.
Jane Addams Senior Caucus, Chicago, IL, $10,000. For general support. 94.
Marklund Childrens Home, Bloomingdale, IL, $15,000. Toward bus. 94.
Maryhaven, Glenview, IL, $20,000. For renovations in Alzheimer's Unit. 94.
Miami Jewish Home and Hospital for the Aged, Miami, FL, $25,000. For training project. 94.
North Shore Senior Center, Northfield, IL, $25,000. For health promotion program. 94.
United Cerebral Palsy of Will County, Joliet, IL, $15,000. For in-home respite and support services. 94.
Visiting Nurse Association of Chicago, Chicago, IL, $20,000. Toward elderly care. 94.

305
Sears Merchandise Group (SMG) Giving Program
c/o Sears Merchandise Group
Dept. 903 (BSC 38-25), Sears Tower 903 BSC 38-23
Chicago 60684 (312) 875-2500
Contact: Paula A. Banks, Dir., Community Rels.

Purpose and activities: Throughout the decades, Sears has conscientiously demonstrated its good corporate citizenship through an active program of community relations including contributions. The company's tradition of philanthropy began in the early 1900's and has been shaped by the changing nature of American society. An early Sears-sponsored animal husbandry program credited with upgrading the quality of livestock for American farmers bears little resemblance to today's advanced job training programs supported by Sears. Today, all Sears contributions are to tax-exempt organizations with 501(c)(3) status. Sears has a special interest in programs that are targeted to its national program priorities: education and family related issues and volunteerism among its associates.
Fields of interest: Museums; Arts/cultural programs; Early childhood education; Child development, education; Elementary school/education; Secondary school/education; Vocational education; Adult education—literacy & basic skills; Reading; Education; Wildlife preservation & protection; Health care; Health associations; Employment; Recreation; Human services; Youth, services; Child development, services; Family services; Aging, centers & services; Women, centers & services; Minorities/immigrants, centers & services; Community development; Voluntarism promotion; Government/public administration; Minorities; Disabled; Aging; Women; Economically disadvantaged.
Types of support: Annual campaigns, donated equipment, donated products.
Limitations: Giving limited to tax exempt organizations serving the local Chicago area or nationally. No support for religious, fraternal, foreign, political, or labor organizations. No grants to individuals, or for advertising in books, brochures, pamphlets, or yearbooks.
Application information: Store General Managers handle giving.
Initial approach: Letter to nearest company facility
Copies of proposal: 1
Deadline(s): None
Board meeting date(s): Periodically; varies by city
Final notification: Varies by city
Number of staff: None.

306
The Siragusa Foundation
919 North Michigan Ave., Suite 2701
Chicago 60611 (312) 280-0833
Contact: John R. Siragusa, Pres.

Trust established in 1950 in IL; incorporated in 1980.
Donor(s): Ross D. Siragusa.‡
Financial data (yr. ended 12/31/95): Assets, $14,647,576 (M); expenditures, $687,679; qualifying distributions, $601,850, including $601,850 for 89 grants (high: $30,000; low: $100; average: $6,762).
Purpose and activities: Emphasis on higher education and medical research; support also for cultural activities, child development programs, education of the handicapped, and care of the elderly.
Fields of interest: Humanities; Arts/cultural programs; Child development, education; Higher education; Adult/continuing education; Education; Environment; Hospitals (general); Health care; Cancer; Heart/circulatory disease; Health organizations; Medical research; Cancer research; Heart/circulatory research; Food services; Human services; Youth, services; Child development, services; Aging, centers & services; Homeless, human services; Disabled; Aging; Economically disadvantaged; Homeless; General charitable giving.
Types of support: General/operating support, equipment, program development, scholarship funds, research, matching funds.
Limitations: Giving primarily in the Midwest, with emphasis on the metropolitan Chicago, IL, area. No grants to individuals, or for endowment funds; no loans.
Publications: Program policy statement, application guidelines.
Application information: Submit proposal only when invited. Application form not required.
Initial approach: Letter
Copies of proposal: 1
Deadline(s): Jan. 15 and Oct. 15
Board meeting date(s): Mar. and Dec.
Final notification: 2 to 3 months
Officer and Directors:* John R. Siragusa,* Pres.; Roy M. Adams, George E. Driscoll, John E. Hicks, Jr., Melvyn H. Schneider, Martha P. Siragusa, Richard D. Siragusa, Ross D. Siragusa, Jr., Sinclair C. Siragusa, James B. Wilson.
Number of staff: 1 full-time professional; 1 full-time support.
EIN: 363100492

307
Square D Foundation
1415 South Roselle Rd.
Palatine 60067
Contact: James R. White, Secy.

Incorporated in 1956 in MI.
Donor(s): Square D Co.
Foundation type: Company-sponsored
Financial data (yr. ended 12/31/95): Assets, $334,277 (M); expenditures, $1,711,519; qualifying distributions, $1,711,519, including $1,711,519 for 298 grants (average: $500-$5,000).
Purpose and activities: Emphasis on community funds and education; support also for hospitals, health agencies, the arts, and employee-related scholarships administered by National Merit Scholarship Corp.
Fields of interest: Arts/cultural programs; Education; Health care; Youth, services; Disabled; Aging; Economically disadvantaged.
Types of support: General/operating support, capital campaigns, building/renovation, professorships, employee matching gifts, employee-related scholarships.
Limitations: Giving primarily in areas of company operations: NC, SC, IA, FL, OH, IL, IN, TN, KY, NE, WI, MO, TX, and CA. No support for organizations already receiving support through United Way, religious organizations, or labor unions. No grants to individuals.
Publications: Application guidelines.
Application information: Submit application to the plant closest to applicant.
Initial approach: Letter; no telephone inquiries
Copies of proposal: 1
Deadline(s): June to Aug. for following fiscal year
Board meeting date(s): As necessary
Final notification: Mar. of fiscal year
Officers and Directors:* W.W. Kurczewski,* Pres.; W.P. Brink, V.P. and Treas.; R.P. Fiorani, V.P. and Treas.; Frank B. Sullivan,* V.P. and Treas.; James R. White, Secy.
Number of staff: 1 part-time support.
EIN: 366054195

308
Irvin Stern Foundation
Boylston Bldg.
116 West Illinois
Chicago 60610 (312) 321-9402
Contact: Jeffrey Epstein, Trustee

Trust established in 1957 in IL.
Donor(s): Irvin Stern.‡
Financial data (yr. ended 09/30/94): Assets, $9,446,478 (M); expenditures, $665,454; qualifying distributions, $583,316, including $552,900 for 45 grants (high: $110,000; low: $1,000; average: $5,000-$25,000).
Purpose and activities: Emphasis on meeting the needs of the Jewish community in the U.S. and Israel; efforts to combat mental illness; vocational training and help for the aged; and improving urban living conditions via neighborhood organizations.
Fields of interest: Vocational education; Education; Mental health/crisis services; Employment; Food services; Human services; Aging, centers & services; Homeless, human services; Community development; Jewish federated giving programs; Public affairs; Jewish agencies & temples; Aging; Homeless.
Types of support: General/operating support, continuing support, annual campaigns, building/renovation, equipment, emergency funds, conferences/seminars, seed money, matching funds.
Limitations: Giving primarily in Chicago, IL. No support for religious or political purposes. No grants to individuals, or for endowment funds, deficit financing, building funds, research, or advertising or program books.
Publications: Application guidelines, program policy statement, 990-PF.
Application information: Application form required.
Initial approach: Letter
Copies of proposal: 1
Deadline(s): Submit proposal preferably in Mar. or Aug.; deadlines Apr. 1 and Sept. 1
Board meeting date(s): Apr. and Oct.
Trustees: E. Allan Epstein, Jeffrey Epstein, Stuart Epstein, Arthur Winter, Dorothy G. Winter, Stanley Winter.
Number of staff: None.
EIN: 366047947

309
Sulzer Family Foundation
1940 West Irving Park Rd.
Chicago 60613 (773) 327-4700
Contact: John J. Hoellen, Pres.

Incorporated in 1956 in IL.
Donor(s): Grace E. Sulzer.‡
Financial data (yr. ended 12/31/93): Assets, $3,955,732 (M); expenditures, $198,724; qualifying distributions, $179,300, including $179,300 for 80 grants (high: $15,000; low: $100; average: $100-$15,000).
Purpose and activities: Giving for education, including higher, secondary, elementary, and adult education; programs for youth and the aged; community development; libraries; and museums and history.
Fields of interest: Museums; History & archaeology; Elementary school/education; Secondary school/education; Higher education; Adult/continuing education; Libraries/library science; Education; Delinquency prevention/services; Youth, services; Aging, centers & services; Community development; Aging.
Types of support: General/operating support, continuing support, scholarship funds.
Limitations: Applications not accepted. Giving limited to the Ravenswood and Lakeview areas of Chicago, IL. No grants to individuals.
Application information: Contributes only to pre-selected organizations.
Board meeting date(s): Nov.
Officers and Directors:* John J. Hoellen,* Pres.; Rev. George Rice,* Secy.; Arthur Telcser,* Treas.; Richard Bjorklund, Robert B. Hoellen.
Number of staff: 1 full-time support.
EIN: 362466016

310
Swiss Benevolent Society of Chicago
c/o Scholarship Committee
P.O. Box 2137
Chicago 60690-2137 (630) 858-7286

Established in 1872 in IL.
Financial data (yr. ended 12/31/94): Assets, $1,271,322 (M); gifts received, $10,186; expenditures, $81,914; qualifying distributions, $61,394, including $48,822 for 39 grants to individuals (high: $2,650; low: $51).
Purpose and activities: To aid individuals of Swiss descent; giving includes scholarships for undergraduate study and relief assistance in case of need or emergency.
Fields of interest: Higher education; Education; Human services; Aging, centers & services; Aging.
Types of support: Scholarship funds, grants to individuals, scholarships—to individuals.
Limitations: Giving primarily in IL and southern WI.
Application information: Application form required.

Initial approach: Letter between Nov. 15 and Feb. 1
Deadline(s): Scholarship applications must be postmarked by Feb. 1
Final notification: No later than May 10 for scholarship winners
Officers: Kurt Engel, Pres.; Erdmann Schmocker, V.P.; Cornelia Ulrich, Secy.; Werner Gartner, Treas.
Directors: Samuel Burkhardt, Ursula Furrer, Valerie Z. Gallagher, Egon R. Jaeggin, Erwin Manenti, Charles L. Michod, Jr., Walter Peyer, Kenneth Schelbert, Erdmann Schmocker.
Number of staff: None.
EIN: 366076395

311
Walgreen Giving Program

200 Wilmot Rd., MS:4DD
Deerfield 60015 (847) 940-2856
Contact: Ruth Crane, Rep., Corp. Rels.

Established in 1901.
Purpose and activities: Supports a variety of programs including: social services, with giving to the United Way and programs for alcohol and drug rehabilitation, underprivileged children and emotionally disturbed children, youth service, race relations and rehabilitation programs; and arts and culture, including theater and symphonies. Individuals and national organizations are considered for funding.
Fields of interest: Theater; Music; Arts/cultural programs; Early childhood education; Child development, education; Secondary school/education; Higher education; Business school/education; Adult/continuing education; Adult education—literacy & basic skills; Reading; Natural resource conservation & protection; Environment; Medical care, rehabilitation; Pharmacology; Health care; Substance abuse, services; Mental health/crisis services; Cancer; Heart/circulatory disease; AIDS; Alcoholism; Health organizations; Cancer research; Heart/circulatory research; AIDS research; Food services; Human services; Children & youth, services; Youth, services; Child development, services; Family services; Aging, centers & services; Minorities/immigrants, centers & services; Homeless, human services; International affairs, goodwill promotion; Race/intergroup relations; Civil rights; Community development; Federated giving programs; Roman Catholic federated giving programs; Jewish agencies & temples; Minorities; Native Americans; Disabled; Aging; Homeless.
Types of support: General/operating support, annual campaigns, capital campaigns, building/renovation, equipment, program development.
Limitations: Giving primarily in headquarters city and major operating areas. No support for international organizations, fraternal, veterans', labor, or religious organizations, political, lobbying, or voter registration organizations, sports teams or events, national headquarters of singe-disease agencies, except those identified through Walgreens' annual special program, additional requests from organizations or institutions already receiving Walgreen Co. grant, scholarship, or in-kind support within the previous 12 months, or organizations that might pose a conflict with the corporation's goals, products, customers, or employees. No grants to individuals, or for hospitals, travel, fundraising events, capital campaigns or projects, or program advertising.
Application information: Trade and Corp. Rels. office handles giving. Application form not required.
Initial approach: Letter or proposal to headquarters. Telephone inquiries and faxes are not accepted
Deadline(s): None
Board meeting date(s): Monthly and as needed
Final notification: 90 days
Number of staff: 2 full-time professional; 2 part-time professional; 1 full-time support; 1 part-time support.

312
Washington Square Health Foundation, Inc.

875 North Michigan Ave., Suite 3516
Chicago 60611 (312) 664-6488
Contact: Howard Nochumson, Exec. Dir.

Established in 1985 in IL.
Donor(s): Henrotin Hospital.
Financial data (yr. ended 09/30/95): Assets, $25,613,604 (M); gifts received, $3,152; expenditures, $1,396,238; qualifying distributions, $1,405,597, including $924,065 for 56 grants (high: $50,000; low: $150; average: $16,501) and $233,800 for 2 program-related investments.
Purpose and activities: "To promote and maintain access to adequate primary health care," through grants for medical and nursing education scholarships, medical research, and direct health care services.
Fields of interest: Medical school/education; Nursing school/education; Nursing care; Nursing home/convalescent facility; Health care; AIDS; Medical research; AIDS research; Domestic violence prevention; Minorities; Disabled; Aging; Women; People with AIDS (PWAs); Gays/lesbians; Immigrants/refugees; Homeless.
Types of support: Equipment, program development, scholarship funds, research.
Limitations: Giving primarily in the Chicago, IL, area. No grants to individuals, or for general operating or administrative expenses, land acquisition, or construction.
Publications: Annual report, application guidelines.
Application information: Application form required.
Initial approach: Pre-application form
Copies of proposal: 4
Deadline(s): June 1 and Dec. 1
Officers and Directors:* Angelo P. Creticos, M.D.,* Pres.; Mrs. Arthur M. Wirtz, Jr.,* V.P.; William B. Friedeman,* Secy.; John C. York,* Treas.; Howard Nochumson, Exec. Dir.; Robert S. Kirby, Howard M. McCue III, Richard B. Patterson, D.P.M., William N. Werner, M.D., Bill G. Wiley.
Number of staff: 2 full-time professional.
EIN: 361210140

313
Wheat Ridge Ministries

One Pierce Place, Suite 250E
Itasca 60143-2634 (630) 766-9066
Contact: Karen Jurgensen, Dir. of Communications
Additional tel.: (800) 762-6748; FAX: (630) 766-9622

Founded in 1905 in CO.
Financial data (yr. ended 06/30/95): Assets, $6,751,423 (L); gifts received, $1,409,686; expenditures, $2,203,336; qualifying distributions, $1,079,511, including $810,939 for 65 grants (high: $60,000; low: $3,000; average: $1,000-$60,000).
Purpose and activities: Provides start up funds for health and healing projects for people of all ages throughout the world. It seeks to assist Lutheran congregations, judicatories, organizations, and other entities by providing seed money for new ministries that serve the whole person. Focus is on short-term projects of one, two, or three years in hopes that these awards help to start new projects which will continue with funding from other sources. Emphasis is on new ministries which can be replicated in other areas and will provide health and hope to those people involved.
Fields of interest: Health care; AIDS; Health organizations; AIDS research; Human services; Youth, services; Aging, centers & services; Homeless, human services; Protestant agencies & churches; Religion; Aging; Homeless; Brazil; India; Philippines; China.
Types of support: Seed money.
Limitations: Giving on an international basis. No grants to individuals, or for deficit financing, capital funding, or endowment or ordinary ongoing operating expenses.
Publications: Occasional report, newsletter, grants list, informational brochure, financial statement, application guidelines.
Application information: Application form required.
Initial approach: Outline of proposal or telephone
Copies of proposal: 2
Deadline(s): Feb. 1 and Aug. 1
Board meeting date(s): May and Nov.
Final notification: May and Nov.
Officers and Directors:* Rev. Norm Eitrheim,* Chair.; Rev. Dr. Thomas R. Zehnder,* Vice-Chair.; Richard W. Bimler,* Pres.; Rev. Bryant Clancy, Jr.,* Secy.; Jerry T. Thompson,* Treas.; Ralph Bohlmann, Gloria Edwards, Gerhard Freche, Mary Wiese Gundelach, Albert Huegli, Erin Johnson, Lita Brusick Johnson, Candace Mueller, Anzara Norton, Dorothea Nuechterlein, Curtis W. Pohl, John E. Puelle, and six additional directors.
Number of staff: 4 full-time professional; 3 full-time support; 1 part-time support.
EIN: 840404924

314
Frederick B. Woods/Molly B. Bodoff Charitable Trust
c/o First National Bank of Chicago
One First National Plaza, Suite 0111
Chicago 60670-0111

Established in 1991 in IL.
Financial data (yr. ended 02/28/95): Assets, $148 (M); gifts received, $125,000; expenditures, $75,911; qualifying distributions, $75,149, including $75,000 for 2 grants (high: $50,000; low: $25,000).
Fields of interest: AIDS; AIDS research; Aging, centers & services; Aging.
Limitations: Applications not accepted. Giving primarily in Chicago, IL and Los Angeles, CA. No grants to individuals.
Application information: Contributes only to pre-selected organizations.
Trustee: First National Bank of Chicago.
EIN: 366923866
Grants for Aging:
Gathering Place, Chicago, IL, $25,000. 95.

INDIANA

315
Bloomington Community Foundation, Inc.
005A Fountain Sq.
Bloomington 47404 (812) 333-9016
Contact: John D. Mulholland, Exec. Dir.

Established in 1990 in IN.
Foundation type: Community
Financial data (yr. ended 12/31/94): Assets, $1,150,000 (M); gifts received, $1,050,000; expenditures, $135,000, including $114,000 for grants.
Fields of interest: Arts/cultural programs; Environment, beautification programs; Health care; Youth, services; Human services; Aging.
Types of support: Program development, seed money, scholarship funds.
Limitations: Giving limited to Monroe County, IN.
Publications: Annual report, newsletter, informational brochure, application guidelines.
Application information: Application form required.
Initial approach: Letter or telephone
Board meeting date(s): Monthly
Officer: John D. Mulholland, Exec. Dir.
Number of staff: 1 part-time support.
EIN: 351811149

316
The Blue River Foundation, Inc.
P.O. Box 938
Shelbyville 46176 (317) 392-7955
Contact: Tom Hession, Pres.

Established in 1988 in IN.
Foundation type: Community
Financial data (yr. ended 12/31/95): Assets, $1,946,068 (M); gifts received, $1,287,450; expenditures, $84,705, including $12,297 for 4 grants and $13,290 for 33 grants to individuals (high: $2,500; low: $175; average: $175-$2,500).
Fields of interest: Theater; Education; Health care, reproductive health; Salvation Army; Aging.
Types of support: Endowment funds, scholarship funds, research, consulting services, grants to individuals, scholarships—to individuals, in-kind gifts, matching funds.
Limitations: Giving limited to Shelby County, IN.
Publications: Annual report, informational brochure, application guidelines.
Application information: Application form required.
Copies of proposal: 1
Deadline(s): 3rd Wednesday of each month for scholarships; Apr. 1, Aug. 1, and Dec. 1 for grants
Board meeting date(s): 3rd Wednesday of each month
Officers and Directors:* Tom Hession,* Pres.; Robert Claxton,* V.P.; Veanna Kessler,* Secy.; Micheal Vaught,* Treas.; Elaine Haehl, Exec. Dir.; Kent Apsley, Larry Browning, Mary Carter, Pete Cunningham, John C. DePrez, Jr., Richard Larkey, Kim Wickizer.
Number of staff: 1 part-time professional; 1 part-time support.
EIN: 351756331

317
Community Foundation of Boone County, Inc.
P.O. Box 92
410 West Oak St., Suite 8A
Zionsville 46077 (317) 873-0210
Contact: Elizabeth A. Casselman, Exec. Dir.
FAX: (317) 873-0219; Additional tel.: (317) 482-0024

Established in 1991 in IN.
Foundation type: Community
Financial data (yr. ended 12/31/95): Assets, $2,144,117 (M); gifts received, $84,832; expenditures, $92,075, including $115,990 for 21 grants (high: $45,010; low: $25) and $15,600 for 14 grants to individuals (high: $3,000; low: $500).
Fields of interest: Arts/cultural programs; Education; Environment; Health care; Domestic violence prevention; Human services; Disabled; Aging; Economically disadvantaged.
Types of support: Emergency funds, program development, scholarship funds, technical assistance, program-related investments/loans, grants to individuals, scholarships—to individuals, matching funds, student loans—to individuals.
Limitations: Giving limited to the Boone County, IN, area. No support for religious or political purposes. No grants to individuals (except for designated scholarship funds).
Publications: Annual report, application guidelines, informational brochure, newsletter.
Application information: Application form not required.
Initial approach: Letter
Copies of proposal: 9
Deadline(s): Mar. 31, June 30, Sept. 30, and Dec. 31
Board meeting date(s): Monthly
Officers and Directors:* Thomas E. Gruhl,* Chair.; Thomas J. Koppelman,* Pres.; G. Byington Pratt, M.D.,* V.P.; Michael J. Andreoli,* Secy.; Ronald L. Lind,* Treas.; Elizabeth A. Casselman, Exec. Dir.; Jean Acton, Paul E. Brooks, Roger L. Burrus, J. David Cook, Rollin M. Dick, Carol Sparks Drake, Kent M. Frandsen, Robert E. Guernsey, H. Pete Hudson, Charles M. Keenan, Margaret A. Larr, Larry W. Metzing, George Morton, Doug Vawter.
Number of staff: 1 part-time professional; 2 part-time support.
EIN: 351829585

318
William Higgins Trust for Avaline Fund
c/o Bank One Trust Group
111 Monument Circle, Suite 1501, P.O. Box 7700
Indianapolis 46277-0115
Application address: Robert A. Duff, National City Bank, Indiana, Lebanon, IN 46052; Tel.: (317) 482-3300

Financial data (yr. ended 10/31/95): Assets, $260,256 (M); expenditures, $138,077; qualifying distributions, $134,907, including $130,884 for 10 grants (high: $116,297; low: $252) and $3,000 for 30 grants to individuals of $100 each.
Fields of interest: Aging, centers & services; Women, centers & services; Aging; Women; Economically disadvantaged.
Types of support: Grants to individuals.
Limitations: Giving limited to residents of IN.
Application information:
Initial approach: Letter
Deadline(s): None
Trustee: Bank One Trust Group.
EIN: 356009209

319
Hook Drug Foundation
P.O. Box 199054
Indianapolis 46219
Contact: Donna Galerman, Secy.

Established in 1969 in IN.
Donor(s): Hook Drugs, Inc.
Foundation type: Company-sponsored
Financial data (yr. ended 12/31/95): Assets, $2,930,640 (M); gifts received, $482,799; expenditures, $210,907; qualifying distributions, $191,280, including $112,625 for 53 grants (high: $30,000; low: $50; average: $10-$20,000).
Purpose and activities: Giving to organizations involved in education, community, cultural, civic and health issues.
Fields of interest: Arts/cultural programs; Higher education; Medical school/education; Education; Pharmacology; Aging, centers & services; Community development; Federated giving programs; Disabled; Aging.
Types of support: General/operating support, scholarship funds.
Limitations: Giving primarily in IN, IL, MO, and OH.

Application information: Application form not required.
Initial approach: Varies with nature of request
Copies of proposal: 1
Deadline(s): None
Board meeting date(s): Jan., Mar., July, and Oct.
Officers and Directors:* James A. Richter,* Pres.; Mark A. Varnau,* V.P.; Donna M. Galerman,* Secy.; Stephen R. Kleifgen,* Treas.; James M. Rogers,* Exec. Dir.; Jeffrey B. Bailey, William B. Byrum, Thomas D. Cochrun, Thomas G. Dingledy, Michael H. Jones, Robert W. Martz, Barbara A. Nelson, Raymond W. Rizzo, Ann Hook Voliva.
Number of staff: 1 part-time support.
EIN: 237046664
Grants for Aging:
Williamsport-Attica Area Senior Center, Williamsport, IN, $500. 95.

320
The Indianapolis Foundation
615 North Alabama St., Rm. 119
Indianapolis 46204 (317) 634-7497
Contact: Kenneth L. Gladish, Ph.D., Exec. Dir.
FAX: (317) 684-0943

Established in 1916 in IN by resolution of trust.
Donor(s): James Proctor,‡ James E. Roberts,‡ Delavan Smith,‡ Charles N. Thompson,‡ Georgeanna Zumpfe.‡
Foundation type: Community
Financial data (yr. ended 12/31/94): Assets, $89,890,070 (M); gifts received, $1,515,574; expenditures, $4,775,808, including $4,035,358 for 113 grants (high: $468,755; low: $1,000; average: $10,000-$50,000).
Purpose and activities: Support for the areas of health, welfare, education, character building, and culture through grants for services to youth and children; health, and the handicapped; family and neighborhood services; civic and cultural programs; and general education.
Fields of interest: Arts/cultural programs; Education; Medical care, rehabilitation; Health care; Mental health/crisis services; Health organizations; Housing/shelter, development; Human services; Children & youth, services; Youth, services; Family services; Aging, centers & services; Community development; Federated giving programs; Government/public administration; Disabled; Aging.
Types of support: General/operating support, annual campaigns, capital campaigns, building/renovation, equipment, land acquisition, emergency funds, program development, seed money, program-related investments/loans, matching funds.
Limitations: Giving limited to Indianapolis and Marion County, IN. No support for religious or sectarian purposes. No grants to individuals, or for endowment funds, long term funding, and post-event funding; generally no loans.
Publications: Annual report (including application guidelines), newsletter, informational brochure.
Application information: Application form required.
Initial approach: Telephone or letter
Copies of proposal: 8
Deadline(s): Consult with program staff
Board meeting date(s): Feb., Apr., June, Sept., and Nov.
Final notification: Immediately following meetings
Officers and Trustees:* Milton O. Thompson,* Chair.; Martha D. Lamkin,* Vice-Chair.; Rexford C. Early,* Secy.; Kenneth L. Gladish, Ph.D., Exec. Dir.; Daniel R. Efroymson, Robert T. Grand, Charles A. Pechette.
Trustee Banks: Bank One, Indianapolis, N.A., Fifth Third Bank of Central Indiana, First of America Bank-Indiana, Huntington National Bank of Indiana, Key Trust Co. of Indiana, N.A., National City Bank, Indiana, NBD Bank, N.A., Union Bank & Trust Co.
Staff: Gregory Lynn, Assoc. Dir.; Rosemary Dorsa, Prog. Officer; Judith Ellyn, Prog. Officer.
Number of staff: 4 full-time professional; 1 part-time professional; 4 full-time support.
EIN: 350868115
Grants for Aging:
Heritage Place of Indianapolis, Indianapolis, IN, $25,000. For associate director to assist in providing programs and services to older adults. 95.
Little Sisters of the Poor, Indianapolis, IN, $57,667. For air conditioning units at Saint Augustine Home for the elderly. 95.

321
Jenn Foundation
P.O. Box 40038
Indianapolis 46240-0038
Contact: Gerald R. Jenn, Pres.

Established in 1963.
Financial data (yr. ended 12/31/95): Assets, $1,731,584 (M); expenditures, $96,715; qualifying distributions, $92,917, including $92,917 for 27 grants (high: $23,100; low: $250).
Fields of interest: Arts/cultural programs; Medical school/education; Hospitals (general); Human services; Christian agencies & churches; Disabled; Aging.
Types of support: Continuing support, capital campaigns.
Limitations: Giving primarily in IN. No grants to individuals.
Application information: Application form not required.
Initial approach: Letter
Deadline(s): None
Board meeting date(s): May and Dec.
Officers and Directors:* Gerald R. Jenn,* Pres.; Robert C. Bruner, Secy.; Clarence Long,* Treas.; Andrew J. Paine, Jr., Jerry Semler.
EIN: 356037030
Grants for Aging:
Alzheimers Association, $5,000. 94.

322
LaGrange County Community Foundation, Inc.
109 East Central Ave., Suite A
P.O. Box 228
LaGrange 46761 (219) 463-4363
Contact: Evelyn J. Evers, Exec. Dir.

Established in 1992 in IN.
Foundation type: Community
Financial data (yr. ended 12/31/95): Assets, $967,501 (L); gifts received, $292,667; expenditures, $148,614, including $82,929 for 35 grants (high: $16,396; low: $168; average: $168-$16,396) and $11,042 for in-kind gifts.
Fields of interest: Arts/cultural programs; Education; Environment; Health care; Children & youth, services; Human services; Community development; Aging.
Limitations: Giving limited to LaGrange County, IN.
Publications: Annual report, grants list, informational brochure (including application guidelines).
Application information: Application form not required.
Initial approach: Write for grant guidelines
Copies of proposal: 6
Deadline(s): Oct. 1 and Apr. 1
Board meeting date(s): 4th Thursday of every month
Final notification: June 1 and Dec. 1
Officers and Directors:* Gene Mory, Jr.,* Pres.; Ned Stump,* V.P.; Robert G. Lee, Jr.,* Secy.; Paul Hostetler, Jr.,* Treas.
Grants Committee: Carol Roberts, Chair.; Bill Huggins, Finance and Investment; Doreen Leer, Mktg. and Development.
Number of staff: 1 part-time professional; 1 part-time support.
EIN: 351834679

323
Cora Lembke Trust
c/o First National Bank
P.O. Box 2147
Valparaiso 46384-2147

Foundation type: Operating
Financial data (yr. ended 09/30/95): Assets, $135,196 (M); expenditures, $12,904; qualifying distributions, $12,904, including $11,400 for 4 grants to individuals (high: $3,600; low: $2,400).
Purpose and activities: Provide assistance to elderly women residents of Porter County, IN.
Fields of interest: Aging, centers & services; Aging.
Types of support: Grants to individuals.
Limitations: Giving limited to Porter County, IN.
Application information:
Initial approach: Letter
Deadline(s): None
Trustee: First National Bank.
EIN: 356043012

324
Eli Lilly and Company Corporate Contributions Program
Lilly Corporate Ctr.
Indianapolis 46285
Contact: Steve Twait, Secy., Eli Lilly and Co. Fdn.

Financial data (yr. ended 12/31/94): Total giving, $105,200,000, including $12,000,000 for 150 grants (high: $2,800,000; low: $500), $8,200,000 for 8,200 employee matching gifts and $85,000,000 for in-kind gifts.

Fields of interest: Museums; Arts/cultural programs; Health care; Mental health/crisis services; Cancer; Heart/circulatory disease; Nerve/muscle/bone disease; Alzheimer's disease; Diabetes; Health organizations.
Types of support: Employee matching gifts, donated equipment, donated products, in-kind gifts.
Limitations: Giving primarily in Indianapolis, IN, and other areas of company operations.
Publications: Corporate giving report (including application guidelines).
Application information: Application form required.
Initial approach: Proposal
Copies of proposal: 1
Deadline(s): None
Board meeting date(s): End of each quarter
Number of staff: 4 full-time professional.

325
Eli Lilly and Company Foundation

Lilly Corporate Ctr.
Indianapolis 46285
Contact: Steve Twait, Secy.

Incorporated in 1968 in IN.
Donor(s): Eli Lilly and Co.
Foundation type: Company-sponsored
Financial data (yr. ended 12/31/94): Assets, $17,988,222 (M); gifts received, $12,000,000; expenditures, $12,123,536; qualifying distributions, $12,095,534, including $6,790,816 for 174 grants (high: $250,000; low: $500; average: $1,000-$25,000) and $5,300,718 for employee matching gifts.
Purpose and activities: Giving primarily for health, civic and public affairs, cultural activities, and education, including higher education, educational programs for minorities, and schools of pharmacy.
Fields of interest: Arts/cultural programs; Education, association; Higher education; Education; Pharmacology; Health care; Health organizations; Human services; Government/public administration; Public affairs; Minorities; African Americans; Latinos; Aging; Women.
Types of support: General/operating support, continuing support, annual campaigns, capital campaigns, equipment, fellowships, employee matching gifts, matching funds.
Limitations: Giving primarily in Indianapolis, IN, and other areas of company operations. No grants to individuals, or for endowment funds, special projects, research, publications, or conferences; no loans.
Publications: Corporate giving report, application guidelines.
Application information: Application form not required.
Initial approach: Proposal
Copies of proposal: 1
Deadline(s): None
Board meeting date(s): Quarterly
Final notification: 3 weeks to 3 months
Officers and Directors:* Stephen A. Stitle,* Pres.; Edward Miller, V.P. and Treas.; Steve Twait, Secy.; James M. Cornelius, Mel Perelman, S.A. Taurel.
Number of staff: 1 full-time professional; 3 full-time support.
EIN: 356202479

326
Frank W. & Joan S. Luerssen Foundation

8226 Parkview
Munster 46321

Established in 1989 in IN.
Donor(s): Frank W. Luerssen, Joan S. Luerssen.
Financial data (yr. ended 12/31/95): Assets, $206,882 (M); expenditures, $25,165; qualifying distributions, $24,585, including $24,585 for 35 grants (high: $9,000; low: $25).
Fields of interest: Arts/cultural programs; Higher education; Education; Youth, services; Federated giving programs; Christian agencies & churches; Aging; Women.
Types of support: General/operating support.
Limitations: Giving primarily in IN.
Trustees: Frank W. Luerssen, Joan S. Luerssen.
EIN: 366894651

327
Mary Jane Luick Trust

c/o American National Trust & Investment Mgmt. Co.
320 South High St.
Muncie 47305-2818
Contact: Judy Polson

Financial data (yr. ended 12/31/95): Assets, $90,056 (M); expenditures, $2,091; qualifying distributions, $913, including $900 for 2 grants to individuals (high: $600; low: $300).
Purpose and activities: To provide help for indigent elderly women of Delaware County, IN.
Fields of interest: Aging; Women; Economically disadvantaged.
Types of support: Grants to individuals.
Limitations: Giving limited to Delaware County, IN.
Application information: Application form not required.
Deadline(s): None
Trustee: American National Trust & Investment Mgmt. Co.
EIN: 356009785

328
The Prophet Sisters Foundation

c/o Fort Wayne National Bank, Trust Dept.
P.O. Box 110
Fort Wayne 46801
Contact: D. Albertson, Trust Officer, Fort Wayne National Bank

Established in 1983 in IN.
Financial data (yr. ended 10/31/95): Assets, $1,582,969 (M); expenditures, $55,086; qualifying distributions, $49,182, including $47,500 for 10 grants (high: $5,000; low: $4,500).
Fields of interest: Adult education—literacy & basic skills; Reading; Human services; Children & youth, services; Aging, centers & services; Women, centers & services; Aging; Women.
Limitations: Giving limited to Fort Wayne, IN. No grants to individuals.
Application information: Application form not required.
Initial approach: Proposal
Deadline(s): None
Trustee: Fort Wayne National Bank.
Number of staff: None.
EIN: 311087791

329
Rieke Corporation Foundation

c/o Norwest Bank Indiana, N.A.
111 East Wayne St., P.O. Box 960
Fort Wayne 46801-6632
Contact: Donald E. Kelly, Trustee
Application address: c/o Rieke Corp., 500 West Seventh St., Auburn, IN 46706-2289; Tel.: (219) 925-3700

Donor(s): Rieke Corp.
Foundation type: Company-sponsored
Financial data (yr. ended 09/30/95): Assets, $731,312 (M); gifts received, $20,000; expenditures, $36,465; qualifying distributions, $28,400, including $28,400 for 10 grants (high: $10,000; low: $200).
Fields of interest: Museums; Libraries/library science; Animal welfare; Human services; Youth, services; Aging, centers & services; Disabled; Aging.
Limitations: Giving limited to Auburn, IN.
Application information:
Initial approach: Letter or telephone
Deadline(s): Aug. 31
Trustees: Donald E. Kelly, Glenn T. Rieke, Mahlon E. Rieke, Norwest Bank Indiana, N.A.
EIN: 510158651

330
Frank L. and Laura L. Smock Foundation

c/o Norwest Bank Indiana, N.A.
P.O. Box 960
Fort Wayne 46801-6632 (219) 461-6451
Contact: Alice Kopfer, V.P., Norwest Bank Indiana, N.A.

Trust established in 1953 in IN.
Donor(s): Laura L. Smock.‡
Financial data (yr. ended 12/31/94): Assets, $9,489,060 (M); expenditures, $507,592; qualifying distributions, $466,880, including $333,335 for 28 grants (high: $85,992; low: $1,080) and $133,545 for 22 grants to individuals (high: $28,088; low: $555).
Purpose and activities: To "promote the health, welfare and happiness of ailing or needy or crippled or blind or elderly and aged men and women of the Presbyterian faith throughout the State of Indiana"; support also for Presbyterian churches and a college.
Fields of interest: Aging, centers & services; Protestant agencies & churches; Disabled; Aging; Economically disadvantaged.
Types of support: Grants to individuals.
Limitations: Giving limited to IN. No grants for general or operating support, capital campaigns, building or endowment funds, or matching gifts; no loans.
Publications: Application guidelines.

Application information: Application form required.
Initial approach: Letter
Deadline(s): None
Board meeting date(s): Monthly
Final notification: 6 weeks
Advisory Committee: Richard Hutchison, John Walley.
Trustee: Norwest Bank Indiana, N.A.
Number of staff: None.
EIN: 356011335

331
William H. Willennar Foundation, Inc.

c/o Fort Wayne National Bank
P.O. Box 110
Fort Wayne 46801-0110 (219) 925-3065
Contact: M.C. Haggarty, Secy.-Treas.

Established in 1962 in IN.
Financial data (yr. ended 06/30/95): Assets, $3,052,728 (M); expenditures, $177,637; qualifying distributions, $155,246, including $149,250 for 15 grants (high: $90,000; low: $1,000).
Purpose and activities: Giving primarily to a hospital, a municipal parks department, and an organization benefiting handicapped children; support also for civic affairs, a council on aging, a community fund, and an automotive heritage association.
Fields of interest: Higher education; Hospitals (general); Aging, centers & services; Community development; Federated giving programs; Disabled; Aging.
Limitations: Giving primarily in IN, with emphasis on Auburn.
Application information:
Initial approach: Letter
Deadline(s): May 1
Board meeting date(s): May 1, Aug. 1, Nov. 1, and Feb. 1
Officers and Trustees:* Alice R. Close,* Pres.; Michael C. Haggarty,* Secy.-Treas.; Fort Wayne National Bank.
Number of staff: 1 part-time professional.
EIN: 356028233
Grants for Aging:
Dekalb County Council on Aging, Auburn, IN, $15,500. 94.
Dekalb County Council on Aging, Auburn, IN, $10,000. 95.

IOWA

332
Samuel & Gussie Bernstein Foundation

c/o James Bernstein
P.O. Box 627
Sioux City 51102

Established in 1989 in IA.
Donor(s): Members of the Bernstein family.
Foundation type: Operating
Financial data (yr. ended 03/31/93): Assets, $378,378 (M); expenditures, $52,386; qualifying distributions, $21,425, including $21,000 for 6 grants (high: $8,350; low: $1,000).
Fields of interest: College; Alzheimer's disease.
Limitations: Applications not accepted. Giving limited to Sioux City, IA.
Application information: Contributes only to pre-selected organizations.
Officers and Directors:* Samuel Bernstein,* Pres.; James Bernstein,* V.P.; Norman Bernstein,* V.P.
EIN: 421335958

333
Demco Charitable Foundation

P.O. Box 189
Boyden 51234 (712) 725-2302
Contact: James E. Koerselman, Pres.

Established in 1988 in IA.
Donor(s): James E. Koerselman, Kenneth G. Mulder, Dethmers Manufacturing Co.
Financial data (yr. ended 06/30/95): Assets, $391,228 (M); gifts received, $85,000; expenditures, $57,342; qualifying distributions, $50,775, including $50,775 for 15 grants (high: $12,275; low: $250).
Fields of interest: Visual arts; Performing arts; Education, fund raising; Higher education; Aging, centers & services; Government/public administration; Aging.
Types of support: General/operating support, annual campaigns, building/renovation, program development, scholarship funds.
Limitations: Giving primarily in northwestern IA. No grants to individuals.
Publications: 990-PF.
Application information: Application form not required.
Initial approach: Proposal
Copies of proposal: 1
Deadline(s): None
Board meeting date(s): Oct.
Officers and Directors:* James E. Koerselman,* Pres.; Kenneth G. Mulder,* V.P. and Secy.
Number of staff: None.
EIN: 421322684
Grants for Aging:
Alzheimers Disease and Related Disorders Association, Sioux City, IA, $250. 94.

334
The Greater Des Moines Foundation

(Formerly Des Moines Community Foundation)
601 Locust, Suite 933
Des Moines 50309-3738 (515) 245-3766
Contact: Monroe J. Colston, Pres.

Community foundation incorporated in 1969 in IA.
Foundation type: Community
Financial data (yr. ended 12/31/95): Assets, $8,200,000 (M); gifts received, $1,200,000; expenditures, $775,000, including $625,000 for 42 grants (high: $46,000; low: $500; average: $5,000) and $20,000 for 4 in-kind gifts.
Purpose and activities: "To provide funds for non-traditional programs with an emphasis on human services causes; support also for the arts and education."
Fields of interest: Arts/cultural programs; Education; Recreation; Human services; Children & youth, services; Child development, services; Aging, centers & services; Women, centers & services; Minorities/immigrants, centers & services; Homeless, human services; Jewish agencies & temples.
Types of support: Building/renovation, emergency funds, seed money, scholarship funds, matching funds.
Limitations: Giving primarily in the greater Des Moines, IA, area. No grants to individuals, or for continuing support.
Publications: Annual report, newsletter, informational brochure (including application guidelines).
Application information: Application form required.
Initial approach: Proposal
Copies of proposal: 4
Deadline(s): 60 days prior to board meeting
Board meeting date(s): Quarterly
Officers and Directors:* Fred Weitz,* Chair.; James Luhrs,* Vice-Chair.; Monroe J. Colston,* Pres.; James W. Hubbell, Jr.,* Treas.; Charles H. Betts, James Cownie, Johnny Danos, Robert Dee, Charles Edwards, Nolden Gentry, Lynn Horak, Ted Hutchison, Ann Kenworthy, David Kruidenier, Donald Lamberti, Myrt Levin, Maddie Levitt, Robert Mannheimer, Liz Newell, Marvin Pomerantz, Richard White.
Trustee: Firstar Bank Iowa, N.A.
Number of staff: 1 full-time professional; 1 part-time professional; 1 part-time support.
EIN: 426139033

335
The Hall-Perrine Foundation, Inc.

(Formerly The Hall Foundation, Inc.)
115 Third St., S.E., No. 803
Cedar Rapids 52401-1222 (319) 362-9079
Contact: Jack B. Evans, Pres.

Incorporated in 1953 in IA.
Donor(s): Members of the Hall family.
Financial data (yr. ended 12/31/95): Assets, $62,057,458 (M); gifts received, $3,000,000; expenditures, $1,820,951; qualifying distributions, $1,507,019, including $1,478,071 for 24 grants (high: $312,000; low: $500; average: $10,000-$100,000).
Purpose and activities: Primary areas of interest include the arts, higher education, social services, community funds, and hospitals. Support also for cultural programs, including fine and performing arts groups, youth agencies, and health services.
Fields of interest: Museums; Theater; Music; Arts/cultural programs; Higher education; Hospitals (general); Health care; Substance abuse, services; Mental health/crisis services; Cancer; Health organizations; Human services; Youth, services; Family services; Aging, centers & services; Disabled; Aging.
Types of support: Capital campaigns, building/renovation, equipment, land acquisition, emergency funds, program development, seed money, matching funds.
Limitations: Giving limited to Linn County, IA. No grants to individuals, or for deficit financing, endowment funds, or fellowships; no loans.
Publications: Informational brochure (including application guidelines).

Application information: Application form required.
Initial approach: Letter
Copies of proposal: 1
Deadline(s): None
Board meeting date(s): Varies
Final notification: After board meetings
Officers and Directors:* William P. Whipple,* Chair.; Jack B. Evans,* Pres.; George C. Foerstner,* V.P.; John G. Lidvall,* V.P.; Darrel A. Morf,* Secy.; Joseph R. Loufek,* Treas.; Dennis L. Boatman, E.J. Buresh, Carleen Grandon, Alex Meyer, Iris E. Muchmore.
Staff: Bethany H. Allsbrook, Prog. Officer.
Number of staff: 1 full-time professional; 1 part-time professional.
EIN: 426057097
Grants for Aging:
Aging Services, Albany, OR, $450,000. To construct and furnish adult day care center. 94.

336
James W. Hubbell, Jr. & Helen H. Hubbell Foundation
c/o Bankers Trust Co., Trust Dept.
P.O. Box 897
Des Moines 50304-0897
Contact: Mindy Nussbaum, Asst. V.P., Bankers Trust Co.
Application address: c/o Bankers Trust Co., 665 Locust St., Des Moines, IA 50309

Established in 1976 in IA.
Donor(s): James W. Hubbell, Jr.
Financial data (yr. ended 06/30/94): Assets, $1,878,396 (M); gifts received, $281; expenditures, $145,944; qualifying distributions, $142,290, including $142,100 for 31 grants (high: $77,400; low: $100).
Fields of interest: Arts/cultural programs; Secondary school/education; Higher education; Reproductive rights; Christian agencies & churches; African Americans; Aging; Women; Economically disadvantaged.
Types of support: General/operating support, continuing support, annual campaigns, capital campaigns, endowment funds, program development, seed money, internships, matching funds.
Limitations: Giving primarily in IA.
Application information:
Initial approach: Letter
Deadline(s): None
Trustees: James W. Hubbell, Jr., Bankers Trust Co.
Number of staff: None.
EIN: 426259130

337
Mid-Iowa Health Foundation
550 39th St., Suite 104
Des Moines 50312 (515) 277-6411
Contact: Kathryn Bradley

Established in 1984 in IA.
Financial data (yr. ended 12/31/94): Assets, $13,553,757 (M); expenditures, $719,780; qualifying distributions, $708,598, including $613,234 for 51 grants (high: $50,000; low: $250).
Purpose and activities: Primary areas of interest include the disadvantaged, the elderly, youth, the handicapped, and health services. Support limited to health-related service projects, including the areas of drug abuse and alcoholism, mental health, nutrition and hunger, nursing, pharmacy, and hospices; giving also for child welfare, the homeless, early childhood and medical education, and capital projects.
Fields of interest: Early childhood education; Medical school/education; Pharmacology; Nursing care; Health care; Substance abuse, services; Mental health/crisis services; Health associations; Alcoholism; Food services; Nutrition; Human services; Children & youth, services; Hospices; Aging, centers & services; Homeless, human services; Disabled; Aging; Economically disadvantaged; Homeless.
Types of support: General/operating support, building/renovation, equipment, program development, scholarship funds, matching funds.
Limitations: Giving limited to Polk County, IA, and seven surrounding counties. No support for hospital programs. No grants for research.
Publications: 990-PF, informational brochure (including application guidelines), application guidelines, grants list.
Application information: Application form required.
Initial approach: Letter or telephone
Copies of proposal: 1
Deadline(s): Feb. 1, May 1, Aug. 1, and Nov. 1
Board meeting date(s): Mar., June, Sept., and Dec.
Final notification: 6 to 8 weeks
Officers and Directors:* Ivan Johnson,* Chair.; Bernard Mercer,* Vice-Chair.; Rex Burns,* Secy.-Treas.; Simon Casady, Donna Drees, Don C. Green, Thomas Jeschke, T. Ward Phillips, F.F. Satterlee.
Number of staff: 1 full-time professional.
EIN: 421235348
Grants for Aging:
Family Counseling Center, Des Moines, IA, $5,000. For ElderCare services. 94.
Heartland Senior Services, Ames, IA, $7,500. For Senior Center program. 94.

338
The Principal Financial Group Corporate Giving Program
711 High St.
Des Moines 50392-0150 (515) 247-5091
Contact: DeAnn Cowman, Contribs. Asst.

Established in 1879 in IA.
Financial data (yr. ended 12/31/95): Total giving, $863,600, including $459,600 for 130 grants (high: $91,250; low: $25; average: $1,000-$5,000), $52,000 for 55 employee matching gifts and $352,000 for in-kind gifts.
Purpose and activities: Support for social services, arts and culture, health, education, and civic and community affairs.
Fields of interest: Visual arts; Museums; Performing arts; Dance; Theater; Arts/cultural programs; Early childhood education; Higher education; Business school/education; Medical school/education; Environment; Health care; AIDS; Health organizations; Medical research; AIDS research; Housing/shelter, development; Family services; Aging, centers & services; Minorities/immigrants, centers & services; Homeless, human services; Civil rights; Urban/community development; Community development; Public policy, research; Government/public administration; Minorities; Aging; Homeless.
Types of support: General/operating support, continuing support, annual campaigns, building/renovation, employee volunteer services, public relations services, use of facilities, employee matching gifts, donated products, in-kind gifts.
Limitations: Giving primarily in IA with emphasis on the Des Moines area; some support for national organizations. No support for athletic, fraternal, religious, denominational, sectarian, trade, industry, professional associations, private foundations, or veterans' groups. No grants to individuals, conference or seminar attendance; festival participation, hospital/health care capital fund drives; or goodwill ads.
Publications: Application guidelines.
Application information: Giving handled by Corp. Rels. Dept. Application form not required.
Initial approach: Request brochure; send requests to headquarters
Copies of proposal: 1
Deadline(s): 4 to 6 weeks prior to contributions meeting
Board meeting date(s): Monthly
Final notification: 6 to 8 weeks

339
The Principal Financial Group Foundation, Inc.
711 High St.
Des Moines 50392-0150 (515) 247-5091
Contact: DeAnn Cowman, Contribs. Asst.

Established in 1987 in IA.
Foundation type: Company-sponsored
Financial data (yr. ended 12/31/95): Assets, $15,749,850 (M); expenditures, $4,374,520; qualifying distributions, $4,374,520, including $3,940,411 for 340 grants (high: $815,000; low: $100) and $434,109 for employee matching gifts.
Purpose and activities: Support for social services, arts and culture, health, education, civic and community affairs, and the United Way of Central IA.
Fields of interest: Performing arts; Theater; Music; Arts/cultural programs; Early childhood education; Higher education; Business school/education; Medical school/education; Education; Environment; Health care; AIDS; Health organizations; Medical research; AIDS research; Housing/shelter, development; Human services; Family services; Aging, centers & services; Minorities/immigrants, centers & services; Urban/community development; Community development; Public policy, research; Government/public administration; Public affairs; Minorities; Aging; Economically disadvantaged; General charitable giving.
Types of support: General/operating support, continuing support, annual campaigns, capital campaigns, building/renovation, program development, employee matching gifts, in-kind gifts.

Limitations: Giving primarily in IA, with emphasis on the Des Moines area. No support for athletic organizations, fraternal organizations, organizations redistributing funds, private foundations, sectarian, religious, or denominational organizations, social organizations, trade, industrial or professional associations, libraries, individual K-12 schools, organizations outside U.S. whose activities are mainly international, or veterans' groups. No grants to individuals, or for conference or seminar attendance, goodwill ads, endowments, festival participation, or hospital or health care capital fund drives.
Publications: Application guidelines, annual report.
Application information: Application form not required.
Initial approach: Proposal
Copies of proposal: 5
Deadline(s): 4 to 6 weeks prior to contributions committee meeting
Board meeting date(s): Approximately once a month
Final notification: 4 to 6 weeks
Officers and Directors:* Theodore Hutchison,* Chair. and Pres.; David Drury,* V.P.; Mary O'Keefe,* V.P.; Richard W. Waugh,* Treas.; Ray Crabtree, Thomas Gaard, Joyce Hoffman.
Number of staff: None.
EIN: 421312301

340
Siouxland Foundation

P.O. Box 2014
Sioux City 51104 (712) 239-3303
Contact: Debbie Hubbard, Exec. Dir.

Established in 1988 in IA.
Foundation type: Community
Financial data (yr. ended 12/31/95): Assets, $1,816,459 (M); gifts received, $89,071; expenditures, $106,500, including $70,301 for 35 grants (high: $6,900; low: $220; average: $250-$5,000) and $700 for 1 grant to an individual.
Fields of interest: Music; Arts/cultural programs; Early childhood education; Child development, education; Medical school/education; Adult/continuing education; Adult education—literacy & basic skills; Reading; Education; Nursing care; Health care; Substance abuse, services; Mental health/crisis services; Alcoholism; Health organizations; Domestic violence prevention; Safety/disasters; Recreation; Human services; Youth, services; Child development, services; Family services; Aging, centers & services; Minorities/immigrants, centers & services; Government/public administration; Minorities; Asians/Pacific Islanders; African Americans; Latinos; Native Americans; Disabled; Aging; Economically disadvantaged; Homeless.
Types of support: General/operating support, building/renovation, equipment, program development, conferences/seminars, seed money, scholarship funds, research.
Limitations: Giving limited to the greater Sioux City, IA, tri-state area (within a 50-mile radius of Sioux City, including NE and SD). No support for religious or political purposes, or for endowment funds, deficit financing, or fundraising campaigns.
Publications: Annual report (including application guidelines), informational brochure, application guidelines.
Application information: Application form required.
Initial approach: Letter or telephone for application procedures
Copies of proposal: 10
Deadline(s): May 15 and Sept. 15
Board meeting date(s): Mar., July, and Nov.
Final notification: By July 31 and Nov. 30
Officers and Directors:* Gretchen R. Hirschbach,* Pres.; Irving F. Jensen, Jr.,* V.P.; John B. Anderson,* Secy.-Treas.; Linda Phillips,* Development Committee Chair.; John W. Aalfs,* Investment Committee Chair.; Lynn Persinger,* Grant Review Committee Chair.; Debbie Hubbard, Exec. Dir.; Douglas Bass, and 22 additional directors.
Number of staff: 1 full-time professional.
EIN: 421323904

341
The Van Buren Foundation, Inc.

c/o Farmers State Bank
Keosauqua 52565 (319) 293-3794
Contact: John O. Manning, Treas.

Incorporated in 1959 in IA.
Donor(s): Ralph S. Roberts.‡
Financial data (yr. ended 12/31/93): Assets, $3,112,035 (M); gifts received, $961; expenditures, $88,556; qualifying distributions, $93,947, including $64,368 for 28 grants (high: $17,000; low: $200), $376 for 6 grants to individuals (high: $215; low: $11) and $28,753 for 1 foundation-administered program.
Purpose and activities: Grants for local community development, aid for the aged, recreation programs, and education.
Fields of interest: Elementary school/education; Nursing school/education; Education; Recreation; Aging, centers & services; Community development; Aging.
Types of support: General/operating support, building/renovation, program development, scholarships—to individuals, student loans—to individuals.
Limitations: Giving limited to Van Buren County, IA.
Application information:
Initial approach: Proposal
Copies of proposal: 1
Deadline(s): None
Board meeting date(s): Twice annually and as needed
Officers and Directors:* Arthur P. Ovrom,* Chair.; Jon Finney,* Vice-Chair.; Davis E. Pollock,* Pres.; Rex Strait,* 1st V.P.; Sandy McLain,* 2nd V.P.; Richard A. Lytle,* Secy.; John O. Manning,* Treas.; Connie Davenport, James A. Dorothy, Mike Gunn, and 7 additional directors.
EIN: 426062589

342
Vermeer Charitable Foundation, Inc.

c/o Vermeer Manufacturing Co.
P.O. Box 200
Pella 50219 (515) 628-3141
Contact: Lois Vermeer, Exec. Secy.

Established in 1977 in IA.
Donor(s): Vermeer Manufacturing Co., Vermeer Sales and Service of Iowa, Vermeer Farms, Inc.
Foundation type: Company-sponsored
Financial data (yr. ended 12/31/95): Assets, $5,516,954 (M); gifts received, $1,251,704; expenditures, $1,154,325; qualifying distributions, $1,149,587, including $1,149,587 for 78 grants (high: $250,000; low: $50; average: $10,000).
Fields of interest: Higher education; Aging, centers & services; Christian agencies & churches; Aging.
Types of support: Building/renovation, seed money.
Limitations: Giving primarily in the Pella, IA, area. No grants to individuals, or for endowment funds, scholarships, fellowships, or matching gifts; no loans.
Application information: Application form required.
Initial approach: Letter
Copies of proposal: 2
Deadline(s): Apr. and Nov.
Board meeting date(s): Dec. and as required
Officers and Directors:* Gary J. Vermeer,* Pres.; Matilda Vermeer,* V.P.; Lois J. Vermeer,* Exec. Secy.; Robert L. Vermeer,* Treas.; Dale Andringa, Mary Andringa.
Number of staff: 2 part-time professional.
EIN: 421087640

343
Wahlert Foundation

c/o FDL Foods, Inc.
P.O. Box 898
Dubuque 52001 (319) 588-5400
Contact: R.H. Wahlert, Pres. and Treas.

Incorporated in 1948 in IA.
Donor(s): Dubuque Packing Co., FDL Foods, Inc., H.W. Wahlert,‡ and officers of the foundation.
Financial data (yr. ended 11/30/94): Assets, $4,699,730 (M); gifts received, $3,460; expenditures, $413,882; qualifying distributions, $309,165, including $309,165 for 45 grants (high: $250,000; low: $500; average: $500-$250,000).
Purpose and activities: Support primarily for higher, secondary, medical and theological education; grants also for health services and hospitals, including medical and cancer research, social service agencies, including drug abuse prevention programs and services for families, the homeless and the handicapped, child welfare programs for minorities, cultural activities, including the arts and museums, Catholic welfare organizations and schools, and agricultural programs and rural development.
Fields of interest: Museums; Arts/cultural programs; Elementary/secondary education; Secondary school/education; Higher education; Medical school/education; Theological school/education; Education; Hospitals

(general); Health care; Substance abuse, services; Cancer; Health organizations; Medical research; Cancer research; Agriculture; Food services; Human services; Children & youth, services; Family services; Aging, centers & services; Minorities/immigrants, centers & services; Homeless, human services; Rural development; Federated giving programs; Roman Catholic federated giving programs; Christian agencies & churches; Roman Catholic agencies & churches; Religion; Minorities; Disabled; Aging; Economically disadvantaged; Homeless; General charitable giving.
Types of support: Continuing support, annual campaigns, capital campaigns, building/renovation, equipment, emergency funds, program development, seed money, scholarship funds.
Limitations: Giving primarily in the metropolitan Dubuque, IA, area. No grants to individuals, or for publications, conferences, or matching gifts; no loans.
Application information: Application form not required.
Initial approach: Proposal
Copies of proposal: 1
Deadline(s): Nov. 30
Board meeting date(s): Dec.
Final notification: Jan. 30
Officers and Trustees:* R.H. Wahlert,* Pres. and Treas.; Alfred E. Hughes,* Secy.; Donald Strausse, Celeste Wahlert, David Wahlert, Donna Wahlert, James Wahlert, Nancy Wahlert, R.C. Wahlert II, Susan Wahlert.
Number of staff: None.
EIN: 426051124

344
Waverly Community Foundation
c/o State Bank of Waverly
P.O. Box 58
Waverly 50677 (319) 352-6000
Contact: Ruth Rodenbeck

Established in 1958 in IA.
Foundation type: Community
Financial data (yr. ended 12/31/94): Assets, $1,584,672 (M); expenditures, $99,997, including $34,300 for 7 grants (high: $25,000; low: $400) and $53,750 for grants to individuals.
Purpose and activities: Support for the aged and scholarships to Bremer County, IA, high school graduates.
Fields of interest: Aging, centers & services; Aging.
Types of support: General/operating support, scholarships—to individuals.
Limitations: Giving limited to residents of Waverly and Bremer County, IA.
Application information:
Initial approach: Letter
Deadline(s): Jan. 1 for grants; Apr. 1 for scholarships
Trustee: Fred Hagemann.
Agent: State Bank of Waverly.
EIN: 426058774

KANSAS

345
Beech Aircraft Foundation
9709 East Central Ave.
Wichita 67201 (316) 676-8785
Contact: Robert B. Welton, Secy.-Treas.

Incorporated in 1966 in KS.
Donor(s): Beech Aircraft Corp.
Foundation type: Company-sponsored
Financial data (yr. ended 12/31/94): Assets, $5,530,678 (M); gifts received, $160,000; expenditures, $454,338; qualifying distributions, $446,126, including $446,126 for 96 grants (high: $108,000; low: $85; average: $75-$10,000).
Purpose and activities: Grants for higher education, community funds, youth agencies, and hospitals; some support for cultural activities, conservation, the handicapped, and the aged.
Fields of interest: Arts/cultural programs; Higher education; Education; Natural resource conservation & protection; Hospitals (general); Youth, services; Aging, centers & services; Federated giving programs; Disabled; Aging.
Types of support: Continuing support, annual campaigns, capital campaigns, building/renovation, program development, publication, seed money, program-related investments/loans, employee matching gifts, employee-related scholarships, exchange programs, matching funds.
Limitations: Giving primarily in communities with company facilities, with emphasis on KS. No grants to individuals (except for employee-related scholarships), or for endowment funds, research, or matching gifts; no loans.
Application information: Application form not required.
Initial approach: Letter
Copies of proposal: 1
Deadline(s): Dec., Mar., June, and Sept.
Board meeting date(s): Jan., Apr., July, and Oct.
Officers and Directors:* Max E. Bleck,* Chair.; Arthur Wegner,* Pres.; Richard Griffiths,* V.P.; Robert B. Welton, Secy.-Treas.; J.A. Elliot, Wey D. Kenny, Wayne Wallace.
Number of staff: None.
EIN: 486125881
Grants for Aging:
Senior Services, Wichita, KS, $5,000. 94.

346
The Cooper-Clark Foundation
c/o Lucille C. Clark
P.O. Box 2707
Liberal 67905-2707 (316) 624-8471
Contact: Jay Hay, Secy.-Treas.

Donor(s): James Clark, Lucille Clark.
Financial data (yr. ended 12/31/95): Assets, $1,260,364 (M); gifts received, $100,000; expenditures, $54,499; qualifying distributions, $49,718, including $47,665 for 23 grants (high: $4,950; low: $500).
Fields of interest: Arts/cultural programs; Elementary/secondary education; Human services; Aging, centers & services; Community development; Aging.
Limitations: Giving primarily in CO and KS. No grants to individuals.
Application information: Application form required.
Deadline(s): None
Officers: Lee Anderson, Pres.; Bob Todd, V.P.; Jay Hay, Secy.-Treas.
Directors: Shirley Anderson, Jim Clark, Lucille Clark, Kay Hay, Sharon Todd.
EIN: 742252034

347
Leo J. Dreiling & Albina Dreiling Charitable Trust
P.O. Box 550
Hays 67601 (913) 625-8327
Contact: Joseph A. Hess, Trustee

Established in 1980 in KS.
Donor(s): Leo J. Dreiling.‡
Financial data (yr. ended 09/30/95): Assets, $4,402,203 (M); expenditures, $252,354; qualifying distributions, $247,383, including $247,383 for 7 grants (high: $102,500; low: $1,000).
Purpose and activities: Giving primarily for education and culture; support also for a rest home.
Fields of interest: Arts/cultural programs; Education; Aging, centers & services; Aging.
Types of support: Building/renovation, scholarship funds.
Limitations: Giving limited to Ellis County, KS. No grants to individuals.
Application information: Application form not required.
Initial approach: Letter
Deadline(s): None
Trustees: Dennis L. Bieker, John G. Dreiling, Norbert R. Dreiling, Joseph A. Hess.
Number of staff: None.
EIN: 480916752

348
Health Concepts Foundation
P.O. Box 47172
Wichita 67201-7172 (316) 685-5311
Contact: Richard W. Stumpf, Secy.-Treas.

Financial data (yr. ended 06/30/95): Assets, $253,797 (M); expenditures, $14,496; qualifying distributions, $12,201, including $9,908 for grants.
Fields of interest: Aging, centers & services; Aging.
Limitations: Giving primarily in Wichita, KS.
Application information:
Initial approach: Letter
Deadline(s): None
Officers and Directors:* Betty Arnold,* Chair.; Calvin Rider, Vice-Chair; Richard W. Stumpf,* Secy.-Treas.; Ernest Crow, M.D., Ann Hunter, Tammy S. Johnson, Frances F. Seidl, R.N.
EIN: 480860225

349
Hutchinson Community Foundation
P.O. Box 298
Hutchinson 67504-0298 (316) 663-5293
Contact: Sandra L. McMullen, Pres.

Established in 1989 in KS.
Foundation type: Community
Financial data (yr. ended 12/31/94): Assets, $4,693,298 (M); gifts received, $1,305,659; expenditures, $682,272, including $637,359 for grants.
Fields of interest: Visual arts; Performing arts; Theater; Arts/cultural programs; Early childhood education; Higher education; Education; Health care; Substance abuse, services; Mental health/crisis services; Health organizations; Housing/shelter, development; Human services; Children & youth, services; Youth, services; Hospices; Aging, centers & services; Civil rights; Community development; Voluntarism promotion; Federated giving programs; Disabled; Aging; Economically disadvantaged; General charitable giving.
Types of support: Seed money, scholarship funds, matching funds.
Limitations: Giving primarily in Reno County, KS.
Publications: Annual report, grants list, newsletter, occasional report, informational brochure, program policy statement, application guidelines.
Application information: Application form required.
Copies of proposal: 7
Deadline(s): Varies
Board meeting date(s): Quarterly
Final notification: Dec.
Officers and Directors:* Jack E. Sutton,* Chair.; Howard J. Carey, Jr.,* Vice-Chair.; Sandra L. McMullen, Pres. and Exec. Dir.; Diane M. Longenecker,* Secy.; Paul W. Dillon,* Treas.; Loren L. Alderson, Richard W. Dillon, R.A. Edwards, James R. Gilliland, Dean K. Johnson, Norman L. Krause, Diane W. Lee, Patrick W. Michaelis, Elizabeth M. Oswald, Virginia H. Rayl, Ruth Ann Sellars, R. Clark Wesley.
Number of staff: 1 part-time professional.
EIN: 481076910

350
The Julia J. Mingenback Foundation, Inc.
c/o Bank IV Kansas, N.A.
One Main Place
McPherson 67460 (316) 241-8000
Contact: Don Steffes, Pres.

Incorporated in 1959 in KS.
Donor(s): E.C. Mingenback.‡
Financial data (yr. ended 12/31/95): Assets, $4,144,395 (M); expenditures, $211,960; qualifying distributions, $125,000, including $125,000 for 4 grants (high: $60,000; low: $20,000).
Fields of interest: Elementary/secondary education; Higher education; Hospitals (general); Aging, centers & services; Religion; Aging.
Types of support: Capital campaigns, building/renovation, equipment.
Limitations: Giving primarily in McPherson County, KS.
Application information:
Initial approach: Letter
Deadline(s): None
Officers: Don C. Steffes, Pres.; Ruth Lancaster, Secy.-Treas.
Directors: James Ketcherside, Edwin T. Pyle.
Trustee: Bank IV Kansas, N.A.
Number of staff: 1 part-time support.
EIN: 486109567

351
Victor Murdock Foundation
c/o Bank IV Kansas, N.A.
P.O. Box 1122
Wichita 67201-9974 (316) 261-4087
Contact: Richard B. Chambers, Asst. V.P. and Trust Officer, Bank IV Kansas, N.A.

Established in 1974 in KS.
Financial data (yr. ended 12/31/95): Assets, $1,092,279 (M); expenditures, $55,357; qualifying distributions, $46,949, including $43,780 for 10 grants (high: $10,707; low: $300) and $500 for 1 grant to an individual.
Fields of interest: Media/communications; Journalism & publishing; Museums; Performing arts; Music; Humanities; History & archaeology; Language & linguistics; Literature; Historic preservation/historical societies; Arts/cultural programs; Early childhood education; Child development, education; Elementary school/education; Secondary school/education; Higher education; Adult education—literacy & basic skills; Libraries/library science; Reading; Education; Speech & hearing centers; Health care; Mental health/crisis services; Health associations; Human services; Children & youth, services; Child development, services; Hospices; Aging, centers & services; Disabled; Aging; Economically disadvantaged; General charitable giving.
Types of support: Building/renovation, equipment, scholarship funds.
Limitations: Giving limited to the Wichita, KS, area. Generally, no grants to individuals.
Application information: Application form not required.
Initial approach: Letter
Copies of proposal: 6
Deadline(s): Mar. 5 and Oct. 5
Board meeting date(s): Apr. and Nov.
Trustees: Fred Berry, Wilson Cadman, Charles Q. Chandler, Victor Delano, Judith Slawson, Bank IV Kansas, N.A.
Number of staff: None.
EIN: 486190755

352
Fidelia E. Plett Charitable Foundation
P.O. Box 513
Inman 67546 (316) 585-6822
Contact: John Balzer, Trustee

Established in 1993 in KS.
Donor(s): Fidelia E. Plett.‡
Financial data (yr. ended 12/31/95): Assets, $675,446 (M); gifts received, $200; expenditures, $37,364; qualifying distributions, $30,068, including $30,068 for 9 grants (high: $5,000; low: $500).
Fields of interest: College; Mental health/crisis services; Offenders/ex-offenders, rehabilitation; Religion; Aging.
Limitations: Giving primarily in Newton, KS.
Application information:
Initial approach: Typewritten proposal
Deadline(s): Nov. 15
Trustees: David K. Balzer, John R. Balzer, Kristina Reimer Balzer, John Gaeddert, Lois Hochstetler, Steve Pankratz, Allen Pauls.
EIN: 481134587

353
Sidwell Charitable Trust
P.O. Box 754
Winfield 67156 (316) 221-4600
Contact: Kay Roberts Light, Dir.

Established in 1989 in KS.
Donor(s): Martell Sidwell.
Foundation type: Operating
Financial data (yr. ended 12/31/95): Assets, $329,307 (M); gifts received, $29,712; expenditures, $20,964; qualifying distributions, $20,773, including $15,577 for 22 grants to individuals (high: $1,953; low: $21).
Purpose and activities: Awards grants to needy residents of Winfield, KS, over age sixty.
Fields of interest: Aging; Economically disadvantaged.
Types of support: Grants to individuals.
Limitations: Giving limited to residents of Winfield, KS.
Application information: Application form required.
Deadline(s): None
Directors: N. Dean Bradbury, Raymond King, Kay Roberts Light.
EIN: 486290978

354
Delos V. Smith Senior Citizens Foundation
c/o Smith Shepherd's Ctr.
101 West First
Hutchinson 67501-5235 (316) 662-0111
Contact: Delos V. Smith, Jr., Treas.

Established in 1977.
Donor(s): Delos V. Smith, Jr.
Foundation type: Operating
Financial data (yr. ended 06/30/95): Assets, $1,363,805 (M); gifts received, $60,582; expenditures, $57,651; qualifying distributions, $57,189, including $215 for 3 grants (high: $100; low: $15; average: $10-$100) and $51,535 for 1 foundation-administered program.
Purpose and activities: The foundation operates a senior center that offers seminars, classes, and recreational activities.
Fields of interest: Continuing education/lifelong learning; Recreation; Aging, centers & services; Aging.
Types of support: Conferences/seminars.
Limitations: Giving primarily in Wichita and Hutchinson, KS.
Application information: Application form not required.

Initial approach: Letter
Deadline(s): None
Board meeting date(s): June
Officers and Directors:* Porter K. Brown,* Pres.; John H. Shaffer,* Secy.; Delos V. Smith, Jr.,* Treas.
Number of staff: 1 full-time professional.
EIN: 480861681

355
K. T. Wiedemann Foundation, Inc.
Ten St. James Place
Wichita 67206
Contact: Douglas S. Pringle, Pres.
Application address: 2842 West Columbine St., Wichita, KS 67204

Incorporated in 1959 in KS.
Donor(s): K.T. Wiedemann Trust.
Financial data (yr. ended 02/28/95): Assets, $310,046 (M); gifts received, $242,646; expenditures, $150,738; qualifying distributions, $141,541, including $104,599 for 11 grants (high: $40,000; low: $1,000; average: $1,000-$40,000).
Fields of interest: Human services; Youth, services; Aging, centers & services; Disabled; Aging.
Types of support: General/operating support, program development.
Limitations: Giving limited to Sedgwick and Butler counties, KS, with emphasis on Wichita. No grants to individuals.
Publications: Application guidelines.
Application information: Application form not required.
Initial approach: 2-page letter
Copies of proposal: 3
Deadline(s): Prior to board meeting dates
Board meeting date(s): Feb. 15, June 15, and Oct. 15
Final notification: Within 2 months of board meeting
Officer and Trustees:* Douglas S. Pringle,* Pres.; Lynne A. Hankins, Bruce A. Pringle, Kenneth W. Pringle.
Number of staff: None.
EIN: 486117541

KENTUCKY

356
J. B. Caldwell Memorial Fund
c/o Farmers National Bank
304 West Main St.
Danville 40422-1814

Financial data (yr. ended 12/31/95): Assets, $532,473 (M); expenditures, $18,992; qualifying distributions, $16,046, including $16,046 for grants.
Purpose and activities: Support for organizations in Boyle County, KY, that provide assistance to needy residents.
Fields of interest: Aging, centers & services; Aging; Economically disadvantaged.
Limitations: Giving limited to Boyle County, KY.
Application information: Applicants should contact Family Services Assn. of Boyle County for information; grants are paid directly to organizations. Application form not required.
Deadline(s): None
Trustee: Farmers National Bank.
EIN: 616092354

357
Homecroft, Inc.
Professional Bldg.
Shepherdsville 40165 (502) 955-6165
Contact: Thomas B. Givhan, Dir.

Established in 1992.
Financial data (yr. ended 02/28/96): Assets, $241,045 (M); expenditures, $17,745; qualifying distributions, $16,995.
Fields of interest: Housing/shelter, development; Aging, centers & services; Aging.
Application information: No grants paid in fiscal 1996.
Initial approach: Letter
Deadline(s): None
Directors: Thomas B. Givhan, William Marshall Lutes, Elise G. Spainhour.
EIN: 611225403

358
Kentucky Social Welfare Foundation
c/o PNC Bank, Kentucky, Inc.
Citizens Plaza, 120 South Main St.
Louisville 40296-0602 (502) 581-2399
Contact: Theodore L. Merhoff, Trust Officer, PNC Bank, Kentucky, Inc.

Established in 1948 in KY.
Donor(s): Martha Davis,‡ Kentucky Social Welfare Foundation Trust Fund.
Financial data (yr. ended 12/31/95): Assets, $948,078 (M); gifts received, $53,903; expenditures, $96,461; qualifying distributions, $89,259, including $84,104 for 14 grants (high: $15,000; low: $2,000).
Purpose and activities: Supports organizations that improve the standard of living and opportunity among poor, sick, unfortunate, and vocationally handicapped residents of KY. Preference given to rural areas, small towns, and areas of special need. Consideration given to social and family services, including child development and welfare, the aged, the handicapped, the disadvantaged, housing programs, and the homeless; health services, drug abuse programs, rehabilitation, mental health, and nutrition; and adult education and literacy programs.
Fields of interest: Adult/continuing education; Adult education—literacy & basic skills; Reading; Medical care, rehabilitation; Health care; Mental health/crisis services; Housing/shelter, development; Human services; Children & youth, services; Family services; Aging, centers & services; Homeless, human services; Rural development; Aging; Homeless.
Types of support: Equipment, program development, conferences/seminars, publication, seed money, scholarship funds, consulting services.
Limitations: Giving primarily in KY. No grants to individuals.
Publications: Informational brochure, application guidelines.
Application information: Application form required.
Copies of proposal: 10
Deadline(s): None
Board meeting date(s): Jan., May, and Oct.
Officers and Trustees:* Sam Neal,* Chair.; Chad Jackson,* Vice-Chair.; T. Jack Eversole, Secy.; Theodore L. Merhoff, Treas.; Linda Gayheart, Alice Lewis, Rev. Michael T. Powers, Roger Recktenwald, Beth Rompf, Dixie Rose.
Number of staff: None.
EIN: 616034264

359
The Mahan Foundation, Inc.
2901 Barrickman Ln.
Goshen 40026 (502) 228-1685
Contact: Ann Smiser, Treas.

Established in 1984 in KY.
Donor(s): Howard B. Mahan.‡
Financial data (yr. ended 12/31/94): Assets, $1,374,607 (M); expenditures, $61,269; qualifying distributions, $60,019, including $60,000 for 34 grants (high: $5,000; low: $1,000).
Fields of interest: Children & youth, services; Aging, centers & services; Christian agencies & churches; Aging.
Limitations: Giving limited to Oldham County, KY.
Application information: Application form not required.
Initial approach: Letter
Copies of proposal: 1
Deadline(s): Dec. 1
Board meeting date(s): 2nd week in Dec.
Officers: Raymond Simpson, V.P.; Jennifer Dick, Secy.; Ann Smiser, Treas.
Directors: Gene Bottorff, William Landis.
Number of staff: None.
EIN: 311087614

360
Mansbach Foundation, Inc.
P.O. Box 1179
Ashland 41105-1179

Donor(s): Gerald Mansbach, Samuel Mansbach.
Financial data (yr. ended 10/31/95): Assets, $1,438,922 (M); gifts received, $660,000; expenditures, $115,159; qualifying distributions, $104,100, including $104,100 for 23 grants (high: $60,000; low: $500).
Fields of interest: Arts/cultural programs; Higher education; Education; Food services; Housing/shelter, development; Human services; Children & youth, services; Jewish federated giving programs; Aging.
Limitations: Applications not accepted. Giving primarily in Ashland, KY. No grants to individuals.
Application information: Contributes only to pre-selected organizations.
Officers: Samuel Mansbach, Pres.; Gerald Mansbach, V.P.; Donald H. Putnam, Secy.; John W. Woods III, Treas.
EIN: 616030981
Grants for Aging:

Sanders Brown Center on Aging, Lexington, KY, $5,000. 95.

361
Kate McClintock Home

c/o Paulette Caywood
848 Bethlehem Rd.
Paris 40361
Application address: Board of Directors, P.O. Box 341, Paris, KY 40361

Classified as a private operating foundation in 1973.
Foundation type: Operating
Financial data (yr. ended 08/31/95): Assets, $194,240 (M); gifts received, $836; expenditures, $22,082; qualifying distributions, $20,600, including $20,600 for 10 grants to individuals (high: $2,700; low: $200).
Purpose and activities: Awards rent supplement to elderly women residents of Bourbon County, KY, who are not receiving state assistance.
Fields of interest: Housing/shelter, development; Aging, centers & services; Women, centers & services; Aging; Women.
Types of support: Grants to individuals.
Limitations: Giving limited to Bourbon County, KY.
Application information: Application form required.
Deadline(s): None
Officers: Henry Prewett, Pres.; Steven W. Elan, Secy.; Paulette Caywood, Treas.
EIN: 610458372

LOUISIANA

362
Baton Rouge Area Foundation

One American Place, Suite 1740
Baton Rouge 70825 (504) 387-6126
Contact: John G. Davies, C.E.O. and Pres.
FAX: (504) 387-6153

Incorporated in 1964 in LA.
Foundation type: Community
Financial data (yr. ended 12/31/94): Assets, $29,421,518 (M); gifts received, $5,132,295; expenditures, $1,852,133, including $1,153,184 for 670 grants (high: $190,472; low: $25) and $30,000 for 1 loan.
Purpose and activities: The foundation funds programs in the areas of arts and humanities, community development, education, environment, human services, health and medical, and religion. Primary areas of interest include elementary and secondary education and health. Preference given to those projects which promise to affect a broad segment of the population or which tend to help a segment of the citzenry who are not being adequately served by the community's resources.
Fields of interest: Arts/cultural programs; Child development, education; Elementary school/education; Secondary school/education; Medical school/education; Nursing school/education; Education; Environment; Health care; Health organizations; Human services; Youth, services; Child development, services; Aging, centers & services; Women, centers & services; Community development; Religion; Disabled; Aging; Women; Economically disadvantaged.
Types of support: Capital campaigns, building/renovation, equipment, endowment funds, emergency funds, program development, seed money, research, matching funds.
Limitations: Giving limited to the Baton Rouge, LA, area, including East Baton Rouge, West Baton Rouge, Livingston, Ascension, Iberville, Pointe Coupee, East Feliciana, and West Feliciana parishes. No grants to individuals, or for continuing support, annual campaigns, deficit financing, scholarships, fellowships, or operating budgets; no loans.
Publications: Annual report (including application guidelines), application guidelines, newsletter, informational brochure.
Application information: Application form required.
Initial approach: Telephone
Copies of proposal: 1
Deadline(s): Feb. 1, May 1, Aug. 1, and Nov. 1; call office for Manship Fund and Arbritton Fund deadlines
Board meeting date(s): Mar., June, Sept., and Dec.
Final notification: 1 week after board meeting
Officers and Directors:* J. Terrell Brown,* Chair.; John G. Davies,* C.E.O. and Pres.; F. Charles McMains, Jr.,* V.P.; Mary Ann Sternberg,* Secy.; William C. Potter,* Treas.; Rosie L. Chaney, Compt.; John W. Barton, and 17 additional directors.
Trustee Bank: Premier Bank, N.A.
Staff: Marcia K. Kantrow, Dir. of Progs.; John L. McKowen, Dir. of Finance.
Number of staff: 7 full-time professional.
EIN: 726030391

363
The Booth-Bricker Fund

830 Union St., Suite 200
New Orleans 70112 (504) 581-2430
Contact: Gray S. Parker, Trustee

Established in 1976 in LA.
Donor(s): John F. Bricker, Nina B. Bricker.‡
Financial data (yr. ended 12/31/93): Assets, $24,590,647 (M); gifts received, $45,000; expenditures, $1,202,553; qualifying distributions, $934,088, including $892,954 for 113 grants (high: $101,050; low: $50).
Fields of interest: Visual arts; Museums; Performing arts; Theater; Historic preservation/historical societies; Arts/cultural programs; Education, fund raising; Elementary/secondary education; Early childhood education; Child development, education; Secondary school/education; Higher education; Theological school/education; Adult education—literacy & basic skills; Libraries/library science; Reading; Education; Environment; Hospitals (general); Speech & hearing centers; Health care; Mental health/crisis services; Cancer; Biomedicine; Health organizations; Medical research; Cancer research; Crime/law enforcement; Food services; Human services; Youth, services; Child development, services; Family services; Aging, centers & services; Homeless, human services; Roman Catholic agencies & churches; Religion; Aging; Economically disadvantaged; Homeless; General charitable giving.
Types of support: Annual campaigns, capital campaigns, building/renovation, equipment, endowment funds, debt reduction, professorships, scholarship funds, research, employee matching gifts, matching funds.
Limitations: Giving primarily in New Orleans, LA. No grants to individuals.
Application information: Application form not required.
Initial approach: Letter or proposal
Deadline(s): None
Board meeting date(s): Quarterly
Officers and Trustees:* John F. Bricker,* Chair.; Donald J. Nalty,* Secy.; Dorothy A. Boyle, Robert L. Goodwin, Henry N. Kuechler III, Gray S. Parker, N.P. Phillips, Jr., John M. Waid, H. Hunter White.
EIN: 720818077

364
The Community Foundation of Shreveport-Bossier

401 Edwards St.
517 Louisiana Tower
Shreveport 71101
Contact: Carol Emanuel, Exec. Dir.

Incorporated in 1961 in LA.
Foundation type: Community
Financial data (yr. ended 12/31/94): Assets, $17,484,728 (M); gifts received, $1,160,386; expenditures, $1,056,928, including $738,733 for 49 grants (high: $100,000; low: $300).
Purpose and activities: Primary areas of interest include health services, literacy, and higher education.
Fields of interest: Arts/cultural programs; Higher education; Adult education—literacy & basic skills; Reading; Education; Health care; Health organizations; Human services; Youth, services; Aging, centers & services; Homeless, human services; Disabled; Aging; Women; Economically disadvantaged; Homeless.
Types of support: Capital campaigns, building/renovation, equipment, program development, conferences/seminars, seed money, scholarship funds, matching funds.
Limitations: Giving limited to the Caddo and Bossier parishes, LA. No grants to individuals.
Publications: Annual report, application guidelines, informational brochure.
Application information: Grant deadlines and meeting dates may change in 1995. Application form required.
Initial approach: Letter of inquiry prior to submitting full grant request
Copies of proposal: 8
Deadline(s): Mar. 31 and Aug. 31
Board meeting date(s): June and Nov.
Final notification: Immediately after board meetings
Officers and Directors:* Joseph L. Hargrove,* Chair.; William C. Peatross,* Vice-Chair.; Sylvia K. Goodman,* Secy.; Quintin T. Hardtner III,* Treas.; L. Frank Moore, W. Clinton Rasberry, Jr., Judge Carl Stewart.

Trustee Banks: Commercial National Bank in Shreveport, Premier Bank, N.A., Whitney National Bank.
Number of staff: 1 full-time professional; 2 full-time support.
EIN: 726022365

MAINE

365
Camden Home for Senior Citizens
c/o Adele Hopkins
66 Washington St.
Camden 04843
Contact: Charles Lowe, Pres.
Application address: Belfast Rd., Camden, ME 04843; Tel.: (207) 236-2014

Established in 1941; classified as a private operating foundation in 1972.
Foundation type: Operating
Financial data (yr. ended 05/31/95): Assets, $1,627,350 (M); gifts received, $1,500; expenditures, $62,571; qualifying distributions, $49,027, including $600 for 2 grants of $300 each and $44,974 for 218 grants to individuals (high: $300; low: $75).
Purpose and activities: Provides heating, food, drugs, rent, real estate taxes, and medical needs to residents of Camden, Rockport, Hope, and Lincolnville, ME.
Fields of interest: Aging, centers & services; Aging; Economically disadvantaged.
Types of support: Grants to individuals.
Limitations: Giving limited to residents of Camden, Rockport, Hope, and Lincolnville, ME.
Application information: Application form required.
Deadline(s): None
Officers: Charles Lowe, Pres.; Sam Jones, V.P.; Adele Hopkins, Secy.-Treas.
EIN: 010248064

366
Emma Belcher Coombs Testamentary Trust
209 Main St.
Freeport 04032 (207) 865-3135
Contact: John L. French, Trustee

Financial data (yr. ended 12/31/95): Assets, $52,090 (M); expenditures, $4,944; qualifying distributions, $4,944, including $2,700 for 16 grants to individuals (high: $450; low: $150).
Purpose and activities: Grants only to residents of Freeport, ME; who are age 65 or older, in financial need, and have no affiliation with the Roman Catholic Church.
Fields of interest: Aging; Economically disadvantaged.
Types of support: Grants to individuals.
Limitations: Giving limited to residents of Freeport, ME.
Application information:
Initial approach: Letter
Deadline(s): Dec. 25
Trustee: John L. French.
EIN: 016014279

367
The Maine Community Foundation, Inc.
210 Main St.
P.O. Box 148
Ellsworth 04605 (207) 667-9735
Contact: Ann Tartre, Prog. Officer
FAX: (207) 667-9738

Incorporated in 1983 in ME.
Foundation type: Community
Financial data (yr. ended 12/31/95): Assets, $20,855,221 (M); gifts received, $3,567,972; expenditures, $2,483,995, including $1,560,955 for grants (high: $500,000; low: $100; average: $500-$5,000) and $192,834 for 233 grants to individuals (high: $3,000; low: $100).
Purpose and activities: Primary areas of interest include the arts, child welfare and youth, the disadvantaged, education, health, and community development.
Fields of interest: Arts/cultural programs; Elementary school/education; Adult/continuing education; Education; Natural resource conservation & protection; Environment; Health care; Health associations; Youth development, services; Human services; Children & youth, services; Aging, centers & services; Community development; Leadership development; Aging; Economically disadvantaged.
Types of support: Program development, conferences/seminars, publication, seed money, technical assistance, scholarships—to individuals, matching funds.
Limitations: Giving limited to ME. No support for religious organizations for religious purposes. No grants to individuals (except for scholarship funds), or for endowment funds, equipment, or annual campaigns for regular operations; grants rarely made for capital campaigns.
Publications: Annual report (including application guidelines), informational brochure, newsletter, program policy statement, application guidelines, grants list.
Application information: Application form required.
Initial approach: Letter or telephone for guidelines
Copies of proposal: 1
Deadline(s): Jan. 15, Apr. 1, July 15, and Oct. 1
Board meeting date(s): 4 times annually
Final notification: 2 months after deadline
Officers and Directors:* Rosalyn Bernstein,* Chair.; Warren Cook, Vice-Chair.; Marion M. Kane, Pres.; Janet Henry, V.P.; Sidney St. F. Thaxter, Clerk; and 23 additional directors.
Staff: Patti D'Angelo, Prog. Officer; Ann Tartre, Prog. Officer; Carole O'Donnell, Financial Officer.
Number of staff: 6 full-time professional.
EIN: 010391479

368
McArthur Home for Aged People Association
c/o Robert Norton
P.O. Box 291
Biddeford 04005

Established in 1974.
Foundation type: Operating
Financial data (yr. ended 10/31/95): Assets, $4,914,524 (M); expenditures, $104,255; qualifying distributions, $181,531, including $74,286 for grants and $107,245 for foundation-administered programs.
Fields of interest: Housing/shelter, aging.
Officers: Carlton Davis, Pres.; Francis Spencer, V.P.; Robert Norton, Treas.; Virginia Carthill, Clerk.
EIN: 010212437

369
Portland Female Charitable Society
c/o Jean E. Leighton
20 Noyes St.
Portland 04103

Financial data (yr. ended 09/30/94): Assets, $141,119 (M); expenditures, $13,815; qualifying distributions, $11,125, including $11,125 for grants to individuals (high: $1,160).
Purpose and activities: Support only to indigent residents of Portland, ME, for health care (including dental care, prescriptions, hearing aids, and glasses), food, or shelter.
Fields of interest: Aging; Economically disadvantaged.
Types of support: Grants to individuals.
Limitations: Giving limited to residents of Portland, ME.
Application information: Application form not required.
Deadline(s): None
Officers and Managers:* Mary Anne Baker,* Pres.; Cecelia Levine,* Secy.; Jean E. Leighton,* Treas.; Sandra Brooks, Phyllis Hutchins, Charlene Libby, Ann McCullum, Mary Alice Reilly, Pat Schaffer, Ruth Stone.
EIN: 010370961

MARYLAND

370
American Occupational Therapy Foundation
c/o P.O. Box 31220
4720 Montgomery Ln.
Bethesda 20824-1220 (301) 652-2682
Contact: Martha Kirkland, Exec. Dir.

Established in 1965 in NY.
Financial data (yr. ended 09/30/94): Assets, $11,553,813 (M); gifts received, $560,617; expenditures, $1,015,275; qualifying distributions, $675,103.
Purpose and activities: Giving primarily for occupational therapy and health, rehabilitation, the disabled, and maintaining independent lifestyles for the elderly.
Fields of interest: Public health, occupational health; Aging, centers & services; Disabled; Aging.
Types of support: Conferences/seminars, fellowships, research, grants to individuals, scholarships—to individuals.
Publications: Annual report, financial statement, informational brochure.

Application information: Application form required.
Initial approach: Letter
Copies of proposal: 2
Board meeting date(s): May and Dec.
Final notification: Varies
Officers: Maralynne D. Mitcham, Ph.D., Pres.; Susan B. Fine, V.P.; Hanna Gruen, Secy.; Byron N. Cohen, Treas.; Martha Kirkland, Exec. Dir.
Directors: Charles Christiansen, Edward Eckenhoff, Lex Frieden, Ann P. Grady, Jim Hinojosa, Ph.D., Rony A. Kozmetsky, Donald F. Lang, Jane Rourk, Leopold G. Selker, Ph.D.
Number of staff: 3 full-time professional; 3 full-time support; 2 part-time support.
EIN: 136189382

371
The Baltimore Community Foundation

The Latrobe Bldg.
Two East Read St., 9th Fl.
Baltimore 21202 (410) 332-4171
Contact: Timothy D. Armbruster, Pres.

Incorporated in 1972 in MD.
Foundation type: Community
Financial data (yr. ended 12/31/94): Assets, $37,150,541 (M); gifts received, $5,033,093; expenditures, $3,791,208, including $2,805,103 for 280 grants (high: $222,300; low: $100; average: $1,000-$10,000), $105,000 for 50 grants to individuals (high: $500; low: $100; average: $100-$500), $4,000 for 1 loan and $600 for 1 in-kind gift.
Purpose and activities: Giving primarily for children and family, cultural, neighborhood, human service, and other community needs. Grants primarily for pilot projects, system-wide solutions, and to increase organizational effectiveness and self-sufficiency.
Fields of interest: Arts education; Arts/cultural programs; Education; Environment; Health care; Mental health/crisis services; Health organizations; Housing/shelter, development; Human services; Youth, services; Family services; Aging, centers & services; Community development; Voluntarism promotion; Government/public administration; Aging.
Types of support: Endowment funds, program development, seed money, technical assistance, consulting services, matching funds.
Limitations: Giving primarily in the Baltimore, MD, area.
Publications: Annual report, newsletter, application guidelines.
Application information: Application form not required.
Initial approach: Letter
Copies of proposal: 1
Deadline(s): 60 days before meetings
Board meeting date(s): 3 times a year
Final notification: Within 2 weeks after meetings
Officers and Trustees:* Edward K. Dunn, Jr.,* Chair.; Calman J. Zamoiski, Jr.,* Vice-Chair.; Timothy D. Armbruster, Pres.; Martha K. Johnston, Secy.; Eddie C. Brown,* Treas.; and 23 additional trustees.
Number of staff: 4 full-time professional; 3 part-time professional; 4 full-time support.
EIN: 237180620

372
Baltimore Gas and Electric Foundation, Inc.

Box 1475
Baltimore 21203 (410) 234-7480
Contact: Malinda B. Small

Established in 1986 in MD.
Donor(s): Baltimore Gas and Electric Co.
Foundation type: Company-sponsored
Financial data (yr. ended 12/31/94): Assets, $3,375,709 (M); gifts received, $1,239,400; expenditures, $2,267,583; qualifying distributions, $2,436,555, including $2,436,555 for 59 grants (high: $725,000; low: $2,000; average: $15,000-$50,000).
Purpose and activities: Support primarily for cultural programs, education, community development, health, and family services. Support also for civic and public affairs, the environment, youth and handicapped services.
Fields of interest: Museums; Arts/cultural programs; Higher education; Adult education—literacy & basic skills; Reading; Education; Environment; Hospitals (general); Health care; Health organizations; Youth, services; Family services; Aging, centers & services; Homeless, human services; Community development; Voluntarism promotion; Federated giving programs; Government/public administration; Public affairs; Disabled; Aging; Homeless.
Types of support: General/operating support, annual campaigns, capital campaigns.
Limitations: Applications not accepted. Giving primarily in MD, with emphasis on the Baltimore area.
Application information: Contributes only to pre-selected organizations.
Board meeting date(s): 4 times a year
Officers and Directors:* C.H. Poindexter,* Chair.; Edward A. Crooke,* Pres.; G.R. Fuhrman, V.P.; C.W. Shivery, Secy.-Treas.; H. Furlong Baldwin, B.B. Byron, J. Owen Cole, D.A. Colussy, J.R. Curtiss, Jerome W. Geckle, F.A. Hrabowski, N. Lampton, George V. McGowan, P.G. Miller, G.L. Russell, Jr., M.D. Sullivan.
Number of staff: 3
EIN: 521452037

373
Nathan & Suzanne Cohen Foundation, Inc.

Two Wyndhurst Ave.
Baltimore 21210
Contact: Wilbert H. Sirota, Secy.
Application address: 36 South Charles St., Baltimore, MD 21201; Tel.: (410) 576-7805

Established in 1988 in MD.
Donor(s): Nathan L. Cohen.‡
Financial data (yr. ended 12/31/95): Assets, $684,103 (M); expenditures, $69,722; qualifying distributions, $67,025, including $67,025 for 10 grants (high: $25,000; low: $1,000).
Purpose and activities: Primary areas of interest include Israel, Jewish welfare funds and other organizations, the arts, health, and education, especially higher education.
Fields of interest: Visual arts; Museums; Performing arts; Theater; Humanities; Arts/cultural programs; Higher education; Education; Hospitals (general); Health care; Health organizations; Human services; Aging, centers & services; Women, centers & services; Homeless, human services; Voluntarism promotion; Jewish federated giving programs; Jewish agencies & temples; Religion; Disabled; Aging; Women; Homeless; General charitable giving; Israel.
Types of support: Continuing support, annual campaigns, capital campaigns, endowment funds, emergency funds, program development, seed money, curriculum development, scholarship funds, research.
Limitations: Giving primarily in Baltimore, MD. No grants to individuals.
Application information:
Initial approach: Letter
Deadline(s): None
Officers: Suzanne F. Cohen, Pres. and Treas.; Wilbert H. Sirota, Secy.
Number of staff: None.
EIN: 521570124

374
The Columbia Foundation

10221 Wincopin Circle
Columbia 21044-2624 (410) 730-7840
Contact: Barbara K. Lawson, Exec. Dir.
FAX: (410) 715-3043

Incorporated in 1969 in MD.
Foundation type: Community
Financial data (yr. ended 12/31/95): Assets, $3,243,470 (M); gifts received, $557,964; expenditures, $413,389, including $287,200 for 49 grants (high: $21,500; low: $800; average: $1,000-$35,000).
Purpose and activities: Grants for health and human services, including programs for youth, the aged, and the disabled; arts and culture, including music, the performing arts, and historic preservation; educational programs; and housing.
Fields of interest: Performing arts; Music; Historic preservation/historical societies; Arts/cultural programs; Education; Health care; Housing/shelter, development; Human services; Children & youth, services; Family services; Aging, centers & services; Disabled; Aging.
Types of support: General/operating support, continuing support, building/renovation, equipment, emergency funds, program development, conferences/seminars, seed money, curriculum development, technical assistance, consulting services, program-related investments/loans, matching funds.
Limitations: Giving limited to Howard County, MD. No support for projects of a sectarian religious nature. No grants to individuals, or for annual campaigns, deficit financing, land acquisition, medical research, or general or special endowments.
Publications: Financial statement, application guidelines, grants list, newsletter, informational brochure (including application guidelines), 990-PF.
Application information: For information on emergency funding, contact the foundation. Project grants are reviewed in Mar. and

operational grants in Nov. Application form required.
Initial approach: Telephone
Copies of proposal: 10
Deadline(s): Feb. for project support; Sept. for operating support
Board meeting date(s): 3rd Wednesday of each month
Final notification: 3 months
Officers and Trustees:* Donald A. Manekin,* Pres.; James R. Moxley, Jr., V.P.; Norma L. Hill,* Secy.; H. Elizabeth Horowitz,* Treas.; Barbara K. Lawson, Exec. Dir.; and 26 additional trustees.
Number of staff: 1 full-time professional; 1 full-time support.
EIN: 520937644

375
Eaton Fund, Inc.
c/o Mercantile-Safe Deposit & Trust Co.
766 Old Hammonds Ferry Rd.
Linthicum 21090
Application address: c/o Donna Davis, Mercantile-Safe Deposit & Trust Co., Two Hopkins Plaza, Baltimore, MD 21201; Tel.: (410) 237-5552

Financial data (yr. ended 12/31/95): Assets, $137,228 (M); gifts received, $14,347; expenditures, $18,147; qualifying distributions, $17,370, including $16,900 for 7 grants to individuals (high: $3,300; low: $1,000).
Purpose and activities: Relief assistance to women aged 60 or older who are residents of Baltimore, MD or its Vicinity and who are unable to provide themselves with the adequate necessities of life. The duration of grants depends on the particular situation and need of the recipient.
Fields of interest: Aging; Women.
Types of support: Emergency funds, grants to individuals.
Limitations: Giving limited to the Baltimore, MD, area.
Application information:
Initial approach: Letter
Deadline(s): None
Officers and Directors:* Mrs. Robert S. Killebrew, Jr.,* Pres.; William J. Evans,* V.P.; Mrs. Redmond Finney,* Secy.; Truman T. Seamans,* Treas.; Mary Burnett.
EIN: 526034106

376
Feldman Family Charitable Foundation, Inc.
9927 South Glen Rd.
Potomac 20854
Contact: Maurice Feldman, Secy.-Treas.

Established in 1979 in MD.
Financial data (yr. ended 04/30/94): Assets, $519,553 (M); gifts received, $116,000; expenditures, $53,107; qualifying distributions, $53,107, including $49,463 for 24 grants (high: $15,000; low: $100).
Fields of interest: Human services; Aging, centers & services; Jewish federated giving programs; Jewish agencies & temples; Aging.
Limitations: Giving primarily in the Washington, DC, area, including MD.
Application information: Application form not required.
Deadline(s): None
Officers and Directors:* Minnie Feldman,* Pres.; Maurice Feldman,* Secy.-Treas.; Pamela Ein.
EIN: 521157486

377
Isador & Fannie Havelock Foundation, Inc.
9505 Reisterstown Rd., Suite 2 South
Owings Mills 21117
Contact: H. Stanley Levy, Pres.
Application address: 2110 Northcliff Dr., Baltimore, MD 21209; Tel.: (410) 664-2225

Financial data (yr. ended 12/31/94): Assets, $460,790 (M); expenditures, $26,000; qualifying distributions, $26,000, including $26,000 for grants.
Fields of interest: Higher education; Theological school/education; Aging, centers & services; Jewish agencies & temples; Aging.
Types of support: General/operating support, scholarship funds.
Limitations: Giving limited to the Baltimore, MD, area.
Application information:
Initial approach: Letter
Deadline(s): None
Officers: H. Stanley Levy, Pres.; Edward R. Levy, V.P. and Secy.; Stephen F. Rosenberg, Treas.
EIN: 521191411

378
Hechinger Foundation
(also known as Sidney L. Hechinger Foundation)
3500 Pennsy Dr.
Landover 20785 (301) 341-0999
Contact: John W. Hechinger, Sr., Trustee

Incorporated in 1955 in DC.
Donor(s): Hechinger Co., members of the Hechinger family.
Foundation type: Company-sponsored
Financial data (yr. ended 06/30/94): Assets, $745,615 (M); gifts received, $600,000; expenditures, $743,808; qualifying distributions, $702,045, including $692,575 for 158 grants (high: $159,000; low: $50; average: $500-$10,000).
Purpose and activities: Emphasis on the performing arts, music, and other cultural programs, Jewish welfare funds, higher education, United Way, and youth and social service agencies, including aid to the handicapped.
Fields of interest: Performing arts; Theater; Music; Arts/cultural programs; Higher education; Education; Health care; Health organizations; Human services; Youth, services; Aging, centers & services; Civil rights; Federated giving programs; Government/public administration; Aging.
Types of support: General/operating support, employee-related scholarships.
Limitations: Giving limited to areas of company operations in Washington, DC, DE, MD, NJ, NY, OH, PA, and VA. No grants to individuals.
Publications: Application guidelines.
Application information: Application form not required.
Initial approach: Proposal
Copies of proposal: 1
Deadline(s): May 31 for scholarships
Board meeting date(s): Continuously
Final notification: 8 to 10 weeks if approved
Manager and Trustees:* S. Ross Hechinger,* Pres.; John W. Hechinger, Sr., John W. Hechinger, Jr.
Number of staff: 1 full-time professional; 1 full-time support; 1 part-time support.
EIN: 526054428
Grants for Aging:
United Seniors Health Cooperative, DC, $500. 94.

379
Katzman Family Foundation
3310 North Leisure World Blvd., No. 701
Silver Spring 20906 (301) 598-2745
Contact: Dr. Howard Katzman, Pres.

Established in 1989.
Donor(s): Howard Katzman, Pearl Katzman.
Financial data (yr. ended 12/31/95): Assets, $372,801 (M); gifts received, $3,700; expenditures, $10,864; qualifying distributions, $16,511, including $9,000 for 5 grants (high: $4,000; low: $1,000).
Fields of interest: Health care; Aging, centers & services; Jewish agencies & temples; Aging.
Limitations: Giving primarily in the Washington, DC, area, including VA and MD.
Application information: Application form not required.
Initial approach: Letter
Deadline(s): None
Board meeting date(s): Nov.
Officers: Howard Katzman, Pres.; Stanley Katzman, V.P.; Marlene Freed, Secy.-Treas.
Trustee: Sidney J. Silver.
Number of staff: None.
EIN: 521639155

380
Leominister-Croft Foundation, Inc.
207 East Redwood St., Suite 802
Baltimore 21202
Contact: L. Gordon Croft, V.P.

Established in 1990 in MD.
Donor(s): Leominister, Inc., L. Gordon Croft.
Foundation type: Company-sponsored
Financial data (yr. ended 12/31/95): Assets, $783,039 (M); expenditures, $38,881; qualifying distributions, $35,550, including $35,550 for 22 grants (high: $25,000; low: $50).
Fields of interest: Education; Human services; Aging, centers & services; Homeless, human services; Disabled; Aging; Economically disadvantaged; Homeless.
Limitations: Giving primarily in Baltimore, MD.
Application information:
Initial approach: Letter
Deadline(s): None

Officers and Trustees:* Kent Gordon Croft,* Pres.; L. Gordon Croft,* V.P.; Jane Aurell Croft,* Secy.
EIN: 521682796

381
Maryland Branch of the Shut-In Society of Baltimore

c/o Allan W. Mund
1311 Glendale Ave.
Baltimore 21239
Contact: Joseph A. Tarr, Treas.

Established in 1908 in MD.
Donor(s): Ida Perry Black.‡
Financial data (yr. ended 12/31/95): Assets, $687,206 (M); gifts received, $133; expenditures, $21,626; qualifying distributions, $14,481, including $13,961 for 5 grants (high: $5,000; low: $461).
Purpose and activities: Grants limited to programs aimed at helping financially deprived, shut-in senior citizens experience recreational activities outside their current environment.
Fields of interest: Recreation; Aging, centers & services; Aging.
Types of support: General/operating support, equipment, program development.
Limitations: Giving limited to MD. No grants to individuals.
Application information:
Initial approach: Brief proposal
Deadline(s): None
Officers and Directors:* Catherine C. Tarr,* Pres.; Irene Heyl,* V.P.; Mrs. William V. Cook,* Recording Secy.; Joseph A. Tarr,* Treas.; Mrs. Charles H. Mund, Allan W. Mund, Carol Smith.
EIN: 526013547

382
The Rouse Company Corporate Contributions

10275 Little Patuxent Pkwy.
Columbia 21044 (410) 992-6375
Contact: Margaret Mauro, Exec. Dir.

Financial data (yr. ended 12/31/94): Total giving, $921,000, including $900,000 for 220 grants (high: $50,000; low: $100), $21,000 for 83 employee matching gifts and $50,000 for 100 foundation-administered programs.
Fields of interest: Performing arts; Humanities; Arts/cultural programs; Higher education; Natural resource conservation & protection; Environment; Housing/shelter, development; Human services; Family services; Hospices; Aging, centers & services; Homeless, human services; Aging; Economically disadvantaged; Homeless.
Types of support: General/operating support, continuing support, annual campaigns, capital campaigns, building/renovation, endowment funds, seed money, scholarship funds, employee volunteer services, program-related investments/loans, donated equipment.
Limitations: Giving primarily in the central MD, area.
Publications: Informational brochure (including application guidelines).
Application information: Company has a staff that only handles contributions. Application form not required.
Initial approach: Letter or telephone to headquarters
Copies of proposal: 1
Deadline(s): None
Board meeting date(s): Every 2 months
Administrators: Margaret P. Mauro, Exec. Dir.; Frances S. Troxler, Contribs. Asst.
Number of staff: 1 full-time professional; 1 part-time support.

383
The Christian and Eleanora Ruppert Home for the Aged

8507 Longfellow Place
Chevy Chase 20815 (301) 652-3345
Contact: Charles E. Frazier, Secy.

Established around 1942.
Financial data (yr. ended 12/31/95): Assets, $1,223,120 (M); expenditures, $57,846; qualifying distributions, $43,500, including $34,000 for 11 grants (high: $5,000; low: $1,000).
Fields of interest: Disasters, search & rescue; Human services; Residential/custodial care; Aging, centers & services.
Limitations: Giving primarily in the greater metropolitan Washington, DC, area. No grants to individuals.
Application information: Application form required.
Deadline(s): None
Officers: J.A. Smith, Pres.; R.C. Frazier, V.P.; B.T. Smith, V.P.; Charles E. Frazier, Secy.
EIN: 530204624

384
Hilda E. & Julius W. Schweinsberg Foundation

Seven Saint Paul St., Suite 1400
Baltimore 21202-1626 (410) 347-8787
Contact: Robert Sloan, Trustee

Financial data (yr. ended 12/31/95): Assets, $590,274 (M); expenditures, $21,871; qualifying distributions, $19,486, including $17,364 for 3 grants (high: $16,014; low: $350).
Fields of interest: Child development, education; Religion; Aging.
Limitations: Giving primarily in MD.
Application information:
Initial approach: Letter
Deadline(s): None
Trustees: John H. Ensor, Robert Sloan.
EIN: 526494445

385
Samuel and Bernice Shapiro Foundation, Inc.

1200 Mercantile Bank & Trust Co.
Two Hopkins Plaza
Baltimore 21201-2930
Contact: Irving Cohn

Established in 1985 in MD.
Donor(s): Bernice Shapiro, Samuel Shapiro.
Financial data (yr. ended 09/30/94): Assets, $306,580 (M); gifts received, $141,944; expenditures, $45,889; qualifying distributions, $42,192, including $42,154 for grants.
Fields of interest: Higher education; Hospitals (general); Medical research; Human services; Aging, centers & services; Jewish federated giving programs; Jewish agencies & temples; Aging.
Limitations: Applications not accepted. Giving primarily in FL and MA. No grants to individuals.
Application information: Contributes only to pre-selected organizations.
Officers: Samuel Shapiro, Pres.; Bernice Shapiro, Secy.-Treas.
EIN: 521464566

386
Albert Shapiro Fund, Inc.

Two Hopkins Plaza, Suite 1200
Baltimore 21201 (410) 385-4099
Contact: Irving Cohen, Secy.-Treas.

Established in 1983 in MD.
Financial data (yr. ended 05/31/94): Assets, $4,644,925 (M); expenditures, $191,296; qualifying distributions, $191,296, including $165,450 for 38 grants (high: $50,000; low: $100).
Purpose and activities: Giving primarily for Jewish organizations, especially welfare funds; support also for cultural programs and a hospital.
Fields of interest: Arts/cultural programs; Hospitals (general); Human services; Aging, centers & services; Jewish federated giving programs; Jewish agencies & temples; Aging.
Limitations: Giving primarily in Baltimore, MD, and Palm Beach, FL. No grants to individuals.
Application information:
Initial approach: Letter
Deadline(s): None
Officers: Albert Shapiro, Pres.; Eileen Shapiro, V.P.; Irving Cohen, Secy.-Treas.
EIN: 521300277

387
Nathan W. Shock and Margaret T. Shock Aging Research Foundation, Inc.

c/o Benjamin Dubin, C.P.A.
7113 Pheasant Cross Dr.
Baltimore 21209
Contact: George T. Baker, Pres.
Application address: 14628 Corona Dr., Silver Spring, MD 20916; Tel.: (301) 384-2948

Established in 1990 in MD.
Donor(s): Nathan W. Shock.‡
Financial data (yr. ended 12/31/94): Assets, $261,437 (M); gifts received, $2,275; expenditures, $12,795; qualifying distributions, $12,353, including $10,000 for grants.
Purpose and activities: Support only for gerontology research.
Fields of interest: Aging, centers & services; Aging.
Limitations: Giving on a national basis.
Application information:
Initial approach: Letter
Deadline(s): Oct. 1

Officers: George T. Baker, Pres.; John H. Shock, V.P.; Joseph B. Shock, Secy.-Treas.
EIN: 521653558

388
The Joseph & Anna Smith Foundation
c/o Joanne C. Smith
10401 Grosvenor Place, No. 1213
Rockville 20852

Financial data (yr. ended 12/31/95): Assets, $323,086 (M); expenditures, $15,650; qualifying distributions, $14,287, including $13,950 for 11 grants (high: $5,000; low: $250).
Fields of interest: Education; Jewish federated giving programs; Jewish agencies & temples; Disabled; Aging.
Limitations: Applications not accepted. Giving primarily in the Washington, DC, area, including MD. No grants to individuals.
Application information: Contributes only to pre-selected organizations.
Trustees: Anne G. Smith, Joanne C. Smith.
EIN: 526037447

389
Leonard P. Steuart Foundation, Inc.
5206 River Rd.
Bethesda 20816
Contact: Harry Martens, Jr., V.P.

Donor(s): Virginia S. Martens.
Financial data (yr. ended 07/31/94): Assets, $313,737 (M); expenditures, $378,164; qualifying distributions, $373,064, including $373,064 for 26 grants (high: $347,414; low: $50).
Fields of interest: Education; Health care; Human services; Aging.
Limitations: Giving primarily in Bethesda, MD, and Washington, DC.
Application information: Application form not required.
Deadline(s): None
Officers: Virginia S. Martens, Pres.; Harry Martens, Jr., V.P.
Directors: Willard C. Kress, Dana Martens, Harry Martens III, John Martens, Leonard Martens, Virginia Martens.
EIN: 526040068
Grants for Aging:
Asbury Methodist Home, Gaithersburg, MD, $347,414. 94.
Asbury Methodist Home, Gaithersburg, MD, $500. 94.

390
The USF&G Foundation, Inc.
100 Light St.
Baltimore 21202 (410) 547-3752
Contact: Sue Lovell, Dir.

Foundation established in 1980 in MD.
Donor(s): United States Fidelity and Guaranty Co.
Foundation type: Company-sponsored
Financial data (yr. ended 12/31/94): Assets, $9,350,567 (M); expenditures, $2,166,168; qualifying distributions, $2,103,491, including $2,103,491 for grants.
Purpose and activities: The mission of the USF&G Foundation is to improve the quality of life at both the local and national level by helping to fund organizations that promote and support education, social welfare, and economic development, with particular focus on the communities served by USF&G and its employees. Emphasis includes health and family services, homelessness, and minorities.
Fields of interest: Elementary school/education; Elementary/secondary education; Education; Hospitals (general); Health care; Health organizations; Domestic violence prevention; Human services; Children & youth, services; Family services; Minorities/immigrants, centers & services; Homeless, human services; Civil rights, disabled; Community development; Minorities; African Americans; Aging; Women; People with AIDS (PWAs); Economically disadvantaged; Homeless.
Types of support: General/operating support, annual campaigns, building/renovation, equipment, emergency funds, program development, curriculum development, internships, employee matching gifts, employee-related scholarships.
Limitations: Giving limited to the U.S. No support for trade and industry associations, political or veterans' organizations, or religious organizations for religious purposes. No grants to individuals (except for employee-related scholarships), or for seed money, emergency funds, deficit financing, land acquisition, matching gifts, research, publications, or conferences; no loans.
Publications: Annual report, grants list, newsletter, informational brochure (including application guidelines).
Application information: Application form required.
Initial approach: Proposal
Copies of proposal: 1
Deadline(s): None
Board meeting date(s): As required
Final notification: 3 to 4 weeks after quarterly meetings
Officers and Trustee:* Norman P. Blake, Jr.,* Pres.; John Hoffen, Secy.; Sue Lovell, Dir.
Number of staff: 1 full-time professional.
EIN: 521197155

391
Anna Emory Warfield Memorial Fund, Inc.
Mercantile Bank & Trust Bldg., Pavilion I
Two Hopkins Plaza
Baltimore 21201 (410) 547-0612
Contact: Mrs. Thelma K. O'Neal, Secy.

Incorporated in 1928 in MD.
Donor(s): S. Davies Warfield.‡
Financial data (yr. ended 12/31/95): Assets, $4,820,125 (M); expenditures, $188,240; qualifying distributions, $177,675, including $750 for 1 grant and $176,925 for 46 grants to individuals (high: $4,225; low: $325; average: $325-$4,225).
Purpose and activities: Organized exclusively to assist aged and dependent women.
Fields of interest: Aging; Women; Economically disadvantaged.
Types of support: Grants to individuals.
Limitations: Giving primarily in the metropolitan Baltimore, MD, area. No grants for capital or endowment funds, general support, matching gifts, scholarships, fellowships, or research; no loans.
Publications: Application guidelines.
Application information: Application form required.
Initial approach: Telephone or letter
Copies of proposal: 1
Deadline(s): None
Board meeting date(s): Apr. and Oct.
Final notification: 2 months
Officers and Trustees:* Charles B. Reeves, Jr.,* Pres.; Braxton D. Mitchell,* V.P.; Thelma K. O'Neal, Secy.; Edward K. Dunn, Jr.,* Treas.; Mrs. W. Page Dame, Jr., Louis W. Hargrave, Mrs. John B. Howard, Mrs. Thomas H. Maddux, Mrs. William F. Schmick, Jr., Mrs. Barry Strudwick, Mrs. Lewis C. Strudwick, Mrs. Guy Warfield.
Number of staff: 1 part-time support.
EIN: 520785672

392
The Harry and Jeanette Weinberg Foundation, Inc.
5518 Baltimore National Pike
Baltimore 21228
Contact: Bernard Siegel, Pres.

Incorporated in 1959 in MD.
Donor(s): Harry Weinberg,‡ and various companies.
Financial data (yr. ended 02/28/95): Assets, $990,900,000 (M); gifts received, $59,700,000; expenditures, $57,900,000; qualifying distributions, $51,229,000, including $51,000,000 for 200 grants (high: $3,000,000; low: $500; average: $5,000-$1,000,000).
Purpose and activities: "To contribute to charitable organizations which will use the distribution to benefit those whose financial resources are less than the financial resources of 50 percent of the members of the relevant community to which such beneficiaries belong."
Fields of interest: Food services; Human services; Aging, centers & services; Homeless, human services; Disabled; Aging; Economically disadvantaged; Homeless.
Types of support: Capital campaigns, building/renovation, endowment funds, matching funds.
Limitations: Applications not accepted. No support for colleges, universities, or museums. No grants to individuals.
Application information: Contributes only to pre-selected organizations.
Board meeting date(s): Periodically
Officers and Directors:* Bernard Siegel,* Pres.; Nathan Weinberg,* V.P. and Secy.; Alvin Awaya,* V.P.; Robert Kelly,* Treas.; Shale D. Stiller.
Number of staff: 3 full-time professional.
EIN: 526037034
Grants for Aging:
Association of Senior Citizens, Denver, CO, $10,000. 95.
Beth Abraham Foundation, Bronx, NY, $110,000. 95.

Beth Abraham Foundation, Bronx, NY, $100,000. 95.
CHAI (Comprehensive Housing Assistance, Inc.), Baltimore, MD, $550,000. 95.
CHAI (Comprehensive Housing Assistance, Inc.), Baltimore, MD, $200,000. 95.
CHAI (Comprehensive Housing Assistance, Inc.), Baltimore, MD, $200,000. 95.
CHAI (Comprehensive Housing Assistance, Inc.), Baltimore, MD, $50,000. 95.
Christmas in April Oahu, Honolulu, HI, $30,000. 95.
Golden Manor Jewish Home for the Aged, San Antonio, TX, $100,000. 95.
Govans Ecumenical Development Corporation, Baltimore, MD, $100,000. 95.
Houston Jewish Geriatric Foundation, Houston, TX, $100,000. 95.
Jewish Association on Aging (JAA), Pittsburgh, PA, $260,000. 95.
Jewish Council for the Aging of Greater Washington, Rockville, MD, $25,000. 95.
Jewish Council for the Aging of Greater Washington, Rockville, MD, $25,000. 95.
Jewish Home and Infirmary of Rochester New York, Rochester, NY, $200,000. 95.
Jewish Home for the Aged, San Francisco, CA, $500,000. 95.
Jewish Home for the Aged, San Francisco, CA, $500,000. 95.
Levindale Hebrew Geriatric Center and Hospital, Baltimore, MD, $25,000. 95.
Meals on Wheels of Lackawanna, Scranton, PA, $176,000. 95.
Metropolitan Jewish Geriatric Center, Brooklyn, NY, $1,000,000. 95.
Milwaukee Jewish Home, Milwaukee, WI, $638,000. 95.
Palolo Chinese Home, Honolulu, HI, $10,000. 95.
River Garden Foundation, Jacksonville, FL, $126,985. 95.
Telespond Senior Services, Scranton, PA, $376,000. 95.

393
The Theophilus & Marie Cover White Memorial Fund

c/o Mercantile-Safe Deposit & Trust Co.
766 Old Hammonds Ferry Rd.
Linthicum 21090
Application address: Donna Davis, Mercantile-Safe Deposit & Trust Co., Two Hopkins Plaza, Baltimore, MD 21201; Tel.: (410) 237-5521

Established in 1987 in MD.
Financial data (yr. ended 12/31/95): Assets, $1,075,859 (M); expenditures, $61,570; qualifying distributions, $51,230, including $51,149 for 5 grants (high: $25,000; low: $6,000).
Purpose and activities: Grants awarded to hospitals for the benefit of elderly persons needing medical assistance.
Fields of interest: Health care; Aging, centers & services; Aging.
Limitations: Giving limited to Baltimore, MD. No grants to individuals.
Application information:
Initial approach: Letter
Deadline(s): None
Trustee: Mercantile-Safe Deposit & Trust Co.
EIN: 526332718

MASSACHUSETTS

394
Andover Home for Aged People

P.O. Box 143
Andover 01810
Contact: Thomas J. Urbelis, Pres.
Application address: Six Eastman Rd., Andover, MA 01810; Tel.: (508) 475-9551

Established in 1983.
Foundation type: Operating
Financial data (yr. ended 09/30/95): Assets, $1,112,522 (M); expenditures, $34,755; qualifying distributions, $26,309, including $24,350 for 6 grants (high: $10,000; low: $350).
Purpose and activities: Support primarily for elderly residents or organizations that support the elderly in Andover, MA.
Fields of interest: Aging, centers & services; Aging.
Types of support: General/operating support, grants to individuals.
Limitations: Giving limited to the Andover, MA, area.
Publications: Annual report, financial statement, grants list.
Application information: Application form not required.
Initial approach: Letter
Copies of proposal: 1
Deadline(s): None
Board meeting date(s): 3rd Tuesday in Sept.
Officers: Thomas J. Urbelis, Pres.; Richard H. Mower, Jr., 1st V.P.; Carlene E. Darby, 2nd V.P.; John R. Petty, Treas.; Judith C. Avery, Clerk.
Number of staff: None.
EIN: 046050619

395
Lewis Dewart Apsley Fund for Aged & Indigent

c/o John J. Irvine, Jr.
233 Lincoln St., P.O. Box 446
Hudson 01749-0446

Financial data (yr. ended 12/31/94): Assets, $320,921 (M); expenditures, $15,318; qualifying distributions, $13,701, including $10,120 for 10 grants (high: $1,200; low: $420) and $1,620 for 1 grant to an individual.
Fields of interest: Aging, centers & services; Christian agencies & churches; Aging; Economically disadvantaged.
Types of support: Grants to individuals.
Limitations: Applications not accepted. Giving limited to Hudson, MA.
Application information: Contributes only to pre-selected organizations.
Officers: Diane C. Buchanan, Secy.; Robert J. Carney, Treas.
Trustee: John J. Irvine, Jr.
EIN: 046061333

396
Ash Charitable Corporation, Inc.

861 Turnpike St.
North Andover 01845 (508) 683-6700
Contact: John T. Pollano, Treas.

Established in 1989 in MA.
Financial data (yr. ended 12/31/94): Assets, $977,037 (M); expenditures, $62,271; qualifying distributions, $57,252, including $49,800 for grants.
Fields of interest: Higher education; Youth development, centers & clubs; Aging, centers & services; Foundations (private grantmaking).
Limitations: Giving primarily in Lawrence, MA. No grants to individuals.
Application information:
Initial approach: Letter or proposal
Deadline(s): None
Officers and Trustees:* Robert H. Goldstein,* Pres.; John T. Pollano,* Treas.; Donald A. George,* Clerk.
EIN: 222994115

397
Association for the Relief of Aged Women of New Bedford

27 South Sixth St.
New Bedford 02740
Contact: Hope Atkinson, Pres.

Established in 1866.
Foundation type: Operating
Financial data (yr. ended 03/31/95): Assets, $8,731,064 (M); gifts received, $3,600; expenditures, $370,909; qualifying distributions, $370,909, including $304,579 for 28 grants to individuals (high: $49,518; low: $220; average: $1,500-$42,000).
Purpose and activities: A private operating foundation; to furnish assistance to and to promote the welfare and relief of elderly women in New Bedford, Dartmouth, and Fairhaven, MA.
Fields of interest: Aging; Women; Economically disadvantaged.
Types of support: Grants to individuals.
Limitations: Giving limited to New Bedford, Dartmouth, and Fairhaven, MA.
Application information: Investigating committee visit to applicant. Application form not required.
Initial approach: Letter or referral from nominating nonprofit agency
Copies of proposal: 1
Deadline(s): None
Board meeting date(s): 1st Monday of each month
Officers and Directors:* Hope Atkinson,* Pres.; Mrs. Don Davies,* Secy.; Mrs. Thornton M. Richards,* Treas.; and 15 additional directors.
Number of staff: None.
EIN: 046056367

398
Charles F. Bacon Trust

c/o Fleet Bank of Massachusetts, N.A.
75 State St.
Boston 02109-1810 (617) 346-2493
Contact: Kerry H. Sullivan, Dir., Grantmaking

Trust established in 1928 in MA.
Donor(s): Charles F. Bacon.‡
Financial data (yr. ended 12/31/94): Assets, $2,598,318 (M); expenditures, $116,065; qualifying distributions, $106,536, including $73,000 for 5 grants (high: $24,000; low: $9,000) and $8,000 for 1 grant to an individual.
Purpose and activities: Areas of interest include family services, minority education, preventative health care, and programs which benefit elderly women.
Fields of interest: Health care; Family services; Minorities; Aging; Women.
Types of support: General/operating support, building/renovation, equipment, seed money, grants to individuals, matching funds.
Limitations: Giving primarily in the greater Boston, MA, area.
Publications: Application guidelines, 990-PF.
Application information: Application form required.
Initial approach: Letter
Copies of proposal: 1
Deadline(s): Feb. 15
Board meeting date(s): Feb.
Final notification: Late Feb.
Trustee: Fleet Bank, N.A.
Number of staff: 4 full-time professional; 1 full-time support.
EIN: 046024467

399
Adelaide Breed Bayrd Foundation
28 Pilgrim Rd.
Melrose 02176 (617) 662-7342
Contact: Russell E. Watts, M.D., Pres.

Incorporated in 1927 in MA.
Donor(s): Frank A. Bayrd,‡ Blanche S. Bayrd.‡
Financial data (yr. ended 12/31/95): Assets, $2,590,030 (M); gifts received, $400,000; expenditures, $468,832; qualifying distributions, $431,343, including $411,700 for 47 grants (high: $20,000; low: $200; average: $1,000-$50,000).
Purpose and activities: To support primarily those activities in which the donor's mother took an active interest. This includes local hospitals, social welfare concerns, libraries, youth oriented programs, and cultural activities. The foundation does not grant individual scholarships but does fund ten scholarships annually through the Malden High School. All grants must in some manner benefit the citizens of Malden.
Fields of interest: Arts/cultural programs; Adult/continuing education; Libraries/library science; Education; Hospitals (general); Health care; Health associations; Human services; Children & youth, services; Family services; Hospices; Aging, centers & services; Community development; Aging; General charitable giving.
Types of support: Annual campaigns, capital campaigns, building/renovation, equipment, emergency funds, program development, scholarship funds.
Limitations: Giving limited to the metropolitan Boston, MA, area, with emphasis on Malden. No support for national or out-of-state organizations or the performing arts. No grants to individuals (except for scholarships supplementary to the will of Blanche Bayrd), or for matching or challenge grants, demonstration projects, conferences, publications, or research; no loans.
Publications: Annual report (including application guidelines).
Application information: Application form not required.
Initial approach: Proposal
Copies of proposal: 1
Deadline(s): Submit proposal preferably in Dec. or Jan.; deadline Apr. 1
Board meeting date(s): 2nd Tuesday in Feb.; special meetings usually held in Apr. or May to consider grant requests
Final notification: Generally in Apr. or May
Officers and Trustees:* Russell E. Watts, M.D.,* Pres.; Susan C. Mansur,* Treas.; Florence C. Burns, C. Henry Kezer, Fred I. Lamson, William H. Marshall, Gaynor K. Rutherford, Jean H. Stearns, H. Allen Stevens.
Number of staff: 1 part-time professional; 1 part-time support.
EIN: 046051258
Grants for Aging:
Melrose Senior Citizens Center, Melrose, MA, $5,000. 95.
Mystic Valley Elder Services, Malden, MA, $10,000. 95.

400
The James Gordon Bennett Memorial Corporation
100 Bertwell Rd.
Lexington 02173
Contact: Carolyn Lee, Pres.
Application address: c/o The New York Times, 229 West 43rd St., New York, NY 10036; Tel.: (212) 556-1250

Incorporated in 1919 in NY.
Donor(s): James Gordon Bennett.‡
Financial data (yr. ended 12/31/94): Assets, $5,159,577 (M); expenditures, $244,804; qualifying distributions, $219,916, including $187,475 for 113 grants to individuals (high: $6,250; low: $300).
Purpose and activities: Direct aid to journalists unable to provide for themselves because of old age, infirmity, or lack of means; limited to employees for ten years or more of a daily newspaper published in New York City, with preference for employees of newspapers in Manhattan; if funds are sufficient, employees of daily newspapers in any borough are eligible, together with their immediate families; any surplus funds to be applied to scholarship aid to children of these persons.
Fields of interest: Journalism & publishing; Human services; Aging, centers & services; Aging; Economically disadvantaged.
Types of support: Grants to individuals, scholarships—to individuals.
Limitations: Giving limited to employees (and their immediate families) of New York City dailies. No grants for building or endowment funds, operating budgets, or special projects.
Publications: Program policy statement, application guidelines.
Application information: Application form required.
Initial approach: Letter
Deadline(s): Mar. 1 for scholarships
Board meeting date(s): May and Dec.
Officers and Directors:* Michael C. Clendenin,* Chair.; Carolyn Lee,* Pres.; Peter Faris,* V.P.; James F. Crain,* Secy.-Treas.
EIN: 136150414

401
Bird Companies Charitable Foundation, Inc.
c/o Bird, Inc.
1077 Pleasant St.
Norwood 02062 (617) 551-0656
Contact: Carol Duffy

Incorporated in 1967 in MA.
Donor(s): Bird & Son, Inc., Bird Machine Co., Inc., Bird Incorporated.
Foundation type: Company-sponsored
Financial data (yr. ended 12/31/93): Assets, $34,665 (M); gifts received, $23,424; expenditures, $19,465; qualifying distributions, $18,588, including $18,452 for 38 grants (high: $5,000; low: $25).
Purpose and activities: The foundation is primarily interested in providing seed money to initiate projects or to explore new ideas. Preference will be given to projects which have the potential to demonstrate solutions to important regional problems and/or positively influence public policy. Areas of national interest: 1) Community Development - Programs involving housing, economic development or citizen participation; 2) Natural Resources - Projects aimed at finding methods to remedy environmental pollution, to ensure environmental or energy conservation or to develop renewable energy resources. Areas of local interest - employee committees: Priority for funding is provided to a scholarship program for qualifying children of Bird Corporation employees, and on an employee gift match basis to those projects which receive volunteer or financial support from Bird employees and which have local sponsorship, interest and involvement. Local grants are not limited to the seed money criterion and may be applied to a variety of financial needs. Particular areas of interest are: 1) Children and Youth- Programs aimed at (a) care for neglected, abused or special needs children; (b) the development of expanded work/vocational education options for disadvantaged youth; 2) Handicapped/Disabled Persons- Programs directed at increasing self-sufficiency or independence from institutionalization for the participants; 3) Elderly- Particularly projects which actively involve older Americans in their implementation or enhance the role of seniors in the local community; 4) Health Care- Programs designed to increase efficiency/reduce cost of local health care, and general support for hospitals used by employees.
Fields of interest: Vocational education; Natural resource conservation & protection; Energy; Environment; Hospitals (general); Health care; Health organizations; Housing/shelter, development; Youth development, citizenship; Human services; Children & youth, services; Youth, services; Aging, centers & services; Community development; Public policy, research; Public affairs, citizen participation; Disabled; Aging; Economically disadvantaged.

Types of support: Seed money.
Limitations: Giving primarily in the Norwood, MA, and Bardstown, KY, areas, and other areas of company operations in AZ, LA, and TX; grants to organizations outside corporate facilities considered when requests address the foundation's national interests. No grants to individuals; or for governmental organizations.
Publications: Program policy statement, application guidelines.
Application information: The foundation allocates its financial resources on a basis which reserves the majority for the grantmaking decisions of its Board of Directors and sets aside specific amounts for distribution by employee committees organized at its corporate installations. Application form not required.
Initial approach: Proposal
Copies of proposal: 1
Final notification: 1 to 6 months
Officers and Directors:* Joseph D. Vechiolla,* Pres.; Frank S. Anthony, Secy.; Joseph M. Grigelevich, Treas.; Robert P. Bass, Jr., Charles S. Bird, Jr., Robert Cooper, Francis J. Dunleavy, John T. Dunlop, Guy W. Fiske, George J. Haufler, Loren R. Watts.
EIN: 237067725

402
Boston Fatherless & Widows Society

c/o Goodwin, Procter & Hoar
Exchange Place, Suite 2200
Boston 02109-2881 (617) 570-1130
Contact: George W. Butterworth III, Treas.

Established in 1817 in MA; incorporated in 1837.
Financial data (yr. ended 11/30/95): Assets, $5,334,581 (M); gifts received, $17,950; expenditures, $270,294; qualifying distributions, $224,826, including $87,000 for grants and $137,826 for grants to individuals (average: $1,000-$3,000).
Purpose and activities: Aid to elderly indigent widows in the greater Boston, MA, area.
Fields of interest: Aging; Women; Economically disadvantaged.
Types of support: General/operating support, grants to individuals.
Limitations: Giving limited to the greater Boston, MA, area.
Application information: Application form not required.
Initial approach: Letter
Deadline(s): None
Officers and Trustees:* Mrs. John S. Clapp, Jr.,* Pres.; Mrs. H. Stephen Kott,* V.P.; Mrs. John R. Johnston,* Secy.; George W. Butterworth III, Treas.; Mrs. Robert B. Bachman, Mrs. Allen N. Clapp, Mrs. E. Raymond Corey, Mrs. Willard S. Levings, Mrs. Robert H. Traylor, Mrs. Robert H. Welsh.
EIN: 046006506

403
The Boston Foundation, Inc.

One Boston Place, 24th Fl.
Boston 02108-4402 (617) 723-7415
Contact: Anna Faith Jones, Pres.
FAX: (617) 589-3616

Established in 1915 in MA by agreement and declaration of trust; incorporated in 1917.
Foundation type: Community
Financial data (yr. ended 06/30/95): Assets, $376,362,750 (M); gifts received, $33,235,064; expenditures, $22,423,605, including $17,078,654 for 1,385 grants (high: $237,000; low: $100; average: $20,000-$40,000).
Purpose and activities: The focus for the foundation's discretionary grantmaking is the Building Family and Community Initiative under which funding priority is given to community building strategies that help children and their families overcome poverty. Support both to programs targeted specifically to the needs of children, youth and families, and broader efforts to develop and strengthen Boston's neighborhoods as vibrant, liveable communities. Broadly stated, the key categories include health, education, jobs/income, housing, active citizenship, and community fabric.
Fields of interest: Arts/cultural programs; Early childhood education; Child development, education; Elementary school/education; Secondary school/education; Adult/continuing education; Adult education—literacy & basic skills; Reading; Education; Health care; Health associations; AIDS; Health organizations; Delinquency prevention/services; Employment; Nutrition; Housing/shelter, development; Youth development, services; Human services; Children & youth, services; Youth, services; Child development, services; Family services; Aging, centers & services; Women, centers & services; Minorities/immigrants, centers & services; Homeless, human services; Race/intergroup relations; Civil rights; Urban/community development; Community development; Voluntarism promotion; Public policy, research; Leadership development; Minorities; Disabled; Aging; Women; Immigrants/refugees; Economically disadvantaged; Homeless.
Types of support: General/operating support, program development, seed money, technical assistance, consulting services, matching funds.
Limitations: Giving from discretionary funds limited to the metropolitan Boston, MA, area. No support for religious purposes, private schools, municipalities, or national or international programs. No grants to individuals, or for medical, scientific, or academic research, books or articles, films, radio, or television programs, equipment, travel, scholarships, fellowships, conferences, or capital campaigns; no loans.
Publications: Annual report, application guidelines, newsletter, occasional report, 990-PF, grants list.
Application information: Accepts NNG Common Grant Application. Application form not required.
Initial approach: Proposal
Copies of proposal: 1
Deadline(s): Mar. 15, June 15, Sept. 15 and Dec. 15
Board meeting date(s): Mar., June, Sept., and Dec.
Final notification: Within 1 or 2 weeks of board meeting
Officers and Distribution Committee:* Frieda Garcia,* Chair.; Ronald A. Homer, Vice-Chair.; Anna Faith Jones, Pres., C.E.O., and Secy.-Treas.; Christine Green, V.P., Progs.; Joan T. Bok, Marianne Bowler, Barbara Dortch-Okara, Robert A. Glassman, Charles Ray Johnson, Edward Masterman, Hanson S. Reynolds, David Rockefeller, Jr., Helen Spaulding.
Trustee Banks: Bank of Boston, Boston Safe Deposit & Trust Co., Fleet Bank of Massachusetts, N.A., Shawmut Bank, N.A., State Street Bank & Trust Co.
Staff: Robert R. Wadsworth, Prog. Dir.; Angel H. Bermudez, Prog. Officer; Glauco Ruesga, Donor Resources Mgr.
Number of staff: 18 full-time professional; 4 part-time professional; 13 full-time support; 1 part-time support.
EIN: 042104021
Grants for Aging:
Boston Aging Concerns, Young and Old United, Boston, MA, $20,000. Toward salary of resident services coordinator for rooming house on Cortez Street. 95.
Boston University, School of Medicine, Boston, MA, $10,000. For Elders Living at Home Program. 95.
Committee to End Elder Homelessness, Boston, MA, $25,000. For expansion of housing development, housing placement and advocacy programs. 95.
Hale-Barnard Corporation, Boston, MA, $10,000. To expand Bill Payer Program to enroll disabled adults. 95.
Massachusetts Senior Action Council, Somerville, MA, $35,000. For organizing and advocacy activities to improve health care and transportation services for Boston area seniors. 95.
Match-Up Interfaith Volunteers, Boston, MA, $10,000. 95.
New England Medical Center, Boston, MA, $25,000. For church-based intergenerational program for grandparents raising their grandchildren. 95.
Rogerson House, Boston, MA, $20,000. 95.
Southwest Boston Senior Services, Roslindale, MA, $15,000. 95.
University of Massachusetts, Boston Gerontology Institute, Boston, MA, $12,000. To publicize results of study of barriers preventing eligible seniors from signing up for Supplemental Social Security Income (SSI). 95.

404
John W. Boynton Fund

c/o State Street Bank & Trust Co.
P.O. Box 351
Boston 02101
Contact: Marilyn E. Wales, V.P., State Street Bank & Trust Co.

Trust established in 1950 in MA.
Donor(s): Dora C. Boynton.‡
Financial data (yr. ended 12/31/94): Assets, $2,743,645 (M); expenditures, $145,335; qualifying distributions, $122,308, including $105,000 for 10 grants (high: $80,000; low: $2,000; average: $2,500).
Purpose and activities: Grants principally to organizations serving low-income elderly; special consideration also to the town of Athol, MA. A limited number of other grants are made

to groups other than the elderly, including youth agencies.
Fields of interest: Human services; Youth, services; Aging, centers & services; Aging.
Types of support: General/operating support, building/renovation, equipment, program development, seed money.
Limitations: Giving limited to Athol and eastern MA. No grants to individuals, or for endowment funds, research, scholarships, fellowships, or matching gifts; no loans.
Publications: Application guidelines, grants list.
Application information: Application form not required.
Initial approach: Proposal
Copies of proposal: 1
Deadline(s): Mar. 15, June 15, Sept. 15, or Dec. 15
Board meeting date(s): Apr., July, Oct., and Jan.
Final notification: 1 month
Trustee: State Street Bank & Trust Co.
Number of staff: 2 part-time support.
EIN: 046036706
Grants for Aging:
South Shore Elder Services, Braintree, MA, $2,500. 94.

405
Bushrod H. Campbell and Adah F. Hall Charity Fund
c/o Palmer & Dodge
One Beacon St., Room 2200
Boston 02108 (617) 573-0176
Contact: Mary Clements Pajak

Trust established in 1956 in MA.
Donor(s): Bushrod H. Campbell,‡ Adah F. Hall.‡
Financial data (yr. ended 05/31/95): Assets, $12,970,616 (M); expenditures, $497,996; qualifying distributions, $426,233, including $373,887 for 88 grants (high: $25,000; low: $1,000; average: $2,000-$6,000).
Purpose and activities: Grants limited to organizations and/or their projects devoted to aid the elderly, population control, and health care. Medical research grants administered through the Medical Foundation. Grants made primarily for services and programs.
Fields of interest: Family planning; Health associations; Medical research; Aging, centers & services; Aging.
Types of support: General/operating support, continuing support, building/renovation, program development, conferences/seminars, seed money, research.
Limitations: Giving limited to the greater Boston, MA, area (within Route 128 and Boston); giving on a national basis to organizations dealing with population control. No grants to individuals, or for annual campaigns, emergency funds, deficit financing, land acquisition, publications, or general endowments; no loans.
Publications: Application guidelines, informational brochure, grants list.
Application information: Application form required.
Initial approach: Telephone or letter
Copies of proposal: 1
Deadline(s): Feb. 1, May 1, Sept. 1, or Nov. 1
Board meeting date(s): Feb., May, Sept., and Nov.
Final notification: By mail only
Trustees: Donald J. Barker, Casimir de Rham, Jr., Arthur B. Page, Curtis Prout.
Number of staff: 1 part-time professional.
EIN: 046013598
Grants for Aging:
Boston Aging Concerns, Young and Old United, Boston, MA, $4,000. For housing program. 95.
Elderlink, Somerville, MA, $4,000. For HouseWorks program. 95.

406
Clipper Ship Foundation, Inc.
c/o Grants Management Assocs.
230 Congress St., 3rd Fl.
Boston 02110 (617) 426-7172
Contact: Suzanne Sack, Fdn. Asst.

Established in 1979 in MA.
Donor(s): David Parmely Weatherhead.‡
Financial data (yr. ended 10/31/95): Assets, $20,909,583 (M); expenditures, $1,085,759; qualifying distributions, $939,375, including $886,398 for 154 grants (high: $62,500; low: $1,000; average: $5,000-$25,000).
Purpose and activities: "Priority given to organizations devoted to helping the homeless, the destitute, the handicapped, children and the aged, or supplying the special needs of minority, low-income individuals and families. Special consideration also given to emergency disaster situations."
Fields of interest: Housing/shelter, development; Human services; Children & youth, services; Aging, centers & services; Minorities/immigrants, centers & services; Homeless, human services; Community development; Public affairs; Minorities; Disabled; Aging; Homeless.
Types of support: General/operating support, continuing support, capital campaigns, emergency funds.
Limitations: Giving primarily in the greater Boston, MA, area. No grants to individuals.
Publications: Annual report (including application guidelines).
Application information: Only 1 proposal per applicant will be considered each calendar year. Application form not required.
Initial approach: Proposal or telephone
Copies of proposal: 1
Deadline(s): Mar. 1, May 1, Aug. 10, and Dec. 1
Board meeting date(s): Every 3 months
Officers and Directors:* Benjamin H. Lacy,* Pres.; John B. Newhall,* V.P.; Suzanne Sack, Secy. and Clerk; Nicholas Carter,* Treas.; Brian S. Kelley, Sarah R. Newbury, George F. Pennington, Mayra Rodriguez-Howard.
Number of staff: 1 part-time professional.
EIN: 042687384
Grants for Aging:
Committee to End Elder Homelessness, Boston, MA, $8,000. 95.
Senior Home Care Services Boston III, Boston, MA, $2,740. 95.

407
Coburn Charitable Society
c/o Pulsifer & Assocs.
P.O. Box 170
Ipswich 01938
Contact: H. Gilman Nichols, Treas.
Application address: Apple St., Essex, MA 01929; Tel.: (508) 768-6985

Financial data (yr. ended 04/30/95): Assets, $1,001,473 (M); gifts received, $1,687; expenditures, $52,697; qualifying distributions, $47,076, including $16,861 for 2 grants (high: $9,861; low: $7,000).
Purpose and activities: Support only for home and residential base care of elderly in Ipswich, MA and adjacent communities.
Fields of interest: Aging, centers & services; Aging.
Limitations: Giving limited to the Ipswich, MA, area. No grants to individuals.
Application information:
Initial approach: Letter
Deadline(s): None
Officers and Trustees:* Ben K. Collins,* Pres.; H. Gilman Nichols,* Treas.; Nathaniel Pulsifer,* Clerk; Stephanie Gaskins, Kathleen Hirbour, Carl Soderland.
EIN: 042104012

408
Community Foundation of Western Massachusetts
1500 Main St., Suite 1800
P.O. Box 15769
Springfield 01115 (413) 732-2858
Contact: Dr. Sandra Eagleton, Pres.

Established in 1991 in MA.
Foundation type: Community
Financial data (yr. ended 03/31/94): Assets, $2,513,376 (M); gifts received, $2,324,082; expenditures, $1,177,089, including $893,000 for grants (average: $8,000).
Fields of interest: Performing arts; Historic preservation/historical societies; Arts/cultural programs; Education, fund raising; Adult/continuing education; Adult education—literacy & basic skills; Libraries/library science; Reading; Education; Natural resource conservation & protection; Environment; Wildlife preservation & protection; Hospitals (general); Family planning; Medical care, rehabilitation; Health care; Substance abuse, services; Cancer; Heart/circulatory disease; AIDS; Health organizations; Cancer research; Heart/circulatory research; AIDS research; Delinquency prevention/services; Crime/law enforcement; Housing/shelter, development; Safety/disasters; Recreation; Human services; Children & youth, services; Youth, services; Aging, centers & services; Women, centers & services; Minorities/immigrants, centers & services; Human rights (international); Civil rights; Community development; Voluntarism promotion; Public policy, research; Public affairs; Minorities; Native Americans; Disabled; Aging; Women; Gays/lesbians; Economically disadvantaged.

Types of support: Capital campaigns, building/renovation, equipment, endowment funds, program development, conferences/seminars, publication, seed money, fellowships, scholarship funds, technical assistance, scholarships—to individuals, matching funds.
Limitations: Giving limited to western MA, with emphasis on Hampden County and Springfield.
Publications: Annual report (including application guidelines), grants list, informational brochure, application guidelines, newsletter.
Application information: Application form required.
Initial approach: Telephone
Copies of proposal: 3
Deadline(s): 1st Monday in Feb., May, Aug., and Nov.
Board meeting date(s): Monthly
Final notification: Within 2 months
Officer: Sandra Eagleton, Pres.
Staff: Brooke Trent, Prog. Officer; Thomas Hidalgo, Education Officer.
Number of staff: 1 full-time professional; 2 part-time professional; 2 full-time support.
EIN: 223089640

409
Sarah A. W. Devens Trust
c/o Rice, Heard & Bigelow, Inc.
50 Congress St., Suite 1025
Boston 02109

Established in 1876 in MA.
Donor(s): Sarah A.W. Devens.‡
Financial data (yr. ended 11/30/95): Assets, $1,410,048 (M); expenditures, $77,047; qualifying distributions, $64,839, including $60,499 for 63 grants to individuals (high: $8,400; low: $175).
Purpose and activities: Giving primarily for elderly economically disadvantaged women.
Fields of interest: Aging, centers & services; Women, centers & services; Aging; Women; Economically disadvantaged.
Types of support: Grants to individuals.
Limitations: Applications not accepted. Giving limited to MA.
Trustees: Edward S. Heard, George H. Stephenson.
EIN: 046291053

410
The Janet G. Elliott Trust
22 Valley Rd.
Needham 02192
Contact: Rev. Allan C. Emery III, Trustee

Established in 1984 in MA.
Donor(s): Janet G. Elliott.‡
Financial data (yr. ended 08/31/95): Assets, $1,142,552 (M); expenditures, $68,137; qualifying distributions, $61,920, including $57,000 for 3 grants (high: $26,500; low: $13,000).
Purpose and activities: Giving primarily for the elderly and indigent elderly by organizations with an evangelistic purpose in the greater Boston area.
Fields of interest: Human services; Aging, centers & services; Christian agencies & churches; Aging; Economically disadvantaged; Homeless.
Types of support: Continuing support.
Limitations: Applications not accepted. Giving primarily in the greater Boston, MA, area. No grants to individuals.
Application information: Contributes grants through evangelistic and evangelical organizations to the elderly who are in need.
Board meeting date(s): June or July
Trustees: Allan C. Emery, Jr., Rev. Allan C. Emery III, Samuel F. Powel IV, Paul E. Toms, Howard A. Williams.
Number of staff: None.
EIN: 066275546
Grants for Aging:
Evangelistic Association of New England, Burlington, MA, $26,500. For elderly care program. 95.

411
Everett Foundation for Aged Persons, Inc.
c/o Boynton & Boynton
535 Boylston St.
Boston 02116-3720

Established in 1902 in MA.
Financial data (yr. ended 12/31/94): Assets, $2,209,594 (M); expenditures, $109,289; qualifying distributions, $83,755, including $71,675 for 7 grants (high: $53,220; low: $1,680).
Purpose and activities: Giving limited to benefit the elderly, including a health counseling clinic and a nursing home.
Fields of interest: Aging, centers & services; Aging.
Limitations: Applications not accepted. Giving primarily in MA. No grants to individuals.
Application information: Contributes only to pre-selected organizations.
Officers and Directors:* Alfred Seaward,* Pres.; Caro M. Grace,* Treas.; George Ahlin, Marjorie L. Dacko, Marie Sapienza, Peter Sapienza, Dana Shattuck, Laura White.
EIN: 042062107

412
Abbie F. Farmer Trust
923 Main St.
Yarmouth Port 02675 (508) 362-5440
Contact: Harold E. Magnuson, Trustee

Financial data (yr. ended 12/31/94): Assets, $7,300 (M); expenditures, $111; qualifying distributions, $111.
Fields of interest: Aging, centers & services; Aging.
Types of support: Grants to individuals.
Limitations: Giving limited to residents of Arlington, MA.
Application information: No grants paid in 1994.
Initial approach: Letter
Deadline(s): None
Trustee: Harold E. Magnuson.
EIN: 046257684

413
Edwin S. Farmer Trust
923 Main St.
Yarmouth Port 02675
Contact: Harold E. Magnuson, Trustee

Financial data (yr. ended 12/31/94): Assets, $288,205 (M); expenditures, $15,153; qualifying distributions, $13,925, including $9,864 for 9 grants to individuals (high: $2,400; low: $109).
Purpose and activities: Support primarily to aged, indigent women and married couples of Arlington, MA.
Fields of interest: Aging; Women.
Types of support: Grants to individuals.
Limitations: Giving limited to Arlington, MA.
Application information:
Initial approach: Letter
Deadline(s): None
Trustee: Harold E. Magnuson.
EIN: 046257543

414
Charles H. Farnsworth Trust
c/o State Street Bank & Trust Co.
P.O. Box 351
Boston 02101
Contact: Marilyn E. Wales, V.P., State Street Bank & Trust Co.

Trust established in 1930; became a charitable trust in 1978.
Donor(s): Charles H. Farnsworth.‡
Financial data (yr. ended 09/30/95): Assets, $18,723,246 (M); expenditures, $877,658; qualifying distributions, $770,479, including $700,752 for 44 grants (high: $120,252; low: $500; average: $10,000-$20,000).
Purpose and activities: To assist elderly persons to live with dignity and independence. Special focus on services which help prevent premature institutionalization. Grants fostering the development of housing for the elderly are also of special interest.
Fields of interest: Housing/shelter, development; Aging, centers & services; Aging.
Types of support: General/operating support, capital campaigns, building/renovation, equipment, program development, seed money, research, technical assistance.
Limitations: Giving limited to the greater Boston, MA, area. No grants to individuals.
Publications: Application guidelines, grants list.
Application information: Application form not required.
Initial approach: Letter of intent
Copies of proposal: 1
Deadline(s): Feb. 15, May 15, Aug. 15, and Nov. 15
Board meeting date(s): Mar., June, Sept., and Dec.
Final notification: Within 1 month of meeting
Trustee: State Street Bank & Trust Co.
Number of staff: 2 part-time support.
EIN: 046096075
Grants for Aging:
Committee to End Elder Homelessness, Boston, MA, $20,000. 95.
Cooperative Elder Services, Concord, MA, $20,000. 95.
Elderlink, Somerville, MA, $20,000. 95.

Hale-Barnard Corporation, Boston, MA, $15,000. 95.
Homeowners Options for Massachusetts Elders (HOME), Boston, MA, $15,000. 95.
Jewish Nursing Home of Chelsea, Women's Auxiliary, Chelsea, MA, $20,000. 95.
Melrose Friends of the Aging, Melrose, MA, $20,000. 95.
Rogerson House, Boston, MA, $30,000. 95.

415
Herbert H. Fletcher Trust
c/o Boston Safe Deposit & Trust Co.
One Boston Place
Boston 02108
Contact: Judith Casey, Asst. V.P., Boston Safe Deposit & Trust Co.

Donor(s): Herbert H. Fletcher.‡
Financial data (yr. ended 08/31/93): Assets, $320,316 (M); expenditures, $18,214; qualifying distributions, $13,662.
Fields of interest: Aging, centers & services; Aging.
Limitations: Giving primarily in the Boston, MA, area.
Application information: Write for application information and deadlines.
Trustee: Boston Safe Deposit & Trust Co.
EIN: 046092529

416
Florence Charitable Trust
99 Lyman Rd.
Chestnut Hill 02167

Established in 1967 in MA.
Financial data (yr. ended 12/31/93): Assets, $295,801 (M); expenditures, $73,579; qualifying distributions, $55,748, including $55,748 for 59 grants (high: $15,000; low: $5).
Fields of interest: Dental school/education; Education; Health care; Health organizations; Human services; Aging, centers & services; Jewish agencies & temples; Aging.
Limitations: Applications not accepted. Giving primarily in MA. No grants to individuals.
Application information: Contributes only to pre-selected organizations.
Trustee: Charlotte Florence.
EIN: 046171728

417
Friends of the Westport Council on Aging, Inc.
P.O. Box N192
Westport 02790

Financial data (yr. ended 12/31/94): Assets, $49,625 (M); expenditures, $5,785; qualifying distributions, $5,785, including $1,655 for grants.
Fields of interest: Aging, centers & services; Aging.
Limitations: Giving primarily in southern MA and RI.
Officers: Elizabeth Derbishire, Pres.; Joan Fradley, V.P.; Janice Trepaner, Secy.; James H. Hudner, Treas.
EIN: 042914504

418
GenRad Foundation
300 Baker Ave.
Concord 01742 (508) 287-7743
Contact: Linda B. Schuler, Trustee

Trust established in 1934 in MA.
Donor(s): GenRad, Inc., Henry Shaw.‡
Financial data (yr. ended 12/31/95): Assets, $1,271,888 (M); expenditures, $152,284; qualifying distributions, $126,523, including $87,449 for grants.
Purpose and activities: Giving primarily for family and social services, the elderly and child welfare, volunteerism, hospitals and health associations, environmental conservation; higher and secondary education, and cultural programs, including museums and the fine and performing arts.
Fields of interest: Visual arts; Museums; Performing arts; Arts/cultural programs; Secondary school/education; Higher education; Education; Natural resource conservation & protection; Environment; Hospitals (general); Mental health/crisis services; Health associations; Human services; Children & youth, services; Family services; Aging, centers & services; Voluntarism promotion; Aging.
Types of support: General/operating support, continuing support, annual campaigns, capital campaigns, building/renovation, endowment funds, program development, seed money.
Limitations: Giving primarily in the Concord, MA, area. No grants to individuals.
Publications: Application guidelines.
Application information: Application form not required.
Initial approach: Telephone for guidelines; proposal limited to 5 pages
Copies of proposal: 1
Deadline(s): None
Board meeting date(s): As needed
Final notification: Generally within 3 months of receipt of proposal
Trustees: James F. Lyons, Raymond F. McNulty, Linda B. Schuler.
Number of staff: 1 full-time professional; 1 part-time support.
EIN: 046043570
Grants for Aging:
Minuteman Home Care Corporation, Lexington, MA, $3,000. 94.

419
German Aid Society of Boston, Inc.
Eight County St.
P.O. Box 207
Walpole 02081
Contact: Gustav Scheer, Agent

Established in 1847.
Financial data (yr. ended 04/30/95): Assets, $771,241 (M); gifts received, $20,225; expenditures, $107,440; qualifying distributions, $101,762, including $49,900 for grants and $37,591 for 15 grants to individuals.
Purpose and activities: Giving material support and assistance in finding employment to Germans and those of German descent in the Boston, MA, area; support also given to nonprofit institutions which serve the same population group, including a nursing care facility for the aged.
Fields of interest: Nursing home/convalescent facility; Human services.
Types of support: General/operating support, grants to individuals.
Limitations: Giving primarily in the Boston, MA, area.
Application information: Applicants must contact society to arrange interview. Application form required.
Initial approach: Letter
Deadline(s): None
Officers: Wolfgang Hieronymus, Pres.; Herbert Pflanz, 1st V.P.; Max Kosin, 2nd V.P.; Lothar David, Recording Secy.; Richard J. Schneiderhan, Financial Secy.; George Baierlein, Treas.
EIN: 046038293

420
Sarah Gillette Services for the Elderly, Inc.
c/o Chapin & Hukowicz
P.O. Box 1308
Westfield 01086-1308
Contact: Gladys Anderson, Pres.

Financial data (yr. ended 06/30/95): Assets, $536,223 (M); gifts received, $92; expenditures, $29,292; qualifying distributions, $27,135, including $27,135 for grants.
Purpose and activities: Support limited to organizations serving elderly residents of Westfield, MA.
Fields of interest: Arts/cultural programs; Health care; Human services; Aging, centers & services; Aging.
Limitations: Giving limited to Westfield, MA.
Application information:
Initial approach: Telephone
Officers and Directors:* Gladys Anderson,* Pres.; Scott Wilcox,* V.P.; Marion Dolan, Secy.; Richard Knight, Treas.; Harry Becker, Ward Carlstrom, Amy McGilpin, Irene Riga, Marie Sharpe, Joseph Sico, Shirley Wiggin.
EIN: 042131415

421
The Nehemias Gorin Foundation
c/o William Gorin
1330 Beacon St.
Brookline 02146 (617) 738-4319

Established in 1964 in MA.
Donor(s): Nehemias Gorin.‡
Financial data (yr. ended 11/30/94): Assets, $3,909,425 (M); gifts received, $1,966,197; expenditures, $578,625; qualifying distributions, $558,352, including $519,000 for 68 grants (high: $100,000; low: $1,000; average: $100-$70,000).
Purpose and activities: Support for health, including hospitals and cancer research; Jewish welfare funds, other Jewish organizations and Israel; higher education; museums and other cultural programs; community funds; and Catholic organizations.

Fields of interest: Museums; Arts/cultural programs; Higher education; Education; Hospitals (general); Health care; Cancer; Health organizations; Cancer research; Human services; Aging, centers & services; Federated giving programs; Jewish federated giving programs; Roman Catholic agencies & churches; Jewish agencies & temples; Disabled; Aging; Israel.
Limitations: Applications not accepted. Giving primarily in MA.
Application information:
Board meeting date(s): Oct. 14
Trustees: Bertha G. Fritz, Stephen Goldenberg, William Gorin, Ida G. Leckart.
Number of staff: None.
EIN: 046119939
Grants for Aging:
Hebrew Rehabilitation Center for Aged, Roslindale, MA, $10,000. 94.

422
Grimes-King Foundation for the Elderly, Inc.

c/o Fiduciary Trust Co.
175 Federal St.
Boston 02110
Contact: Susan R. Gunderson, Treas.

Established in 1964 in MA.
Donor(s): Rice, Heard & Bigelow, Inc.
Financial data (yr. ended 11/30/95): Assets, $1,848,388 (M); gifts received, $3,051; expenditures, $85,378; qualifying distributions, $80,557, including $76,500 for 8 grants (high: $15,000; low: $2,000).
Purpose and activities: Support primarily for social services and community development benefiting elderly women of color living in Boston, MA; emphasis is on housing.
Fields of interest: Housing/shelter; Human services; Aging, centers & services; Minorities/immigrants, centers & services; Community development; Minorities; Aging.
Types of support: General/operating support.
Limitations: Giving limited to Boston, MA. No grants to individuals.
Application information:
Initial approach: Letter
Deadline(s): None
Board meeting date(s): Late spring
Officers and Directors:* Laura B. Morris,* Pres.; Newell Cook, 1st V.P.; Margaret McKinney, 2nd V.P.; Susan R. Gunderson, Treas.; Ruth-Arlene W. Howe,* Clerk; Leonard W. Johnson, and 14 additional directors.
EIN: 046070226
Grants for Aging:
Elders Living at Home, $10,000. 95.
Little Brothers Friends of the Elderly, Boston, MA, $2,000. 95.
Massachusetts Senior Action Council, Somerville, MA, $15,000. 95.

423
Maria Hayes Home for Aged Persons, Inc.

P.O. Box 402
Natick 01760

Classified as a private operating foundation in 1977.
Foundation type: Operating
Financial data (yr. ended 12/31/93): Assets, $572,271 (M); gifts received, $7,768; expenditures, $31,515; qualifying distributions, $29,754, including $28,500 for 2 grants (high: $15,000; low: $13,500).
Fields of interest: Hospitals (general); Aging, centers & services; Aging.
Limitations: Applications not accepted. Giving limited to Natick, MA. No grants to individuals.
Application information: Contributes only to pre-selected organizations.
Officers: Karl A. Bremner, Pres.; Joseph F. Everett, V.P.; Dight W. Crain, Secy.; Richard H. Potter, Jr., Treas.
EIN: 042103798

424
Home for Aged Men in the City of Brockton

c/o Creedon & Creedon
One Centre St.
Brockton 02401

Trust established in MA.
Donor(s): Horace Howard,‡ Daniel W. Field Trust.
Foundation type: Operating
Financial data (yr. ended 03/31/95): Assets, $3,776,011 (M); gifts received, $5,569; expenditures, $70,427; qualifying distributions, $37,000, including $37,000 for 5 grants (high: $10,000; low: $2,500).
Purpose and activities: A private operating foundation; awards grants for homes for the aged and hospitals to encourage development of the facilities' public assistance programs.
Fields of interest: Hospitals (general); Aging, centers & services; Aging.
Limitations: Applications not accepted. Giving primarily in MA. No grants to individuals.
Application information: Contributes only to pre-selected organizations.
Officers: John F. Creedon, Pres.; Robert Prince, Treas.; Ida Caggiano, Clerk.
EIN: 042103796

425
The Hyams Foundation, Inc.

175 Federal St., 14th FL.
Boston 02110 (617) 426-5600
Contact: Elizabeth B. Smith, Exec. Dir.
FAX: (617) 426-5696

Godfrey Hyams Trust and Sarah A. Hyams Fund established in 1921 and 1929 in MA respectively.
Donor(s): Godfrey M. Hyams,‡ Sarah A. Hyams.‡
Financial data (yr. ended 12/31/95): Assets, $91,907,944 (M); expenditures, $4,569,249; qualifying distributions, $3,364,371, including $3,364,371 for 218 grants (high: $70,000; low: $1,200; average: $15,000-$20,000).
Purpose and activities: Giving for the benefit of low-income residents through support primarily of neighborhood-based programs; support also for other social service, youth service, community organizing, advocacy, and community development purposes, and for expenses for summer youth programs. Priority program areas initiated since 1984 include housing, refugee services, racial, ethnic and cultural diversity, and neighborhood safety.
Fields of interest: Adult/continuing education; Family planning; Substance abuse, services; AIDS; Alcoholism; Domestic violence prevention; Housing/shelter, development; Human services; Youth, services; Family services; Homeless, human services; Race/intergroup relations; Urban/community development; Community development; Asians/Pacific Islanders; African Americans; Latinos; Native Americans; Disabled; Aging; People with AIDS (PWAs); Gays/lesbians; Immigrants/refugees; Economically disadvantaged.
Types of support: General/operating support, continuing support, program development, technical assistance, program-related investments/loans, matching funds.
Limitations: Giving primarily in Boston, Cambridge, Chelsea, Lynn, and Somerville, MA. No support for municipal, state, or federal agencies; institutions of higher learning for standard educational programs; religious organizations for sectarian religious purposes; or national or regional health organizations; support for medical research is being phased out. No grants to individuals, or for endowment funds, hospital capital campaigns, fellowships, publications, conferences, or films or videos.
Publications: Annual report, grants list, informational brochure (including application guidelines).
Application information: Application form not required.
Initial approach: Proposal, no more than 10 pages
Copies of proposal: 1
Deadline(s): None
Board meeting date(s): 10 times a year between Sept. and June
Final notification: 1 to 6 months
Officers and Trustees:* John H. Clymer,* Chair.; Elizabeth B. Smith, Exec. Dir.; Barbara Casey, James Jennings, Meizhu Lui, Deborah Prothrow-Stith, Roslyn M. Watson.
Number of staff: 3 full-time professional; 1 part-time professional; 2 full-time support; 1 part-time support.
Grants for Aging:
Boston Aging Concerns, Young and Old United, Boston, MA, $12,500. For operating support. 94.
Community Servings, Dorchester, MA, $10,000. For renovations and equipment. 94.

426
Edward Bangs Kelley and Elza Kelley Foundation, Inc.

243 South St.
P.O. Drawer M
Hyannis 02601 (508) 775-3117
Contact: Henry L. Murphy, Jr., Admin. Mgr., or Rebecca Jason

Incorporated in 1954 in MA.
Donor(s): Edward Bangs Kelley,‡ Elza deHorvath Kelley.‡

Financial data (yr. ended 12/31/95): Assets, $3,963,927 (M); gifts received, $2,650; expenditures, $174,447; qualifying distributions, $156,504, including $85,674 for 24 grants (high: $15,000; low: $150) and $47,900 for 93 grants to individuals (high: $2,000; low: $75; average: $250-$4,000).
Purpose and activities: To promote health and welfare of inhabitants of Barnstable County, MA; grants for higher education, including scholarships, and particularly for medical and paramedical education; support also for health and hospitals, hospices, prevention of drug and alcohol abuse, child development and youth agencies, the elderly, libraries, the environment, marine sciences, and cultural programs, including museums, fine arts, theater, and the performing arts.
Fields of interest: Visual arts; Museums; Performing arts; Theater; Arts/cultural programs; Child development, education; Higher education; Medical school/education; Libraries/library science; Education; Environment; Hospitals (general); Health care; Substance abuse, services; Alcoholism; Health organizations; Youth, services; Child development, services; Hospices; Aging, centers & services; Marine science; Aging.
Types of support: General/operating support, capital campaigns, building/renovation, equipment, land acquisition, emergency funds, program development, conferences/seminars, publication, seed money, scholarship funds, research, technical assistance, scholarships—to individuals, matching funds.
Limitations: Giving limited to Barnstable County, MA. No grants to individuals (except for scholarships), or for annual campaigns, deficit financing, land acquisition, endowment funds, exchange programs, fellowships, publications, or conferences; no loans.
Publications: Annual report (including application guidelines).
Application information: Application form required.
Initial approach: Letter, followed by proposal
Copies of proposal: 6
Deadline(s): Apr. 30 for scholarships; no deadline for grants; grants considered Apr., July, and Oct. if greater than $2,500
Board meeting date(s): Jan., Apr., July, and Oct.
Final notification: 3 weeks
Officers and Directors:* Milton L. Penn,* Pres.; Henry L. Murphy, Jr.,* V.P.; Thomas S. Olsen,* Treas.; Mary Louise Montgomery,* Clerk; John F. Aylmer, Jocelyn Bowman, Palmer Davenport, Townsend Hornor, John M. Kayajan, Kenneth S. MacAffer, Jr., Stephen L. Malaquias, M.D., Joshua A. Nickerson, Jr., Charles N. Robinson, Barbara H. Sheaffer.
Number of staff: 1 part-time professional.
EIN: 046039660

427
Knowlton Foundation for the Elderly, Inc.
c/o Elden E. Bjurling
Seven Abbott St.
Gardner 01440
Contact: John R. Tinker, Pres.
Application address: 132 Pearl St., Gardner, MA 01440; Tel.: (508) 632-2641

Established in 1980 in MA.
Financial data (yr. ended 03/31/95): Assets, $874,592 (M); expenditures, $57,699; qualifying distributions, $45,915, including $42,200 for grants.
Purpose and activities: Aid and assistance is restricted to the elderly in the greater Gardner, MA, area.
Fields of interest: Libraries/library science; Hospitals (general); Nursing care; Aging, centers & services; Aging.
Types of support: General/operating support, grants to individuals.
Limitations: Giving limited to the greater Gardner, MA, area.
Application information:
Initial approach: Informal letter
Deadline(s): None
Officers and Directors:* John R. Tinker,* Pres.; Nancy Anderson,* V.P.; Stephen A. Brooks,* V.P.; Nancy Hawke,* Secy.; Elden E. Bjurling,* Treas.; Grethe Anderholm, Joseph Forte, Janet Guzzetta, Ethel L. Kendall, Margaret Miller, Martha Mossman, Rocco Raduazo, Leo R. Reponen, Donald Stuart, Richard Tourigny.
EIN: 046060834

428
Henry B. Martin Fund, Inc.
c/o Russell, Brier & Co.
50 Congress St., Rm. 900
Boston 02109

Financial data (yr. ended 12/31/94): Assets, $1,098,705 (M); gifts received, $14,800; expenditures, $79,526; qualifying distributions, $70,110, including $6,000 for 3 grants (high: $4,000; low: $1,000) and $52,525 for 46 grants to individuals (high: $2,000; low: $175).
Purpose and activities: Support limited to needy, elderly citizens and to organizations that either now or previously have had a relationship to Milton, MA.
Fields of interest: Elementary/secondary education; Aging, centers & services; Aging.
Types of support: General/operating support, grants to individuals.
Limitations: Applications not accepted. Giving limited to Milton, MA.
Officers and Directors:* John T. Hemenway, Pres.; David H. Morse,* Treas.; Enid W. Chapman, Nick A. Grace, Bonnie M. Healy, Harley F. Laing.
EIN: 046031995

429
The New England Corporate Giving Program
501 Boylston St.
Boston 02116-3700 (617) 578-2119
Contact: Bryan K. Spence, Public Affairs Consultant

Financial data (yr. ended 12/31/95): Total giving, $487,500, including $457,500 for 150 grants (high: $15,000; low: $1,000; average: $1,000-$5,000) and $30,000 for 25 in-kind gifts.
Purpose and activities: Supports charitable, educational, cultural, civic and health organizations. Special emphasis given to programs aimed at females, minorities, elderly, youth and community social services organizations.
Fields of interest: Arts/cultural programs; Vocational education; Health care; Health organizations; Human services; Youth, services; Aging, centers & services; Women, centers & services; Minorities/immigrants, centers & services; Minorities; Aging; Women.
Types of support: General/operating support, capital campaigns, employee volunteer services, use of facilities, donated equipment, matching funds.
Limitations: Giving primarily in Boston, MA, area. No grants for religious or political organizations, films, or individuals.
Application information: Public Affairs Dept. handles giving. Application form not required.
Initial approach: Telephone call to headquarters
Copies of proposal: 1
Deadline(s): None
Board meeting date(s): Quarterly
Administrator: Bryan K. Spence, Contribs. Administrator.
Number of staff: 1 full-time professional.

430
Joseph Nickerson Trust
c/o Boston Safe Deposit & Trust Co.
One Boston Place
Boston 02108 (617) 722-7340
Contact: Judith Casey, Asst. V.P., Boston Safe Deposit & Trust Co.

Donor(s): Joseph Nickerson.‡
Financial data (yr. ended 08/31/94): Assets, $207,662 (M); expenditures, $18,387; qualifying distributions, $14,501, including $13,500 for 4 grants (high: $6,000; low: $2,500).
Purpose and activities: Support for organizations which benefit needy residents of Brewster, MA.
Fields of interest: Human services; Aging, centers & services; Aging.
Limitations: Giving limited to the Brewster, MA, area. No grants to individuals.
Application information: Write for application guidelines and information.
Trustee: Boston Safe Deposit & Trust Co.
EIN: 046093086

431
Amelia Peabody Charitable Fund
201 Devonshire St.
Boston 02110-1401 (617) 451-6178
Contact: Jo Anne Borek, Exec. Dir.

Established in 1974.
Donor(s): Amelia Peabody,‡ Eaton Foundation.
Financial data (yr. ended 12/31/95): Assets, $124,514,337 (M); expenditures, $6,100,000;

qualifying distributions, $5,664,600, including $5,664,600 for grants (high: $1,000,000; low: $3,000; average: $5,000-$25,000).
Purpose and activities: Grants primarily for hospitals, medical research, health and family services, higher education, the environment, and culture, including museums.
Fields of interest: Museums; Arts/cultural programs; Higher education; Education; Natural resource conservation & protection; Environment; Hospitals (general); Health care; Substance abuse, services; Health organizations; Medical research; Human services; Youth, services; Aging, centers & services; Homeless, human services; Disabled; Aging; Economically disadvantaged; Homeless; General charitable giving.
Types of support: Capital campaigns, building/renovation, equipment, endowment funds, research.
Limitations: Giving primarily in MA. No support for tax-supported municipal or government organizations or religious groups. No grants to individuals, or for salaries or operating expenses.
Publications: Application guidelines.
Application information: Application form not required.
Initial approach: Letter with proposal
Copies of proposal: 1
Deadline(s): None
Board meeting date(s): 3 times annually
Officer and Trustees:* Jo Anne Borek,* Exec. Dir.; Richard A. Leahy, J. Elisabeth Rice, Patricia E. Rice.
Number of staff: 1 full-time professional; 1 part-time professional.
EIN: 237364949

432
The Perpetual Benevolent Fund
c/o BayBank
39 Main St.
Watertown 02172 (617) 894-6500
Contact: Marjorie M. Kelley, Secy.

Charitable trust established in 1932 in MA; activated in 1957.
Donor(s): Nathan P. Cutler,‡ William H. Cutler,‡ Howard A. Haney.‡
Financial data (yr. ended 08/31/95): Assets, $4,727,604 (M); gifts received, $380,000; expenditures, $245,918; qualifying distributions, $152,992, including $53,000 for 13 grants (high: $10,000; low: $1,000; average: $5,000-$10,000) and $99,992 for grants to individuals (average: $300-$500).
Purpose and activities: To assist local needy individuals. Individuals are referred by health, welfare, hospitals, or other organizations; support also for child welfare, social services, the homeless and disadvantaged, and restricted funds for the elderly.
Fields of interest: Human services; Children & youth, services; Aging, centers & services; Homeless, human services; Aging; Economically disadvantaged; Homeless.
Types of support: Continuing support, emergency funds, grants to individuals, matching funds.
Limitations: Giving limited to Newton, Waltham, and adjacent communities in MA. No grants for scholarships.
Publications: Application guidelines.
Application information: Formal applications submitted through social service agencies, including schools, hospitals, health, and welfare depts. Proposals accepted for restricted funds for the elderly. Each application reviewed on the basis of need, low-income, one-time crisis, emergency, and other priority factors. Application form required.
Initial approach: Telephone or proposal
Copies of proposal: 1
Deadline(s): None
Board meeting date(s): Annually, in Nov.
Final notification: 1 week
Officers and Fund Committee:* Norman E. MacNeil,* Chair.; Marjorie M. Kelley, Secy. and Administrator; John Bihldorff, Mrs. Champe A. Fisher, Mrs. Maurice E. Keenan, Edward P. Leibensperger, Mrs. Giles E. Mosher, Jr., James J. Sidd, M.D.
Trustee: BayBank.
Number of staff: 1 full-time professional.
EIN: 237011723

433
Raytheon Company Corporate Giving Program
141 Spring St.
Lexington 02173 (617) 862-6600
Contact: Janet Taylor, Mgr., Corp. Contribs.

Financial data (yr. ended 12/31/92): Total giving, $5,500,000, including $5,000,000 for 1,000 grants (high: $100,000; low: $100; average: $5,000) and $500,000 for 4,000 employee matching gifts.
Purpose and activities: "Raytheon funds organizations dedicated to improving service in four areas: quality of education; quality of care; quality of opportunity; and quality of life. Assuring quality services, building on proven success, meeting community needs, helping to build the management capacity of nonprofit organizations, and supporting innovative problem-solving - these are the ways that the company seeks to be involved in its local communities. Raytheon Company believes it has a responsibility to be an active member of its communities - by providing resources and expertise." Grant size varies, depending on the scope of the project and the company's relationship to it. Multiple year grants will be considered for capital purposes. The range of one-year grants is $500 to $20,000; typical size is $5,000. Multi-year commitments paid over 3-5 years range from $10,000 to $250,000. Requests for product donations of kitchen and laundry appliances and marine electronics will be considered in lieu of, or as a supplement to, cash grants.
Fields of interest: Museums; Arts/cultural programs; Education, fund raising; Engineering school/education; Education; Natural resource conservation & protection; Environment; Human services; Youth, services; Aging, centers & services; Women, centers & services; Minorities/immigrants, centers & services; Mathematics; Engineering & technology; Engineering; Science; Minorities; Disabled; Aging; Women; Economically disadvantaged.
Types of support: General/operating support, capital campaigns, building/renovation, equipment, program development, technical assistance, employee matching gifts, donated equipment, donated products.
Limitations: Giving limited to local organizations in plant communities and to regional organizations benefiting plant communities. No support for religious, political, athletic, fraternal, or veterans' organiaztions, disease-specific organizations, independent elementary and secondary schools, organizations with primarily international activities, productions for public broadcasting, or private foundations. No grants to individuals, or for basic research projects, operating support for United Way affiliates, or organizations whose applications have been denied within the past 12 months.
Publications: Application guidelines, corporate report, informational brochure.
Application information: Raytheon has a staff that only handles contributions. Application form not required.
Initial approach: Write to the Manager of Human Resources at the local Raytheon facility or send to headquarters; telephone inquiries discouraged and formal interviews not always possible; follow-up contact will be made by Raytheon as needed.
Deadline(s): Mar. 31, June 30, and Sept. 30
Final notification: Generally within 6 months; volume of requests may delay notification
Number of staff: 1 full-time professional; 1 part-time support.

434
Charlotte M. Robbins Trust
c/o State Street Bank & Trust Co.
P.O. Box 351, M-10
Boston 02101
Contact: Cheryl D. Curtin, V.P., State Street Bank & Trust Co.
Application address: c/o State Street Bank & Trust Co., 225 Franklin St., Boston, MA 02110

Financial data (yr. ended 12/31/94): Assets, $294,122 (M); expenditures, $21,461; qualifying distributions, $19,563, including $16,653 for 13 grants to individuals (high: $3,000; low: $70).
Purpose and activities: Support for aged couples and aged women who are residents of Ayer, Groton, Shirley, Littleton and Harvard, MA.
Fields of interest: Aging; Women.
Types of support: Grants to individuals.
Limitations: Giving limited to residents of Ayer, Groton, Shirley, Littleton, and Harvard, MA.
Application information:
Initial approach: Letter
Deadline(s): None
Trustee: State Street Bank & Trust Co.
EIN: 046096044

435
Roehr Family Foundation, Inc.
c/o Michael K. Schaefen
185 Devonshire St., Suite 720
Boston 02110-1407

Established in 1986 in MA.
Financial data (yr. ended 06/30/95): Assets, $1,602,357 (M); expenditures, $89,115;

qualifying distributions, $73,500, including $73,500 for 12 grants (high: $20,000; low: $1,000).
Fields of interest: Education; Food services; Housing/shelter, development; Camps; Human services, mind/body enrichment; Aging, centers & services.
Limitations: Applications not accepted. Giving primarily in MA. No grants to individuals.
Application information: Contributes only to pre-selected organizations.
Trustees: Cynthia R. Anthony, Carolyn A. Roehr, Marcia A. Roehr, Mary E. Roehr.
EIN: 222777634
Grants for Aging:
Vintage, Pittsburgh, PA, $15,000. 95.
Vintage, Pittsburgh, PA, $10,000. 94.

436
Sophia F. Romero Trust
c/o First National Bank of Boston
P.O. Box 1861
Boston 02105

Established in 1953 in MA.
Financial data (yr. ended 04/30/95): Assets, $2,105,811 (M); expenditures, $108,376; qualifying distributions, $90,038, including $88,000 for 6 grants (high: $4,000; low: $1,500).
Purpose and activities: Support limited to aiding the elderly through social services and health care.
Fields of interest: Health care, home services; Human services, Aging, centers & services; Aging.
Limitations: Applications not accepted. Giving limited to Bristol County, MA. No grants to individuals.
Application information: Contributes only to pre-selected organizations.
Trustee: First National Bank of Boston.
EIN: 046029538
Grants for Aging:
Dighton Council on Aging, Dighton, MA, $10,500. 95.

437
Sailors' Snug Harbor of Boston
c/o T.L. Condon and Co.
225 Water St., Suite 501
Plymouth 02360 (617) 426-7172
Contact: Gloria Oldsman
Application address: c/o Grants Management Assocs., 230 Congress St., Boston, MA 02110

Established in 1852 in MA.
Financial data (yr. ended 04/30/95): Assets, $4,907,693 (M); gifts received, $1,617; expenditures, $256,937; qualifying distributions, $220,048, including $187,330 for 28 grants (high: $15,000; low: $2,000).
Purpose and activities: Giving for the health and welfare of the aged, sailors, and others; grants to institutions for the relief and support of aged sailors.
Fields of interest: Health care; Health organizations; Human services; Family services; Aging, centers & services; Marine science; Aging; Economically disadvantaged.
Limitations: Giving primarily in the Boston, MA, area. No grants to individuals.
Application information: Application form not required.
Initial approach: Proposal
Deadline(s): In time for approval at board meetings
Board meeting date(s): Nov. 15, Feb. 15, and Apr. 15
Officers and Trustees:* William Bancroft,* Pres.; George B. Motley,* V.P.; Francis B. Lothrop, Jr.,* Treas.; Arthur Page,* Clerk; Charles K. Cobb, Jr., G. Lincoln Dow, Joseph E. Eaton, Charles R. Eddy, Lincoln B. Hansel, Frances Lawrence, Lisa S. Lewis, Stephen Little, Robert W. Loring, Everett Morss, Jr., John A. Perkins, Charles E. Rogerson II, Thomas Rogerson, G. West Saltonstall, William L. Saltonstall, Jo-Ann Watson, Benjamin Williams, Thomas B. Williams, Jr.
EIN: 042104430
Grants for Aging:
Boston Aging Concerns, Young and Old United, Boston, MA, $15,000. 94.
Boston Aging Concerns, Young and Old United, Boston, MA, $8,500. 95.
Boston University Medical Center/The University Hospital, Boston, MA, $10,000. For Elders Living at Home program. 95.
Committee to End Elder Homelessness, Boston, MA, $6,500. 94.
Elderlink, Somerville, MA, $10,000. 94.
Massachusetts Senior Action Council, Somerville, MA, $6,000. 94.
Match-Up Interfaith Volunteers, Boston, MA, $10,000. 95.

438
Salem Female Charitable Society
c/o Fiduciary Trust Co.
175 Federal St.
Boston 02110
Contact: Rosamond Dennis, Treas.
Application address: 33 Warren St., Salem, MA 01970

Financial data (yr. ended 04/30/95): Assets, $611,904 (M); gifts received, $102; expenditures, $23,167; qualifying distributions, $19,968, including $19,200 for 20 grants to individuals (high: $1,800; low: $50).
Purpose and activities: Awards to aged and indigent women in the Salem, MA, area. Award is forfeited if recipient moves from the area.
Fields of interest: Aging, centers & services; Aging; Women.
Types of support: Grants to individuals.
Limitations: Giving limited to female residents of Salem, MA, and vicinity.
Application information:
Initial approach: Letter
Deadline(s): None
Officers and Directors:* Mrs. T. McLeon Griffin,* 1st Directress; Rosamond Dennis,* Treas.; Mrs. Stillman G. Davis,* Clerk; Mrs. W. Channing Bacall, Eleanor Broodhead, Jane A. Phillips, Mrs. Stephen Phillips, Mrs. Alfred P. Putnam, Rebecca D. Putnam, Ruth R. Ropes, Martha Sanders, Mrs. Richard Stevens.
EIN: 046014190

439
Sanders Fund, Inc.
50 Congress St., Rm. 800
Boston 02109
Contact: Marge Finigan

Established in 1921.
Donor(s): Chas Sanders.‡
Financial data (yr. ended 12/31/94): Assets, $2,789 (M); gifts received, $122,886; expenditures, $126,888; qualifying distributions, $126,018, including $111,260 for 19 grants (high: $22,000; low: $500) and $14,758 for 8 grants to individuals (high: $4,000; low: $577).
Purpose and activities: Giving to programs serving the homeless.
Fields of interest: Family services; Aging, centers & services; Homeless, human services; Aging; Homeless.
Types of support: General/operating support.
Limitations: Applications not accepted. Giving limited to Boston, Cambridge, and Salem, MA.
Application information: Unsolicited requests for funds not considered.
Board meeting date(s): Dec.
Officers and Directors:* William L. Saltonstall,* Pres.; George Lewis,* Treas.; Dudley H. Willis,* Clerk.
EIN: 042265212

440
Trustees of Sears and Other Funds
Trinity Church, Copley Sq.
Boston 02106 (617) 536-0944
Contact: Sarah W. Wilcox, Treas.

Financial data (yr. ended 02/28/95): Assets, $1,472,939 (M); expenditures, $93,469; qualifying distributions, $84,557, including $79,500 for 20 grants (high: $16,000; low: $1,000).
Purpose and activities: Giving primarily for Episcopalian churches and services.
Fields of interest: Education; Human services; Aging, centers & services; Protestant agencies & churches; Aging.
Limitations: Giving primarily in Boston, MA. No grants to individuals.
Application information:
Initial approach: Proposal
Deadline(s): None
Officers and Trustees:* David S. Lee,* Pres.; Sarah W. Wilcox,* Treas.; John Bigelow, James D. Colt, John H. Finley III, Frieda Garcia, Edward S. Heard, E. Miles Herter,* Rev. Thomas B. Kennedy, John Lowell, Guido R. Perera, Jr., Stokley P. Towles.
EIN: 046040032
Grants for Aging:
Sherrill House, Jamaica Plain, MA, $2,000. 95.

441
Frank R. and Elizabeth Simoni Foundation, Inc.
c/o Victor F. Coletti
434 Providence Hwy.
Norwood 02062

Established in 1992 in MA.
Donor(s): Frank R. Simoni.

Financial data (yr. ended 12/31/94): Assets, $1,225,961 (M); expenditures, $51,799; qualifying distributions, $51,799, including $50,000 for 9 grants (high: $20,000; low: $1,000).
Fields of interest: Education; Health care; Residential/custodial care; Aging, centers & services; Mentally disabled, centers & services; Disabled.
Limitations: Applications not accepted. Giving primarily in MA. No grants to individuals.
Application information: Contributes only to pre-selected organizations.
Officers and Directors:* Frank R. Simoni, Pres.; Victor Coletti,* V.P.; Elizabeth M. Simoni, Treas.; Robert B. MacDonald, Jr., Clerk; Ann M. MacDonald.
EIN: 043109508

442
Almira N. Simons Trust
c/o First National Bank of Boston
P.O. Box 1861
Boston 02105
Application address: c/o Wellesley Council on Aging, 219 Washington St., Wellesley, MA 02181

Financial data (yr. ended 09/30/93): Assets, $712,472 (M); expenditures, $52,435; qualifying distributions, $29,410, including $27,529 for 27 grants (high: $6,500; low: $12) and $739 for 3 grants to individuals (high: $484; low: $25).
Purpose and activities: Giving for indigent residents of Wellesley, MA, over 60 years of age.
Fields of interest: Aging, centers & services; Aging; Economically disadvantaged.
Types of support: Grants to individuals.
Limitations: Giving limited to residents of Wellesley, MA.
Application information: Application form not required.
Deadline(s): None
Trustee: Bank of Boston.
EIN: 046008364

443
Smith-Denison Foundation
c/o Brown Brothers, Harriman & Co.
40 Water St.
Boston 02109 (617) 742-1818
Contact: Clifford A. Clark, Trustee

Donor(s): Mary Smith Denison.
Financial data (yr. ended 05/31/95): Assets, $683,211 (M); expenditures, $51,625; qualifying distributions, $44,033, including $44,000 for grants.
Fields of interest: Libraries/library science; Aging, centers & services.
Application information: Application form not required.
Deadline(s): None
Trustees: Clifford A. Clark, Mary Smith Denison.
EIN: 112848979

444
Spero Charitable Foundation
850 Rear Providence Hwy.
Dedham 02026-6822
Contact: Louis Spero, Trustee

Established in 1968 in MA.
Donor(s): Louis Spero.
Financial data (yr. ended 12/31/93): Assets, $1,441,898 (M); gifts received, $75,000; expenditures, $139,016; qualifying distributions, $136,616, including $136,616 for grants.
Fields of interest: Arts/cultural programs; Child development, education; Higher education; Business school/education; Hospitals (general); Health care; Cancer; Heart/circulatory disease; Health organizations; Cancer research; Heart/circulatory research; Human services; Children & youth, services; Youth, services; Child development, services; Aging, centers & services; Homeless, human services; Community development; Federated giving programs; Roman Catholic federated giving programs; Jewish federated giving programs; Government/public administration; Jewish agencies & temples; Minorities; Aging; Homeless; General charitable giving; Israel.
Types of support: General/operating support.
Limitations: Applications not accepted. Giving primarily in MA. No grants to individuals.
Application information: Contributes only to pre-selected organizations.
Trustee: Louis Spero.
EIN: 046183682

445
Artemas W. Stearns Trust
70 East St.
Methuen 01844-4597 (508) 687-0151
Contact: Clifford E. Elias, Esq., Trustee
Applications must also be sent to: Vincent Morton, Jr., 14 Sunset Rock Rd., Andover, MA 01810; Marsha E. Rich, Esq., 59 Lucerne Dr., Andover, MA 01810; Eileen Khoury, 49 Boxford St., Lawrence, MA 01843; Rev. Joachim Lally, 365 Haverhill St., Lawrence, MA 07840

Trust established in 1896 in MA.
Donor(s): Artemas W. Stearns.‡
Financial data (yr. ended 12/31/95): Assets, $3,829,000 (M); expenditures, $230,000; qualifying distributions, $172,700, including $172,700 for 24 grants (high: $25,000; low: $1,000; average: $10,000).
Purpose and activities: Support for organizations which service and benefit the deserving poor and indigent aged people, including hospitals, community projects, and secondary schools.
Fields of interest: Secondary school/education; Education; Hospitals (general); Human services; Aging, centers & services; Community development; Aging.
Types of support: General/operating support, annual campaigns, building/renovation, equipment, emergency funds, program development, publication, scholarship funds.
Limitations: Giving limited to the greater Lawrence, MA, area. No grants to individuals, or for endowment funds or matching gifts; no loans.
Publications: 990-PF, application guidelines.
Application information: Application form not required.
Initial approach: Letter or proposal
Copies of proposal: 5
Deadline(s): Jan. 31
Board meeting date(s): Quarterly
Trustees: Clifford E. Elias, Eileen M. Khoury, Rev. Joachim Lally, Vincent P. Morton, Jr., Marsha E. Rich.
Number of staff: 1 part-time professional; 1 part-time support.
EIN: 042137061
Grants for Aging:
Family Service Association of Greater Lawrence, Lawrence, MA, $5,000. For elderly services. 94.

446
The Abbot and Dorothy H. Stevens Foundation
P.O. Box 111
North Andover 01845 (508) 688-7211
Contact: Elizabeth A. Beland, Administrator

Trust established in 1953 in MA.
Donor(s): Abbot Stevens.‡
Financial data (yr. ended 12/31/95): Assets, $14,740,089 (M); expenditures, $735,418; qualifying distributions, $835,418, including $680,888 for 87 grants (high: $75,000; low: $100; average: $2,000-$8,000) and $100,000 for 1 program-related investment.
Fields of interest: Museums; Humanities; Historic preservation/historical societies; Arts/cultural programs; Medical school/education; Education; Natural resource conservation & protection; Health care; Health organizations; Domestic violence prevention; Human services; Youth, services; African Americans; Latinos; Disabled; Aging; Immigrants/refugees; Economically disadvantaged.
Types of support: General/operating support, continuing support, capital campaigns, building/renovation, equipment, endowment funds, seed money, technical assistance, program-related investments/loans, matching funds.
Limitations: Giving limited to MA, with emphasis on the greater Lawrence area. No support for national organizations, or for state or federal agencies. No grants to individuals, or for annual campaigns, deficit financing, exchange programs, internships, professorships, scholarships, or fellowships.
Publications: Program policy statement, application guidelines.
Application information: Application form not required.
Initial approach: Proposal
Copies of proposal: 1
Deadline(s): None
Board meeting date(s): Monthly except July and Aug.
Final notification: 1 week following board meetings
Trustees: Phebe S. Miner, Christopher W. Rogers, Samuel S. Rogers.
Number of staff: None.
EIN: 046107991

447
The Nathaniel and Elizabeth P. Stevens Foundation

P.O. Box 111
North Andover 01845 (508) 688-7211
Contact: Elizabeth A. Beland, Administrator

Trust established in 1943 in MA.
Donor(s): Nathaniel Stevens.‡
Financial data (yr. ended 12/31/95): Assets, $11,445,642 (M); expenditures, $648,388; qualifying distributions, $648,388, including $576,499 for 79 grants (high: $84,000; low: $100; average: $2,000-$10,000) and $9,425 for 22 employee matching gifts.
Fields of interest: Museums; Historic preservation/historical societies; Arts/cultural programs; Medical school/education; Education; Natural resource conservation & protection; Hospitals (general); Health care; Health organizations; Domestic violence prevention; Housing/shelter, development; Human services; Minorities/immigrants, centers & services; Minorities; African Americans; Latinos; Disabled; Aging; Immigrants/refugees; Economically disadvantaged.
Types of support: General/operating support, continuing support, capital campaigns, building/renovation, equipment, land acquisition, endowment funds, emergency funds, program development, conferences/seminars, seed money, technical assistance, consulting services, program-related investments/loans, matching funds.
Limitations: Giving limited to MA, with emphasis on the greater Lawrence area. No support for national organizations, or for state or federal agencies. No grants to individuals, or for deficit financing, exchange programs, internships, lectureships, research, professorships, scholarships, fellowships, or annual campaigns; no loans.
Publications: Application guidelines, program policy statement.
Application information: Application form not required.
Initial approach: Proposal
Copies of proposal: 1
Deadline(s): None
Board meeting date(s): Monthly except July and Aug.
Final notification: 2 months
Trustees: Joshua L. Miner IV, Phebe S. Miner, Samuel S. Rogers.
Number of staff: None.
EIN: 042236996
Grants for Aging:
Northern Essex Elder Transport, Amesbury, MA, $5,000. 94.

448
Swift Charity, Inc.

c/o Russell, Brier & Co.
50 Congress St., Rm. 900
Boston 02109

Financial data (yr. ended 12/31/95): Assets, $733,837 (M); gifts received, $1,000; expenditures, $50,043; qualifying distributions, $42,315, including $4,000 for 1 grant and $27,378 for 25 grants to individuals (high: $2,000; low: $278).
Purpose and activities: Provide grants to needy elderly individuals and organizations which have or previously had a relationship to the town of Milton, MA.
Fields of interest: Aging; Economically disadvantaged.
Types of support: Grants to individuals.
Limitations: Applications not accepted. Giving limited to Milton, MA.
Officers and Directors:* John T. Hemenway,* Pres.; David H. Morse,* Secy.-Treas.; Enid W. Chapman, Nicholas A. Grace, Bonnie M. Healy, Harley F. Laing.
EIN: 046052150

449
TJX Foundation

(Formerly Zayre Foundation, Inc.)
c/o TJX Companies, Inc.
770 Cochituate Rd., Route 2E
Framingham 01701 (508) 390-3199
Contact: Carla Bertonazzi, Corp. Community Rels.

Incorporated in 1966 in MA.
Donor(s): The TJX Companies, Inc.
Foundation type: Company-sponsored
Financial data (yr. ended 01/28/95): Assets, $202,248 (M); gifts received, $900,000; expenditures, $790,829; qualifying distributions, $790,294, including $790,294 for 173 grants (high: $111,744; low: $150; average: $1,000-$5,000).
Purpose and activities: Primary areas of interest include social services, child welfare, the elderly, the handicapped, and education.
Fields of interest: Arts/cultural programs; Higher education; Education; Health care; Human services; Children & youth, services; Aging, centers & services; Women, centers & services; Minorities/immigrants, centers & services; Homeless, human services; Minorities; Disabled; Aging; Women; Economically disadvantaged; Homeless.
Limitations: Giving limited to areas of company operations in the greater Boston, MA, community. No support for political groups or fraternal organizations. No grants to individuals.
Publications: Annual report, application guidelines.
Application information: Application form not required.
Copies of proposal: 1
Deadline(s): None
Board meeting date(s): Twice a year
Officers and Directors:* Bernard Cammarata,* Pres.; Richard Lesser,* V.P.; Donald Campbell,* Treas.
Number of staff: 1 full-time professional; 2 full-time support.
EIN: 042399760
Grants for Aging:
Baypath Senior Citizens Service, Southboro, MA, $500. 94.
Boston Aging Concerns, Young and Old United, Boston, MA, $2,000. 95.
Council of Elders, Roxbury, MA, $500. 95.

450
Harold and Anna S. Ullian Charitable Foundation

c/o Lane & Altman
101 Federal St.
Boston 02110-1800 (617) 345-9800
Contact: Steven A. Meyer, Trustee

Established in 1990 in MA.
Financial data (yr. ended 10/31/94): Assets, $242,274 (M); gifts received, $3,643; expenditures, $27,646; qualifying distributions, $27,646, including $27,100 for grants.
Fields of interest: Hospitals (general); Jewish agencies & temples; Aging.
Limitations: Giving primarily in MA.
Application information:
Initial approach: Letter
Deadline(s): None
Trustees: Steven A. Meyer, Robert Snider.
EIN: 043107591

451
George C. Wadleigh Foundation, Inc.

(Formerly George C. Wadleigh Home for Aged Men, Inc.)
P.O. Box 226
Groveland 01834
Contact: Edmund J. Cote, Jr., Pres.

Established in 1981 in MA.
Donor(s): George C. Wadleigh.‡
Financial data (yr. ended 12/31/95): Assets, $7,571,360 (M); expenditures, $382,092; qualifying distributions, $324,322, including $319,736 for 13 grants (high: $62,100; low: $4,000).
Purpose and activities: Grants primarily to organizations benefiting the aged in the greater Haverhill, MA, area; giving also for the benefit of the indigent of Haverhill, MA.
Fields of interest: Human services; Aging, centers & services; Aging.
Limitations: Giving primarily in the greater Haverhill, MA, area. No grants to individuals, or for general operating expenses, or research.
Publications: Annual report, application guidelines.
Application information: Application form not required.
Initial approach: Letter
Copies of proposal: 1
Deadline(s): Aug. 30
Board meeting date(s): 2nd Tuesday of Feb., May, Aug., and Nov.
Final notification: Dec.
Officers and Directors:* Edmund J. Cote, Jr.,* Pres.; A. Bruce McGregor,* Secy.; Richard Cammett,* Treas.; Kenneth Fowle, David Hindle, Donald Ruhl, Charles Traver, Zoe Veasey.
Number of staff: 1 part-time professional.
EIN: 042720087

452
Widows' Society in Boston

581 Boylston St.
Boston 02116 (617) 536-7951
Contact: Jackie Husid, Exec. Dir.

Established in 1816 in MA.
Foundation type: Operating
Financial data (yr. ended 10/31/95): Assets, $2,983,968 (M); gifts received, $1,900; expenditures, $165,969; qualifying distributions, $160,259, including $125,224 for grants to individuals.
Purpose and activities: A private operating foundation; support for widowed, divorced, or single women who are over 60 years old and in need of financial aid.
Fields of interest: Aging, centers & services; Women, centers & services; Aging; Women; Economically disadvantaged.
Limitations: Giving limited to applicants living within 25 miles of the State House in Boston, MA.
Publications: Annual report.
Application information: Application form not required.
Initial approach: Referrals from public and social organizations
Deadline(s): None
Officers: Mrs. Donald Newman, Secy.; Richard V. Howe, Treas.
Directors: Susan G. Loring, Mrs. Samuel E. Shaw II.
Number of staff: 1 part-time professional.
EIN: 042306840

453 Greater Worcester Community Foundation, Inc.

44 Front St., Suite 530
Worcester 01608-1782 (508) 755-0980
Contact: Ms. Ann T. Lisi, Exec. Dir.

Incorporated in 1975 in MA.
Foundation type: Community
Financial data (yr. ended 12/31/95): Assets, $44,146,249 (M); gifts received, $1,798,285; expenditures, $2,497,835, including $1,760,617 for 260 grants (high: $100,000; low: $200; average: $1,000-$10,000) and $129,220 for 100 grants to individuals (high: $7,000; low: $200; average: $500-$2,000).
Purpose and activities: "To support programs that improve the quality of life for residents of the greater Worcester area."
Fields of interest: Humanities; Arts/cultural programs; Dental school/education; Medical school/education; Nursing school/education; Education; Environment; Health care; Health organizations; Medical research; Abuse prevention; Housing/shelter, development; Youth development; Human services; Youth, services; Family services; Aging, centers & services; Homeless, human services; Community development; Government/public administration; Public affairs; African Americans; Disabled; Aging; People with AIDS (PWAs); Economically disadvantaged; Homeless.
Types of support: Building/renovation, program development, seed money, scholarship funds, technical assistance, program-related investments/loans, scholarships—to individuals, matching funds.
Limitations: Giving limited to Worcester County, MA, and contiguous towns. No grants to individuals (except for designated scholarship funds); generally no grants for general operating expenses, capital improvements, or endowment campaigns.
Publications: Annual report, application guidelines, newsletter.
Application information: Submit 2 copies of Foundation's Summary of Application Form plus 2 copies of complete proposal. Scholarships are for residents of Worcester County, MA, only. Application form required.
Initial approach: Telephone or letter
Copies of proposal: 2
Deadline(s): Jan. 1, Apr. 1, and Sept. 1 for organizations; Mar. 15 for scholarships
Board meeting date(s): Jan., Mar., June, Sept., Nov., and as required
Final notification: 3 months
Officers and Directors:* Sumner B. Tilton, Jr.,* Pres.; David K. Woodbury,* V.P.; Sarah B. Garfield,* Treas.; Ann T. Lisi, Exec. Dir.; Michael D. Brockelman,* Clerk; Zoila Torres Feldman,* Member-at-Large; Carol L. Seager,* Distrib. Comm. Chair.; Christopher Bramley, Stacey DeBoise, Ross K. Dik, N. Lynn Eckert, M.D., Barbara Greenberg, Joseph Hagan, James H. Harrington, Monica Escobar Lowell, John W. Lund, John M. Nelson, Vincent F. O'Rourke, Jr., Melvin M. Rosenblatt, Margaret W. Traina.
Distribution Committee: Robert Bachelder, Veronica Mancini Griffin, Patricia Lewis, John W. Lund, Mary Melville, Richard C. Van Nostrand.
Staff: Amanda Flores-Witte, Prog. Officer; Jay S. Sherwin, Prog. Officer; Cynthia C. Taylor, Scholarship Coord.
Number of staff: 4 full-time professional; 1 part-time professional; 2 full-time support; 1 part-time support.
EIN: 042572276
Grants for Aging:
Massachusetts Senior Action Council, Somerville, MA, $10,000. For community organizing and advocacy program led by senior citizens. 94.

MICHIGAN

454 Ann Arbor Area Community Foundation

(Formerly Ann Arbor Area Foundation)
201 South Main, Suite 801
Ann Arbor 48104-2113 (313) 663-0401
Contact: Cheryl Elliott, Prog. Dir.
FAX: (313) 663-3514

Incorporated in 1963 in MI.
Foundation type: Community
Financial data (yr. ended 12/31/95): Assets, $9,704,261 (M); gifts received, $386,000; expenditures, $353,366, including $279,997 for 38 grants (high: $25,000; low: $600; average: $500-$7,500) and $53,000 for 57 grants to individuals.
Purpose and activities: Support for innovative programs and projects encompassing charity, civic affairs, culture, health and human services, ecology, historic preservation, and education.
Fields of interest: Visual arts; Performing arts; Theater; Arts/cultural programs; Higher education; Education; Natural resource conservation & protection; Environment; Health care; Health associations; Domestic violence prevention; Human services; Children & youth, services; Family services; Aging, centers & services; Homeless, human services; Community development; Aging; Homeless.
Types of support: Emergency funds, program development, conferences/seminars, publication, seed money, scholarship funds, research, matching funds.
Limitations: Giving limited to the Ann Arbor, MI, area. No support for religious or sectarian purposes; or for advocacy or political purposes. No grants to individuals (except from designated funds), or for operating budgets, construction projects, computer hardware equipment, continuing support, annual campaigns, deficit financing, fundraising purposes, land acquisition, endowment funds, consulting services, technical assistance, fellowships; no loans or program-related investments.
Publications: Annual report (including application guidelines), program policy statement, application guidelines, informational brochure (including application guidelines), newsletter.
Application information: Application form required.
Initial approach: Telephone
Copies of proposal: 11
Deadline(s): Feb., May, and Oct. for grants; Sept. for youth projects
Board meeting date(s): Jan., Mar., May, July, Sept., and Nov.
Final notification: 60 days
Officers and Trustees:* Dennis Pearsall,* Chair.; Judith Nold,* Secy.; William Hermann,* Treas.; Carol Amster, Phil Bowen, Brian Campbell, David Clyde, Joseph Dulin, Rosalie Edwards, Patricia Garcia, Judith Goodman, Sheldon Markel, M.D., Chris McKenny, Barbara Meadows, Hon. Melinda Morris, Douglas Weber, David Wierman.
Number of staff: 2 part-time professional; 1 full-time support.
EIN: 386087967
Grants for Aging:
Catholic Social Services, Grand Rapids, MI, $15,000. To expand Grandparents As Parents Program. 94.
Child and Family Services of Washtenaw County, Ann Arbor, MI, $12,000. For preliminary planning to relocate Adult Day Care Center to permanent location. 94.
Neighborhood Senior Services, Ann Arbor, MI, $12,500. To stabilize and expand medical access transportation and accompaniment program to Ann Arbor residents. 94.
Packard Community Clinic, Ann Arbor, MI, $10,000. Toward medicines, medical supplies and specialists visits for low-income senior population. 94.
Washtenaw County Council on Aging, Ann Arbor, MI, $10,000. For expansion of Senior Connection crisis line. 94.

455 Berrien Community Foundation, Inc.

515 Ship St., Suite 210
St. Joseph 49085-0092 (616) 983-3304

Contact: Margaret Poole, Exec. Dir.
FAX: (616) 983-4939

Incorporated in 1952 in MI.
Foundation type: Community
Financial data (yr. ended 12/31/94): Assets, $4,448,113 (M); gifts received, $277,259; expenditures, $205,681, including $115,136 for 42 grants (high: $16,775; low: $875).
Purpose and activities: Primary areas of interest include youth, education, family issues, and general charitable giving.
Fields of interest: Museums; Music; Humanities; Historic preservation/historical societies; Arts/cultural programs; Elementary school/education; Secondary school/education; Adult education—literacy & basic skills; Libraries/library science; Reading; Education; Environment; Health care; Substance abuse, services; Health associations; Health organizations; Nutrition; Safety/disasters; Recreation; Youth development; Human services; Youth, services; Aging, centers & services; Homeless, human services; Community development; Voluntarism promotion; Engineering & technology; Science; Public affairs; Disabled; Aging; Homeless; General charitable giving.
Types of support: Endowment funds, program development, seed money, scholarship funds, in-kind gifts, matching funds.
Limitations: Giving limited to Berrien County, MI. No support for sectarian religious purposes. No grants to individuals, or for consulting services, technical assistance, operating funds, deficit financing, or annual fund drives; no loans or program-related investments.
Publications: Annual report, application guidelines, program policy statement, financial statement.
Application information: Application guidelines available on request. 20 copies of application required for youth-oriented projects only. Application form required.
Initial approach: Telephone
Copies of proposal: 1
Deadline(s): Sept. 1 for winter meeting; Mar. 1 for spring meeting
Board meeting date(s): Quarterly
Final notification: 6 weeks to 2 months
Officers and Trustees:* Larry Bubb,* Pres.; Marily Schanze,* V.P.; Mark A. Miller,* Secy.; Allan J. Westmaas,* Treas.; Margaret Poole,* Exec. Dir.; B. David Allen, Nadra Kissman, Kay Delle Koch, Marion Preston, Malcolm S. Ross, Larry Schuler, Stephen Sizer, John Steimle, Jeff Upton.
Staff: Judy Loeffler, Prog. Mgr.; Susan Burns, Admin. Asst.
Number of staff: 1 full-time professional; 1 part-time professional; 1 full-time support.
EIN: 386057160

456
The Blodgett Foundation
2740 Littlefield, N.E.
Grand Rapids 49506

Established in 1994 in MI.
Financial data (yr. ended 12/31/95): Assets, $1,144,366 (M); expenditures, $122,506; qualifying distributions, $110,170, including $106,180 for 61 grants (high: $25,000; low: $200).
Fields of interest: Higher education; Human services; Youth, services; Aging, centers & services; Christian agencies & churches.
Limitations: Applications not accepted. Giving primarily in MI. No grants to individuals.
Application information: Contributes only to pre-selected organizations.
Director: Edith I. Blodgett.
EIN: 383202330

457
The Bugas Fund
P.O. Box 1882
Jackson 49204-1882 (517) 787-1800

Established in 1956 in MI.
Financial data (yr. ended 11/30/95): Assets, $1,671,227 (M); expenditures, $85,698; qualifying distributions, $70,273, including $66,000 for 9 grants (high: $25,000; low: $1,000).
Purpose and activities: Giving primarily for health associations, including hospitals and an association for diabetes; support also for social services.
Fields of interest: Hospitals (general); Health care; Health associations; Alzheimer's disease; Diabetes; Alzheimer's disease research; Human services.
Limitations: Applications not accepted. Giving primarily in MI. No grants to individuals.
Application information: Contributes only to pre-selected organizations.
Board meeting date(s): Early Nov.
Officers: Patricia Bugas Harris, Pres.; John S. Bugas, Jr., V.P.; Beverly A. Newton, Secy.; Terry S. Moats, Treas.
Number of staff: None.
EIN: 386067261
Grants for Aging:
Alzheimers Disease Research Center, Ann Arbor, MI, $25,000. 95.

458
Buhr Foundation
c/o Robert L. Johnson
4777 West Liberty Rd.
Ann Arbor 48103

Established in 1953 in MI.
Donor(s): Buhr Machine Tool Co.
Financial data (yr. ended 12/31/95): Assets, $1,502,659 (M); gifts received, $3,000; expenditures, $63,131; qualifying distributions, $57,650, including $52,875 for 15 grants (high: $6,000; low: $965).
Fields of interest: Adult/continuing education; Hospitals (general); Human services; Family services; Aging, centers & services; General charitable giving; Aging.
Types of support: Capital campaigns, building/renovation.
Limitations: Applications not accepted. Giving limited to the Ann Arbor, MI, area. No grants to individuals, or for operating funds.
Application information: Contributes only to pre-selected organizations.
Board meeting date(s): Nov. 15
Officers and Trustees:* Martha B. Hahn,* Pres.; Wilbur K. Pierpont,* V.P.; Richard J. Buhr,* Secy.; Robert L. Johnson,* Treas.; James D. Buhr.
Number of staff: None.
EIN: 386072288
Grants for Aging:
Lincoln Senior Citizen Program, Golden Ages Club, Ypsilanti, MI, $3,250. 95.
Neighborhood Senior Services, Ann Arbor, MI, $3,000. 94.
United Methodist Retirement Homes, Chelsea, MI, $5,000. For endowment fund. 95.

459
Cadillac Area Community Foundation
P.O. Box 102
Cadillac 49601 (616) 775-9911
Contact: Robert J. VanDellen, Exec. Dir.
Application address: 107 1/2 North Mitchell St., Cadillac, MI 49601

Established in 1988 in MI.
Foundation type: Community
Financial data (yr. ended 12/31/95): Assets, $1,295,000 (M); gifts received, $35,000; expenditures, $73,500, including $56,427 for 16 grants (high: $10,000; low: $500).
Purpose and activities: Giving primarily to the arts, community development, education, health, and youth.
Fields of interest: Arts/cultural programs; Early childhood education; Elementary school/education; Education; Natural resource conservation & protection; Environment; Health care; Substance abuse, services; Health associations; Health organizations; Recreation; Human services; Youth, services; Hospices; Aging, centers & services; Homeless, human services; Community development; Federated giving programs; Economics; Aging; Homeless.
Types of support: General/operating support, building/renovation, equipment, endowment funds, emergency funds, program development, publication, seed money, curriculum development, research, technical assistance, matching funds.
Limitations: Giving limited to the greater Cadillac, MI, area.
Publications: Application guidelines, occasional report, informational brochure, program policy statement, annual report.
Application information: Application form required.
Copies of proposal: 15
Deadline(s): Mar. 31 and Aug. 31
Board meeting date(s): Monthly
Final notification: 45 days after deadline
Officer: Robert J. VanDellen, Exec. Dir.
Directors: John Bishop, Lee Brown, Tom Harris, Richard Heydenberk, Regan O'Neill, Dennis Renander, Melissa Sjogren, Frederick Sprague, Ronald Swanson.
Number of staff: 1 part-time professional.
EIN: 382848513

460
The Clarence & Grace Chamberlin Foundation
600 Woodbridge Place
Detroit 48226-4302 (313) 567-1000

Contact: John L. King, Pres.

Incorporated in 1941 in MI.
Donor(s): Clarence P. Chamberlin,‡ Grace Chamberlin.‡
Financial data (yr. ended 12/31/94): Assets, $1,182,375 (M); expenditures, $94,645; qualifying distributions, $73,800, including $73,800 for 44 grants (high: $5,000; low: $300).
Fields of interest: Education; Medical care, rehabilitation; Health care; Human services; Children & youth, services; Youth, services; Family services; International relief; Federated giving programs; African Americans; Disabled; Aging; Women; Economically disadvantaged; Homeless.
Types of support: General/operating support, continuing support, program development, seed money, curriculum development, scholarship funds.
Limitations: Giving primarily in Detroit, MI. No grants to individuals or for building funds.
Application information: Application form not required.
Initial approach: Letter with proposal
Copies of proposal: 1
Deadline(s): None
Board meeting date(s): Apr. for camp grants; Dec.
Officers: John L. King, Pres.; Roger H. Fitch, V.P.; Dennis M. Mitzel, Secy.-Treas.
Number of staff: None.
EIN: 386062061

461
Chrysler Corporate Giving Program
12000 Chrysler Dr.
Highland Park 48288-1919 (810) 512-2501
Contact: Ms. Lynn A. Feldhouse, Mgr., or Kim-Lan Trinh, Administrator

Established in 1953.
Financial data (yr. ended 12/31/95): Total giving, $5,000,000.
Purpose and activities: Support for education, especially secondary education, leadership development, including Junior Achievement, employment training, economic development, minority affairs, and community funds. Chrysler also has an Assets Donation Program in which the corporation donates vehicles and auto parts to high schools and vocational schools for the training of auto mechanics and technicians. Through generous contributions to the United Way and by getting involved in their communities, the people of Chrysler addressed a variety of needs in 1994.
Fields of interest: Arts/cultural programs; Elementary school/education; Secondary school/education; Vocational education; Higher education; Business school/education; Engineering school/education; Adult education—literacy & basic skills; Reading; Education; Health care; Substance abuse, services; AIDS; Alcoholism; Health organizations; AIDS research; Crime/law enforcement; Employment; Food services; Youth development, services; Youth, services; Family services; Aging, centers & services; Minorities/immigrants, centers & services; Homeless, human services; Voluntarism promotion; Federated giving programs; Engineering; Economics; Leadership development; Minorities; Aging; Homeless.
Types of support: General/operating support, continuing support, equipment, emergency funds, program development, fellowships, scholarship funds, employee volunteer services, employee matching gifts, employee-related scholarships, donated equipment, donated products, in-kind gifts, matching funds.
Limitations: Giving primarily in headquarters city and major operating areas, including MI, IN, MO, IL, NY, OH, DE, AL, and TX. No grants to individuals, or for endowments, or research; no vehicle donations (except through Assets Donation Program).
Publications: Corporate report, corporate giving report, application guidelines, annual report.
Application information: Application form not required.
Initial approach: Letter to headquarters
Copies of proposal: 1
Deadline(s): None
Board meeting date(s): As soon as possible
Final notification: 4 months
Administrators: Lynn A. Feldhouse, Mgr.; Kim-Lan Trinh, Administrator; Yvonne Williams, Admin. Analyst.
Number of staff: 2 full-time professional; 1 full-time support.

462
The Chutney Foundation, Inc.
377 Fisher Rd.
Grosse Pointe Farms 48230

Established in 1991 in MI.
Donor(s): Cora Buhl Barbour.
Financial data (yr. ended 12/31/94): Assets, $120,064 (M); gifts received, $40,515; expenditures, $33,600; qualifying distributions, $31,600, including $31,600 for grants.
Fields of interest: Hospitals (general); Philanthropy/voluntarism; Aging.
Limitations: Giving primarily in MT.
Application information:
Initial approach: Letter
Deadline(s): June 30
Directors: Lawrence DeLong Buhl, Elizabeth B. Cocchiarella, Land M. Lindbergh, John O. Mudd, William A. Reynolds, M.D.
EIN: 810468480

463
Community Foundation of Monroe County
105 East Front
Monroe 48161 (313) 242-1976
Contact: Kathy Duvall, Acting Interim Exec. Dir.

Established in 1979 in MI.
Foundation type: Community
Financial data (yr. ended 03/31/94): Assets, $610,000 (M); gifts received, $419,000; expenditures, $149,455, including $93,957 for 27 grants (high: $26,985; low: $50; average: $500-$5,000) and $1,259 for 3 grants to individuals (high: $720; low: $139; average: $100-$1,000).
Fields of interest: Performing arts; Theater; Music; History & archaeology; Historic preservation/historical societies; Arts/cultural programs; Elementary school/education; Higher education; Adult education—literacy & basic skills; Reading; Education; Natural resource conservation & protection; Environment; Health care; Substance abuse, services; Health organizations; Food services; Housing/shelter, development; Human services; Children & youth, services; Youth, services; Aging, centers & services; Minorities/immigrants, centers & services; Homeless, human services; Community development; Voluntarism promotion; Public affairs; Minorities; Disabled; Aging; Economically disadvantaged; Homeless; General charitable giving.
Types of support: General/operating support, capital campaigns, building/renovation, equipment, program development, seed money, scholarship funds, technical assistance, consulting services, scholarships—to individuals, matching funds.
Limitations: Giving limited to Monroe County, MI. No grants to individuals (except through designated scholarship funds); no loans.
Publications: Financial statement, grants list, newsletter, application guidelines, informational brochure.
Application information: Application form required.
Initial approach: Letter or telephone
Copies of proposal: 7
Deadline(s): Jan. 1, Mar. 1, May 1, July 1, Sept. 1, and Nov. 1
Board meeting date(s): Last Tuesday in Jan., Mar., May, July, Sept., and Nov.
Officers and Directors:* Thomas Matthes,* Pres.; Carolyn Solomon,* V.P.; Mary Daume,* Secy.; Richard Bare,* Treas.; and 17 additional directors.
Number of staff: None.
EIN: 382236628

464
J. F. Ervin Foundation
3893 Research Park Dr.
P.O. Box 1168
Ann Arbor 48106 (313) 769-4600
Contact: Harriet A. Birch, Pres.

Established in 1953 in MI.
Donor(s): J.F. Ervin.‡
Financial data (yr. ended 12/31/95): Assets, $1,945,401 (M); expenditures, $89,428; qualifying distributions, $84,785, including $81,000 for 33 grants (high: $10,000; low: $1,000).
Purpose and activities: To assist in local needs; primary areas of interest include child welfare and development, delinquency, the elderly, and health services.
Fields of interest: Humanities; Arts/cultural programs; Child development, education; Hospitals (general); Health care; Substance abuse, services; Delinquency prevention/services; Children & youth, services; Child development, services; Aging, centers & services; Homeless, human services; Aging; Homeless.
Types of support: General/operating support, continuing support, annual campaigns, program development.

Limitations: Giving limited to Ann Arbor and Adrian, MI. No grants to individuals, or for scholarships; no loans.
Publications: Annual report (including application guidelines).
Application information: Application form not required.
Initial approach: Proposal in letter form
Copies of proposal: 1
Deadline(s): None
Board meeting date(s): Quarterly beginning in Mar.
Officers and Trustees:* Harriet A. Birch,* Pres.; John E. Pearson,* 1st V.P.; Susan K. Lovejoy,* V.P.; James E. Stephenson,* V.P.; William R. Kulenkamp,* Secy.; Mary Kay Pearson,* Treas.
Number of staff: 2 part-time support.
EIN: 386053755
Grants for Aging:
Neighborhood Senior Services, Ann Arbor, MI, $2,000. 95.
Washtenaw County Council on Aging, Ann Arbor, MI, $1,500. 95.

465
George R. and Elise M. Fink Foundation

377 Fisher Rd., Suite C-5
Grosse Pointe 48230 (313) 886-8451
Contact: Elyse F. Jones, Pres.

Incorporated in 1955 in MI.
Donor(s): George R. Fink,‡ Elise M. Fink.‡
Financial data (yr. ended 11/30/95): Assets, $1,975,188 (M); expenditures, $129,375; qualifying distributions, $109,802, including $103,700 for 10 grants (high: $25,000; low: $900; average: $100-$52,000).
Purpose and activities: Giving primarily to the community for secondary education, Protestant church support and church-related institutions.
Fields of interest: Secondary school/education; Children & youth, services; Aging, centers & services; Protestant agencies & churches.
Types of support: General/operating support.
Limitations: Giving primarily in MI. No grants to individuals, or for scholarships or fellowships; no loans.
Publications: 990-PF.
Application information: Application form not required.
Initial approach: Proposal
Copies of proposal: 1
Deadline(s): Quarterly
Board meeting date(s): Mar., June, Sept., and Dec.
Officers and Trustees:* Elyse F. Jones,* Pres.; John M. Fink,* V.P.; Lynn G. Carpenter,* Treas.
Number of staff: 1 part-time support.
EIN: 386059952
Grants for Aging:
Adult Well Being Services, Detroit, MI, $15,000. 95.

466
Four County Foundation

155 Rawles St.
Box 118
Romeo 48065-0118 (810) 752-4484
Contact: Peggy Hamilton, Exec. Dir.

Established in 1987 in MI.
Foundation type: Community
Financial data (yr. ended 12/31/95): Assets, $3,436,736 (M); gifts received, $108,375; expenditures, $222,586, including $121,311 for 91 grants (high: $10,000; low: $125; average: $2,000-$5,000) and $13,095 for 24 grants to individuals (high: $1,000; low: $150; average: $500-$1,000).
Fields of interest: Education; Health care; Health organizations; Youth, services; Aging, centers & services; Aging.
Types of support: Continuing support, program development, seed money, matching funds.
Limitations: Giving limited to southeast Lapeer, northwest Macomb, northeast Oakland, and southwest St. Clair counties, MI. Generally no grants to individuals, or for operating expenses.
Publications: Annual report, financial statement, application guidelines, informational brochure, newsletter.
Application information: Application form required.
Initial approach: Letter of inquiry
Copies of proposal: 10
Deadline(s): Jan. 1, Apr. 1, July 1, and Oct. 1
Board meeting date(s): 4th Thursday monthly
Final notification: Within 30 days
Officers: John Ligon, Pres.; Edmund L. Risch, V.P.; Kathleen Eubank, Secy.; John S. Bishop, Treas.; Peggy Hamilton, Exec. Dir.
Number of staff: 1 full-time professional; 1 part-time support.
EIN: 382736601

467
The Fremont Area Foundation

108 South Stewart
Fremont 49412 (616) 924-5350
Contact: Elizabeth Cherin, Exec. Dir.
FAX: (616) 924-5391;
E-mail: faf@ncats.newaygo.mi.us

Incorporated in 1951 in MI.
Foundation type: Community
Financial data (yr. ended 12/31/95): Assets, $137,264,344 (M); gifts received, $1,653,934; expenditures, $5,440,000, including $3,816,724 for 420 grants (high: $633,000; low: $10; average: $10-$633,000), $18,275 for 20 grants to individuals (high: $2,000; low: $200; average: $200-$2,000) and $325,800 for 2 foundation-administered programs.
Purpose and activities: "The foundation has established six broad funding categories: 1) Newaygo County Community Services: to sustain operations of this autonomous agency established for the delivery of general social welfare services and educational programs; 2) Community Development: to strengthen the municipal activities of villages, cities, governmental units, and other related organizations; 3) Education: to augment and promote the special projects of schools, libraries, and other organizations for instruction and training, and for scholarships to promote higher education and learning in specialized programs; 4) Arts and Culture: to support activities that promote appreciation of and participation in artistic expression such as music, theater, dance, sculpture, and painting; 5) Human Services: to foster the delivery of services and the operation of programs to help meet basic human needs and to support the provision of rehabilitative services; and 6) Health Care: made to health care providers and other related organizations for activities designed to promote optimal well-being and to provide health-related education. The foundation is also interested in supporting programs that address the particular needs of youth and older adults (aged)."
Fields of interest: Visual arts; Performing arts; Arts/cultural programs; Libraries/library science; Education; Medical care, rehabilitation; Health care; Substance abuse, services; Health organizations; Human services; Children & youth, services; Youth, services; Family services; Aging, centers & services; Community development; Government/public administration; Aging; Economically disadvantaged.
Types of support: General/operating support, building/renovation, equipment, emergency funds, program development, seed money, scholarship funds, consulting services, program-related investments/loans, scholarships—to individuals, matching funds.
Limitations: Giving primarily in Newaygo County, MI. No grants to individuals (except for scholarships from specified funds of the foundation), or for endowments, contingencies, reserves, or deficit financing; no loans.
Publications: Annual report, application guidelines, informational brochure, financial statement, grants list.
Application information: Application form required.
Initial approach: Letter or telephone to arrange interview
Copies of proposal: 10
Deadline(s): Feb. 15, May 15, and Sept. 15, except for emergencies
Board meeting date(s): Bimonthly
Final notification: 3 months
Officers and Trustees:* Donald J. Bont,* Pres.; James H. McCormick,* V.P.; Robert L. Jordan,* Treas.; Elizabeth Cherin, Exec. Dir.; Forrest Bowman, Carl Dekuiper, Lana A. Ford, Jack Hendon, Robert Kjolhede, Eric W. Rudert, Mary Schafer, Norma A. Schuiteman, Linda Shively, Josephine Toliver, Donald VanSingel, Lon Vredeveld.
Staff: Kathy Huschke, Sr. Prog. Officer.
Number of staff: 9 full-time professional; 1 part-time support.
EIN: 381443367
Grants for Aging:
Catholic Human Development, Grand Rapids, MI, $43,787. For operating support for Newaygo County Foster Grandparent Program. 94.
Catholic Human Development, Grand Rapids, MI, $17,500. For Newaygo County Foster Grandparent Program. Grant made through United Way of Newaygo County. 94.
Gerber Memorial Hospital, Fremont, MI, $14,000. For Continu-Care-Respite services. 94.
Newaygo County Commission on Aging, White Cloud, MI, $55,538. For Senior Services Coordinator position. 94.

Newaygo District Health Department No. 5, White Cloud, MI, $14,000. For respite services. 94.

Newaygo Medical Care Facility, Fremont, MI, $10,300. For dining room furnishings. Grant made though United Way of Newaygo County. 94.

468
The Rollin M. Gerstacker Foundation

P.O. Box 1945
Midland 48641-1945 (517) 631-6097
Contact: E.N. Brandt, V.P. and Secy.

Incorporated in 1957 in MI.
Donor(s): Eda U. Gerstacker,‡ Carl A. Gerstacker.‡
Financial data (yr. ended 12/31/95): Assets, $94,061,002 (M); gifts received, $499,055; expenditures, $4,224,837; qualifying distributions, $4,103,307, including $4,103,307 for 116 grants (high: $624,000; low: $1,000; average: $5,000-$30,000).
Purpose and activities: To assist community projects, with emphasis on the aged and youth; grants also for higher education, health care, medical research, and hospitals.
Fields of interest: Higher education; Hospitals (general); Health care; Mental health/crisis services; Health organizations; Human services; Youth, services; Aging, centers & services; Government/public administration; Aging.
Types of support: General/operating support, continuing support, annual campaigns, capital campaigns, building/renovation, equipment, land acquisition, endowment funds, emergency funds, seed money, research, matching funds.
Limitations: Giving primarily in MI and OH. No grants to individuals, or for scholarships or fellowships; no loans.
Publications: Annual report.
Application information: Application form not required.
Initial approach: Letter
Copies of proposal: 1
Deadline(s): May 15 and Nov. 15
Board meeting date(s): June and Dec.
Final notification: 1 month
Officers and Trustees:* Gail E. Lanphear,* Pres.; E.N. Brandt,* V.P. and Secy.; Esther S. Gerstacker,* V.P.; Alan W. Ott,* Treas.; Alexio R. Baum, Gilbert A. Currie, Frank Gerace, Lisa J. Gerstacker, Paul F. Oreffice, Jean U. Popoff, William D. Schuette, William S. Stravropoulus.
Number of staff: None.
EIN: 386060276
Grants for Aging:
Alzheimers Disease and Related Disorders Association, Ann Arbor, MI, $10,000. 94.

469
Gilmore Foundation

c/o Old Kent Bank
300 Old Kent Bank Bldg.
Grand Rapids 49503
Contact: Mark Mitchel, Dir.
Application address: c/o Old Kent Bank, P.O. Box 4019, Kalamazoo, MI 40097

Trust established in 1956 in MI.
Donor(s): Irving S. Gilmore.
Financial data (yr. ended 12/31/94): Assets, $22,589 (M); gifts received, $85,068; expenditures, $87,398; qualifying distributions, $85,608, including $78,806 for 35 grants to individuals (high: $7,480; low: $444).
Purpose and activities: Limited primarily to benevolence grants to low-income individuals residing in local area who are unable to care for themselves due to physical limitations or advanced age.
Fields of interest: Aging, centers & services; Aging; Economically disadvantaged.
Types of support: Grants to individuals.
Limitations: Giving primarily in the Kalamazoo, MI, area.
Application information: Application form required.
Deadline(s): None
Directors: Craig Kobylik, Theodore F. McCarty, Mark Mitchell.
Trustee: Old Kent Bank.
Number of staff: None.
EIN: 386052803

470
The Grand Rapids Foundation

209-C Waters Bldg.
161 Ottawa, N.W.
Grand Rapids 49503-2703 (616) 454-1751
Contact: Marcia Rapp, Prog. Dir.

Established in 1922 in MI by resolution and declaration of trust.
Foundation type: Community
Financial data (yr. ended 06/30/95): Assets, $69,411,689 (M); gifts received, $1,409,244; expenditures, $3,277,582, including $2,345,124 for 126 grants (high: $250,000; low: $500; average: $500-$250,000), $183,353 for 304 grants to individuals (high: $2,500; low: $250; average: $250-$2,500), $155,830 for 5 foundation-administered programs and $200,000 for 1 program-related investment.
Purpose and activities: To provide support for projects or causes designed to benefit the people and the quality of life in Grand Rapids and its surrounding communities, through grants for social needs, youth agencies, cultural programs, health, recreation, neighborhood development, the environment, and education, including scholarships for Kent County residents to attend selected colleges.
Fields of interest: Museums; Performing arts; Theater; Humanities; Historic preservation/historical societies; Arts/cultural programs; Child development, education; Higher education; Reading; Education; Environment; Substance abuse, services; Mental health/crisis services; AIDS; Alcoholism; Health organizations; Employment; Nutrition; Housing/shelter, development; Recreation; Youth development, services; Human services; Children & youth, services; Youth, services; Child development, services; Family services; Hospices; Aging, centers & services; Women, centers & services; Minorities/immigrants, centers & services; Homeless, human services; Civil rights, immigrants; Civil rights, minorities; Civil rights, disabled; Civil rights, women; Civil rights, aging; Civil rights, gays/lesbians; Reproductive rights; Race/intergroup relations; Community development; Voluntarism promotion; Leadership development; Minorities; Asians/Pacific Islanders; African Americans; Native Americans; Disabled; Aging; Women; People with AIDS (PWAs); Gays/lesbians; Immigrants/refugees; Economically disadvantaged; Homeless.
Types of support: Capital campaigns, building/renovation, equipment, land acquisition, program development, seed money, scholarship funds, technical assistance, program-related investments/loans, employee-related scholarships, scholarships—to individuals, matching funds.
Limitations: Giving limited to Grand Rapids, MI, and surrounding communities. No support for religious organizations, hospitals, K-12 schools, child care centers, or nursing homes/retirement facilities. No grants to individuals (except for scholarships), or for continued operating support, annual campaigns, travel expenses, medical or scholarly research, deficit financing, endowment funds, computers, or vehicles; no student loans; no funds for films, videos, conferences, or venture capital for competitive profit-making activities.
Publications: Annual report, informational brochure, newsletter, application guidelines.
Application information: The student loan program has been discontinued; new loans will not be made. Application form required.
Initial approach: Letter or telephone
Copies of proposal: 5
Deadline(s): Submit scholarship applications between Jan. 1 and Apr. 15; deadline for all other applications is 12 weeks preceding board meeting
Board meeting date(s): Varies
Final notification: June 15 for scholarships; 1 month for other requests
Officer: Diana R. Sieger, Pres.
Trustees: Robert L. Hooker, Chair.; Dirk C. Hoffius, Vice-Chair.; Ann M. Cooper, Thomas R. Hilliker, James E. McKay, Shirley K. Perkins, Charles L. Royce, David J. Wagner, Casey Wondergem.
Trustee Banks: Michigan National Bank, NBD Bank, Old Kent Bank.
Number of staff: 5 full-time professional; 1 part-time professional; 3 full-time support.
EIN: 382877959

471
Granger Foundation

P.O. Box 22187
Lansing 48909-2187 (517) 393-1670
Contact: Alton L. Granger, Trustee

Established in 1978.
Donor(s): Granger Associates, Granger Construction Co., and members of the Granger family.
Financial data (yr. ended 06/30/95): Assets, $10,751,395 (M); gifts received, $1,012,786; expenditures, $355,268; qualifying distributions, $332,666, including $330,338 for 40 grants (high: $50,000; low: $450; average: $5,000-$10,000).
Fields of interest: Substance abuse, services; Human services; Children & youth, services; Family services; Aging, centers & services; Federated giving programs; Protestant federated giving programs; Protestant agencies &

churches; Roman Catholic agencies & churches; Disabled; Aging; Economically disadvantaged; General charitable giving.
Types of support: Annual campaigns, capital campaigns.
Limitations: Giving primarily in MI. No grants to individuals.
Publications: Annual report, 990-PF, program policy statement, application guidelines.
Application information: Application form required.
Initial approach: Letter
Copies of proposal: 4
Deadline(s): None
Board meeting date(s): Semiannually
Trustees: Alton L. Granger, Donna M. Granger, Janice M. Granger, Jerry P. Granger, Lynne C. Granger, Ronald K. Granger.
Number of staff: None.
EIN: 382251879
Grants for Aging:
Geriatric Assessment Center, Baton Rouge, LA, $7,388. 95.

472
Luella Hannan Memorial Home
4750 Woodward Ave.
Detroit 48201 (313) 833-1300
Contact: Ellen Kayrod, Exec. Dir.

Established in 1925 in MI.
Donor(s): William Hannan,‡ Luella Hannan.‡
Foundation type: Operating
Financial data (yr. ended 11/30/94): Assets, $17,960,430 (M); expenditures, $923,354; qualifying distributions, $858,978, including $6,078 for 2 grants (high: $3,500; low: $2,578) and $852,900 for 2 foundation-administered programs.
Fields of interest: Aging, centers & services; Aging.
Limitations: Applications not accepted. Giving primarily in the City of Detroit and Wayne, Oakland, and Macomb counties, MI. No grants to individuals.
Application information: Contributes only to pre-selected organizations.
Officers and Trustees:* Harold Berry,* Pres.; W.C. Osborn, Jr.,* V.P. and Treas.; Zena Baum,* V.P.; Gretchen Elston,* V.P.; Richard H. Austin,* Secy.; Ellen Kayrod, Exec. Dir.; Mrs. Powell L. Cozart, Rev. Nicholas Hood, George E. Parker III, Joel D. Steinberg, Brent S. Treist.
Number of staff: 1 full-time professional; 1 part-time professional; 7 full-time support.
EIN: 381358386

473
Health Education Foundation
(Formerly Michigan Foundation for Medical & Health Education)
120 West Saginaw
East Lansing 48823 (517) 337-1351
Contact: Dawn M. Reha, Exec. Secy.

Financial data (yr. ended 11/30/94): Assets, $549,142 (M); gifts received, $6,550; expenditures, $31,111; qualifying distributions, $29,572, including $24,613 for 8 grants (high: $9,003; low: $150) and $500 for 1 grant to an individual.
Purpose and activities: To "stimulate support and/or initiate lay or professional education, research programs, and projects in the field of health; encourage the advancement of healthy lifestyles, the prevention, diagnosis or cure of disease, and the care of the sick; provide a vehicle for Michigan State Medical Society to foster humanitarian public service in health education and research, and to provide support for physicians who suffer impairment; develop and administer fund for the support of health education and research; and provide a resource for the management and distribution of signature funds or bequests designated for special health education and research projects."
Fields of interest: Medical school/education; Education; Health care; Health organizations; Aging, centers & services.
Types of support: Research, grants to individuals.
Limitations: Giving limited to MI.
Publications: Application guidelines.
Application information:
Initial approach: Proposal
Copies of proposal: 1
Deadline(s): None
Officers and Trustees:* Robert E. Paxton, M.D., Pres.; William E. Madigan,* V.P.; Dawn M. Reha, Exec. Secy.; Kevin A. Kelly, Secy.; Henry M. Domzalski, M.D.,* Treas.; Busharat Ahmad, M.D., Thomas J. Archambeau, M.D., Gilbert Bluhm, M.D., Anna H. Broecker, M.D., Nancy Crandall, John W. Hall, M.D., Vivian M. Lewis, M.D., W. Peter McCabe, M.D., Suzanne H. Pederson, Rev. Bertram Vermeulen, Richard D. Weber.
Number of staff: 1 shared staff
EIN: 386069432

474
Hillsdale County Community Foundation
P.O. Box 276
52 East Bacon St.
Hillsdale 49242-0276 (517) 439-5101
Contact: Jim McCall, Exec. Dir.

Established in 1991 in MI.
Foundation type: Community
Financial data (yr. ended 12/31/95): Assets, $2,723,875 (M); gifts received, $209,520; expenditures, $97,164, including $20,312 for 13 grants (high: $15,000; low: $90), $8,612 for 16 grants to individuals (high: $600; low: $90) and $6,120 for in-kind gifts.
Fields of interest: Visual arts; Performing arts; Theater; Arts/cultural programs; Education, association; Early childhood education; Child development, education; Elementary school/education; Higher education; Libraries/library science; Education; Natural resource conservation & protection; Environment; Animal welfare; Hospitals (general); Health care; Health organizations; Delinquency prevention/services; Crime/law enforcement; Employment; Food services; Recreation; Youth development, services; Human services; Children & youth, services; Youth, services; Child development, services; Family services; Hospices; Aging, centers & services; Community development; Voluntarism promotion; Biological sciences; Economics; Leadership development; Public affairs; Aging; Economically disadvantaged.
Types of support: Annual campaigns, publication, seed money, scholarship funds, scholarships—to individuals, matching funds.
Limitations: Giving limited to Hillsdale County, MI.
Publications: Annual report, financial statement, newsletter, informational brochure (including application guidelines), application guidelines.
Application information: Application form required.
Initial approach: Telephone or in person
Copies of proposal: 3
Deadline(s): May 15 and Nov. 15; Mar. 1, June 30, and Oct. 31 for youth grants
Board meeting date(s): Monthly
Final notification: Within 2 months
Officer: Jim McCall, Exec. Dir.
Number of staff: 3 part-time professional.
EIN: 383001297
Grants for Aging:
Hillsdale County Senior Center, Hillsdale, MI, $1,600. For Free Street Too performing ensemble. 94.

475
James and Lynelle Holden Fund
802 East Big Beaver
Troy 48083-1404
Contact: Herbert J. Wilson, Pres.

Incorporated in 1941 in MI.
Donor(s): James S. Holden,‡ Lynelle A. Holden.‡
Financial data (yr. ended 10/31/95): Assets, $7,382,480 (M); expenditures, $1,022,197; qualifying distributions, $934,751, including $895,500 for 26 grants (high: $400,000; low: $3,000; average: $2,500-$35,000).
Purpose and activities: Support for medical research, including medical schools and hospitals; aid to youth agencies, minority and underprivileged children, higher education, and care of the aged; grants also for cultural programs.
Fields of interest: Arts/cultural programs; Higher education; Medical school/education; Hospitals (general); Medical research; Children & youth, services; Aging, centers & services; Minorities/immigrants, centers & services; Minorities; Aging.
Types of support: General/operating support, continuing support, annual campaigns, building/renovation, equipment, fellowships, scholarship funds, research, matching funds.
Limitations: Giving primarily in MI, with emphasis on Detroit. No grants to individuals, or for endowment funds; no loans.
Application information: Application form not required.
Initial approach: Letter or proposal
Copies of proposal: 1
Deadline(s): None
Board meeting date(s): Jan., Apr., July, and Oct.
Final notification: Several weeks
Officers and Trustees:* Herbert J. Wilson,* Pres.; Arthur Kaufmann,* Treas.; George H. Vitta, Herbert E. Weston.
Number of staff: 1 full-time professional; 1 part-time professional.
EIN: 386052154

476
Holland Community Foundation, Inc.

One West 8th St.
Holland 49423 (616) 396-6590
Contact: William Vanderbilt, Exec. Dir.
(FAX): (616) 394-7059

Incorporated in 1951 in MI.
Foundation type: Community
Financial data (yr. ended 12/31/95): Assets, $4,997,785 (M); gifts received, $1,415,733; expenditures, $240,500, including $161,779 for grants (average: $500-$41,000).
Purpose and activities: To support cultural, educational, human services, youth activities, and the preservation and conservation of historical and cultural resources.
Fields of interest: Art conservation; Historic preservation/historical societies; Arts/cultural programs; Education; Human services; Children & youth, services; Aging.
Types of support: Annual campaigns, capital campaigns, building/renovation, equipment, land acquisition, program development, seed money, curriculum development, matching funds.
Limitations: Giving limited to the Holland, MI, area. No grants to individuals, or for building or endowment funds, operating budgets, research, scholarships, fellowships, or matching gifts, or computers.
Publications: Informational brochure, annual report.
Application information: Application form required.
Initial approach: Letter or telephone
Copies of proposal: 10
Deadline(s): Jan. 15
Board meeting date(s): Feb., Apr., Aug., and Nov.
Final notification: Apr. 30
Officers and Distribution Committee:* James E. Townsend, Pres.; Kenneth Pierce, V.P.; Ronald Dalman, 2nd V.P.; Gordon J. Van Wylen, V.P., Development; Robert L. Sterken,* Secy.; Harvey J. Buter, Treas.; William Vanderbilt, Exec. Dir.
Trustees: Char Amante, John Bouws, Thomas J. Bratt, Sr., Donna Brooks, William P. DeLong, Janice Graham, Jackie Leary Hoover, Walter Jones, Paul A. Kuiper, Lawrence B. Lee, Carolyn Marquis, Edward H. Marsilje, Carol Myers, Lupita Reyes, Barry Werkman, Ella Weyman.
Number of staff: 2 part-time support.
EIN: 386095283

477
India Foundation

2601 Cochise Ln.
Okemos 48864
Contact: Shrikumar Poddar, Pres.

Established in 1970.
Donor(s): Shrikumar Poddar, Mayurika Poddar.
Financial data (yr. ended 12/31/94): Assets, $2,347,833 (M); expenditures, $165,467; qualifying distributions, $138,622, including $111,058 for 8 grants (high: $75,000; low: $658).
Purpose and activities: Support primarily for East Indian religious and charitable organizations.
Fields of interest: Education; Gun control; Domestic violence prevention; Civil rights, aging; Religion; Asians/Pacific Islanders; Native Americans; Immigrants/refugees; Economically disadvantaged; Homeless.
Types of support: Conferences/seminars, technical assistance, in-kind gifts, matching funds.
Limitations: Giving primarily in MI. No grants to individuals.
Application information: Application form not required.
Initial approach: Letter
Copies of proposal: 1
Deadline(s): Apr. 1 and Aug. 1
Board meeting date(s): Semiannually in June and Sept.
Officers: Shrikumar Poddar, Pres. and Treas.; Mayurika Poddar, V.P.; Eleanor Finn, Secy.
Number of staff: None.
EIN: 237300230

478
W. K. Kellogg Foundation

One Michigan Ave. East
Battle Creek 49017-4058 (616) 968-1611
Contact: Nancy A. Sims, Mgr., Grant Proposals
FAX: (616) 968-0413

Incorporated in 1930 in MI.
Donor(s): W.K. Kellogg,‡ W.K. Kellogg Foundation Trust.
Financial data (yr. ended 08/31/95): Assets, $6,034,576,655 (M); expenditures, $267,615,586; qualifying distributions, $234,243,090, including $213,268,038 for 1,356 grants (high: $10,000,000; low: $71; average: $5,000-$1,000,000), $7,825,089 for 354 grants to individuals (high: $73,625; low: $20), $1,598,654 for employee matching gifts and $11,551,309 for foundation-administered programs.
Purpose and activities: The W.K. Kellogg Foundation was established in 1930 "to help people help themselves through the practical application of knowledge and resources to improve their quality of life and that of future generations." The foundation targets its grants toward specific focal points or areas. These include: health; food systems and rural development; youth and education, and higher education; and philanthropy and volunteerism. When woven throughout these areas, funding also is provided for leadership; information systems/technology; efforts to capitalize on diversity; and family, neighborhood, and community development programming. Grants are concentrated in the United States, Latin America and the Caribbean, and Southern Africa.
Fields of interest: Early childhood education; Elementary school/education; Secondary school/education; Higher education; Health sciences school/education; Adult/continuing education; Education; Health care, support services; Health care; Health organizations; Agriculture; Agriculture/food; Youth development, services; Youth, services; Aging, centers & services; Minorities/immigrants, centers & services; Community development, neighborhood development; Rural development; Community development; Voluntarism promotion; Computer science; International studies; Leadership development; Minorities; African Americans; Aging; Caribbean; Southern Africa; Latin America.
Types of support: Seed money, fellowships, employee matching gifts.
Limitations: Giving primarily in the U.S., Latin America and the Caribbean, and Southern Africa; support also for international fellowship programs in other countries. No support for religious purposes. No grants to individuals (except through fellowship programs), or for building or endowment funds, research, development campaigns, films, equipment, publications, conferences, or radio and television programs unless they are an integral part of a project already being funded; no grants for operating budgets, annual campaigns, emergency funds, deficit financing, land acquisition, or renovation projects; no loans.
Publications: Annual report (including application guidelines), informational brochure (including application guidelines), newsletter, occasional report.
Application information: Proposals must conform to specified program priorities. Application form not required.
Initial approach: Pre-proposal letter (1 to 2 pages)
Copies of proposal: 1
Deadline(s): None
Board meeting date(s): Monthly
Officers and Trustees:* William C. Richardson, Ph.D.,* Pres. and C.E.O.; Gregory A. Lyman, Sr. V.P. and Corp. Secy.; William W. Fritz, V.P., Finance and Treas.; Karen R. Hollenbeck, V.P., Administration; Richard M. Foster, V.P., Progs.; Gail D. McClure, V.P., Progs.; Dan E. Moore, V.P., Progs.; Gloria R. Smith, V.P., Progs.; Jack K. Mawdsley, Interim V.P., Prog.; Shirley D. Bowser, Chris T. Christ, Dorothy A. Johnson, William E. LaMothe, Russell G. Mawby, Wenda Weekes Moore, Robert L. Raun, Howard F. Sims, Jonathan T. Walton.
Staff: Jana Arriagada Riedemann, Prog. Dir.; Bobby W. Austin, Prog. Dir.; Leah M. Austin, Prog. Dir.; C. Patrick Babcock, Prog. Dir.; Tyrone R. Baines, Prog. Dir. and Dir., Youth Initiatives Prog.; John A. Beineke, Prog. Dir.; Joyce A. Brown, Prog. Dir.; Thomas A. Bruce, Prog. Dir.; John C. Burkhardt, Prog. Dir.; Heliodoro Diaz Cisneros, Prog. Dir.; Bruce M. Darr, Prog. Dir. and Dir., Battle Creek Progs.; Robert A. DeVries, Prog. Dir. & Dir., Intl. Study Grants; Antonio Gomez, Prog. Dir.; Guillermina Hernandez-Gallegos, Prog. Dir.; Oran B. Hesterman, Prog. Dir.; Mary M. Hlalele, Prog. Dir.; Susan Jenkins, Prog. Dir.; Marcos Kisil, Prog. Dir. and Dir., Latin American Progs.; Christine M. Kwak, Prog. Dir.; Robert F. Long, Prog. Dir.; Larraine R. Matusak, Prog. Dir., Leadership Scholar; Marvin H. McKinney, Prog. Dir.; Gloria T. Meert, Prog. Dir.; Judith Watson Olson, Prog. Dir.; Joel J. Orosz, Prog. Dir.; Betty J. Overton, Prog. Dir. & Dir., Higher Education; Delores A. Parker, Prog Dir.; Ronald W. Richards, Prog. Dir.; Rosana Rodriguez, Prog. Dir.; Blas Santos, Prog. Dir.; John R. Seita, Prog. Dir.; Gerald K. Smith, Prog. Dir.; Roger H. Sublett, Prog. Dir. & Dir., Kellogg Natl. Fell. Prog.; Francisco B. Tancredi, Prog. Dir.; Frank C. Taylor, Prog. Dir. & Assoc. Dir. Kellogg Intl. Lead. Prog.; Andres A. Thompson, Prog. Dir.;

Thomas L. Thorburn, Prog. Dir.; Henrie M. Treadwell, Prog. Dir.; Steven Uranga McKane, Prog. Dir.; Valora Washington, Prog. Dir.; Freddye Webb-Petett, Prog. Dir. & Dir., Kellogg Intl. Leadership Prog.; Robert A. Blanchard, Dir., Administration; Timothy L. Dechant, Dir., Technology; Thomas C. Fritz, Dir., Internal Audit; Robert E. Hencey, Dir., Special Projects; Karla J. Kretzschmer, Dir., Human Resources; Karen E. Lake, Dir., Communications; Ricardo A. Millett, Dir., Evaluation; Christina D. Hammond, Mgr., Grant Commitments; Nancy A. Sims, Mgr., Grant Proposals; Roslyn McCallister Brock, Prog. Assoc.; Valorie J. Johnson, Prog. Assoc.; Phyllis D. Meadows, Prog. Assoc.; Steven E. Peffers, Prog. Assoc.; Kay Randolph-Back, Prog. Assoc.; Michelle M. Reece, Prog. Assoc.; Paul D. Vander Velde, Prog. Assoc.; Alice M. Warner, Prog. Assoc.
Number of staff: 105 full-time professional; 2 part-time professional; 158 full-time support; 4 part-time support.
EIN: 381359264
Grants for Aging:
Burnham Brook Center, River Edge Senior Center, Battle Creek, MI, $15,050. To improve opportunities and service delivery for senior citizens in Calhoun County by supporting the development of the Burnham Brook Center. Grant brings total of Foundation assistance for this project to $4,615,050. This grant was made because of the Foundation's responsibility as a corporate member of the Greater Battle Creek Area. Foundation would not make such a grant in any other community. 95.
Center for Human Services, Bethesda, MD, $30,000. To improve success of school-aged children from disadvantaged neighborhoods by replicating successful intergenerational model program. Grant made because of Foundation's response to special programming opportunities. It is unlikely Foundation would make such a grant otherwise. 95.
ShareCare of Leelanau, Suttons Bay, MI, $23,600. To improve health of elderly through independent living program for seniors that integrates and coordinates countywide community services by a nurse/care manager. Grant was made because of Foundation's response to special programming opportunities. It is unlikely Foundation would make such a grant otherwise. 95.
Tonatierra Community Development Institute, Phoenix, AZ, $70,000. To strengthen families through programs that help preserve intergenerational ties. Grant made because of Foundation's response to special programming opportunities. It is unlikely Foundation would make such a grant otherwise. 95.
Wayne State University, Detroit, MI, $94,000. To develop self-management training program for grandparents who are raising children. Grant made as part of Foundation's emergent programming. A very limited number of such grants will be made. 95.

479
Elizabeth E. Kennedy Fund
110 Miller Ave., No. 300
Ann Arbor 48104-1339 (313) 761-3780
Contact: John S. Dobson, Secy.

Incorporated in 1954 in MI.
Donor(s): Elizabeth E. Kennedy.
Financial data (yr. ended 12/31/95): Assets, $4,518,756 (M); expenditures, $190,186; qualifying distributions, $170,400, including $170,400 for 28 grants (high: $14,000; low: $900; average: $1,000-$10,000).
Purpose and activities: Emphasis on higher and other education, the arts, archaeology, conservation and the environment, health, family planning, medical research, and mental health; preference is to provide seed money.
Fields of interest: History & archaeology; Arts/cultural programs; Education, research; Higher education; Education; Natural resource conservation & protection; Environment; Family planning; Health care; Mental health/crisis services; Health associations; Medical research; Aging, centers & services; Minorities; Aging.
Types of support: Capital campaigns, building/renovation, equipment, land acquisition, program development, seed money, scholarship funds, research.
Limitations: Giving limited to MI, with emphasis on the less populated areas of the state. No grants to individuals.
Publications: Annual report (including application guidelines), 990-PF, application guidelines.
Application information: Application form not required.
Initial approach: Letter
Copies of proposal: 5
Deadline(s): None
Board meeting date(s): July and Dec.
Officers and Trustees:* Ann K. Irish,* Pres.; Joan K. Slocum,* V.P.; John S. Dobson,* Secy.; James Gamble,* Treas.; James A. Kennedy, Jr., Susan Kennedy, William W. Slocum.
Number of staff: None.
EIN: 386063463
Grants for Aging:
Neighborhood Senior Services, Ann Arbor, MI, $7,500. For safety devices for senior citizens. 95.

480
Key Bank National Association Corporate Giving Program
(Formerly Society Bank, Michigan Corporate Giving Program)
100 South Main St.
Ann Arbor 48104 (313) 994-5555
Contact: Spencer Swank, Sr. V.P.

Fields of interest: Visual arts; Performing arts; Humanities; Arts/cultural programs; Higher education; Education; Animal welfare; Hospitals (general); Health care; Cancer; Biomedicine; Health organizations; Medical research; Cancer research; Employment; Housing/shelter, development; Safety/disasters; Recreation; Human services; Youth, services; Aging, centers & services; Minorities/immigrants, centers & services; Homeless, human services; Business & industry; Community development; Federated giving programs; Government/public administration; Minorities; Disabled; Aging; Homeless; General charitable giving.
Types of support: General/operating support, continuing support, annual campaigns, capital campaigns, building/renovation, program development, conferences/seminars, scholarship funds.
Limitations: Giving primarily in areas of company operations.
Application information:
Initial approach: Send requests to company headquarters in care of Administration Dept.
Number of staff: None.

481
Harry B. & Anna Korman Foundation
c/o Larry Zietz, Gittleman, Paskel et al.
2472 Northwestern Hwy.
Southfield 48075
Contact: Harry B. Korman, Pres.

Established in 1956.
Donor(s): Harry B. Korman.
Financial data (yr. ended 12/31/95): Assets, $978,107 (M); expenditures, $82,871; qualifying distributions, $67,000, including $67,000 for 5 grants (high: $25,500; low: $3,000).
Fields of interest: Higher education; Cancer; Cancer research; Aging, centers & services; Jewish agencies & temples; Aging.
Application information:
Initial approach: Letter
Deadline(s): None
Officers and Directors:* Harry B. Korman, Pres.; Anna Korman,* V.P.; Lawrence D. Zietz,* Secy.; Ingeborg Schuetz,* Treas.; Helen Braverman.
EIN: 386078083

482
The Metro Health Foundation
333 West Fort St., Suite 1370
Detroit 48226-3134 (313) 965-4220
Contact: Glenn F. Kossick, Exec. Dir.

Incorporated in 1986 in MI.
Financial data (yr. ended 12/31/94): Assets, $6,635,749 (M); expenditures, $467,932; qualifying distributions, $408,194, including $283,254 for 44 grants (high: $25,000; low: $50; average: $5,000-$25,000) and $17,290 for foundation-administered programs.
Purpose and activities: "Dedicated to helping metropolitan Detroit organizations meet the community's health care needs. Grants support a wide variety of health related services for people of all ages. Collaborative programs which make comprehensive, primary health care accessible to at-risk urban groups are a priority." Areas of primary interest include: teenage pregnancy crisis; health care transportation for the elderly and homeless; in-home health-care assistance; medically related assistance to the homeless; health-care equipment and medical supplies in limited amounts, preferably for underfunded organizations; medical education in special situations in the tri-county Detroit area; and start-up and support money for projects such as AIDS, epilepsy, cancer, heart disease, leukemia, and other major ills of substantial public

concern. Note: AIDS-related grants are made through Michigan AIDS Fund.
Fields of interest: Nursing school/education; Health care; AIDS; Health organizations; Gun control; Domestic violence prevention; Children & youth, services; Aging, centers & services; Homeless, human services; Reproductive rights; African Americans; Disabled; Aging; Women; Economically disadvantaged; Homeless.
Types of support: General/operating support, equipment, emergency funds, publication, seed money, internships, scholarship funds, matching funds.
Limitations: Giving limited to the metropolitan tri-county, Detroit, MI, area. No support for religious organizations or government agencies (except by specific Board action). No grants to individuals, or for building campaigns; no loans.
Publications: Annual report (including application guidelines), 990-PF.
Application information: Application form required.
Initial approach: Telephone for application and to discuss proposal idea
Copies of proposal: 5
Deadline(s): Aug. 1 and Dec. 1
Board meeting date(s): Oct. and Feb.
Final notification: Within 90 days
Officers and Trustees:* Richard L. Justice,* Pres.; Lillie Tabor,* V.P.; Frank B. Walker, M.D.,* Treas.; Glenn F. Kossick,* Exec. Dir.; Judith Bean, Ph.D., Cheryl Chandler, Raymond Cochran, Doris M. Fell, Jaqueline Martin, Gloria Robinson, Randy Walainis.
Number of staff: 1 full-time professional; 1 full-time support.
EIN: 382100939

483
Prince Foundation
One Prince Ctr.
Holland 49423

Established in 1977.
Donor(s): Edgar D. Prince, Elsa D. Prince, Prince Corp.
Financial data (yr. ended 06/30/95): Assets, $47,802,370 (M); gifts received, $2,702,579; expenditures, $3,304,809; qualifying distributions, $3,262,006, including $3,155,086 for 40 grants (high: $630,000; low: $118; average: $5,000-$100,000).
Purpose and activities: Giving to Christian organizations, churches, and schools; support also for a senior citizens center.
Fields of interest: Elementary/secondary education; Aging, centers & services; Christian agencies & churches; Religion; Aging.
Types of support: General/operating support.
Limitations: Applications not accepted. Giving primarily in MI. No grants to individuals.
Application information: Contributes only to pre-selected organizations.
Officers: Elsa D. Prince, Pres.; Elisabeth De Vos, V.P.; Eileen Ellens, V.P.; Erik D. Prince, V.P.; Emilie Wierda, V.P.; Robert Haveman, Secy.-Treas.
EIN: 382190330

484
Harvey M. Rice Charitable Trust
210 Orange Lake
Bloomfield Hills 48302

Established in 1990 in MI.
Donor(s): Harvey M. Rice.
Financial data (yr. ended 06/30/94): Assets, $668,242 (M); gifts received, $149,328; expenditures, $27,731; qualifying distributions, $27,732, including $22,300 for grants.
Fields of interest: Human services, special populations; Roman Catholic agencies & churches; Religion; Aging.
Limitations: Applications not accepted. Giving primarily in MI.
Application information: Contributes only to pre-selected organizations.
Officers: Dave Thomas, Pres.; John Solecki, Treas.
EIN: 382936753

485
Southfield Community Foundation
26000 Evergreen Rd.
Southfield 48037 (810) 354-9617
Contact: Susan E. Ellis, Exec. Dir.
Additional address: P.O. Box 2055, Southfield, MI 48037

Established in 1989 in MI.
Foundation type: Community
Financial data (yr. ended 06/30/95): Assets, $92,926 (M); gifts received, $125,625; expenditures, $143,837, including $56,600 for grants (high: $9,000; low: $250).
Fields of interest: Arts/cultural programs; Education; Youth development; Children & youth, services; Race/intergroup relations; Community development; Aging.
Types of support: Annual campaigns.
Limitations: Giving limited to the Southfield, MI, area. No support for religious purposes, endowments, building campaigns, deficit financing, films, or for general operating support. No grants to individuals.
Publications: Annual report, 990-PF, application guidelines, informational brochure (including application guidelines), financial statement.
Application information: Application form required.
Initial approach: Letter requesting application form
Copies of proposal: 1
Deadline(s): Nov. 1, Apr. 1, and Aug. 1
Board meeting date(s): 3rd Monday in Jan., Mar., May, July, Sept., and Nov.
Final notification: Following board meeting
Directors: Robert R. Block, Rosalind Cooperman, Marlene Davis, Edgar Fenton, George Francis III, David Fukuzawa, William Hoffman, Richard Marburger, Joseph F. McCarthy, Chuck Stokes, James Zick.
Number of staff: 1 full-time professional.
EIN: 382918048

486
Mary Thompson Foundation
c/o Comerica Bank
P.O. Box 75000, M/C 3302
Detroit 48275
Application address: c/o Mrs. Douglas F. Roby, Jr., P.O. Box 568, St. Clair Shores, MI 48080-9998

Established in 1942.
Financial data (yr. ended 12/31/95): Assets, $3,337,127 (M); expenditures, $219,323; qualifying distributions, $177,142, including $174,571 for 16 grants (high: $40,000; low: $2,281).
Fields of interest: Aging, centers & services; Aging.
Limitations: Giving limited to MI.
Application information: Application form required.
Initial approach: Letter
Deadline(s): None
Officers and Trustees:* Mrs. William D. Dahling, Pres.; Mrs. E. Irving Book,* V.P.; Antoinette P. Book,* Secy.; Mrs. Ferdinand Cinelli,* Treas.; Mrs. Douglas F. Roby, Jr.,* Grant Chair.; Mrs. Charles W. Adams, Mrs. John D. Bayne, Mrs. George E. Cartmill, Mrs. Vernor Davis, Mrs. Henry T. Ewald, Jr., Mrs. Martin S. Hayden, Mrs. William H. Ledyard, Mrs. John H. Longley, Mrs. David Viger.
Comerica Bank.
Number of staff: None.
EIN: 381359097

487
Harold and Grace Upjohn Foundation
c/o Mall Plaza, Suite 90
157 South Kalamazoo Mall
Kalamazoo 49007 (616) 344-2818
Contact: Floyd L. Parks, Secy.-Treas.

Incorporated in 1958 in MI.
Donor(s): Grace G. Upjohn.‡
Financial data (yr. ended 10/31/95): Assets, $8,357,035 (M); expenditures, $393,516; qualifying distributions, $356,638, including $341,993 for 30 grants (high: $30,000; low: $1,000).
Purpose and activities: Grants primarily "to promote scientific research for the alleviation of human suffering; to care for the sick, aged, and helpless whose private resources are inadequate; to conduct research for and otherwise assist in the improvement of living, moral and working conditions; to promote the spread of education and to provide scholarships for deserving young men and women; to promote and aid in the mental, moral, intellectual and physical improvement, assistance and relief of the poor, indigent or deserving inhabitants of the U.S., regardless of race, color or creed."
Fields of interest: Arts/cultural programs; Higher education; Environment; Family services; Aging, centers & services; Community development, neighborhood development.
Types of support: Program development, seed money, scholarship funds, research.
Limitations: Giving primarily in the greater Kalamazoo, MI, area. No grants to individuals, or for operating budgets or annual campaigns.

Publications: Annual report, program policy statement, application guidelines.
Application information: Application form required.
Initial approach: Call or write for application form and instructions
Copies of proposal: 1
Deadline(s): Apr. 1 and Sept. 1
Board meeting date(s): Spring and fall
Final notification: 30 days after board meeting
Officers and Trustees:* Florence Upjohn Orosz,* Pres.; Christopher U. Light,* V.P.; Floyd L. Parks, Secy.-Treas.; Janet J. Deal, Mary U. Meader, Jon L. Stryker.
EIN: 386052963
Grants for Aging:
Senior Services, Pauline Allen Nutrition Center, Kalamazoo, MI, $25,000. 95.

488
Frank S. and Mollie S. VanDervoort Memorial Foundation

c/o Comercia Bank
P.O. Box 75000, M/C 3302
Detroit 48275
Contact: Ann L. Gessert, Secy.
Application address: 4646 Okemos Rd., Okemos, MI 48864; Tel.: (517) 349-7232

Established in 1970 in MI.
Donor(s): Frank S. VanDervoort,‡ Mollie S. VanDervoort.‡
Financial data (yr. ended 06/30/95): Assets, $1,509,946 (M); expenditures, $84,572; qualifying distributions, $68,314, including $62,098 for 19 grants (high: $13,000; low: $500).
Purpose and activities: To assist worthy indigent older people and crippled children by funding requests through appropriate operating agencies.
Fields of interest: Human services; Children & youth, services; Aging, centers & services; Disabled; Aging; Economically disadvantaged.
Limitations: Giving limited to Ingham County, MI.
Application information: Application form not required.
Initial approach: Proposal
Copies of proposal: 3
Deadline(s): None
Board meeting date(s): Monthly
Officers and Board Members:* Robert A. Fisher,* Pres.; Helen H. Deliyanne,* V.P.; Ann L. Gessert,* Secy.
Agent: Comerica Bank.
EIN: 386190789
Grants for Aging:
East Lansing Older Peoples Program, East Lansing, MI, $3,800. 94.
Mobile Meals, East Lansing, MI, $7,000. 95.
Mobile Meals, Lansing, MI, $7,000. 94.
Sixty Plus, Lansing, MI, $4,500. 95.
Tri-County Office on Aging, Lansing, MI, $13,000. 94.
Tri-County Office on Aging, Lansing, MI, $13,000. 95.

489
Young Woman's Home Association of Detroit

349 Notre Dame
Grosse Pointe 48230 (313) 822-9512
Contact: Debbie Tischler
Application address: 1009 Audubon Rd., Grosse Pointe, MI 48230; Tel.: (313) 885-9311; Additional tel.: (313) 823-1509

Established in 1877 in MI.
Donor(s): Jessie Castle Roberts Trust.
Financial data (yr. ended 03/31/95): Assets, $1,411,043 (M); gifts received, $42,205; expenditures, $69,461; qualifying distributions, $65,483, including $64,125 for 41 grants (high: $3,500; low: $500).
Purpose and activities: Grants made to organizations benefiting women and children in MI.
Fields of interest: Arts/cultural programs; Child development, education; Hospitals (general); Substance abuse, services; Health associations; Human services; Children & youth, services; Youth, services; Child development, services; Family services; Aging, centers & services; Women, centers & services; Homeless, human services; Disabled; Aging; Women; Economically disadvantaged; Homeless.
Types of support: Continuing support, building/renovation, equipment, emergency funds, program development, curriculum development.
Limitations: Giving primarily in MI. No grants to individuals.
Application information: Application form required.
Deadline(s): Sept. 1 and Mar. 1
Board meeting date(s): 3rd Tuesday of each month from Sept. through June
Final notification: Apr. or Oct.
Officers and Trustees:* Mrs. Howard Tischler,* Pres.; Mrs. Richard T. Walsh,* V.P.; Mrs. Charles Endicott,* Corresponding Secy.; Mrs. Frank K. Zinn,* Recording Secy.; Mrs. Arthur H. Engstrom,* Treas.; and 16 additional trustees.
Number of staff: None.
EIN: 381360595
Grants for Aging:
Lutheran Social Services of Michigan, Detroit, MI, $1,000. For Calvary Center program. 95.
Renaissance Home Health Care, Detroit, MI, $2,500. 95.
Renaissance Home Health Care, Detroit, MI, $2,000. 94.
World Medical Relief, Detroit, MI, $2,500. For prescriptions for female senior citizens. 94.

MINNESOTA

490
American Express Minnesota Foundation

c/o IDS Financial Services
IDS Tower 10, Tax Dept. Unit 1163
Minneapolis 55440 (612) 671-3321
Contact: Marie Tobin, Community Rels. Specialist
Application Tel.: (612) 671-5874

Established in 1987 in MN.
Donor(s): IDS Financial Corp.
Foundation type: Company-sponsored
Financial data (yr. ended 12/31/94): Assets, $0 (M); gifts received, $723,384; expenditures, $872,326; qualifying distributions, $872,326, including $872,326 for 3,367 employee matching gifts.
Purpose and activities: Main emphasis on cultural diversity and national heritage programs, higher education, employment and training, and child welfare. The foundation looks for programs that provide high-quality services, serve children and families, offer direct services to the public, find innovative solutions to community problems, involve IDS employees, and fit within the company's primary focus areas. Priority will be given to specific projects (as opposed to general operating support), to projects supported by public/private partnerships, to efforts that involve IDS beyond grant support (e.g., business/school/parent coalitions), and to distinctive projects where company involvement can make a noticeable difference. The IDS Matching Program matches IDS employees' individual gifts to various nonprofit organizations.
Fields of interest: Visual arts; Museums; Performing arts; Dance; Theater; Music; Historic preservation/historical societies; Arts/cultural programs; Early childhood education; Child development, education; Higher education; Adult/continuing education; Education; AIDS; AIDS research; Employment; Human services; Children & youth, services; Youth, services; Child development, services; Family services; Aging, centers & services; Women, centers & services; Minorities/immigrants, centers & services; Homeless, human services; Community development; Voluntarism promotion; Economics; Minorities; Native Americans; Aging; Women; Economically disadvantaged; Homeless.
Types of support: General/operating support, program development, employee matching gifts.
Limitations: Giving primarily in MN. No support for religious, political, fraternal, or sports organizations, medical research, or hospitals. No grants to individuals, or for books, magazines, endowments, capital campaigns, benefits, or charitable dinners.
Publications: Corporate giving report (including application guidelines), 990-PF.
Application information: Application form not required.
Initial approach: Proposal
Copies of proposal: 1
Deadline(s): Jan. 15 for culture; Apr. 15 for education and employment; and July 15 for community service programs
Board meeting date(s): Quarterly
Final notification: Within 6 to 8 weeks
Officers and Directors:* Pamela J. Moret, Pres.; Susan L. Gethin, V.P.; Colleen C. Curran, Secy.; Morris Goodwin, Jr.,* Treas.; Karl J. Breyer, James E. Choat, Samuel E. Kasuske, Susan D. Kinder, Suzanne M. Roberts, Marty R. Shugarts, Stephen W. Swenson.

Number of staff: 3 full-time professional; 1 part-time professional.
EIN: 411607944

491
Otto Bremer Foundation

445 Minnesota St., Suite 2000
St. Paul 55101-2107 (612) 227-8036
Contact: John Kostishack, Exec. Dir.
FAX: (612) 227-2522

Trust established in 1944 in MN.
Donor(s): Otto Bremer.‡
Financial data (yr. ended 12/31/95): Assets, $200,318,354 (M); expenditures, $8,440,089; qualifying distributions, $8,652,618, including $7,432,494 for 502 grants (high: $150,000; low: $500; average: $1,200-$25,000) and $494,945 for 10 program-related investments.
Purpose and activities: Emphasis on rural poverty and combating racism. Support also for post-secondary education, human services, health, religion, and community affairs.
Fields of interest: Early childhood education; Child development, education; Higher education; Libraries/library science; Education; Family planning; Health care; Mental health/crisis services; Health organizations; Delinquency prevention/services; Domestic violence prevention; Legal services; Nutrition; Housing/shelter, development; Youth development, citizenship; Human services; Children & youth, services; Youth, services; Child development, services; Hospices; Women, centers & services; Minorities/immigrants, centers & services; Homeless, human services; Peace; Human rights (international); Civil rights, immigrants; Civil rights, minorities; Civil rights, disabled; Civil rights, women; Civil rights, aging; Civil rights, gays/lesbians; Race/intergroup relations; Civil rights; Rural development; Community development; Voluntarism promotion; Public affairs, citizen participation; Public affairs; Minorities; Asians/Pacific Islanders; African Americans; Latinos; Native Americans; Disabled; Aging; Women; People with AIDS (PWAs); Gays/lesbians; Immigrants/refugees; Economically disadvantaged; Homeless.
Types of support: General/operating support, continuing support, building/renovation, equipment, emergency funds, program development, conferences/seminars, seed money, internships, technical assistance, program-related investments/loans, matching funds.
Limitations: Giving limited to cities in MN, ND, and WI where there are Bremer Bank affiliates, and to organizations addressing poverty in the city of St. Paul. No support for national health organizations. No grants to individuals, or for endowment funds, medical research, or professorships.
Publications: Annual report (including application guidelines).
Application information: Application form not required.
Initial approach: Letter or telephone
Copies of proposal: 1
Deadline(s): Submit proposal at least 3 months before funding decision is desired
Board meeting date(s): Monthly
Final notification: 3 months
Officer: John Kostishack,* Exec. Dir.
Trustees: Charlotte S. Johnson, William H. Lipschultz, Daniel Reardon, Robert Reardon.
Staff: Karen Starr, Sr. Prog. Officer; Lynda Miner, Grants Mgr.
Number of staff: 3 full-time professional; 1 part-time professional.
EIN: 416019050
Grants for Aging:
Adult Abuse Community Services, Grand Forks, ND, $20,000. To sustain services to victims of family violence, sexual assault and other personal injuries. 95.
Alvarado, City of, Alvarado, MN, $10,000. For repairs to Senior Citizen-Community Center. 95.
Bethesda Pleasantview Nursing Home, Willmar, MN, $10,000. To renovate activity kitchen to be used by elderly residents of Bethesda Heritage Home. 95.
Catholic Family Service, Fargo, ND, $10,000. For guardianship program for mentally ill and elderly populations in Minot. 95.
Catholic Services for the Elderly, Saint Paul, MN, $15,000. For matching grant for construction of adult day care center. 95.
Dakota Area Resources and Transportation for Seniors (DARTS), West Saint Paul, MN, $10,000. To establish client centered continuum of health care that connects social and health service programs in efficient manner. 95.
Dunn County Interfaith Volunteer Caregivers, Menomonie, WI, $25,000. To develop homeless shelter for region. 95.
Earthstar Project, Saint Paul, MN, $25,000. For Earthstar Program which serves Native American elders. 95.
Indian Family Services, Minneapolis, MN, $15,000. For transportation services to elders. 95.
Minnesota Senior Federation, Saint Paul, MN, $20,000. To improve health care access in Willmar area. 95.
Minot Commission on Aging, Minot, ND, $35,000. For equipment for Region II Senior Services Providers food delivery program. 95.
White Earth Reservation Tribal Council, White Earth, MN, $36,000. To construct water and sewer systems for housing for low-income elders. 95.
White Earth Reservation Tribal Council, White Earth, MN, $21,000. For appliances for elderly housing. 95.

492
Ceridian Corporate Giving Program

(Formerly Control Data Public Affairs Department)
8100 34th Ave. South
Bloomington 55425 (612) 853-5082
Contact: Norma Anderson, V.P., Devel. Resources
URL: http://www.ceridian.com/charitable.html

Purpose and activities: Ceridian's philanthropic focus is on cutting-edge Work and Life Balancing Programs for employees. "Programs that help employees better balance the often conflicting demands of job and non-work interests are becoming increasingly important to employees everywhere." Areas covered include, but are not limited to, public policy advocacy, employee/dependent care, employee assistance, employee/eldercare, working parent support, and work/life stress reduction. The company seeks to contribute to emerging, innovative, and creative undertakings in this area. In addition, through the community action Field Program, grants are awarded to organizations for which employees volunteer.
Fields of interest: Education; Employment; Family services; Aging, centers & services; Aging.
Types of support: Program development, employee volunteer services, use of facilities, donated products, in-kind gifts.
Limitations: Giving primarily in headquarters and company locations. No support for political organizations, or religious organizations for religious purposes.
Publications: Program policy statement.
Application information: Application form not required.
Initial approach: Letter to Public Affairs
Copies of proposal: 1
Deadline(s): None
Final notification: 2 to 3 weeks
Number of staff: 3 full-time professional; 1 full-time support.

493
Doherty, Rumble & Butler Foundation

2800 Minnesota World Trade Ctr.
30 East Seventh St.
St. Paul 55101 (612) 291-9333
Contact: Thomas A. Berreman, Secy.

Established in 1979 in MN.
Donor(s): Doherty, Rumble & Butler, P.A.
Foundation type: Company-sponsored
Financial data (yr. ended 12/31/93): Assets, $13,386 (M); gifts received, $76,245; expenditures, $72,946; qualifying distributions, $72,923, including $72,900 for 58 grants (high: $11,200; low: $100).
Fields of interest: Film/video; Visual arts; Museums; Performing arts; Dance; History & archaeology; Arts/cultural programs; Higher education; Law school/education; Education; Hospitals (general); Legal services; Housing/shelter, development; Human services; Children & youth, services; Youth, services; Family services; Aging, centers & services; Community development; Native Americans; Disabled; Aging; Economically disadvantaged.
Types of support: General/operating support, annual campaigns, capital campaigns, seed money.
Limitations: Giving primarily in the Minneapolis-St. Paul, MN, metropolitan area. No grants to individuals; no loans.
Application information: Application form not required.
Initial approach: Proposal
Deadline(s): None
Board meeting date(s): Usually, once every 2 months
Officer and Directors:* Thomas A. Berreman,* Secy.; William J. Cosgriff, Terrance A. Costello, Marc J. Manderscheid, Elizabeth Hoene Martin, Daniel C. Mott, Lori Wiese-Parks.
Number of staff: None.
EIN: 411353915

494
Ecolab Corporate Contributions Program

c/o Ecolab Inc.
Ecolab Center
St. Paul 55102 (612) 293-2259
Contact: Lois J. West, Dir., Community and Public Rels.

Financial data (yr. ended 12/31/94): Total giving, $1,176,000, including $1,176,000 for grants (high: $164,032; average: $500-$12,000).
Purpose and activities: "We want to make a difference. In tough economic times, we believe it is especially important to invest in our communities because they are our future. By helping them become healthy and vital, we ensure our well-being." The company's operating and capital grants serve the categories of education, community development, health and human services, and arts and culture. However, Ecolab channels its resources primarily to agencies and programs that give disadvantaged groups and individuals the tools they need to become self-sufficient. The corporate contributions program addresses company concerns through charitable contributions, creative programming, and employee volunteerism.
Fields of interest: Arts/cultural programs; Child development, education; Education; Health care; Health organizations; Human services; Child development, services; Aging, centers & services; Women, centers & services; Minorities/immigrants, centers & services; Homeless, human services; Community development; Minorities; Aging; Women; Homeless.
Types of support: General/operating support, capital campaigns, endowment funds, employee volunteer services, employee matching gifts.
Limitations: Giving primarily in the St. Paul-Minneapolis area in MN; support also in Garland, TX, Joliet, Il, Woodbridge, NJ, Beloit, WI, and Atlanta, GA. No support for sectarian or denominational religious organizations unless funds are to be used in direct interest of the whole community, political or lobbying organizations, or industry, trade or professional association memberships. No grants to individuals, or for fundraisers, loans, investments, luncheons, ticket purchases, or advertisements.
Publications: Application guidelines.
Application information:
Initial approach: Letter
Deadline(s): July 1
Number of staff: 1 full-time professional; 1 part-time support.

495
General Mills Foundation

P.O. Box 1113
Minneapolis 55440 (612) 540-7891
Contact: Reatha Clark King, Pres. and Exec. Dir.
FAX: (612) 540-4925; Internet and E-mail: mills999@mail.genmills.com

Incorporated in 1954 in MN.
Donor(s): General Mills, Inc.
Foundation type: Company-sponsored
Financial data (yr. ended 05/31/95): Assets, $54,310,223 (M); gifts received, $9,000,000; expenditures, $16,289,017; qualifying distributions, $16,098,887, including $15,147,285 for 700 grants (high: $1,070,217; average: $10,000-$100,000) and $951,602 for 2,031 employee matching gifts.
Purpose and activities: Grants for higher and secondary education, social services, United Ways, community funds, health, and civic and cultural activities.
Fields of interest: Media/communications; Museums; Performing arts; Dance; Theater; Music; Humanities; Arts/cultural programs; Early childhood education; Child development, education; Elementary school/education; Secondary school/education; Higher education; Adult/continuing education; Adult education—literacy & basic skills; Libraries/library science; Reading; Education; Hospitals (general); Health care; Substance abuse, services; Cancer; AIDS; Alcoholism; Health organizations; Cancer research; AIDS research; Legal services; Crime/law enforcement; Employment; Food services; Nutrition; Housing/shelter, development; Youth development, services; Human services; Youth, services; Child development, services; Family services; Hospices; Aging, centers & services; Women, centers & services; Minorities/immigrants, centers & services; Homeless, human services; Race/intergroup relations; Urban/community development; Community development; Voluntarism promotion; Federated giving programs; Leadership development; Minorities; Native Americans; Disabled; Aging; Women; Economically disadvantaged; Homeless.
Types of support: General/operating support, capital campaigns, program development, conferences/seminars, scholarship funds, employee matching gifts, employee-related scholarships, in-kind gifts, matching funds.
Limitations: Giving primarily in areas of major parent company operations. No support for religious purposes, recreation, or national or local campaigns to eliminate or control specific diseases. No grants to individuals, or, generally, for endowments, research, publications, films, advertising, athletic events, testimonial dinners, workshops, symposia, travel, fundraising events, or deficit financing; no loans.
Publications: Corporate giving report (including application guidelines), informational brochure, application guidelines, annual report.
Application information: Application form is available from the foundation office but is not required. Preliminary telephone calls or personal visits discouraged. Application form not required.
Initial approach: Proposal with brief cover letter
Copies of proposal: 1
Deadline(s): None
Board meeting date(s): 4 times a year and as required
Final notification: 8 weeks
Officers and Trustees:* S.W. Sanger, Chair.; Reatha Clark King,* Pres. and Exec. Dir.; David A. Nasley, V.P.; A.P. Sullivan, Jr., Secy.; David B. Van Benschoten, Treas.; Leslie M. Frecon, Charles W. Gaillard, Michael A. Peel.
Staff: Suzanne E. Fuller-Terrill, Sr. Prog. Officer and Assoc. Dir.
Number of staff: 2 full-time professional; 3 full-time support.
EIN: 416018495
Grants for Aging:
Big Brothers/Big Sisters of Greater Tri-Cities, Johnson City, TN, $40,000. For intergenerational mentoring program. 95.
Birth, Education, Training, Acceptance (BETA), Orlando, FL, $27,500. For home visits program. 95.
Claretian Associates Neighborhood Development Office, Chicago, IL, $10,000. To establish Villa Guadalupe Social Service program. 95.
National Retiree Volunteer Coalition, Minneapolis, MN, $10,000. For operating support. 95.
Powderhorn Community Council, Minneapolis, MN, $20,000. For Shared Living Residency project. 95.
Sabathani Community Center, Minneapolis, MN, $20,000. For senior citizens and youth programs. 95.
Seminole County Better Living for Seniors, Longwood, FL, $10,000. For meals for rural elderly. 95.
Seniors First, Orlando, FL, $15,000. For operating support. 95.
Store to Door, Saint Paul, MN, $10,000. For operating support. 95.

496
Hanna R. Kristianson Trust

211 South Newton
Albert Lea 56007
Application address: Richard J. Haug, Trustee, Clarks Grove, MN 56016; Tel.: (507) 256-4415

Foundation type: Operating
Financial data (yr. ended 12/31/94): Assets, $118,551 (M); expenditures, $11,729; qualifying distributions, $10,420, including $5,184 for 13 grants to individuals (high: $1,166; low: $19).
Purpose and activities: Grants to residents of Freeborn County, MN, who are over 50 years of age.
Fields of interest: Aging.
Types of support: Grants to individuals.
Limitations: Giving limited to residents of Freeborn County, MN.
Application information: Application form not required.
Deadline(s): None
Trustees: Richard J. Haug, Ila Hibbard, Robert Pleiss.
EIN: 416209010

497
Mardag Foundation

600 Norwest Ctr.
St. Paul 55101 (612) 224-5463
Contact: Paul A. Verret, Secy.

Established in 1969 in MN.
Donor(s): Agnes E. Ober.‡
Financial data (yr. ended 12/31/94): Assets, $31,076,762 (M); expenditures, $1,508,813; qualifying distributions, $1,147,462, including $1,147,462 for 70 grants (high: $105,000; low: $3,500; average: $3,000-$100,000).
Purpose and activities: The foundation is committed to enhancing and improving the

quality of life in Minnesota. Their focus is on children, the elderly and other at-risk populations, education, and the arts. Where appropriate, the foundation will be an active participant with others in grantmaking programs and will be proactive in addressing issues as well as responsive to applications for grants.
Fields of interest: Arts/cultural programs; Child development, education; Elementary school/education; Adult education—literacy & basic skills; Reading; Education; Natural resource conservation & protection; Human services; Youth, services; Child development, services; Aging, centers & services; Minorities; Aging.
Types of support: General/operating support, program development, seed money, matching funds.
Limitations: Giving limited to MN. No support for sectarian religious programs or federated campaigns. No grants to individuals, or for annual campaigns, endowment funds, conservation, medical research, scholarships, fellowships, or generally for continuing support.
Publications: Annual report, 990-PF, program policy statement, application guidelines.
Application information: Application form not required.
Initial approach: Letter or proposal
Copies of proposal: 1
Deadline(s): None
Board meeting date(s): Apr., Aug., and Nov.
Final notification: 90 days
Officers and Directors:* Thomas G. Mairs,* Pres.; Gayle M. Ober, V.P.; Paul A. Verret, Secy.; Richard B. Ober, Treas.; James E. Davidson, Dolores Henderson, Katherine V. Lilly, Timothy M. Ober.
Number of staff: None.
EIN: 411698990
Grants for Aging:
Alzheimers Disease and Related Disorders Association, Metro Chapter, Bloomington, MN, $10,000. Toward expansion of Family Service Project to Saint Paul area. 94.
Faribault Area Senior Citizens, Faribault, MN, $20,000. Toward kitchen equipment. 94.
Mankato State University, Mankato, MN, $12,100. Toward Minnesota Area Geriatric Education Center of Southern Minnesota. 94.
North End South Como Block Nurse Program, Saint Paul, MN, $10,000. Toward volunteer nursing services. 94.
Presbyterian Homes, Arden Hills, MN, $25,000. Toward renovation of Lakeview Residence. 94.

498
Medtronic Corporate Giving Program
7000 Central Ave., N.E.
Minneapolis 55432 (612) 574-4000
Contact: Penny Hunt, Dir., Community Affairs and Fdn.
Toll-free number: (800) 328-2518. Additional addresses: Metronic Cardiopulmonary Div., 4633 East LaPalma Ave., Anaheim, CA 92807; Tel.: (714) 779-3700; Medtronic Electromedics and HemoTec, 18501 East Plaza Dr., Parker, CO 80134; Tel.: (303) 840-4000; Medtronic Heart Valve Div., 18011 South Mitchell, Irvine, CA 92714; Tel.: (619) 474-3943; Medtronic Interventional Vascular, 9410 Carroll Park Dr., San Diego, CA 92121; Tel.: (619) 458-6400; Metronic Interventional Vascular, 37A Cherry Hill Dr., Danvers, MA 01923; Tel. (508) 777-0042; Medtronic Micro-Rel, Inc., 2343 West Tenth Place, Tempe, AZ 85281; (602) 968-6411; Medtronic Med Rel, Inc., P.O. Box 8687, Humacao, PR 00661; Tel.: (809) 852-0276; Medtronic Puerto Rico, Inc., Carretera 149 KM 56.3, Call Box 6001, Villalba, PR 00766; Tel.: (809) 847-3500; Medtronic Milaca, Inc., 900 Sixth Ave., NE, Milaca, MN 56353; Tel.: (320) 983-2531

Financial data (yr. ended 04/30/94): Total giving, $5,058,000, including $358,000 for grants (high: $10,000; low: $250; average: $500) and $4,700,000 for in-kind gifts.
Purpose and activities: "Medtronic believes in sharing its success in business with the communities in which we reside. Over the years we have learned that our operations flourish in healthy and vibrant communities. That's one reason we commit more than two percent of our U.S. taxable income to results-oriented community programs. We also have come to realize that successful communities would not be possible without the active participation of our employees, and we encourage employee involvement in community affairs programs." In 1990 the company began developing a long-range plan for the community affairs program which includes cash donations, employee involvement in volunteer activities, special community projects, and product and equipment donations. Medtronic also helps its communities by utilizing minority vendors and participates in the Minority Purchasing Council. The United Way is supported by company and employee contributions. In all its giving, the company stresses programs that benefit people of color and economically disadvantaged people and that use older adults as resources. Generally 90 percent of cash donations stem from Medtronic Foundation and 10 percent from the company.
Fields of interest: Education; Health care; Health organizations; Human services; Aging, centers & services; Minorities/immigrants, centers & services; Community development; Minorities; Aging; Economically disadvantaged.
Types of support: Employee volunteer services, donated equipment, donated products.
Limitations: Giving limited to Medtronic communities. Generally no support for programs operated by a single hospital, or lobbying, political, or religious activities, or fraternal organizations. Generally no grants for endowment campaigns, fundraising, programs requesting multi-year commitments, or for clinics, research, or social events.
Application information: In Minneapolis/St. Paul, write to headquarters; requests from other areas should be directed to the local facility's manager who after review will forward them to headquarters. Decision making committees are comprised of 9 board members and other company and community representatives.
Initial approach: Letter
Final notification: 60 days
Number of staff: 1 full-time professional; 2 part-time professional; 1 full-time support.

499
The Medtronic Foundation
7000 Central Ave., N.E.
Minneapolis 55432 (612) 574-3024
Contact: Penny Hunt, Dir.

Established in 1979 in MN.
Donor(s): Medtronic, Inc.
Foundation type: Company-sponsored
Financial data (yr. ended 04/30/95): Assets, $1,224,093 (M); gifts received, $3,900,000; expenditures, $3,705,469; qualifying distributions, $3,207,728, including $2,954,822 for 240 grants (high: $422,000; low: $50; average: $1,000-$20,000) and $231,995 for employee matching gifts.
Purpose and activities: Priority given to programs for people of color, the economically disadvantaged, or projects that use older adults as resources.
Fields of interest: Arts/cultural programs; Elementary school/education; Secondary school/education; Higher education; Education; Health care; Health associations; Health organizations; Human services; Voluntarism promotion; Federated giving programs; Science; Biological sciences; Minorities; Aging; Economically disadvantaged; Canada; Europe; Africa; Asia; Middle East.
Types of support: General/operating support, continuing support, annual campaigns, program development, seed money, scholarship funds, employee matching gifts.
Limitations: Giving primarily in areas of company operations, including Phoenix and Tempe, AZ; Parker, CO; the Twin Cities-Seven County metro, MN, area; Anaheim, Irvine, and San Diego, CA; Danvers, MA; Grand Rapids, MI; and Humacao and Villalba, PR, or to national organizations having an effect on these areas; international giving in Medtronic communities. Generally no support for primarily social organizations, religious, political, or fraternal activities, health research, or treatment or substance abuse programs. No grants to individuals, or for deficit financing, research, travel, fundraising events, advertising, conferences, or multiple-year commitments; grants seldom for capital or endowment funds.
Publications: Corporate giving report (including application guidelines), grants list.
Application information: Requests from the Twin Cities to be sent to MN address; requests from other Medtronic communities to be sent to local manager. Application form required.
Initial approach: Proposal with letter
Copies of proposal: 1
Deadline(s): Feb. 15, Apr. 15, July 15, and Oct. 15
Board meeting date(s): June, Sept., Dec., and Apr.
Final notification: At least 60 days

Officers and Directors:* Janet S. Fiola,* Chair.; Art Collins, Vice-Chair.; Jackie Eastwood, Secy.; Tom Rooney, Treas.; Walter Cuevas, Mike Kallok, Bonnie Labosky, Ray Lavoie, John Meslow, Stan Myrum, Marcea Staten, Steve Tranter.
Staff: Penny Hunt, Dir., Community Affairs; Kay O'Keefe, Consultant, STAR Program; Darralu Lindholm, Consultant, Community Affairs.
Number of staff: 1 full-time professional; 1 full-time support.
EIN: 411306950
Grants for Aging:
Anoka County Community Health and Human Services Department, Anoka, MN, $16,500. For Anoka County Prenatal Abuse Project and health promotion for older adults. 95.
Cooperative Older Adult Ministry (COAM), Minneapolis, MN, $10,000. For AGEWELL program for older adults. 95.
Dakota Area Resources and Transportation for Seniors (DARTS), West Saint Paul, MN, $25,000. For community health care project. 95.
Good Neighbor Foundation, Saint Paul, MN, $10,000. For Health Promotion in the Streets project. 95.
Living at Home Block Nurse Program, Saint Paul, MN, $24,000. For program support. 95.
Minnesota Senior Federation, Saint Paul, MN, $15,000. For Senior Partners Care program and Discovery Fest '94. 95.
Saint Olaf Residence, Minneapolis, MN, $10,000. For start-up support for adult day care program. 95.
Senior Resources, Minneapolis, MN, $10,000. For Anoka County Senior Linkage Line and TeleFriends Program. 95.
YWCA of Minneapolis, Minneapolis, MN, $14,000. For Wellness Plus seniors' program. 95.

500
The Minneapolis Foundation

A200 Foshay Tower
821 Marquette Ave. South
Minneapolis 55402 (612) 339-7343
Contact: Emmett D. Carson, Pres.
Application address for the Minnesota Nonprofits Assistance Fund: Susan Kenny Stevens, Administrator, Hamline Park Plaza, 570 Asbury St., Suite 207, St. Paul, MN 55104; FAX: (612) 672-3846

Incorporated in 1915 in MN.
Foundation type: Community
Financial data (yr. ended 03/31/95): Assets, $148,734,675 (M); gifts received, $7,007,253; expenditures, $12,290,233, including $8,622,383 for 365 grants (high: $203,500; low: $185; average: $7,500-$35,000).
Purpose and activities: The foundation believes that the well-being of each citizen is connected to that of every other and that the vitality of any community is determined by the quality of those relationships. With this principle in mind, the foundation's purpose is to join with others to strengthen the community, in measurable and sustainable ways, for the benefit of all citizens, especially those who are disadvantaged. The foundation is committed to be an effective resource developer and a responsible steward of those resources, an active grantmaker and convener addressing crucial community needs, and a constructive catalyst changing systems to serve people better.
Fields of interest: Early childhood education; Child development, education; Education; Health care; Domestic violence prevention; Human services; Children & youth, services; Youth, services; Child development, services; Family services; Women, centers & services; Civil rights, immigrants; Civil rights, minorities; Civil rights, disabled; Civil rights, women; Civil rights, aging; Civil rights, gays/lesbians; Race/intergroup relations; Civil rights; Community development; Public policy, research; Minorities; Asians/Pacific Islanders; African Americans; Latinos; Native Americans; Disabled; Aging; Women; People with AIDS (PWAs); Gays/lesbians; Immigrants/refugees; Economically disadvantaged; Homeless.
Types of support: General/operating support, continuing support, building/renovation, equipment, emergency funds, program development, seed money, technical assistance, program-related investments/loans.
Limitations: Giving primarily in MN, with emphasis on the Minneapolis-St. Paul, seven-county metropolitan area. No support for national campaigns, religious organizations for religious purposes, veterans' or fraternal organizations, or organizations within umbrella organizations. No grants to individuals, or for annual campaigns, deficit financing, building or endowment funds, land acquisition, matching gifts, scholarships, fellowships, research, publications, conferences, courtesy advertising, benefit tickets, telephone solicitations, or memberships.
Publications: Annual report, newsletter, application guidelines, informational brochure (including application guidelines).
Application information: Application form required.
Initial approach: Applicant should request guidelines for the appropriate fund
Copies of proposal: 1
Deadline(s): Applicant should request guidelines for the appropriate fund Mar. 15 and Sept. 15
Board meeting date(s): Quarterly; distribution committee meets 4 times a year
Final notification: Approximately 4 months after deadlines
Officers and Trustees:* Conley Brooks, Jr.,* Chair.; Michele Keith,* Vice-Chair.; Emmett D. Carson, Pres. and C.E.O.; Stuart Appelbaum, V.P., Development; George Garnett, V.P., Programs; Flo Wiger,* Secy.; Anthony Genia, Sr.,* Treas.; and 29 additional trustees.
Trustee Banks: First Bank, N.A., Norwest Bank Minnesota, N.A.
Staff: Genie Dixon, Prog. Officer; Ronald J. Hick, Prog. Officer; Karen Kelley-Ariwoola, Prog. Officer; Brian Malloy, Prog. Officer.
Number of staff: 13 full-time professional; 7 full-time support.
EIN: 416029402
Grants for Aging:
Episcopal Community Services, Minneapolis, MN, $10,000. For development of parenting classes, respite care and mentoring connections for participants in Parents Anonymous programs. 95.
Minnesota Senior Federation, Saint Paul, MN, $15,000. For operating support for senior health programs. 95.
Powderhorn Community Council, Minneapolis, MN, $30,000. For capital support for shared living residence for low-income senior citizens. 95.
Saint Olaf Residence, Minneapolis, MN, $30,000. For capital support for equipment and van for adult day care center. 95.
Walker Cityview, Minneapolis, MN, $19,300. For capital support for renovation of fourth floor of facility. 95.
West Suburban Adult Day Center, Open Circle, Minneapolis, MN, $25,000. For capital support to purchase and renovate program space. 95.

501
Minnesota Mining and Manufacturing Foundation, Inc.

(also known as 3M Foundation, Inc.)
3M Center, Bldg. 591-30-02
St. Paul 55144-1000
Contact: Richard E. Hanson, V.P.
FAX: (612) 737-3061

Incorporated in 1953 in MN.
Donor(s): Minnesota Mining and Manufacturing Co.
Foundation type: Company-sponsored
Financial data (yr. ended 12/31/94): Assets, $13,755,213 (M); gifts received, $10,366,500; expenditures, $8,993,704; qualifying distributions, $8,420,788, including $7,274,176 for 377 grants (high: $1,485,786; low: $75; average: $500-$10,000) and $1,146,612 for employee matching gifts.
Purpose and activities: Primary areas of interest include community funds, higher and vocational education, educational programs for minorities, the performing arts, drug abuse programs, and the elderly. Support also for human services, including programs for alcohol abuse, the disabled and disadvantaged, women and youth, rehabilitation, civic involvement, and preventive health care.
Fields of interest: Performing arts; Dance; Theater; Arts/cultural programs; Early childhood education; Child development, education; Vocational education; Higher education; Business school/education; Engineering school/education; Education; Natural resource conservation & protection; Environment; Dental care; Medical care, rehabilitation; Health care; Substance abuse, services; Cancer; Heart/circulatory disease; Alcoholism; Health organizations; Medical research; Cancer research; Heart/circulatory research; Crime/law enforcement; Food services; Human services; Youth, services; Child development, services; Aging, centers & services; Women, centers & services; Minorities/immigrants, centers & services; Homeless, human services; Business & industry; Community development; Federated giving programs; Physical/earth sciences; Chemistry; Computer science; Engineering; Biological sciences; Economics; Government/public administration; Minorities; Native Americans; Disabled; Aging; Women; Homeless.

Types of support: General/operating support, annual campaigns, emergency funds, program development, fellowships, internships, scholarship funds, research, employee matching gifts, employee-related scholarships, in-kind gifts, matching funds.
Limitations: Giving primarily in the 127 locations where the company has facilities in AL, CA, GA, IL, IN, IA, KY, MA, MI, MN, MS, MO, NE, NJ, NC, ND, OH, OK, OR, PA, SC, SD, TX, UT, VA, WA, WV, and WI. No support for projects of specific religious denominations or sects, athletic events, or conduit agencies. No grants to individuals, or for capital or endowment funds, loans or investments, advocacy and lobbying efforts, fundraising events and associated advertising, travel, publications unrelated to foundation-funded projects, seed money, purchase of equipment not manufacutured by 3M, deficit financing, or conferences.
Publications: Corporate giving report (including application guidelines), informational brochure (including application guidelines).
Application information: Application form required.
Initial approach: Letter or personal visit by appointment
Copies of proposal: 1
Deadline(s): At least 8 weeks prior to month in which board meets
Board meeting date(s): Mar., Aug., and Dec.
Final notification: 3 months
Officers and Directors:* Richard A. Lidstad,* Pres.; Richard E. Hanson,* V.P.; Cynthia F. Kleven, Secy.; Janet L. Yeomans, Treas.; J. Marc Adam, Ronald O. Baukol, William E. Coyne, Livio D. DeSimone, Richard E. Hanson, Barbara W. Kaufmann, William J. McLellan, W. George Meredith, Ronald A. Mitsch, Raymond C. Richelsen, L. James Schoenwetter, John J. Ursu.
Number of staff: None.
EIN: 416038262
Grants for Aging:
Dakota Area Resources and Transportation for Seniors (DARTS), West Saint Paul, MN, $10,000. 94.
Meals on Wheels of Saint Paul, Saint Paul, MN, $13,582. 94.

502
Ordean Foundation
501 Ordean Bldg.
424 West Superior St.
Duluth 55802 (218) 726-4785
Contact: Stephen A. Mangan, Exec. Dir.

Incorporated in 1933 in MN.
Donor(s): Albert L. Ordean,‡ Louise Ordean.‡
Financial data (yr. ended 12/31/95): Assets, $31,740,724 (M); expenditures, $1,659,071; qualifying distributions, $1,172,740, including $1,132,623 for grants (high: $176,800; average: $178-$145,800) and $13,967 for foundation-administered programs.
Purpose and activities: To administer and furnish relief and charity for the local poor, including the aged and homeless; to make grants to local organizations performing services or providing facilities in certain areas of health and youth activities, including rehabilitation, drug and alcohol and juvenile delinquency programs, and mental illness institutions.
Fields of interest: Education; Medical care, rehabilitation; Health care; Substance abuse, services; Mental health/crisis services; Alcoholism; Health organizations; Delinquency prevention/services; Food services; Housing/shelter, development; Human services; Youth, services; Family services; Aging, centers & services; Homeless, human services; Disabled; Aging; Economically disadvantaged; Homeless.
Types of support: General/operating support, continuing support, building/renovation, equipment, program development, scholarship funds, technical assistance, program-related investments/loans, matching funds.
Limitations: Giving limited to Duluth and contiguous cities and townships in St. Louis County, MN. No support for direct religious purposes. No grants to individuals (directly), or for endowment funds, travel, conferences, seminars or workshops, benefits, dinners, research, including biomedical research, deficit financing, national fundraising campaigns, or to supplant government funding.
Publications: Annual report (including application guidelines), grants list, 990-PF.
Application information: Accepts Minnesota Common Grant Application Form. Application form not required.
Initial approach: Telephone, letter, or proposal
Copies of proposal: 12
Deadline(s): 15th of each month
Board meeting date(s): 3rd Wednesday of each month
Final notification: Within 1 day of board meeting
Officers and Directors:* Charles M. Bell,* Pres.; Rita D. Hutchens,* V.P.; James F. Westman,* Secy.; Charles E. House,* Treas.; Stephen A. Mangan, Exec. Dir.; James N. Abelsen, Patrick D. Francisco, Bonita T. Nelson, Jon L. Welles, Marjorie T. Whitney.
Staff: Joe E. Everett, Prog. Dir.; Donna M. Morris, Office Mgr.
Number of staff: 2 full-time professional; 2 part-time support.
EIN: 410711611

503
Otter Tail Power Company Corporate Giving Program
215 South Cascade St.
Fergus Falls 56537 (218) 739-8200
Contact: John MacFarlane, Pres. and C.E.O.

Financial data (yr. ended 12/31/94): Total giving, $400,000, including $320,000 for grants, $40,000 for employee matching gifts and $40,000 for in-kind gifts.
Purpose and activities: Giving for arts and culture; the elderly; child welfare; community development; the disadvantaged; the environment; the handicapped; mental health; volunteerism; recreation; minorities; health, including cancer; welfare; education, including secondary and business; and civic activities. Also gives through in-kind donations.
Fields of interest: Visual arts; Museums; Performing arts; Music; Historic preservation/historical societies; Arts/cultural programs; Education, fund raising; Child development, education; Secondary school/education; Business school/education; Libraries/library science; Education; Environment; Hospitals (general); Health care; Mental health/crisis services; Cancer; Heart/circulatory disease; Health organizations; Cancer research; Heart/circulatory research; Crime/law enforcement; Recreation; Youth development, services; Human services; Children & youth, services; Child development, services; Hospices; Aging, centers & services; Minorities/immigrants, centers & services; Community development; Voluntarism promotion; Government/public administration; Leadership development; Minorities; Disabled; Aging; Economically disadvantaged; General charitable giving.
Types of support: Continuing support, annual campaigns, building/renovation, equipment, endowment funds, conferences/seminars, employee volunteer services, use of facilities, sponsorships, employee matching gifts, donated equipment, in-kind gifts, matching funds.
Limitations: Giving primarily in home and division offices in MN, ND, and SD.
Application information: The office of the C.E.O. handles giving. Application form not required.
Initial approach: Letter
Final notification: 1 to 4 weeks
Number of staff: None.

504
The Jay and Rose Phillips Family Foundation
(Formerly The Phillips Foundation)
Ten 2nd St., N.E., No. 200
Minneapolis 55413 (612) 623-1654
Contact: Patricia A. Cummings, Exec. Dir.

Incorporated in 1944 in MN.
Donor(s): Jay Phillips,‡ and members of the Phillips family.
Financial data (yr. ended 12/31/94): Assets, $91,595,712 (M); gifts received, $243,024; expenditures, $4,706,572; qualifying distributions, $4,061,371, including $3,690,111 for 310 grants (high: $200,000; low: $50; average: $1,000-$10,000).
Purpose and activities: Giving primarily for health, services for the handicapped, Jewish religious organizations and welfare funds, education, and social services.
Fields of interest: Arts/cultural programs; Higher education; Medical school/education; Education; Hospitals (general); Health care; Health organizations; Domestic violence prevention; Human services; Family services; Civil rights, immigrants; Civil rights, minorities; Civil rights, disabled; Civil rights, women; Civil rights, aging; Civil rights, gays/lesbians; Reproductive rights; Jewish federated giving programs; Jewish agencies & temples; Asians/Pacific Islanders; African Americans; Latinos; Native Americans; Disabled; Aging; Women; People with AIDS (PWAs); Gays/lesbians; Immigrants/refugees; Economically disadvantaged; Homeless.
Types of support: General/operating support, annual campaigns, capital campaigns, building/renovation, equipment, program

development, seed money, scholarship funds, research.
Limitations: Giving primarily in MN. No support for religious organizations for sectarian purposes. No grants to individuals, or for endowment funds.
Publications: Annual report, application guidelines.
Application information: Application form not required.
Initial approach: Letter or telephone
Copies of proposal: 1
Deadline(s): None
Board meeting date(s): As required
Final notification: 90 to 120 days
Officers and Trustees:* Morton B. Phillips,* Co-Chair.; Rose Phillips,* Co-Chair.; Patricia A. Cummings, Exec. Dir.; Erik P. Bernstein, Paula Bernstein, William Bernstein, Jack I. Levin, John P. Levin, Suzan Levin, Edda J. Phillips, Pauline Phillips.
Staff: Sharon L. Burt, Grants Administrator.
Number of staff: 2 full-time professional; 1 full-time support.
EIN: 416019578
Grants for Aging:
Alzheimers Disease and Related Disorders Association, Los Angeles, CA, $10,000. For general operating support. 94.
Beth Israel at Shalom Park, Aurora, CO, $20,000. For Urinary Incontinence Retraining Program and psychological counseling service. 94.
Jewish Community Center, Denver, CO, $50,000. For Jay and Rose Phillips Senior Social Hall. 94.
Jewish Community Center, Denver, CO, $26,330. For senior adult department. 94.
Jewish Family Service of Colorado, Denver, CO, $140,073. For older adults services department. 94.
Sholom Foundation, Saint Paul, MN, $100,000. For Sholom Home West Phillips Endowment. 94.
Sholom Foundation, Saint Paul, MN, $18,128. For Sholom Home West general operating support. 94.
Sholom Home, Saint Paul, MN, $63,327. For Sholom Home Auxiliary. 94.

505
Margaret Rivers Fund
c/o First National Bank
P.O. Box 197
Stillwater 55082
Contact: David F. Pohl, Pres.

Incorporated in 1948 in MN.
Donor(s): Robert E. Slaughter.‡
Financial data (yr. ended 12/31/94): Assets, $23,475,464 (M); gifts received, $2,405,649; expenditures, $1,231,609; qualifying distributions, $1,139,082, including $1,108,856 for 207 grants (high: $80,000; low: $250).
Purpose and activities: Grants primarily for hospitals, church support, youth agencies, aid to the handicapped, and care of the aged; support also for cultural programs and conservation.
Fields of interest: Arts/cultural programs; Natural resource conservation & protection; Hospitals (general); Youth, services; Aging, centers & services; Christian agencies & churches; Disabled; Aging.
Types of support: General/operating support.
Limitations: Giving primarily in MN. No grants to individuals.
Application information: Application form not required.
Initial approach: Letter
Deadline(s): None
Board meeting date(s): Monthly
Officers and Trustees:* David F. Pohl,* Pres. and Treas.; Robert G. Briggs,* V.P.; Lawrence Severson, Secy.
EIN: 416017102

506
Rochester Area Foundation
1815 N.W. 14th St.
Rochester 55901 (507) 282-0203
Contact: Steve Thornton, Exec. Dir.
FAX: (507) 282-4938

Established in 1944 in MN by resolution of trust.
Foundation type: Community
Financial data (yr. ended 12/31/95): Assets, $4,807,516 (M); gifts received, $583,107; expenditures, $288,615, including $145,730 for 19 grants (high: $25,000; low: $110).
Purpose and activities: To help launch new projects which represent innovative approaches to community needs, support special purposes of established organizations, promote volunteer and citizen involvement in the community, respond to current human needs in community, and support projects without other sources of support; giving in areas of health, education, human services, and development and assistance of community affairs.
Fields of interest: Arts/cultural programs; Child development, education; Higher education; Education; Environment; Housing/shelter, development; Human services; Child development, services; Aging, centers & services; Minorities/immigrants, centers & services; Civil rights; Community development; Voluntarism promotion; Government/public administration; Public affairs; Minorities; Disabled; Aging.
Types of support: Emergency funds, seed money, technical assistance, consulting services, program-related investments/loans, matching funds.
Limitations: Giving limited to Olmsted County, MN. No support for religious organizations for sectarian purposes. No grants to individuals, or for endowment funds, annual campaigns, operating budgets, continuing support, land acquisition, deficit financing, scholarships, fellowships, or research.
Publications: Annual report, application guidelines, newsletter, informational brochure (including application guidelines).
Application information: Application form required.
Initial approach: Pre-application form
Copies of proposal: 1
Deadline(s): Jan. 1, May 1, and Sept. 1
Board meeting date(s): Feb., Apr., May, Aug., Sept., Oct., Nov., and Dec.
Final notification: 4 months
Officers and Trustees:* Jane Campion,* Chair.; Dan Berndt, Vice-Chair.; Paul Olander,* Vice-Chair.; David Griffin,* Secy.; Lance Davenport,* Treas.; Michael Bue, Dorothy Callahan, Alan De Boer, Rev. Lester J. Horntvedt, Ronald Seeger, Sheryl Tasher, Alan O. Tuntland, John Withers.
Number of staff: 1 full-time professional; 1 full-time support.
EIN: 416017740

507
The Simmet Foundation
1645 Red Rock Rd.
P.O. Box 288
Newport 55055 (612) 735-9660
Contact: Bob Simmet, Secy.

Established in 1989 in MN.
Donor(s): John P. Simmet, Nancy A. Simmet, Patricia M. Simmet, Peter C. Simmet, Robert P. Simmet, Christine A. Simmet, John L. Simmet.
Financial data (yr. ended 12/31/95): Assets, $206,000 (M); gifts received, $10,000; expenditures, $28,000; qualifying distributions, $28,000, including $28,000 for 14 grants (high: $5,000; low: $1,000; average: $1,000-$5,000).
Fields of interest: Education; Natural resource conservation & protection; Health care; Human services; Children & youth, services; Family services; Aging, centers & services; Women, centers & services; Disabled; Aging.
Types of support: General/operating support, equipment, emergency funds, program development, research.
Limitations: Giving primarily in MN, with emphasis on the metropolitan Twin Cities area and Crow Wing County.
Publications: Application guidelines.
Application information: Grants are for a 1-year period. Application form required.
Initial approach: Proposal
Copies of proposal: 1
Deadline(s): Oct. 1
Board meeting date(s): Oct. or Nov.
Final notification: Jan. of following year
Officers and Directors:* Margaret Simmet, Pres.; Joan M. Stewart,* V.P.; Robert P. Simmet,* Secy.; John P. Simmet,* Treas.; Susan M. Seiwart, Christine A. Simmet, Mary C. Simmet, Mary M. Simmet, Nancy A. Simmet, Patricia M. Simmet.
Number of staff: None.
EIN: 411643809

508
Southwest Minnesota Foundation
(Formerly Southwest Minnesota Initiative Fund)
P.O. Box 130
881 Prentice Ave.
Granite Falls 56241 (320) 564-3060
Additional tel.: (800) 594-9480; FAX: (320) 564-3391

Established in 1986 in MN.
Financial data (yr. ended 06/30/95): Assets, $16,704,810 (L); gifts received, $2,671,164; expenditures, $1,104,524, including $248,829 for grants and $1,672,550 for loans.
Purpose and activities: The mission of the fund is to serve the socio-economic needs of the territory through innovative programs. In concert with the people of the southwest community, the fund builds partnerships among people within and beyond the territory, nourishes strengths gained through experience,

and overcomes or diminishes barriers between people, and between people and opportunity. The fund's focus areas are (a) Business Finance, which promotes greater economic diversity and new wealth, (b) Community Cultural Alliance, which increases stability and expands investment in the community, (c) Strengthening the Family, which positively affects relationships of parents and children, and (d) the Paul and Alma Schwan Aging Trust Fund, which improves and enriches the lives of the area's aging population. The fund offers grants (not exceeding $20,000) and loans (not exceeding $100,000); both types of support may be used to fund up to 50 percent of a project's cost.
Fields of interest: Family services; Aging, centers & services; Race/intergroup relations; Economic development; Business & industry; Community development; Aging.
Types of support: General/operating support, continuing support, program development, conferences/seminars, technical assistance, program-related investments/loans, matching funds.
Limitations: Giving limited to Big Stone, Chippewa, Cottonwood, Jackson, Kandiyohi, Lac Qui Parle, Lincoln, Lyon, McLeod, Meeker, Murray, Nobles, Pipestone, Redwood, Renville, Rock, Swift, and Yellow Medicine counties in southwestern MN.
Publications: Annual report, newsletter, informational brochure (including application guidelines), application guidelines, program policy statement.
Application information: Application form required.
Initial approach: Letter of inquiry
Copies of proposal: 1
Deadline(s): 15th of preceding month
Board meeting date(s): 4th Wednesday of each month
Final notification: After Exec. Board meeting
Officers and Trustees:* Alicia Johnson,* Chair.; Joan Ratzloff, Vice-Chair.; Jim Bakken, Gary Becker, Connie Crowell, Larry Graf, Dennis Klute, Mr. Berdette Schoep, Elwood Throndrud.
Staff: Karen Nieuwbeerta, Admin. Assistant; Barb Carroll, C.F.O.; Becky Clayton, Business Finance Officer; Judy Larson, Aging Trust Fund Officer; Karen Jacobson, Strengthening the Family Officer; Kimberly Johnson, Business Finance Prog. Assistant; Brenda Arne, Grant Prog. Assistant.
Number of staff: 9 full-time professional.
EIN: 411555592

509
Alex and Mollie Tankenoff Foundation

(Formerly Alex G. Tankenoff Foundation)
1111 Third Ave. South, Suite 440
Minneapolis 55404-1003 (612) 371-0123
Contact: Gary L. Tankenoff, Trustee

Established in 1944.
Donor(s): Gary L. Tankenoff, James C. Tankenoff, Scott M. Tankenoff.
Financial data (yr. ended 12/31/94): Assets, $1,122,745 (M); expenditures, $59,347; qualifying distributions, $58,634, including $58,410 for 104 grants (high: $30,500; low: $10).
Fields of interest: Theater; Arts/cultural programs; Environment; Family planning; Health care; Mental health/crisis services; Cancer; Heart/circulatory disease; Health organizations; Cancer research; Heart/circulatory research; Gun control; Domestic violence prevention; Children & youth, services; Family services; Aging, centers & services; Minorities/immigrants, centers & services; Homeless, human services; Human rights (international); Race/intergroup relations; Reproductive rights; Civil rights; Jewish federated giving programs; Jewish agencies & temples; Minorities; Disabled; Aging; Economically disadvantaged; Homeless; General charitable giving; Israel.
Types of support: General/operating support, continuing support, annual campaigns, capital campaigns, building/renovation.
Limitations: Giving primarily in the Twin Cities, MN, area. No grants to individuals.
Application information: Application form required.
Trustees: Gary L. Tankenoff, James C. Tankenoff, Scott M. Tankenoff.
Number of staff: None.
EIN: 416032235
Grants for Aging:
Senior Resources, Minneapolis, MN, $1,000. 94.

510
James R. Thorpe Foundation

5201 Eden Circle, Suite 202
Minneapolis 55436 (612) 929-1093
Contact: Edith D. Thorpe, Pres., or Jane M. Stamstad, Exec. Dir.

Incorporated in 1974 in MN.
Donor(s): James R. Thorpe.‡
Financial data (yr. ended 11/30/95): Assets, $8,000,000 (M); expenditures, $467,800; qualifying distributions, $433,674, including $402,200 for 103 grants (high: $15,000; low: $1,000; average: $3,000-$5,000).
Purpose and activities: Primary areas of interest include the disadvantaged, youth, the elderly, education, and cultural programs. Giving for social service agencies and higher and secondary education; support also for community health care and AIDS services.
Fields of interest: Performing arts; Arts/cultural programs; Education; Environment; Health care; Mental health/crisis services; AIDS; Housing/shelter, development; Human services; Children & youth, services; Family services; Aging, centers & services; Homeless, human services; Disabled; Aging; Economically disadvantaged.
Types of support: General/operating support, capital campaigns, equipment, program development, internships, scholarship funds.
Limitations: Giving limited to Hennepin County, MN. No grants to individuals, or for continuing support, emergency or endowment funds, deficit financing, land acquisition, matching gifts, publications, seminars, benefits, or conferences; no loans.
Publications: Annual report.
Application information: Application form not required.
Initial approach: Telephone or letter of inquiry (no more than 8 pages)
Copies of proposal: 1
Deadline(s): Mar. 1 and Sept. 1
Board meeting date(s): May and Nov.
Final notification: 1 week
Officers and Directors:* Edith D. Thorpe,* Pres.; Leonard M. Addington,* V.P.; Mary C. Boos,* V.P.; Elizabeth A. Kelly,* V.P.; Samuel A. Cote,* Secy.; Samuel S. Thorpe III,* Treas.; Jane M. Stamstad, Exec. Dir.
Number of staff: 1 part-time professional.
EIN: 416175293

511
Wedum Foundation

6860 Flying Cloud Dr.
Eden Prairie 55344 (612) 944-5547
Contact: Mayo Johnson, Pres.

Established in 1959 in MN.
Donor(s): Maynard C. Wedum,‡ John A. Wedum.
Financial data (yr. ended 12/31/93): Assets, $6,249,158 (M); expenditures, $559,013; qualifying distributions, $299,685, including $247,527 for 12 grants (high: $160,000; low: $100) and $1,640 for 4 grants to individuals (high: $720; low: $200).
Fields of interest: Business school/education; Education; Wildlife preservation & protection; Health associations; Alcoholism; Human services; Youth, services; Aging, centers & services; Rural development; Community development; Voluntarism promotion; Computer science; Aging.
Types of support: Land acquisition, conferences/seminars, seed money, program-related investments/loans, scholarships—to individuals, matching funds.
Limitations: Giving primarily in the Alexandria, MN, area.
Publications: 990-PF.
Application information: Student aid support beyond existing programs available through local "Dollars for Scholars" units. Application form required.
Copies of proposal: 1
Deadline(s): None
Board meeting date(s): Fall
Final notification: Late fall
Officers: Mayo Johnson, Pres. and Treas.; John A. Wedum, V.P. and Managing Dir.; Gary Slette, V.P.; Mary Beth Wedum, Secy.
Number of staff: 1 part-time professional; 1 part-time support.
EIN: 416025661

512
Woman's Christian Association

10249 Yellow Circle Dr., Suite 101
Minnetonka 55343 (612) 932-9032
Contact: Karen Reamer

Established in 1866 in MN.
Financial data (yr. ended 12/31/94): Assets, $8,512,203 (M); gifts received, $2,113; expenditures, $493,078; qualifying distributions, $407,098, including $171,600 for 30 grants (high: $10,000; low: $2,000; average: $1,000-$12,000) and $104,576 for 1 foundation-administered program.

Purpose and activities: Primary area of interest is for programs helping women achieve or sustain self-sufficiency.
Fields of interest: Children & youth, services; Family services; Aging, centers & services; Human services; Women.
Types of support: General/operating support, capital campaigns, building/renovation, emergency funds, scholarship funds.
Limitations: Giving limited to MN. No support for private foundations, political or veterans' organizations, religious organizations for religious purposes, national medical associations, pro-life/pro-choice programs, or organizations affiliated with the foundation. No grants to individuals, or for annual fund drives for medical research, previously incurred deficits; no multi-year awards.
Publications: Application guidelines.
Application information: Application form required.
Initial approach: Letter, FAX, or telephone to request application form
Copies of proposal: 1
Deadline(s): May 15 and Nov. 15
Board meeting date(s): 1st Friday of each month
Final notification: 2 to 4 months following deadline dates
Officer and Director:* Marjorie Garwood,* Pres.
Number of staff: 1 full-time professional; 1 full-time support.
EIN: 410694712

MISSOURI

513
The Claudia Bloodworth Company
c/o Thomas Fineman
626 Cynthia St.
Poplar Bluff 63901-5010 (573) 686-3040
Contact: Diane Mitchell, Exec. Dir.

Established in 1991 in MO.
Donor(s): Linda Bloodworth-Thomason.
Foundation type: Operating
Financial data (yr. ended 12/31/93): Assets, $4,101,325 (M); gifts received, $4,542,421; expenditures, $175,455; qualifying distributions, $284,440.
Purpose and activities: Primarily awards scholarships to female students at Three Rivers Community College, Poplar Bluff, MO; support also for programs benefiting women, children and youth, and the elderly.
Fields of interest: Higher education; Youth development, services; Youth, services; Human services; Aging; Women.
Types of support: Scholarship funds, scholarships—to individuals.
Limitations: Giving limited to MO.
Application information: No grants paid in 1993.
Initial approach: Letter
Deadline(s): Mar. for scholarships
Officer: Mary Lou Brown, Exec. Dir.; Millicent Colingsworth, Exec. Dir.; Diane Mitchell, Exec. Dir.
EIN: 431574170

514
The Milford and Lee Bohm Charitable Foundation
7730 Carondelet, Suite 411
St. Louis 63105
Contact: Milford Bohm, Trustee, and Leona Bohm, Trustee

Established in 1989 in MO.
Donor(s): Milford Bohm, Leona Bohm.
Financial data (yr. ended 12/31/94): Assets, $2,953,281 (M); expenditures, $305,870; qualifying distributions, $284,642, including $284,642 for 37 grants (high: $102,000; low: $100).
Purpose and activities: Giving primarily to Jewish organizations, including welfare funds; support also for an affiliated fund for the elderly, a community fund, and cultural organizations.
Fields of interest: Arts/cultural programs; Human services; Aging, centers & services; Federated giving programs; Jewish federated giving programs; Jewish agencies & temples; Aging.
Limitations: Applications not accepted. Giving primarily in St. Louis, MO. No grants to individuals.
Publications: Annual report.
Trustees: Leona Bohm, Milford Bohm.
Number of staff: None.
EIN: 436355629

515
Ina Calkins Board
c/o Boatmen's First National Bank of Kansas City
P.O. Box 419038
Kansas City 64183 (816) 691-7481
Contact: David P. Ross, Sr. V.P.

Established in 1930 in MO.
Donor(s): Ina Calkins Trust.
Financial data (yr. ended 12/31/94): Assets, $141,940 (M); gifts received, $205,337; expenditures, $200,908; qualifying distributions, $198,101, including $172,331 for 8 grants (high: $120,234; low: $3,500) and $25,070 for 16 grants to individuals (high: $7,500; low: $240).
Purpose and activities: Emphasis on a social service agency; grants also for youth agencies and child welfare.
Fields of interest: Human services; Aging, centers & services; Aging; Economically disadvantaged.
Types of support: General/operating support, grants to individuals.
Limitations: Giving limited to Kansas City, MO.
Publications: 990-PF, program policy statement, application guidelines.
Application information:
Initial approach: Letter (no more than 3 pages)
Copies of proposal: 1
Deadline(s): Submit proposal 1 month before board meets
Board meeting date(s): Jan. 1, Apr. 1, July 1, and Oct. 11
Trustee: Boatmen's First National Bank of Kansas City.
Number of staff: 1 shared staff
EIN: 446088022
Grants for Aging:
Visiting Nurse Association of Greater Kansas City, Kansas City, MO, $120,234. For homemaker's program. 94.

516
Dunn Family Foundation
929 Holmes St.
Kansas City 64106-2682 (816) 474-8600
Contact: Ardyth L. Wendte, Secy.

Established in 1981 in MO.
Financial data (yr. ended 06/30/94): Assets, $5,117 (M); gifts received, $5,000; expenditures, $2,928; qualifying distributions, $2,925.
Fields of interest: Education; Health care; Health organizations; Aging, centers & services; Minorities/immigrants, centers & services; Community development; Roman Catholic agencies & churches; Minorities; Disabled; Aging.
Types of support: General/operating support, building/renovation, equipment.
Limitations: Giving limited to the greater metropolitan Kansas City, MO, area. No support for the visual or performing arts. No grants to individuals, or for research, endowments, travel, conferences, or telethons.
Publications: Informational brochure (including application guidelines).
Application information:
Initial approach: 1- to 2-page letter
Deadline(s): None
Board meeting date(s): Quarterly
Officers and Directors:* William H. Dunn,* Chair.; Stephen D. Dunn,* V.P. and Treas.; Terrence P. Dunn,* V.P.; William H. Dunn, Jr.,* V.P.; Ardyth L. Wendte, Secy.
EIN: 431244010

517
The Catherine Manley Gaylord Foundation
314 North Broadway, Rm. 1230
St. Louis 63102
Contact: Donald E. Fahey, Trustee

Trust established about 1959 in MO.
Donor(s): Catherine M. Gaylord.‡
Financial data (yr. ended 06/30/95): Assets, $5,163,819 (M); expenditures, $323,123; qualifying distributions, $305,282, including $209,723 for 68 grants (high: $39,405; low: $100; average: $3,000).
Purpose and activities: Giving primarily for Protestant and Roman Catholic church support, youth and child welfare agencies, civic affairs, social services, and music and art.
Fields of interest: Music; Arts/cultural programs; Higher education; Human services; Children & youth, services; Government/public administration; Protestant agencies & churches; Roman Catholic agencies & churches; Minorities; African Americans; Aging.
Types of support: General/operating support, continuing support, annual campaigns, building/renovation, equipment, emergency funds, program development, publication, seed money, matching funds.

Limitations: Applications not accepted. Giving primarily in the metropolitan St. Louis, MO, area. No grants to individuals; no loans.
Publications: Annual report, program policy statement, application guidelines.
Application information:
Board meeting date(s): Monthly
Trustees: Donald E. Fahey, Leigh Gerdine, Glenn K. Robbins II.
Number of staff: 1 full-time professional; 1 part-time support.
EIN: 436029174
Grants for Aging:
Franciscan Missionary Brothers of the Sacred Heart, Eureka, MO, $10,000. For nursing home programs deficit reduction. 95.
Franciscan Missionary Brothers of the Sacred Heart, Eureka, MO, $9,600. For Saint Josephs Hill Infirmary and Price Memorial Home. 94.

518
Carrie Elligson Gietner Foundation, Inc.
424 North Kirkwood Rd.
St. Louis 63122
Contact: Mrs. Althea Wilson, Secy.

Financial data (yr. ended 12/31/94): Assets, $2,022,711 (M); expenditures, $296,941; qualifying distributions, $281,800, including $281,800 for grants.
Purpose and activities: Giving primarily to provide for the elderly and infirmed.
Fields of interest: Hospitals (general); Nursing care; Human services; Aging, centers & services; Aging.
Types of support: General/operating support, scholarship funds.
Limitations: Giving primarily in St. Louis, MO. No grants to individuals.
Application information:
Initial approach: Letter
Deadline(s): None
Officers: Oliver Gutman, Pres.; George Von Hoffman, Jr., V.P.; Althea H. Wilson, Secy.
Directors: Herbert Buchman, Delbert Miller, Jr.
EIN: 431404189

519
Allen P. & Josephine B. Green Foundation
P.O. Box 523
Mexico 65265 (573) 581-5568
Contact: Walter G. Staley, Jr., Secy.-Treas.

Trust established in 1941 in MO.
Donor(s): Allen P. Green,‡ Josephine B. Green.‡
Financial data (yr. ended 12/31/94): Assets, $5,990,554 (M); expenditures, $408,447; qualifying distributions, $282,815, including $269,000 for 40 grants (high: $25,000; low: $1,000).
Purpose and activities: Giving for human services, with emphasis on child development and the family, women, and the elderly; health services, including rehabilitation programs for drug and alcohol abuse, cancer care, and nursing; arts and humanities, especially fine and performing arts groups and historic preservation; education, including early childhood, elementary and secondary, adult and vocational, theological and medical and other higher educational institutions, and libraries; community development and civic affairs; and environmental conservation and animal welfare.
Fields of interest: Performing arts; History & archaeology; Historic preservation/historical societies; Arts/cultural programs; Early childhood education; Child development, education; Elementary school/education; Secondary school/education; Vocational education; Higher education; Theological school/education; Adult/continuing education; Adult education—literacy & basic skills; Libraries/library science; Reading; Natural resource conservation & protection; Environment; Animal welfare; Medical care, rehabilitation; Nursing care; Health care; Mental health/crisis services; Eye disease; Health organizations; Eye research; Delinquency prevention/services; Nutrition; Human services; Children & youth, services; Youth, services; Child development, services; Hospices; Aging, centers & services; Women, centers & services; Aging; Women; Economically disadvantaged.
Types of support: Capital campaigns, building/renovation, equipment, endowment funds, emergency funds, program development, conferences/seminars, seed money, scholarship funds, matching funds.
Limitations: Giving primarily in the Mexico, MO, area; no giving outside the continental U.S. No grants to individuals, or for operating budgets; no loans.
Publications: Annual report.
Application information: Application form not required.
Initial approach: Letter
Copies of proposal: 1
Deadline(s): Apr. 1 or Oct. 1
Board meeting date(s): May and Nov.
Final notification: 1 month
Officers and Directors:* George C. Willson III,* Pres.; A.D. Bond III,* V.P.; Walter G. Staley, Jr.,* Secy.-Treas.; Christopher S. Bond, Robert R. Collins, Carl D. Fuemmeler, Martha S. Marks, James F. McHenry, Robert E. McIntosh, Nancy White, Robert A. Wood.
Number of staff: 1 part-time support.
EIN: 436030135
Grants for Aging:
Cardinal Ritter Institute, Adult Day Care Center, Saint Louis, MO, $20,000. For bus. 94.

520
Independence Community Foundation
Commerce Bank Bldg.
300 North Osage
Independence 64050 (816) 836-8189
Contact: Robert F. Glaser, Exec. Dir.

Community foundation incorporated in 1982 in MO; in 1994 merged with the Independence Regional Health Center Foundation.
Foundation type: Community
Financial data (yr. ended 01/31/96): Assets, $3,000,000 (M); gifts received, $629,002; expenditures, $369,388, including $162,000 for 30 grants (high: $15,000; low: $500; average: $500-$15,000).
Purpose and activities: Giving primarily for arts and cultural programs and historic preservation; higher, youth, and adult education; job training and employment; community development, infrastructure and housing; social services for the aged, at-risk youth, and families; violence prevention; community health programs; child care; transportation; and leadership development.
Fields of interest: Arts/cultural programs; Education; Health care; Crime/law enforcement; Employment; Human services; Youth, services; Family services; Community development; Aging.
Types of support: General/operating support, continuing support, program development, seed money, scholarship funds, research, in-kind gifts, matching funds.
Limitations: Giving limited to eastern Jackson County, MO. No support for religious purposes. No grants to individuals.
Publications: Annual report, informational brochure, application guidelines.
Application information: Application form not required.
Initial approach: Letter (no more than 2 pages) on letterhead
Copies of proposal: 9
Deadline(s): Contact foundation for specific dates
Board meeting date(s): Quarterly
Officers and Directors:* Robert W. Watkins, Ph.D.,* Chair.; Barbara J. Potts,* Vice-Chair.; Robert J. Reeds,* Secy.; R. Duane Holder,* Treas.; Robert F. Glaser, Exec. Dir.; Shirley Baker, James Barbour, Mike Chappelow, Paul Consiglio, Byron Constance, Karen Downey, Helen French, F.E. (Pat) Hansen, Rick Hemmingsen, Robert Henley, Paul Herzog, Thomas G. Holzbaur, Norman Humphrey, Jr., Ed Kerins, J. Scott King, C. William Kramer, K. Martin Kuny, Joseph Lammers, Allen L. Lefko, Michael Martin, George Matteson, William J. McDonald, Don Potter, Maurice Russell, Wallace B. Smith, Steve Sturm, Norman E. Swails, Beverly Norman Weishar, Paul Weston, Karen White, Terry C. Williams, D.D.S., Gerald E. Winship, Roger Yarrington, Ph.D.
Number of staff: 2 full-time professional; 1 part-time professional.
EIN: 431482136

521
The Leader Foundation
7711 Carondelet Ave., 10th Fl.
St. Louis 63105-3388
Contact: Edwin G. Shifrin, V.P.

Established in 1944.
Financial data (yr. ended 01/31/95): Assets, $2,743,601 (M); expenditures, $276,379; qualifying distributions, $254,876, including $87,253 for 9 grants (high: $17,920; low: $2,000) and $143,483 for 30 grants to individuals (high: $12,658; low: $114).
Purpose and activities: Giving only to needy ex-employees and their dependents of the Stix, Baer & Fuller Co. and to charitable organizations.
Fields of interest: Health care; Health associations; Family services; Aging, centers & services; Aging; Economically disadvantaged.
Types of support: Continuing support, program development, grants to individuals.

Limitations: Giving primarily in St. Louis, MO.
Publications: 990-PF.
Application information: Application form not required.
Initial approach: Letter
Copies of proposal: 1
Deadline(s): None
Board meeting date(s): May and Nov.
Officers and Directors:* Donald E. Ray,* Pres.; Edwin G. Shifrin,* V.P.; Steven M. Rafsky,* Secy.-Treas.; Philip Marlo, Patricia A. Reaves.
Number of staff: None.
EIN: 436036864
Grants for Aging:
Alzheimers Disease and Related Disorders Association, Saint Louis, MO, $14,000. 94.
Alzheimers Disease and Related Disorders Association, Saint Louis, MO, $10,000. 95.
Community Aging Corporation, $15,000. 94.
Elderly Services, $3,000. 94.
Gateway Older Adult Legal Services, Saint Louis, MO, $2,000. 95.

522
Stanley and Lucy Lopata Foundation
c/o Lopata, Hoffman, Flegel & Co.
500 Washington Ave., Suite 1204
St. Louis 63101
Contact: Monte Lopata, Trustee

Established in 1968.
Donor(s): Stanley Lopata, Lucy Lopata.
Financial data (yr. ended 12/31/93): Assets, $4,309,213 (M); gifts received, $197,716; expenditures, $262,969; qualifying distributions, $243,059, including $243,059 for grants.
Purpose and activities: Giving primarily for Jewish welfare funds and temple support; support also for cultural institutions, and a university and other educational institutions, including a science museum.
Fields of interest: Museums; Arts/cultural programs; Higher education; Education; Human services; Jewish federated giving programs; Jewish agencies & temples; Disabled; Aging; Homeless; General charitable giving.
Types of support: General/operating support, annual campaigns, capital campaigns, endowment funds, emergency funds, program development.
Limitations: Giving primarily in St. Louis, MO. No grants to individuals.
Application information: Application form not required.
Copies of proposal: 1
Board meeting date(s): June 15, Dec. 15, and as needed
Officer: Stanley Lopata, Mgr.
Trustees: Lucy Lopata, Monte L. Lopata.
Number of staff: None.
EIN: 436099972

523
Lutheran Charities Foundation of St. Louis
709 South Laclede Station Rd.
St. Louis 63119-4911 (314) 961-0344
Contact: Fred Bleeke, Pres.
FAX: (314) 968-5590

Established in 1985 in MO.
Financial data (yr. ended 12/31/95): Assets, $59,271,362 (M); expenditures, $4,379,725; qualifying distributions, $331,911.
Purpose and activities: The foundation provides indirect care to a wide range of people. Grants are awarded to congregations, agencies, and organizations that provide health and healing care of the total person (physical, intellectual, emotional, and spiritual), within the family, church, and community, to Lutherans and others in the St. Louis, MO, area. Specific areas of interest include youth and older adults, victims of violence and abuse, the homeless, the hungry, the mentally ill, the physically ill, the developmentally and physically disabled, the indigent, children and adults with HIV or AIDS, flood victims, capital projects enabling health and healing programs or projects, handicapped accessibility projects, and programmatic outreach services of Lutheran congregations.
Fields of interest: Mental health/crisis services; Domestic violence prevention; Housing/shelter, homeless; Youth development, religion; Youth, services; Family services; Family services, domestic violence; Human services, mind/body enrichment; Senior continuing care community; Aging, centers & services; Mentally disabled, centers & services; Protestant agencies & churches; Disabled; Aging; People with AIDS (PWAs); Economically disadvantaged; Homeless.
Types of support: Endowment funds.
Limitations: Giving limited to the St. Louis, MO, area. No grants to individuals, or for ordinary operating expenses or deficit financing.
Publications: Annual report, financial statement, grants list, newsletter, informational brochure (including application guidelines).
Application information: Denied proposals may be resubmitted once; Special application form required for Partnership Grants. Application form required.
Initial approach: Concept paper (no more than 500 words)
Copies of proposal: 3
Deadline(s): Mar. 1, June 1, Nov. 1 for submission of concept papers, Apr. 1, Aug. 1, and Dec. 1 for proposals (Regular Grants); Aug. 1 (Partnership Grants); no deadline for Immediate Response Grants
Board meeting date(s): Feb., Mar., May, June, Sept., Oct., and Nov.
Final notification: June for Apr. submissions; Oct. for Aug. submissions; Feb. for Dec. submissions; and Sept. for Partnership Grants
Officers and Directors:* Herbert F. Eggerding, Jr.,* Chair.; Barbara J. Reitz,* Vice-Chair.; Fred Bleeke, Pres.; Dr. Elmer Belsha,* Secy.; Benjamin L. Berry, David Binder, Charles H. Burmeister, Rev. Alan M. Erdman, John W. Gerber, Rev. Vernon D. Gundermann, Allan A. Huning, Beverly J. McCray, Harold A. Melser, Barbara J. Selders, Rev. Jonathan P. Stein, Norman J. Tice.
Staff: Kyle Struckmann, Dir. of Community Rels.; Debbie Larkin, Secy.; Jan Doggendorf, Admin. Asst.
Number of staff: 1 full-time professional; 1 part-time professional; 1 full-time support; 1 part-time support.
EIN: 431379359

524
Mallinckrodt Medical, Inc. Community Partnership Program
P.O. Box 5840
675 McDonnell Blvd.
St. Louis 63134 (314) 895-2000
Contact: Betsy Kippenberger, Community Rels. Specialist

Established in 1991.
Financial data (yr. ended 06/30/94): Total giving, $770,000, including $697,000 for grants (high: $250,000; low: $1,000) and $73,000 for 250 employee matching gifts.
Purpose and activities: Support for programatic, grassroots efforts and capital campaigns focusing on employee concerns, health initiatives, civic progress, emergency services, and youth education.
Fields of interest: Visual arts; Performing arts; Theater; Humanities; Arts/cultural programs; Early childhood education; Child development, education; Elementary school/education; Secondary school/education; Higher education; Medical school/education; Adult education—literacy & basic skills; Reading; Education; Environment; Health care; Substance abuse, services; Health associations; Cancer; AIDS; Health organizations; Medical research; Cancer research; AIDS research; Delinquency prevention/services; Housing/shelter, development; Human services; Children & youth, services; Youth, services; Child development, services; Family services; Aging, centers & services; Women, centers & services; Homeless, human services; Human rights (international); Community development; Voluntarism promotion; Mathematics; Engineering & technology; Science; Economics; Aging; Women; Economically disadvantaged; Homeless; Canada; Europe; Netherlands; Ireland; Italy; Germany; Sweden; Mexico; Japan.
Types of support: Continuing support, annual campaigns, capital campaigns, program development, conferences/seminars, research, technical assistance, employee volunteer services, loaned talent, employee matching gifts, donated equipment, donated products, in-kind gifts, matching funds.
Limitations: Giving in the U.S., Canada, Europe, Mexico, and Japan. No support for religious, fraternal, or athletic organizations.
Publications: Corporate report, program policy statement, corporate giving report (including application guidelines), application guidelines, newsletter, informational brochure (including application guidelines).
Application information: Send requests to headquarters or nearest company facility. Application form required.
Initial approach: Site visits
Copies of proposal: 1
Deadline(s): Mar., June, Sept., Dec.
Board meeting date(s): Quarterly
Final notification: Immediately following quarterly meeting
Number of staff: 1 full-time professional; 1 full-time support.

525
Joseph & Elsie McBride Charitable Foundation, Inc.

11 McBride & Son Corporate Center Dr.
Chesterfield 63005 (314) 537-2000
Contact: Pat Kiehl

Established in 1984 in MO.
Donor(s): McBride & Sons Enterprises.
Foundation type: Company-sponsored
Financial data (yr. ended 04/30/94): Assets, $387,637 (M); gifts received, $43,241; expenditures, $37,937; qualifying distributions, $28,422, including $28,422 for 110 grants (high: $3,384; low: $40).
Fields of interest: Adult education—literacy & basic skills; Reading; Education; Medical care, rehabilitation; Health care; Substance abuse, services; Mental health/crisis services; Cancer; Cancer research; Food services; Human services; Children & youth, services; Youth, services; Family services; Aging, centers & services; Homeless, human services; Religious federated giving programs; Transportation; Disabled; Economically disadvantaged; Homeless; General charitable giving.
Types of support: General/operating support, equipment, scholarship funds.
Application information: Application form required.
Deadline(s): None
Board meeting date(s): 2nd Monday of each month
Officers and Directors:* Richard C. McBride, Sr., Chair.; Richard R. Gastorf, Pres.; Richard T. Sullivan, Jr.
Number of staff: 1
EIN: 431353387

526
The McGee Foundation

4800 Main St., Suite 458
Kansas City 64112-2510 (816) 931-1515
Contact: Joseph J. McGee, Jr., Pres.

Incorporated in 1951 in MO.
Donor(s): Joseph J. McGee,‡ Mrs. Joseph J. McGee,‡ Frank McGee,‡ Mrs. Frank McGee,‡ Louis B. McGee,‡ Old American Insurance Co., Thomas McGee and Sons, Joseph J. McGee, Jr., Julie McGee.
Financial data (yr. ended 12/31/95): Assets, $8,521,299 (M); expenditures, $387,642; qualifying distributions, $362,067, including $350,850 for 33 grants (high: $50,000; low: $500; average: $10,632).
Purpose and activities: Giving primarily in four areas: "1) to care for the sick, aged, and helpless; 2) to encourage and provide means for the development and advancement of education and educational facilities; 3) to encourage and provide means and facilities for education and training of persons that their lives may be more useful to themselves and others; and 4) to make gifts to other benevolent, charitable, religious, or educational institutions either for specific purposes for their general support."
Fields of interest: Education; Health care; Youth, services; Roman Catholic agencies & churches; Aging.
Types of support: General/operating support, continuing support, capital campaigns, building/renovation, equipment, program development, scholarship funds.
Limitations: Giving limited to the greater Kansas City, MO, area. No support for the visual or performing arts, historic preservation, community development or rehabilitation, public information programs, united appeals, walkathons or telethons, or national organizations with wide support. No grants to individuals, or for endowment funds, research, publications, or conferences; no loans or multiple year grants.
Publications: Application guidelines.
Application information: Application form not required.
Initial approach: Letter
Copies of proposal: 1
Deadline(s): None
Board meeting date(s): Mar., June, Sept., and Dec.
Final notification: 6 weeks
Officers and Directors:* Joseph J. McGee, Jr.,* Pres.; Thomas F. McGee,* V.P.; Thomas R. McGee,* Secy.-Treas.; Virginia L. Coppinger, Mrs. Bernard J. Duffy, Jr., Robert A. Long, Thomas R. McGee, Jr.
Advisory Board: Sheila M. Lillis, Simon P. McGee.
Number of staff: 1 part-time support.
EIN: 446006285

527
The Jack & Helyn Miller Foundation

1055 Broadway
Kansas City 64105-1595
Contact: Kathleen Hermes, Prog. Officer

Established in 1967.
Donor(s): Jack Miller,‡ Helyn Miller.‡
Financial data (yr. ended 12/31/93): Assets, $7,056,076 (M); expenditures, $423,620; qualifying distributions, $404,509, including $404,509 for 19 grants (high: $150,000; low: $1,000; average: $3,900-$150,000).
Fields of interest: Arts/cultural programs; Health care; Children & youth, services; Aging.
Limitations: Giving primarily in the bi-state metropolitan Kansas City area. No grants to individuals.
Application information: Application form not required.
Initial approach: Letter
Deadline(s): Jan. and Aug.
Board meeting date(s): Apr. and Oct.
Officers and Directors:* Harold S. Melcher,* Pres. and Treas.; Robert J. Margolin,* V.P.; Abraham E. Margolin,* Secy.; James E. Anderson.
Number of staff: 1
EIN: 436070986

528
Oppenstein Brothers Foundation

911 Main St., Suite 100
P.O. Box 13095
Kansas City 64199-3095 (816) 234-8671
Contact: Sheila K. Rice, Prog. Officer

Trust established in 1975 in MO.
Donor(s): Michael Oppenstein.‡
Financial data (yr. ended 03/31/96): Assets, $23,415,515 (M); expenditures, $1,039,552; qualifying distributions, $867,000, including $867,000 for 96 grants (average: $1,000-$80,000).
Purpose and activities: Grants primarily for social services and early childhood, elementary, secondary, adult, vocational and higher education, emphasizing the prevention of illness and abuse, and programs which enhance the ability of individuals to remain or become self-sufficient; some support for community and leadership development, family planning and services, social services and welfare agencies, Jewish welfare organizations, programs for youth, minorities, the handicapped, disadvantaged, mentally ill, homeless and elderly, and arts education.
Fields of interest: Museums; Performing arts; Theater; Arts/cultural programs; Early childhood education; Child development, education; Elementary school/education; Secondary school/education; Higher education; Adult/continuing education; Adult education—literacy & basic skills; Libraries/library science; Reading; Education; Medical care, rehabilitation; Health care; Substance abuse, services; Mental health/crisis services; AIDS; Alcoholism; Health organizations; AIDS research; Delinquency prevention/services; Employment; Nutrition; Housing/shelter, development; Youth development, services; Human services; Children & youth, services; Youth, services; Child development, services; Family services; Aging, centers & services; Minorities/immigrants, centers & services; Homeless, human services; Urban/community development; Community development; Voluntarism promotion; Jewish federated giving programs; Leadership development; Jewish agencies & temples; Minorities; Disabled; Aging; Economically disadvantaged; Homeless.
Types of support: General/operating support, capital campaigns, building/renovation, emergency funds, program development, conferences/seminars, seed money, curriculum development, consulting services, matching funds.
Limitations: Giving limited to the metropolitan Kansas City, MO, area. No support for medical research. No grants to individuals, or for annual campaigns, building funds or expansion, scholarships, fellowships, medical equipment, or generally for endowment funds; limited operating funds for United Way or Jewish Federation supported agencies; no loans.
Publications: Multi-year report, informational brochure (including application guidelines).
Application information: Application form not required.
Initial approach: Telephone or letter
Copies of proposal: 1
Deadline(s): Submit proposal with complete information 3 weeks prior to board meetings; no set deadline
Board meeting date(s): Usually bimonthly
Final notification: 2 to 4 months
Disbursement Committee: John A. Morgan, Chair.; Mary Bloch, Laura Kemper Fields, Roger T. Hurwitz, Estelle Sosland.
Trustee: Commerce Bank of Kansas City, N.A.
Staff: Sheila K. Rice, Prog. Officer.

Number of staff: None.
EIN: 436203035
Grants for Aging:
Palestine Senior Citizens Activity Center, Kansas City, MO, $20,000. 94.

529
Roosevelt Financial Group, Inc.
900 Roosevelt Pkwy.
St. Louis 63017 (314) 532-6205
Contact: David L. Dilthey

Purpose and activities: To fulfill Roosevelt's responsibility as a corporate citizen through contributions to organizations or projects that benefit the communities in which the Bank operates, a Contributions Committee has been established to disburse funds consistent with the guidelines outlined below. The Committee reviews all requests on a monthly basis and either approves or denies the request based on these guidelines.
Fields of interest: Education; Housing/shelter; Aging, centers & services; Human services; Public affairs; Aging.
Types of support: Annual campaigns, capital campaigns, scholarship funds, sponsorships, employee matching gifts, matching funds.
Limitations: Giving primarily in headquarters and company locations.
Application information: Marketing Dept. handles giving. Application form not required.
Initial approach: Send requests to headquarters
Copies of proposal: 1
Board meeting date(s): Monthly

530
Roy W. Slusher Charitable Foundation
c/o Mercantile Bank of Springfield
P.O. Box 10327
Springfield 65808-0327 (417) 882-9090
Contact: Charles A. Fuller, Jr., Mgr.

Established in 1988 in MO.
Financial data (yr. ended 02/28/95): Assets, $3,166,065 (M); expenditures, $285,914; qualifying distributions, $155,780, including $155,780 for 32 grants (high: $20,000; low: $500).
Purpose and activities: Funding to meet the needs of disadvantaged youth and their families and to increase the quality of life for the elderly through the following broad areas: educational scholarships, broad national health issues, youth camps and programs, senior citizens programs, and public radio and television.
Fields of interest: Media/communications; Hospitals (general); Housing/shelter, homeless; Children & youth, services; Aging, centers & services; International relief; Christian agencies & churches; Aging.
Types of support: General/operating support, building/renovation, seed money, scholarship funds.
Limitations: Giving primarily in MO. No grants to individuals, or for routine operating needs, annual fundraising, or endowments.
Application information: Application form required.
Copies of proposal: 3
Deadline(s): Feb. 15 and Aug. 15
Board meeting date(s): Mar. and Sept.
Officer: Charles A. Fuller, Jr., Mgr.
Trustee: Mercantile Bank of Springfield.
Number of staff: None.
EIN: 436339151

531
Victor E. Speas Foundation
c/o Boatmen's First National Bank of Kansas City
14 West Tenth St.
Kansas City 64183 (816) 691-7481
Contact: David P. Ross, Sr. V.P., Boatmen's First National Bank of Kansas City

Trust established in 1947 in MO.
Donor(s): Effie E. Speas,‡ Victor E. Speas,‡ Speas Co.
Financial data (yr. ended 12/31/94): Assets, $24,671,408 (M); expenditures, $1,400,178; qualifying distributions, $1,199,682, including $1,165,684 for 48 grants (high: $145,000; low: $1,300; average: $5,000-$20,000) and $4,000 for 2 loans to individuals.
Purpose and activities: Giving restricted to improving the quality of health care in the Kansas City, MO, area. Support mainly for medically-related higher education, including loans for medical students at the University of Missouri at Kansas City, preventive health care, and medical research; grants also for agencies serving the health care needs of the elderly, youth, and the handicapped.
Fields of interest: Medical school/education; Hospitals (general); Dental care; Medical care, rehabilitation; Health care; Substance abuse, services; Mental health/crisis services; Cancer; Heart/circulatory disease; AIDS; Alcoholism; Medical research; Cancer research; Heart/circulatory research; AIDS research; Safety/disasters; Children & youth, services; Youth, services; Hospices; Aging, centers & services; Women, centers & services; Voluntarism promotion; Disabled; Aging; Women.
Types of support: General/operating support, capital campaigns, building/renovation, equipment, emergency funds, program development, seed money, research, matching funds, student loans—to individuals.
Limitations: Giving limited to Jackson, Clay, Platte, and Cass counties, MO. No grants for endowment funds or scholarships (except to medical students at the University of Missouri at Kansas City); no loans.
Publications: 990-PF, program policy statement, application guidelines.
Application information: Application form not required.
Initial approach: Letter (no longer than 3 pages)
Copies of proposal: 1
Deadline(s): None
Board meeting date(s): Bimonthly
Final notification: 2 months
Trustee: Boatmen's First National Bank of Kansas City.
Number of staff: 1 full-time professional.
EIN: 446008340

532
St. Louis Community Foundation
222 South Central Ave., Suite 203
St. Louis 63105-3509 (314) 725-9893
Contact: Tullia Hamilton, Exec. Dir.

Established in 1915 in MO.
Foundation type: Community
Financial data (yr. ended 12/31/95): Assets, $26,544,198 (M); gifts received, $4,257,998; expenditures, $2,341,338, including $1,857,690 for 402 grants (high: $1,050,713; low: $25; average: $2,500-$7,500) and $27,285 for 14 grants to individuals (high: $3,800; low: $500; average: $500-$2,500).
Purpose and activities: Primary areas of interest include the arts, community development, education, health services, the environment, and human services. Purposes include, but are not limited to, the promotion of education, social and scientific research, the care of the sick, aged, infirm, and handicapped, the care of children, the improvement of living, working, recreation, and environmental conditions or facilities, cultural programs, and other such charitable, educational, and social purposes that will assist the betterment of the mental, moral, social, and physical conditions of the inhabitants of the St. Louis metropolitan area. Priority given to projects that 1) represent new approaches to meeting needs; 2) enable people to move to self-reliance; 3) increase effectiveness of established organizations; 4) address underlying causes; or 5) represent collaborative efforts.
Fields of interest: Visual arts; Performing arts; Arts/cultural programs; Education; Natural resource conservation & protection; Environment; Health care; Human services; Children & youth, services; Youth, services; Family services; Aging, centers & services; Women, centers & services; Community development; Engineering & technology; Science; Disabled; Aging; Women; Economically disadvantaged.
Types of support: Program development, seed money, scholarship funds, employee-related scholarships.
Limitations: Giving primarily in the metropolitan St. Louis, MO, area. No support for sectarian religious programs, or private elementary or secondary schools. No grants to individuals (except through scholarship funds), or for deficit financing, or endowment or building funds; grants for operating expenses only during an organization's start-up.
Publications: Annual report, newsletter, application guidelines.
Application information: Contact foundation for application guidelines. Application form required.
Initial approach: Letter
Copies of proposal: 1
Deadline(s): Dec., Mar., and June
Board meeting date(s): Bimonthly
Final notification: Usually within 1 week of board meetings
Officers and Directors:* Susan B. Musgrave,* Chair.; Eugene J. Gabianelli,* Vice-Chair.; Leigh Gerdine,* Vice-Chair.; Charles A. Stewart, Jr.,* Treas.; Tullia Hamilton, Exec. Dir.; Clarence C. Barksdale, Belle A. Cori, David Cornfield, Mark A. Dow, Clarence Harmon, Ruth K. Jacobson,

William B. McMillan, Marvin E. McMillian, Kathryn Nelson, Charles A. Newman, Glenn J. Sheffield, Donald H. Strett, Josephine C. Throdahl, Franklin F. Wallis, Jane Woods-Miller.
Trustee Banks: A.G. Edwards Trust Co., Boatmen's National Bank of St. Louis, Commerce Bank of St. Louis, N.A., Guaranty Trust Co. of Missouri, Magna Trust Co., Mark Twain Bank, Mercantile Bank of St. Louis, N.A., Merrill Lynch Trust Co.
Number of staff: 2 full-time professional; 1 part-time professional; 1 full-time support.
EIN: 436023126

533
Sam and Ida Turken Charitable Foundation

575 Fee Fee Rd., Suite 204
Maryland Heights 63043
Contact: Mark Turken, V.P.

Established in 1986 in MO.
Donor(s): Harry Turken.
Financial data (yr. ended 12/31/94): Assets, $541,913 (M); gifts received, $10,546; expenditures, $29,188; qualifying distributions, $29,188, including $27,000 for grants to individuals.
Fields of interest: Higher education; Alzheimer's disease.
Types of support: Research, scholarships—to individuals.
Limitations: Giving primarily in MO and TN.
Application information: Application form required.
Deadline(s): None
Officers: Harry Turken, Pres.; Mark Turken, V.P.; Meyer Turken, Secy.-Treas.
EIN: 431431267

534
Union Electric Company Charitable Trust

1901 Chouteau Ave.
P.O. Box 149, Mail Code 100
St. Louis 63166 (314) 554-2902
Contact: Ms. Carlin Scanlan, Mgr., Corp. Communications, Union Electric Co.

Trust established in 1944 in MO.
Donor(s): Union Electric Co.
Foundation type: Company-sponsored
Financial data (yr. ended 12/31/95): Assets, $11,634,999 (M); gifts received, $4,000,000; expenditures, $1,839,977; qualifying distributions, $1,839,977, including $1,789,361 for 62 grants (high: $675,000; low: $1,500; average: $5,000-$25,000) and $50,616 for employee matching gifts.
Purpose and activities: Current emphasis is on education (especially higher education), services for youth and the elderly, and the environment. Giving also for community funds, social service agencies, arts and cultural programs, including music and dance, community development, and public policy; employee-related scholarships administered by the National Merit Scholarship Corp.
Fields of interest: Museums; Performing arts; Music; Education, fund raising; Early childhood education; Child development, education; Secondary school/education; Higher education; Adult education—literacy & basic skills; Libraries/library science; Reading; Education; Natural resource conservation & protection; Energy; Environment; Food services; Housing/shelter, development; Human services; Children & youth, services; Youth, services; Child development, services; Aging, centers & services; Minorities/immigrants, centers & services; Homeless, human services; Urban/community development; Business & industry; Community development; Voluntarism promotion; Federated giving programs; Engineering & technology; Science; Public policy, research; Public affairs; Minorities; Aging; Economically disadvantaged; Homeless; General charitable giving.
Types of support: General/operating support, continuing support, annual campaigns, capital campaigns, building/renovation, equipment, emergency funds, program development, scholarship funds, research, employee matching gifts, employee-related scholarships, in-kind gifts, matching funds.
Limitations: Giving limited to company locations in IL and MO. No support for religious, political, or veterans' organizations or social groups. No grants to individuals, or for endowment funds; no loans.
Publications: Corporate report (including application guidelines), corporate giving report, application guidelines.
Application information: Application form not required.
Initial approach: Letter
Copies of proposal: 1
Deadline(s): None
Board meeting date(s): 2 or 3 times a year
Final notification: 60 to 90 days
Trustees: Charles W. Mueller, Chair. and C.E.O.; Boatmen's Trust Co.
Number of staff: 1 full-time professional; 1 part-time professional; 1 full-time support.
EIN: 436022693

535
Union Electric Company Corporate Giving Program

1901 Chouteau Ave.
P.O. Box 149, Mail Code 100
St. Louis 63166 (314) 554-2902
Contact: Ms. Carlin Scanlan, Mgr., Corp. Communications, Union Electric Co.

Established in 1944 in MD.
Financial data (yr. ended 12/31/94): Total giving, $2,146,003, including $1,878,216 for 57 grants (high: $640,000; low: $2,000; average: $5,000-$25,000), $53,869 for 58 employee matching gifts and $213,918 for 122 in-kind gifts.
Purpose and activities: At Union Electric, the company's goal is to be the best it can in all phases of its operations. That means more than just doing a good job in business, it also means working to improve the quality of life in the communities the company serves. Union Electric has a long tradition of corporate community involvement, and company employees also have an impressive record of community service. The company's charitable contributions policy states that the recognition of charitable needs, which is viewed as a basic part of good citizenship, must necessarily be a responsible interest of Union Electric.
Fields of interest: Arts/cultural programs; Higher education; Engineering school/education; Education; Natural resource conservation & protection; Energy; Environment; Youth development, services; Human services; Children & youth, services; Aging, centers & services; Voluntarism promotion; Federated giving programs; Engineering & technology; Engineering; Minorities; Aging; Economically disadvantaged.
Types of support: General/operating support, annual campaigns, capital campaigns, building/renovation, equipment, endowment funds, emergency funds, program development, scholarship funds, research, technical assistance, employee volunteer services, use of facilities, sponsorships, employee matching gifts, employee-related scholarships, donated equipment, in-kind gifts.
Limitations: Giving primarily in the St. Louis, MO, area and operating locations. No support for political organizations or candidates, or social, religious, fraternal, veterans', social or similar organizations. No grants to individuals, or for electric or natural gas service.
Publications: Informational brochure (including application guidelines), corporate giving report (including application guidelines), application guidelines.
Application information: Company has a staff that only handles contributions. Application form not required.
Initial approach: Proposal on organization letterhead; send to headquarters
Copies of proposal: 1
Deadline(s): None
Board meeting date(s): Applications reviewed as received
Final notification: 60 to 90 days after receipt
Administrators: M. Patricia Barrett, V.P., Corp. Communications; Carlin Scanlan, Mgr., Corp. Communications.
Number of staff: 2 full-time professional; 1 full-time support.

MONTANA

536
Beaverhead Foundation

(Formerly Parkview Acres Convalescent & Nursing Home, Inc.)
P.O. Box 528
Dillon 59725
Contact: Gayle Murray, Pres.
Application address: South Nevada, Dillon, MT 59725; Tel.: (406) 683-4036

Financial data (yr. ended 02/28/94): Assets, $409,394 (M); expenditures, $15,785; qualifying distributions, $15,268, including $14,856 for 4 grants (high: $7,500; low: $700).
Fields of interest: Aging, centers & services; Aging.
Limitations: Giving primarily in Beaverhead County, MT. No grants to individuals.

Application information:
Initial approach: Proposal
Deadline(s): None
Officers and Directors:* Gayle Murray,* Pres.; Margaret Hagenbarth,* V.P.; W. Cecil Jones,* Secy.; Harold Peterson,* Treas.
EIN: 810294449

537
Gladys E. Knowles Charitable Memorial Trust
c/o First Trust Co. of Montana, N.A.
P.O. Box 30678
Billings 59115
Contact: Helen M. Hancock, V.P. and Trust Officer, First Trust Co. of Montana, N.A.

Established in 1983 in MT.
Financial data (yr. ended 12/31/94): Assets, $1,876,493 (M); expenditures, $101,610; qualifying distributions, $85,015, including $80,263 for grants.
Fields of interest: Higher education; Hospitals (general); Aging, centers & services; Protestant agencies & churches; Aging.
Limitations: Applications not accepted. Giving primarily in MT. No grants to individuals.
Application information: Contributes only to pre-selected organizations.
Trustee: First Trust Co. of Montana, N.A.
EIN: 810423029

538
Dennis & Phyllis Washington Foundation, Inc.
(Formerly Dennis R. Washington Foundation, Inc.)
P.O. Box 7067
Missoula 59807-7067 (406) 523-1300
Contact: Russell J. Ritter, Pres.
Additional tel.: (406) 449-6510

Established in 1988 in MT.
Donor(s): Montana Rail Link, Montana Resources, Washington Contractors Group Inc., Envirocon Inc., Modern Machinery Co., Western Transport.
Foundation type: Company-sponsored
Financial data (yr. ended 12/31/93): Assets, $6,010,233 (M); gifts received, $622,400; expenditures, $311,171; qualifying distributions, $284,635, including $284,635 for 196 grants (high: $25,000; low: $85).
Purpose and activities: Priorities for grant consideration are youth-oriented programs and education focusing on the needs of the underprivileged and less fortunate located in those communities serviced by the Washington Companies.
Fields of interest: Visual arts; Performing arts; Theater; Higher education; Business school/education; Education; Hospitals (general); Family planning; Substance abuse, services; Delinquency prevention/services; Food services; Youth development, centers & clubs; Youth, services; Family services; Aging, centers & services; Women, centers & services; Federated giving programs; Aging; Women; Economically disadvantaged.
Types of support: Continuing support, annual campaigns, capital campaigns, building/renovation.
Limitations: Giving limited to areas of company operations. No support for religious organizations, war veterans' and fraternal service organizations, or national health organizations. No grants to individuals, or for general endowment funds, computer-related projects, fundraising events, conferences or seminars, or travel expenses; no loans.
Publications: Newsletter, application guidelines, informational brochure (including application guidelines).
Application information: Application form required.
Initial approach: Letter
Copies of proposal: 1
Deadline(s): None
Board meeting date(s): Quarterly; grants committee meets monthly
Final notification: Within 30 to 45 days of receiving applications
Officers and Directors:* Russell J. Ritter,* Pres.; Helen B. Miller, V.P.; James A. Broulette, Secy.; Deborah M. Brown, Treas.; William H. Brodsky, Frank Gardner, Helen Miller, Dorn Parkinson.
Number of staff: 1 part-time professional; 1 part-time support.
EIN: 363606913

NEBRASKA

539
Paul and Oscar Giger Foundation, Inc.
c/o Fraser, Stryker, Vaughn, Meusey, Olson, Boyer & Bloch, P.C.
500 Energy Plaza, 409 South 17th St.
Omaha 68102-2663 (402) 341-6000
Contact: John K. Boyer, Esq.

Established in 1985 in NE.
Donor(s): Ruth Giger.‡
Financial data (yr. ended 12/31/94): Assets, $1,913,948 (M); expenditures, $121,445; qualifying distributions, $96,201, including $78,000 for 13 grants (high: $25,000; low: $500).
Purpose and activities: The four major areas of interest are: musical endeavors and music education; natural resources; Christian-related giving; and senior citizens.
Fields of interest: Music; Natural resource conservation & protection; Christian agencies & churches; Aging.
Limitations: Giving limited to the Omaha, NE, area. No support for private foundations. No grants to individuals.
Application information: Application form required.
Initial approach: Letter requesting application
Copies of proposal: 4
Deadline(s): May 15 and Oct. 1
Board meeting date(s): Quarterly
Officers: Frank A. Blazek, Pres.; Beverly Ingram, V.P.; Janet Acker, Secy.
EIN: 470682708

540
Bernard K. & Norma F. Heuermann Foundation
P.O. Box 228
Aurora 68818
Contact: John B. Atkins, Treas.
Application address: c/o Norwest Bank Nebraska, N.A., Trust Dept., P.O. Box 3959, Omaha, NE 68103

Established in 1991 in NE.
Donor(s): Bernard K. Heuermann, Norma F. Heuermann.
Financial data (yr. ended 07/31/94): Assets, $3,187,214 (M); gifts received, $3,053; expenditures, $80,609; qualifying distributions, $73,359, including $65,450 for 6 grants (high: $21,368; low: $2,000; average: $1,000-$25,000).
Fields of interest: Education; Agriculture; Children, services; Mentally disabled, centers & services; Disabled; Aging.
Types of support: Endowment funds, fellowships, research.
Limitations: Giving limited to NE. No grants to individuals.
Publications: Application guidelines.
Application information: Application form not required.
Initial approach: 2-page proposal
Copies of proposal: 3
Deadline(s): May 1
Board meeting date(s): Summer, fall, and spring
Final notification: July
Officers and Directors:* Bernard K. Heuermann,* Pres.; Norma F. Heuermann,* V.P.; Charles L. Whitney,* Secy.; John B. Atkins,* Treas.
Number of staff: None.
EIN: 470748466

541
Hazel R. Keene Trust
c/o Fremont National Bank & Trust Co., Trust Dept.
P.O. Box 169
Fremont 68025 (402) 721-1050
Contact: Joe Twidwell

Established in 1986 in NE.
Donor(s): Hazel Keene.
Financial data (yr. ended 06/30/93): Assets, $2,136,065 (M); expenditures, $204,054; qualifying distributions, $100,000, including $100,000 for 18 grants (high: $50,000; low: $500).
Purpose and activities: Primary areas of interest include community development, the elderly, child welfare, and early childhood education. Giving for social services, adult and other education, health, agriculture and animal welfare, the arts, and historic preservation.
Fields of interest: Arts/cultural programs; Early childhood education; Education; Natural resource conservation & protection; Health care; Health organizations; Crime/law enforcement; Agriculture; Nutrition; Recreation; Human services; Children & youth, services; Youth, services; Aging, centers & services; Community development; Federated giving programs; Disabled; Aging; Economically disadvantaged.

Types of support: General/operating support, capital campaigns, building/renovation, endowment funds, publication, seed money, curriculum development, scholarship funds, matching funds.
Limitations: Giving limited to Fremont and Dodge County, NE. No grants to individuals.
Publications: Annual report, financial statement.
Application information: Grants must directly serve residents of Fremont and Dodge County, NE. Application form required.
Initial approach: Letter
Copies of proposal: 2
Deadline(s): May 1
Board meeting date(s): May 30
Final notification: June 30
Trustees: Elnor Dunn, John Kerrigan, Stan Lundstrom, Fremont National Bank & Trust Co.
Number of staff: None.
EIN: 476144486

542
Lincoln Community Foundation, Inc.
(Formerly Lincoln Foundation, Inc.)
215 Centennial Mall South, Rm. 200
Lincoln 68508-1813 (402) 474-2345
Contact: Kim Carlson, Prog. Dir.

Incorporated in 1955 in NE.
Foundation type: Community
Financial data (yr. ended 12/31/94): Assets, $24,594,327 (M); expenditures, $2,311,820, including $906,273 for grants, $100,825 for grants to individuals and $312,000 for 1 foundation-administered program.
Purpose and activities: To enrich the quality of life in the greater Lincoln, NE, area by responding to emerging and changing needs and sustaining existing organizations and institutions through grants for education, culture, health, social services, economic development, and civic affairs in Lincoln/Lancaster County, NE. Primary areas of interest include family issues, children's issues, older adults, environmental enhancement, higher education, and basic needs.
Fields of interest: Child development, education; Higher education; Environment; Human services; Child development, services; Family services; Aging, centers & services; Aging.
Types of support: General/operating support, building/renovation, emergency funds, program development, seed money, scholarship funds, research, matching funds.
Limitations: Giving limited to the Lincoln-Lancaster County, NE, area. No support for religious purposes. No grants to individuals, (except for scholarships), or for endowments, routine operating expenses, large capital expenditures, budget deficits, or projects with long future commitments.
Publications: Annual report, program policy statement, application guidelines, newsletter, informational brochure.
Application information: Application form required.
Initial approach: Telephone or letter requesting application form
Copies of proposal: 1
Deadline(s): May 1 and Nov. 1
Board meeting date(s): 3rd Thursday of July and Jan.
Final notification: Day of board meeting
Officers and Directors:* Jean S. Jeffrey,* Chair.; James Griesen,* Vice-Chair.; Dawson Dowty, Pres.; Brad Korell,* Secy.; Thomas E. Henning,* Treas.; Robert Allington, Mollie Anderson, Harold Clarke, Linda Crump, Jay Dunlap, Ron Ecklund, Lana Flagtwet, Joel Gajardo, Virginia G. Johnson, Marc LeBaron, James Linderholm, JoAnn Martin, Marilyn Moore, Robert Moyer, Lorraine Pallesen, Julie Pokorny, Harry P. Seward III, Linda Steinman, Jim Strand.
Staff: Kim Carlson, Prog. Dir.
Number of staff: 3 full-time professional; 1 part-time professional; 1 full-time support; 1 part-time support.
EIN: 470458128

543
Henry A. Stalp & Ramona F. Stalp Foundation
1598 River Rd.
West Point 68788

Established in 1993 in NE.
Donor(s): Henry A. Stalp.
Financial data (yr. ended 12/31/94): Assets, $103,391 (M); gifts received, $5,000; expenditures, $13,476; qualifying distributions, $13,476, including $13,000 for 5 grants (high: $5,000; low: $2,000).
Fields of interest: Education; Nursing home/convalescent facility; Christian agencies & churches.
Limitations: Applications not accepted. Giving limited to NE.
Application information: Contributes only to pre-selected organizations.
Directors: Earl Scudder, Jr., Henry A. Stalp, Ramona F. Stalp, Cleo Toelle.
EIN: 363662988

NEVADA

544
Dermody Properties Foundation
P.O. Box 7438
Reno 89510 (702) 333-6745
Contact: Paula Anne Smith Dermody, Secy.

Established in 1987 in NV.
Donor(s): Dermody Properties, Inc.
Foundation type: Company-sponsored
Financial data (yr. ended 12/31/94): Assets, $6 (M); gifts received, $19,660; expenditures, $19,777; qualifying distributions, $19,777, including $18,660 for 29 grants (high: $2,500; low: $100).
Fields of interest: Arts/cultural programs; Early childhood education; Child development, education; Higher education; Business school/education; Education; Natural resource conservation & protection; Health care; Human services; Youth, services; Child development, services; Family services; Aging, centers & services; Federated giving programs; Aging; Economically disadvantaged.
Types of support: Endowment funds, program development, seed money, scholarship funds.
Limitations: Giving limited to NV. No grants to individuals.
Publications: Informational brochure.
Application information:
Initial approach: Proposal
Deadline(s): Oct. 1
Board meeting date(s): Quarterly
Final notification: Dec. 31
Officers: Michael C. Dermody, Pres.; Paula Anne Smith Dermody, Secy.; Bruce D. Storey, Treas.
Number of staff: 1 part-time support.
EIN: 943086271

545
The Hall Family Foundation
P.O. Box 1479
Minden 89423-1479
Contact: Joanne Hall, Secy.-Treas.

Established in 1983 in NV.
Donor(s): Joanne Hall.
Financial data (yr. ended 12/31/95): Assets, $7,459,722 (M); gifts received, $1,750,000; expenditures, $190,388; qualifying distributions, $178,011, including $164,350 for 30 grants (high: $20,000; low: $350).
Purpose and activities: Giving primarily for higher education, conservation of wilderness areas, cancer research and a facility that provides temporary lodging for families of cancer patients on a cost-free basis, and a child welfare organization; support also for health, including medical education, and the biological sciences, and nursing.
Fields of interest: Performing arts; Music; Arts/cultural programs; Higher education; Education; Natural resource conservation & protection; Environment; Hospitals (general); Family planning; Speech & hearing centers; Nursing care; Health care; Substance abuse, services; Health associations; Cancer; Heart/circulatory disease; AIDS; Alcoholism; Biomedicine; Medical research; Cancer research; Heart/circulatory research; AIDS research; Human services; Children & youth, services; Aging, centers & services; Biological sciences; Disabled; Aging; Economically disadvantaged.
Types of support: General/operating support, continuing support, building/renovation, emergency funds, research, matching funds.
Limitations: Applications not accepted. Giving primarily in CA and NV. No grants to individuals.
Publications: 990-PF.
Application information: Contributes only to pre-selected organizations.
Officers and Directors:* Arthur E. Hall,* Chair.; Joanne Hall,* Secy.-Treas.; William H.T. Bush, Whitney S. Hall.
EIN: 880193741

546
The Lincy Foundation
4835 Koval Ln.
Las Vegas 89109
Contact: James D. Aljian, Pres.

Established in 1989 in CA.
Financial data (yr. ended 09/30/95): Assets, $68,283,982 (M); expenditures, $11,776,244;

qualifying distributions, $11,776,244, including $11,747,406 for 175 grants (high: $1,000,000; low: $2,000; average: $20,000-$100,000).
Purpose and activities: Support primarily for Armenian charities.
Fields of interest: Arts/cultural programs; Medical research; Aging, centers & services; International relief; Religion; Aging.
Limitations: Giving primarily in CA. No grants to individuals.
Application information: Application form not required.
Initial approach: Letter or proposal
Deadline(s): None
Officers and Directors:* James D. Aljian, Chair. and Pres.; Alex Yemenidjian, V.P.; Anthony Mandekic, Secy. and C.F.O.; Kirk Kerkorian, Walter M. Sharp.
EIN: 954238697
Grants for Aging:
Alzheimers Disease and Related Disorders Association, Chicago, IL, $50,000. 95.
Alzheimers Disease and Related Disorders Association, Las Vegas, NV, $15,000. 95.
California Home for the Aged, Fresno, CA, $100,000. 95.
NorCal Armenian Home, Burlingame, CA, $25,000. 95.
Senior Health and Peer Counseling Center, Santa Monica, CA, $25,000. 95.

547
Nevada Community Foundation, Inc.
1660 East Flamingo
Las Vegas 89119 (702) 892-2326
Contact: Douglas Beckley, Exec. Dir.

Established in 1988 in NV.
Foundation type: Community
Financial data (yr. ended 12/31/94): Assets, $1,709,214 (M); gifts received, $14,772; expenditures, $99,145, including $30,850 for 6 grants (high: $12,500; low: $500).
Fields of interest: Adult/continuing education; Adult education—literacy & basic skills; Reading; Education; Medical care, rehabilitation; Health care; Substance abuse, services; Mental health/crisis services; Cancer; Heart/circulatory disease; AIDS; Health organizations; Cancer research; Heart/circulatory research; AIDS research; Food services; Youth development, citizenship; Human services; Children & youth, services; Youth, services; Family services; Aging, centers & services; Women, centers & services; Minorities/immigrants, centers & services; Homeless, human services; Community development; Federated giving programs; Government/public administration; Public affairs, citizen participation; Minorities; Disabled; Aging; Women; Economically disadvantaged; Homeless; General charitable giving.
Types of support: General/operating support, capital campaigns, equipment, emergency funds, program development, conferences/seminars, publication, seed money, scholarship funds, technical assistance, matching funds.
Limitations: Giving limited to the Las Vegas, NV, area.
Publications: Annual report, 990-PF, financial statement.
Application information: Application form not required.
Initial approach: Letter
Copies of proposal: 1
Deadline(s): None
Board meeting date(s): Quarterly
Final notification: Fall
Officer: Douglas Beckley, Exec. Dir.
Directors: Gard Jameson, Chair.; Jeffrey Burr, James Cashman III, Margaret Crockett, Marti Cruden, Mark Dreschler, Daniel Goldfarb, Ellsworth Heiman, Robin Joyce, Scott MacTaggart, Monte Miller, Dick Oshins, Don Pitchford, George L. Ralphs, Scott Ruthe, Deborah Stout, Richard H. Taggart, Orest Taraban, Keith Thomas.
Number of staff: 1 part-time professional.
EIN: 880241420

548
William N. and Myriam Pennington Foundation
(Formerly William N. Pennington Foundation)
441 West Plumb Ln.
Reno 89509 (702) 333-9100
Contact: Kent Green, Cont.

Established in 1989 in NV.
Donor(s): William N. Pennington.
Financial data (yr. ended 12/31/95): Assets, $5,417,126 (M); expenditures, $244,326; qualifying distributions, $240,581, including $229,429 for 5 grants (high: $180,000; low: $4,000) and $9,050 for 3 grants to individuals (high: $4,050; low: $2,500).
Purpose and activities: Giving primarily for education, health, and medical research.
Fields of interest: Higher education; Medical school/education; Hospitals (general); Medical care, rehabilitation; Cancer; Medical research; Human services; Children & youth, services; Disabled; Aging; Economically disadvantaged.
Types of support: General/operating support, building/renovation, equipment, scholarships—to individuals.
Limitations: Giving primarily in NV.
Publications: 990-PF (including application guidelines), financial statement.
Application information: Application form not required.
Initial approach: Proposal
Copies of proposal: 1
Deadline(s): Oct. 1
Board meeting date(s): Nov. or Dec.
Officers: William N. Pennington, Chair.; Raymond C. Avansino, Jr., Secy.; Richard P. Banis, Treas.
Trustees: John Mackell, Myriam Pennington.
Number of staff: None.
EIN: 943096845

549
Nell J. Redfield Foundation
P.O. Box 61
1755 East Plumb Ln., Suite 212
Reno 89504 (702) 323-1373
Contact: Gerald C. Smith, Dir.

Established in 1982 in NV.
Donor(s): Nell J. Redfield.‡
Financial data (yr. ended 12/31/95): Assets, $8,178,612 (M); gifts received, $5,279,492; expenditures, $1,012,837; qualifying distributions, $953,471, including $953,471 for 45 grants (high: $160,000; low: $1,400).
Purpose and activities: Support primarily for the advancement of health care, medical research, and the care of handicapped children; support also for the aged, education, and religion.
Fields of interest: Education; Health care; Health associations; Medical research; Aging, centers & services; Religion; Disabled; Aging.
Types of support: Building/renovation, equipment, endowment funds, scholarship funds.
Limitations: Giving primarily in Reno, NV.
Application information: Application form required.
Initial approach: Letter
Deadline(s): Jan. 15 through June 1
Directors: Iris G. Brewerton, Betty Alyce Jones, Helen Jeane Jones, Gerald C. Smith, Kenneth G. Walker.
Trustee: Farmers & Merchants Trust Co.
EIN: 237399910
Grants for Aging:
Foster Grandparent Program, Sparks, NV, $14,000. For at-risk youth tutoring program. 95.
Senior Alliance, $13,500. For home delivery program. 95.

550
The Gary and Joan Zimmerman Foundation
4625 South Procyon, No. 201
Las Vegas 89103

Established in 1991 in CA.
Donor(s): Joan Goodman Zimmerman, Gary A. Zimmerman.
Financial data (yr. ended 12/31/95): Assets, $1,222,161 (M); gifts received, $177,570; expenditures, $40,315; qualifying distributions, $40,010, including $40,010 for grants (high: $27,855).
Fields of interest: Arts/cultural programs; Nursing home/convalescent facility; Jewish federated giving programs; Jewish agencies & temples; Aging.
Limitations: Applications not accepted.
Application information: Contributes only to pre-selected organizations.
Directors: Gary A. Zimmerman, Joan Goodman Zimmerman.
EIN: 943148874

NEW HAMPSHIRE

551
Foundation for Seacoast Health
P.O. Box 4606
Portsmouth 03802-4606 (603) 433-3008
Contact: Susan Bunting, Exec. Dir.
FAX: (603) 433-2036

Incorporated in 1984 in NH as the Portsmouth Hospital Foundation; name changed in 1986 to Foundation for Seacoast Health.
Financial data (yr. ended 12/31/95): Assets, $50,195,474 (M); expenditures, $1,963,860; qualifying distributions, $1,411,482, including $1,274,232 for 64 grants (high: $281,395; low: $500) and $137,250 for 47 grants to individuals (high: $7,500; low: $1,000).
Purpose and activities: To support, develop, and promote health care in five areas: infants/children; adolescents; the elderly; through the discretionary fund for research and development, and health education and information, including drug abuse, AIDS, family planning and services; and through scholarships for local students pursuing health-related fields of study. Giving also for volunteerism, hospices, and nursing.
Fields of interest: Medical school/education; Family planning; Nursing care; Health care; Substance abuse, services; AIDS; Health organizations; AIDS research; Children & youth, services; Youth, services; Family services; Hospices; Aging, centers & services; Voluntarism promotion; Aging.
Types of support: Program development, seed money, technical assistance, scholarships—to individuals, matching funds.
Limitations: Giving limited to Portsmouth, Rye, New Castle, Greenland, Newington, and North Hampton, NH; and Kittery, Eliot, and York, ME. No grants to individuals (except through the foundation scholarship program), or for operating expenses, deficit financing, or travel.
Publications: Annual report (including application guidelines), newsletter, application guidelines, occasional report.
Application information: Application form not required.
Initial approach: Letter (no more than 2 pages)
Copies of proposal: 2
Deadline(s): Feb. 1 for scholarships; last day of month for discretionary fund; Mar. 15 for infant/child/adolescent health; June 1 for general health; Oct. 1 for women's health
Board meeting date(s): 1st Tuesday of Mar., May, Aug., and Nov.; annual meeting, 3rd Tuesday in Apr.
Final notification: Apr. for scholarships; 1 month for discretionary funds; May for infant/child/adolescent health; Aug. for general health; Nov. for women's health
Officers and Trustees:* Kenneth L. Chute,* Pres.; Thomas M. Keane,* V.P.; William Henson,* Treas.; Susan R. Bunting, Exec. Dir.; Robert A. Allard, Peter L. Bergeron, Eileen D. Foley, Wendy A. McLaughlin, M.D.
Number of staff: 2 full-time professional; 1 full-time support.
EIN: 020386319
Grants for Aging:
Community Council of Senior Citizens, Portsmouth, NH, $24,570. For office space at City Hall. 95.
Community Council of Senior Citizens, Portsmouth, NH, $24,570. 94.
Visiting Nurse Association, Portsmouth Regional, Portsmouth, NH, $30,000. For Adult Day Program at Feaster Building. 95.
YMCA, Seacoast Family, Portsmouth, NH, $15,000. For staff training and expansion of senior citizen exercise programs to include programs for handicapped. 94.
York School Department, York, ME, $35,097. For development of collaborative intergenerational health promotion program with York Senior Center and York Hospital. 95.

552
Kingsbury Fund
c/o Kingsbury Corp.
80 Laurel St.
Keene 03431-7020 (603) 352-5212
Contact: James E. O'Neil, Jr., Exec. Trustee

Trust established in 1952 in NH.
Donor(s): Kingsbury Corp.
Foundation type: Company-sponsored
Financial data (yr. ended 12/31/94): Assets, $2,937,845 (M); gifts received, $40,000; expenditures, $174,017; qualifying distributions, $143,057, including $118,125 for 168 grants (high: $20,000; low: $10; average: $2,000), $21,000 for 11 grants to individuals (high: $2,000; low: $1,000) and $3,540 for 29 employee matching gifts.
Purpose and activities: Giving for higher and other education, including scholarships for children of employees; support also for youth agencies and social services and other charitable activities.
Fields of interest: Dance; Arts/cultural programs; Education, association; Education, research; Education, fund raising; Early childhood education; Child development, education; Elementary school/education; Higher education; Adult/continuing education; Education; Natural resource conservation & protection; Environment; Youth development, citizenship; Human services; Youth, services; Child development, services; Aging, centers & services; Community development; Federated giving programs; Government/public administration; Public affairs, citizen participation; Aging.
Types of support: Capital campaigns, equipment, program development, seed money, employee matching gifts, employee-related scholarships, matching funds.
Limitations: Giving limited to Keene, Cheshire County, and the Monadnock region of NH.
Application information: Application form for scholarships only.
Deadline(s): Mar. 30 for scholarships
Board meeting date(s): Spring, summer, and fall
Trustees: James E. O'Neil, Jr., Exec. Trustee; John S. Cookson, Charles J. Hanrahan, James L. Koontz, Priscilla K. Maynard, Jeffery Toner.
EIN: 026004465

553
Mascoma Savings Bank Foundation
c/o Mascoma Savings Bank
67 North Park St.
Lebanon 03766-1317 (603) 448-3650
Contact: Clark A. Griffiths, Chair.
Application address: P.O. Box 435, Lebanon, NH 03766-0435

Established in 1988 in NH.
Donor(s): Mascoma Savings Bank.
Foundation type: Company-sponsored
Financial data (yr. ended 12/31/94): Assets, $1,231,803 (M); gifts received, $250; expenditures, $69,164; qualifying distributions, $62,663, including $62,595 for grants.
Purpose and activities: Grants for a community land trust and a medical center; support also for community development, the disadvantaged, welfare, and general charitable giving, including the arts, adult education, the aged, programs concerning the environment and conservation, animal welfare, hospices, and the homeless.
Fields of interest: Arts/cultural programs; Adult/continuing education; Natural resource conservation & protection; Environment; Animal welfare; Hospitals (general); Human services; Hospices; Aging, centers & services; Homeless, human services; Community development; Aging; Economically disadvantaged; Homeless; General charitable giving.
Types of support: General/operating support, continuing support, annual campaigns, capital campaigns, building/renovation, equipment, land acquisition, endowment funds, program development, seed money, matching funds.
Limitations: Giving primarily in Lebanon, West Lebanon, Enfield, Canaan, Hanover, Meriden, Plainfield, and Lyme, NH, and Hartford, Norwich, and Thetford, VT. No grants to individuals.
Publications: Grants list, application guidelines, informational brochure.
Application information: Application form not required.
Initial approach: Letter (no telephone calls)
Copies of proposal: 1
Deadline(s): Apr. 1 and Oct. 1
Board meeting date(s): Varies
Final notification: 10 weeks
Officer and Trustees:* Clark Griffiths,* Chair. and Secy.; Patricia Brown, Raymond Lagasse, Jacqueline Lary.
Manager: Charter Trust Co.
Number of staff: None.
EIN: 222816632

554
Abbie F. Mosley Trust
c/o First NH Investment Svcs.
P.O. Box 1017
Concord 03302-1017

Established in 1991 in NH.
Donor(s): Abbie F. Mosley.‡
Financial data (yr. ended 05/31/93): Assets, $1,709,770 (M); expenditures, $75,424; qualifying distributions, $64,128, including $61,000 for grants.
Fields of interest: Hospitals (general); American Red Cross; YM/YWCAs & YM/YWHAs; Aging, centers & services; Women, centers & services.
Limitations: Applications not accepted. Giving primarily in Concord, NH.
Application information: Contributes only to pre-selected organizations.
Trustee: First NH Bank, N.A.
EIN: 223126410

555
The Lenna Wilson Perry Foundation, Inc.
Nine Capitol St.
P.O. Box 1256
Concord 03302-1256 (603) 224-2341
Contact: David F. Conley, Chair.

Established 1987 in NH.
Financial data (yr. ended 06/30/95): Assets, $775,165 (M); expenditures, $45,634; qualifying distributions, $43,677, including $25,000 for 1 grant and $18,602 for 3 grants to individuals (high: $13,240; low: $1,692).
Purpose and activities: Support for organizations providing medical, social or economic assistance to the elderly; also awards scholarships to local area residents pursuing degrees in medicine, nursing, and forestry.
Fields of interest: Medical school/education; Nursing care; Aging, centers & services; Aging.
Types of support: Scholarships—to individuals.
Limitations: Giving limited to NH; giving for scholarships limited to Jaffrey, Greenville, Sharon, and Rindge, NH.
Application information: Application form required for scholarships.
Deadline(s): May 16
Officers: David F. Conley, Chair.; Susan J. Harwood, Secy.; Gale F. Hennessey, Treas.
EIN: 222753638

556
Elizabeth Dinsmore Pillsbury Memorial Trust Fund
c/o Margaret McCormack
70 West St.
Milford 03055

Financial data (yr. ended 12/31/95): Assets, $16,665 (M); expenditures, $848; qualifying distributions, $800, including $800 for 28 grants to individuals (high: $50; low: $25).
Purpose and activities: Financial assistance is given to the elderly and uncomplaining poor of Milford, NH; no direct applications from individuals are accepted.
Fields of interest: Aging, centers & services; Aging; Economically disadvantaged.
Types of support: Grants to individuals.
Limitations: Applications not accepted. Giving limited to residents of Milford, NH.
Application information: Recipients are recommended by nursing home directors, clergy, and/or visiting nurses.
Officers and Trustees:* John E. Ruonala,* Chair.; Charlene Dooley,* Secy.; Margaret S. McCormack,* Treas.; Richard Bianchi, Gloria Maguire.
EIN: 237122062

NEW JERSEY

557
Acorn Alcinda Foundation, Inc.
c/o R.J. Kennedy
One Warwick Circle
Springfield 07081

Established in 1984 in VA.
Donor(s): Robert J. Kennedy.
Financial data (yr. ended 05/31/94): Assets, $2,362,151 (M); gifts received, $193,464; expenditures, $121,387; qualifying distributions, $104,365, including $102,500 for 23 grants (high: $42,500; low: $500).
Purpose and activities: Support for organizations which 1) promote scientific research, advancement, and knowledge in wood chemistry, forestry, and tree farming; or 2) assist in developing means and procedures for the recovery, training, and education of the elderly who have become disabled as the result of strokes, heart attacks, or disease.
Fields of interest: Natural resource conservation & protection; Environment; Medical care, rehabilitation; Health associations; Aging, centers & services; Aging.
Types of support: General/operating support.
Limitations: Applications not accepted. Giving primarily on the East Coast. No grants to individuals.
Application information: Contributes only to pre-selected organizations.
Officers and Directors:* Robert J. Kennedy,* Pres. and Treas.; Kit C. Kennedy,* V.P. and Secy.; Jan B. Kennedy,* V.P.
EIN: 541303250

558
AlliedSignal Corporate Contributions Program
101 Columbia Rd.
Morristown 07962-2245 (201) 455-5877
Contact: Alan S. Painter, V.P. and Exec. Dir., Corp. Affairs
Application address: P.O. Box 2245, Morristown, NJ 07962-2245

Financial data (yr. ended 12/31/95): Total giving, $1,000,000, including $1,000,000 for grants ().
Purpose and activities: Most contributions are made through the foundation. The corporation, however, does award some grants. These grants include educational grants, charitable and community awards of less than $1,000 and grants to organizations that do not qualify under IRS 501(c)(3) status.
Fields of interest: Arts/cultural programs; Vocational education; Education; Youth, services; Aging, centers & services; Women, centers & services; Minorities/immigrants, centers & services; Urban/community development; Community development; Engineering & technology; Science; International studies; Government/public administration; Minorities; Aging; Women.
Types of support: Annual campaigns, equipment, research, technical assistance.
Limitations: Giving primarily in headquarters city and major operating locations,including NJ, MD, VA, FL, SC, TN, IN, MO, MI, CA, and AZ. No support for church-related programs. No grants to individuals, or for endowments or loans.
Application information:
Initial approach: Query letter; send requests to nearest company facility
Copies of proposal: 1
Deadline(s): Best time to apply is between July and Aug.
Board meeting date(s): Ongoing as needed
Final notification: Applicant will receive notice only if request is approved

559
AlliedSignal Foundation
(Formerly Allied Corporation Foundation)
101 Columbia Rd.
Morristown 07962-2245
Contact: Alan S. Painter, V.P. and Exec. Dir.
Application address: P.O. Box 2245, Morristown, NJ 07962-2245

Incorporated in 1963 in NY; in 1982 absorbed Bunker Ramo Foundation; in 1984 absorbed Bendix Foundation; merged and incorporated in 1982 in NJ as Allied Corporation Foundation; in 1987 name changed to AlliedSignal Foundation.
Donor(s): AlliedSignal Inc.
Foundation type: Company-sponsored
Financial data (yr. ended 12/31/95): Assets, $0 (M); gifts received, $9,027,042; expenditures, $9,198,577; qualifying distributions, $9,198,577, including $7,558,538 for 800 grants (high: $100,000; low: $1,000; average: $2,000-$50,000) and $1,640,039 for 2,200 employee matching gifts.
Purpose and activities: Support primarily for education, including fellowship and scholarship aid to colleges and universities that are a major source of future employees for the community; grants also for community funds, health, aging, human services, youth agencies, urban affairs, and cultural programs in communities where AlliedSignal has its operations.
Fields of interest: Arts/cultural programs; Elementary school/education; Secondary school/education; Higher education; Business school/education; Engineering school/education; Adult/continuing education; Human services; Youth, services; Community development; Engineering & technology; Engineering; Science; Minorities; Aging.
Types of support: General/operating support, continuing support, annual campaigns, building/renovation, equipment, fellowships, scholarship funds, employee matching gifts.
Limitations: Giving primarily in areas of company operations. No support for church-related programs, special interest groups (such as labor or veterans) unless activity benefits entire community, political organizations, or for international organizations. No grants to individuals, or for endowment funds; no loans.
Application information: The foundation only considers proposals that are submitted through and recommended by AlliedSignal Plant locations. Application form not required.
Initial approach: Letter
Copies of proposal: 1
Deadline(s): Sept. 1

Board meeting date(s): Dec.
Final notification: Only if approved
Officers and Directors:* Lawrence A. Bossidy,* Chair.; Peter M. Kreindler,* Pres.; Alan S. Painter, V.P. and Exec. Dir.; Nancy Garvey, Treas.; Isaac R. Barpal, John W. Barter, Daniel P. Burnham, Fred M. Poses, Paul R. Schindler, James E. Sierk, Richard Wallman.
Number of staff: None.
EIN: 222416651

560
The Albert A. Arditti Foundation, Inc.
c/o United National Bank
1130 Route 22 East, P.O. Box 6000
Bridgewater 08807-0010
Contact: Dirs.
Application address: P.O. Box 4506, Warren, NJ 07060

Established in 1966 in NY.
Financial data (yr. ended 12/31/95): Assets, $524,204 (M); expenditures, $24,050; qualifying distributions, $23,350, including $21,400 for 16 grants (high: $15,000; low: $50).
Fields of interest: Education; Mental health/crisis services; Health associations; Medical research; Aging, centers & services; Christian agencies & churches; Jewish agencies & temples; Religion; Aging.
Limitations: Giving primarily in NJ, NY, and NC.
Application information:
Initial approach: Letter
Deadline(s): None
Officers and Directors:* Arthur A. Arditti,* Pres.; Andrew Arditti, V.P.; Alison Simioni,* Secy.; Shirley Arditti,* Treas.
Number of staff: None.
EIN: 136208776

561
AT&T Company Corporate Giving Program
295 North Maple Ave.
Basking Ridge 07920 (212) 841-4657
Contact: Gary Doran, District Mgr.
University Equipment Prog.: Room 2F-111, P.O. Box 3044, 1100 E. Warrenville Rd., Naperville, IL 60566-7044

AT&T Foundation and AT&T Corporate Contributions Program established in 1984.
Financial data (yr. ended 12/31/95): Total giving, $5,100,000, including $600,000 for 40 in-kind gifts.
Purpose and activities: "For more than one hundred years, AT&T has been steadfastly committed to public service and social responsibility. From the beginning, we've recognized that our business interests are entwined with the well-being of our society. As a result, AT&T has developed an ethic of not just doing well, but doing good. At the heart of our corporate citizenship is a set of beliefs. We believe in innovation - in taking risks and trying new approaches. We believe in diversity - that we are richer when we embrace our differences, and learn from them. We believe in equality - that everyone should have an equal opportunity to achieve success and independence. We believe in human development - that investing in the talents and potential of people is the key to a better society. We believe in involvement - that people working together can make a difference." In addition to giving cash and equipment, the company also supports nonprofit organizations through employee volunteerism.
Fields of interest: Performing arts; Dance; Theater; Music; Historic preservation/historical societies; Arts/cultural programs; Child development, education; Higher education; Engineering school/education; Education; Energy; Environment; Hospitals (general); Health care; Health organizations; Employment; Human services; Youth, services; Child development, services; Family services; Aging, centers & services; Women, centers & services; Minorities/immigrants, centers & services; Federated giving programs; Engineering & technology; Engineering; Science; Minorities; Aging; Women.
Types of support: Employee volunteer services, use of facilities, donated equipment, in-kind gifts.
Limitations: Giving primarily in areas of company operations except for national organizations.
Publications: Informational brochure, biennial report.
Application information: National organizations, or universities, or organizations in New York City should write to NY office; local organizations should write for list of regional Contributions Coordinators. Application form not required.
Initial approach: Letter of inquiry no more than 3 pages; send requests to nearest company facility
Copies of proposal: 1
Deadline(s): None
Number of staff: 1 full-time professional; 8 part-time professional; 1 full-time support; 2 part-time support.

562
The Beer Foundation
131 Brayton St.
Englewood 07631
Contact: M.L. Beer, Trustee

Established about 1965 in NJ.
Financial data (yr. ended 06/30/95): Assets, $455,211 (M); expenditures, $63,923; qualifying distributions, $63,700, including $63,700 for 14 grants (high: $25,000; low: $250).
Fields of interest: Early childhood education; Theological school/education; Medical care, rehabilitation; Human services; Aging, centers & services; Jewish federated giving programs; Jewish agencies & temples; Aging.
Limitations: Applications not accepted. Giving primarily in NJ. No grants to individuals.
Application information: Contributes only to pre-selected organizations.
Trustees: Lovey G. Beer, Murray L. Beer.
EIN: 226073903
Grants for Aging:
Jewish Home and Rehabilitation Center of New Jersey, Jersey City, NJ, $11,000. 94.
Jewish Home and Rehabilitation Center of New Jersey, Jersey City, NJ, $6,000. 95.

563
The Edward & Edna Beron Charitable Foundation
c/o Michael A. Hyett, Esq.
3430 Atlantic Ave.
Atlantic City 08401

Established in 1985 in FL.
Financial data (yr. ended 12/31/93): Assets, $1,025,256 (M); gifts received, $10,000; expenditures, $118,899; qualifying distributions, $113,725, including $112,725 for 11 grants (high: $48,000; low: $100).
Fields of interest: Museums; Aging, centers & services; Jewish federated giving programs; Jewish agencies & temples.
Limitations: Applications not accepted. Giving primarily in FL, NJ, PA, and NY.
EIN: 592276327

564
The Elizabeth Foundation
c/o Lum, Hoens, Abeles, Conant & Danzis
58 Chatham Rd.
Short Hills 07078
Contact: William B. Lum, Exec. Dir.

Incorporated in 1974 in NJ.
Donor(s): The Fund for New Jersey.
Financial data (yr. ended 03/31/95): Assets, $119,173 (M); expenditures, $78,087; qualifying distributions, $52,835, including $35,000 for 3 grants (high: $15,000; low: $5,000).
Fields of interest: Theater; Environment; Human services; Children & youth, services; Aging, centers & services; Community development; Aging.
Limitations: Giving primarily in SC. No grants to individuals.
Application information: Application form not required.
Initial approach: Letter
Deadline(s): None
Officers: Melinda G. Atwood, Pres.; Marcelle Skepelhorn, Secy.; William Boyce Lum, Exec. Dir.
EIN: 237379321
Grants for Aging:
Council on Aging of Jasper County, Hardeeville, SC, $16,000. 94.

565
First Fidelity Bancorporation Giving Program
550 Broad St.
Newark 07102 (201) 565-3200
Contact: Jerome Greco, Sr. V.P., Div. of Public Affairs/Govt.

Centralized in 1990.
Financial data (yr. ended 12/31/92): Total giving, $3,629,441, including $3,549,441 for grants (high: $125,000; low: $25; average: $25-$5,000) and $80,000 for 15 employee matching gifts.
Purpose and activities: "First Fidelity Bancorporation's commitment to community reinvestment is clearly defined and communicated through our subsidiaries to all of our neighborhoods. Each subsidiary is

responsible for vigorous compliance with the corporation's stated goals. These goals include: determining the credit needs of community residents, including low- and moderate-income individuals and families; developing special loan products and services that positively impact the communities' less affluent neighborhoods; instituting specially targeted forms of marketing presentations to ensure widespread dissemination of the availability of relevant credit services and programs; and protecting the soundness and viability of the Bank and its communities, as well as the financial best interest of its customers by insisting on the credit worthiness of all borrowers."
Fields of interest: Performing arts; Humanities; Arts/cultural programs; Education, research; Education, fund raising; Elementary school/education; Higher education; Adult education—literacy & basic skills; Libraries/library science; Reading; Education; Hospitals (general); Health care; Health organizations; Housing/shelter, development; Recreation; Human services; Youth, services; Family services; Aging, centers & services; Homeless, human services; Urban/community development; Community development; Roman Catholic federated giving programs; Government/public administration; Public affairs; Aging; Economically disadvantaged; Homeless; Haiti.
Types of support: Annual campaigns, capital campaigns, endowment funds, conferences/seminars, scholarship funds, technical assistance, employee matching gifts.
Limitations: Giving primarily in headquarters and company locations.
Publications: Corporate report, informational brochure (including application guidelines).
Application information: Application form not required.
Initial approach: Proposal to headquarters; requests/proposal received in the Public Affairs Office by region; written proposal/documentation must be submitted
Copies of proposal: 1
Board meeting date(s): Varies
Final notification: 1 to 4 weeks
Administrators: Jerome D. Greco, Sr. V.P. and Dir., Public Affairs; Fleeta J. Barnes, V.P.; Daniel Newell, V.P.; Kurt Zwikl, V.P.
Number of staff: 11 full-time professional; 1 part-time professional; 7 full-time support.

566
Fox Foundation
P.O. Box 708
Newfield 08344 (609) 697-9226
Contact: Rex S. Fox, Trustee, or Mark B. Fox, Trustee

Established in 1956 in NJ.
Financial data (yr. ended 12/31/95): Assets, $1,865,880 (M); gifts received, $410,930; expenditures, $55,402; qualifying distributions, $54,298, including $54,298 for 85 grants (high: $9,930; low: $50).
Fields of interest: Arts/cultural programs; Hospitals (general); Health care; Health associations; Medical research; Recreation; Children & youth, services; Federated giving programs; Christian agencies & churches; African Americans; Disabled; Aging; Gays/lesbians; Economically disadvantaged; Homeless; General charitable giving.
Types of support: Annual campaigns, endowment funds, scholarship funds, research.
Limitations: Giving primarily in NJ. No grants to individuals.
Publications: Annual report, biennial report, corporate giving report, grants list.
Application information: Application form not required.
Initial approach: Letter
Copies of proposal: 1
Deadline(s): None
Trustees: Mark B. Fox, Rex S. Fox.
Number of staff: None.
EIN: 226057667

567
Grotta Foundation for Senior Care
P.O. Box 189
Maplewood 07079 (201) 761-4900
Contact: Susan R. Friedman, Exec. Dir.

Established in 1993 in NJ.
Financial data (yr. ended 06/30/94): Assets, $6,412,156 (M); gifts received, $5,855; expenditures, $505,753; qualifying distributions, $505,753, including $318,000 for grants (high: $80,000; low: $4,600; average: $1,000-$35,000).
Purpose and activities: Giving primarily to programs that enhance the quality of life for elderly people and their families in New Jersey.
Fields of interest: Aging.
Types of support: Program development, conferences/seminars, publication, seed money, research, technical assistance, matching funds.
Limitations: Giving primarily in Essex, Morris, and Union counties, NJ. No grants to individuals, or for capital or endowment funds, general operating expenses, or deficit financing.
Publications: Informational brochure (including application guidelines).
Application information: Application form required.
Initial approach: Telephone to request guidelines
Copies of proposal: 11
Deadline(s): Sept. 15 and Feb. 25
Board meeting date(s): 3 times a year
Final notification: 5 months
Officers and Directors:* Stephen Greene,* Pres.; Steven Bernstein,* V.P.; Ken Jaffe,* V.P.; Eleanor Lazarus,* Secy.; Nancy Kridel,* Treas.; Susan R. Friedman, Exec. Dir.; Myles Adelman, Nancy Berkley, Nancy Bernstein, Candy Blau, Belinda Eichler, Joseph Gorrell, Murray Granet, Betty Greene, Jane Grotta, Ginnie Grumbach, Lois Hull, Allan Janoff, Arthur Levy, Andrew Liss, Florette Lowy, Sue Nimaroff, Judy Peskin, Nancy Scher, Susan Zucker.
Number of staff: 1 part-time professional.
EIN: 221500655

568
The Hackett Foundation, Inc.
33 Second St.
Raritan 08869 (908) 231-8252
Contact: Ms. Alice T. Hackett, Grants Chair.

Incorporated in 1975 in NY.
Donor(s): William J. Hackett.‡
Financial data (yr. ended 12/31/95): Assets, $15,545,764 (M); expenditures, $1,231,341; qualifying distributions, $1,000,670, including $842,466 for 35 grants (high: $460,000; low: $1,852; average: $1,000-$20,000).
Purpose and activities: Grants primarily to Catholic missions in the U.S. and Third World countries; also giving locally to Catholic social service agencies, nursing homes, hospitals, and schools for the handicapped.
Fields of interest: Human services; Aging, centers & services; Roman Catholic federated giving programs; Roman Catholic agencies & churches; Aging; Developing countries.
Types of support: Equipment.
Limitations: Giving primarily in NJ, NY, and PA; giving nationally and in Third World countries for Catholic missions. No grants to individuals, or for land acquisition, endowment funds, matching gifts, scholarships, fellowships, research, demonstration projects, publications, salaries, or conferences; no loans.
Publications: Annual report (including application guidelines).
Application information: Application form required.
Initial approach: Letter requesting application form
Copies of proposal: 1
Deadline(s): 10th of every month
Board meeting date(s): 2nd Friday of every month
Final notification: 60 days
Officers and Trustees:* R. Kevin Hackett,* Pres. and Treas.; Denis Hackett,* V.P.; Alice T. Hackett,* Secy. and Grants Chair.; Rev. Denis P. Hackett, Sister Patricia Mary Hackett.
Number of staff: 2 full-time professional.
EIN: 132840750
Grants for Aging:
Little Sisters of the Poor, Jeanne Jugan Residence, Bronx, NY, $13,500. For security doors. 94.
Saint Josephs Home for the Elderly of the Little Sisters of the Poor, Totowa, NJ, $10,687. For mattresses and tables. 94.

569
The Hyde and Watson Foundation
437 Southern Blvd.
Chatham 07928 (201) 966-6024
Contact: Robert W. Parsons, Jr., Pres.

The Lillia Babbitt Hyde Foundation incorporated in 1924 in NY; The John Jay and Eliza Jane Watson Foundation incorporated in 1949; consolidation of two foundations into Hyde and Watson Foundation in 1983.
Donor(s): Lillia Babbitt Hyde,‡ Eliza Jane Watson.‡
Financial data (yr. ended 12/31/95): Assets, $75,721,933 (M); expenditures, $4,128,507; qualifying distributions, $3,688,162, including $3,219,140 for 247 grants (high: $100,000; low: $2,100; average: $3,000-$25,000).
Purpose and activities: Support primarily for capital projects of lasting value which tend to increase quality, capacity or efficiency of a grantee's programs or services, such as purchase or relocation of facilities, facility improvements, capital equipment, instructive materials

development, and certain medical research areas. Broad fields include health, education, religion, social services, arts, and humanities. A substantial proportion of grant funds each year will be allocated to projects for which the foundation's support makes a major contribution.
Fields of interest: Performing arts; Humanities; Arts/cultural programs; Education, fund raising; Early childhood education; Child development, education; Elementary school/education; Secondary school/education; Medical school/education; Education; Natural resource conservation & protection; Environment; Hospitals (general); Medical care, rehabilitation; Health care; Substance abuse, services; Mental health/crisis services; Cancer; AIDS; Health organizations; Medical research; Cancer research; AIDS research; Human services; Children & youth, services; Youth, services; Child development, services; Family services; Aging, centers & services; Minorities/immigrants, centers & services; Homeless, human services; Protestant federated giving programs; Religion; Minorities; Disabled; Aging; Economically disadvantaged; Homeless.
Types of support: Capital campaigns, building/renovation, equipment, land acquisition, debt reduction, emergency funds, research, technical assistance, matching funds.
Limitations: Giving includes the metropolitan New York, NY, region and primarily Essex, Union and Morris counties in NJ; No giving outside the U.S. No grants to individuals, or generally for operating budgets, continuing support, annual campaigns, general endowments, deficit financing, scholarships, or fellowships.
Publications: Annual report (including application guidelines), program policy statement, application guidelines.
Application information: Application format required if proposal is considered by grants committee.
Initial approach: Letter
Copies of proposal: 1
Deadline(s): Submit preliminary letter of appeal by Feb. 15 for spring meeting and by Sept. 15 for fall meeting. Appeals are evaluated on an ongoing basis; therefore, early submission of appeals is encouraged
Board meeting date(s): Apr./May and Nov./Dec.
Final notification: After grant or board meeting
Officers and Trustees:* John W. Holman, Jr.,* Chair.; Robert W. Parsons, Jr.,* Pres.; Roger B. Parsons,* V.P. and Secy.; Hunter W. Corbin,* V.P.; H. Corbin Day,* Treas.; Elizabeth R. Curry, William V. Engel, David G. Ferguson, Kate B. Wood.
Staff: Nancy A. Allocco, Grants Administrator.
Number of staff: 7 full-time professional.
EIN: 222425725
Grants for Aging:
Alzheimers Disease and Related Disorders Association, Parsippany, NJ, $15,700. For copier equipment. 94.
Cancer Care of New Jersey, Maplewood, NJ, $15,000. For equipment to establish toll-free counseling line for New Jersey cancer patients and their families. 94.
Partnership for the Homeless, NYC, NY, $10,000. For alteration and modernization of Peter's Place, drop-in center to enhance capacity and effectiveness of programs for elderly, homeless individuals. 94.
Village Center for Care, NYC, NY, $10,000. For construction of Rivington House facility to enhance programs of long-term care for people with AIDS. 94.

570
The Robert Wood Johnson Foundation

P.O. Box 2316
Princeton 08543-2316 (609) 452-8701
Contact: Edward H. Robbins, Proposal Mgr.

Incorporated in 1936 in NJ; became a national philanthropy in 1972.
Donor(s): Robert Wood Johnson.‡
Financial data (yr. ended 12/31/94): Assets, $3,754,153,612 (M); expenditures, $168,717,478; qualifying distributions, $166,923,118, including $135,496,065 for 969 grants, $365,890 for employee matching gifts and $6,398,670 for 4 foundation-administered programs.
Purpose and activities: The foundation is devoted exclusively to health and health care and concentrates its grantmaking in four areas: assuring access to basic health services; improving the way services are organized and provided for people with chronic health conditions; reducing the harm caused by substance abuse; and helping the nation address the problem of rising health care costs.
Fields of interest: Child development, education; Medical school/education; Hospitals (general); Dental care; Health care, cost containment; Nursing care; Health care; Substance abuse, services; Mental health/crisis services; Health organizations; Children & youth, services; Youth, services; Child development, services; Family services; Aging, centers & services; Homeless, human services; Minorities; Native Americans; Disabled; Aging; Homeless.
Types of support: Program development, seed money, research, program-related investments/loans, matching funds.
Limitations: Giving limited to the U.S. No support for international activities, programs or institutions concerned solely with a specific disease, or basic biomedical research. No grants to individuals, or for ongoing general operating expenses, endowment funds, capital costs, including construction, renovation, or equipment, or research on unapproved drug therapies or devices.
Publications: Annual report (including application guidelines), informational brochure, application guidelines, occasional report, newsletter, grants list.
Application information: Application form not required.
Initial approach: Letter
Copies of proposal: 1
Deadline(s): None
Board meeting date(s): Quarterly
Final notification: 6 to 12 months
Officers and Trustees:* Sidney F. Wentz,* Chair.; Steven A. Schroeder, M.D.,* Pres.; Lewis G. Sandy, Exec. V.P.; J. Warren Wood III, V.P., General Counsel and Secy.; John Gilliam, V.P. and Treas.; Peter Goodwin, V.P., Financial Monitoring; Frank Karel III, V.P. for Communications; Ruby P. Hearn, V.P.; Paul S. Jellinek, V.P.; Nancy J. Kaufman, V.P.; James R. Knickman, V.P.; Edward C. Andrews, Jr., M.D., James E. Burke, Robert E. Campbell, David R. Clare, Rheba de Tornyay, Lawrence G. Foster, Linda Griego, John J. Heldrich, John J. Horan, Hon. Thomas H. Kean, Edward E. Matthews, Jack W. Owen, Franklin D. Raines, Norman Rosenberg, M.D., John H. Steele.
Staff: Nancy L. Barrand, Sr. Prog. Officer; Michael P. Beachler, Sr. Prog. Officer; Joel C. Cantor, ScD., Sr. Prog. Officer; Marjorie A. Gutman, Ph.D., Sr. Prog. Officer; Robert G. Hughes, Ph.D., Sr. Prog. Officer; Marguerite Johnson Rountree, Sr. Prog. Officer; Annie Lea Shuster, Sr. Prog. Officer; Beth A. Stevens, Ph.D., Sr. Prog. Officer; Eric P. Coleman, Prog. Officer; Andrea S. Gerstenberger, ScD., Prog. Officer; Rosemary Gibson, Prog. Officer; Janet Heroux, Prog. Officer; Rush L. Russell, Prog. Officer.
Number of staff: 43 full-time professional; 1 part-time professional; 77 full-time support; 5 part-time support.
EIN: 226029397
Grants for Aging:
AIDS Family Services, Buffalo, NY, $25,000. To replicate Faith in Action: Interfaith Volunteer Caregivers Program, designed to develop interfaith caregiving projects for people of all ages with chronic health conditions. 94.
Allegheny Valley Association of Churches, Natrona Heights, PA, $25,000. To replicate Faith in Action: Interfaith Volunteer Caregivers Program, designed to develop interfaith caregiving projects for people of all ages with chronic health conditions. 94.
Alliance for the Mentally Ill, Mid-Valley, Albany, OR, $25,000. To replicate Faith in Action: Interfaith Volunteer Caregivers Program, designed to develop interfaith caregiving projects for people of all ages with chronic health conditions. 94.
Allied Silver Spring Interfaith Services for Seniors Today, Silver Spring, MD, $25,000. To replicate Faith in Action: Interfaith Volunteer Caregivers Program, designed to develop interfaith caregiving projects for people of all ages with chronic health conditions. 94.
Ark of Refuge, San Francisco, CA, $25,000. To replicate Faith in Action: Interfaith Volunteer Caregivers Program, designed to develop interfaith caregiving projects for people of all ages with chronic health conditions. 94.
Beatitudes Center for Developing Older Adult Resources, Phoenix, AZ, $202,784. For matching grant as part of Local Initiative Funding Partners Program-Phase II focusing on initiatives in Chronic Health Conditions. 94.
California Association for Health Services at Home Foundation, Sacramento, CA, $140,650. For uniform health database and patient classification. 94.
Catholic Social Services, Owosso, MI, $25,000. To replicate Faith in Action: Interfaith Volunteer Caregivers Program, designed to develop interfaith caregiving projects for people of all ages with chronic health conditions. 94.
Center for Health and Long-Term Care Research, Waltham, MA, $49,326. Toward understanding geographic variation in use of Medicaid and Medicare home care services. 94.

Church of the Holy Comforter, Burlington, NC, $25,000. To replicate Faith in Action: Interfaith Volunteer Caregivers Program, designed to develop interfaith caregiving projects for people of all ages with chronic health conditions. 94.
Council on Aging of the Midlands, Columbia, SC, $199,762. For matching grant as part of Local Initiative Funding Partners Program-Phase II focusing on initiatives in Chronic Health Conditions. 94.
East Hill Foursquare Church, Gresham, OR, $25,000. To replicate Faith in Action: Interfaith Volunteer Caregivers Program, designed to develop interfaith caregiving projects for people of all ages with chronic health conditions. 94.
Ecumenical Outreach Project, Clarksville, PA, $25,000. To replicate Faith in Action: Interfaith Volunteer Caregivers Program, designed to develop interfaith caregiving projects for people of all ages with chronic health conditions. 94.
First Baptist Church, Hornell, NY, $25,000. To replicate Faith in Action: Interfaith Volunteer Caregivers Program, designed to develop interfaith caregiving projects for people of all ages with chronic health conditions. 94.
First Congregational Church, Memphis, TN, $25,000. To replicate Faith in Action: Interfaith Volunteer Caregivers Program, designed to develop interfaith caregiving projects for people of all ages with chronic health conditions. 94.
First Presbyterian Church of Miami, Miami, FL, $25,000. To replicate Faith in Action: Interfaith Volunteer Caregivers Program, designed to develop interfaith caregiving projects for people of all ages with chronic health conditions. 94.
Florida Department of Elder Affairs, Tallahassee, FL, $217,249. For State Initiatives in Long-Term Care, program aimed at reform of long-term care financing and service delivery systems and development of strategies to broaden access to long-term care coverage. 94.
Friedens Evangelical Church, Port Washington, WI, $25,000. To replicate Faith in Action: Interfaith Volunteer Caregivers Program, designed to develop interfaith caregiving projects for people of all ages with chronic health conditions. 94.
Grace Episcopal Church, Middletown, NY, $25,000. To replicate Faith in Action: Interfaith Volunteer Caregivers Program, designed to develop interfaith caregiving projects for people of all ages with chronic health conditions. 94.
Highlands Community Services Board, Bristol, VA, $25,000. To replicate Faith in Action: Interfaith Volunteer Caregivers Program, designed to develop interfaith caregiving projects for people of all ages with chronic health conditions. 94.
Hope House of Saint Croix Valley, Stillwater, MN, $25,000. To replicate Faith in Action: Interfaith Volunteer Caregivers Program, designed to develop interfaith caregiving projects for people of all ages with chronic health conditions. 94.
Inter-Faith Ministries, Wichita, KS, $25,000. To replicate Faith in Action: Interfaith Volunteer Caregivers Program, designed to develop interfaith caregiving projects for people of all ages with chronic health conditions. 94.
Interfaith Network for Volunteer Caregiving, Waukesha, WI, $25,000. To replicate Faith in Action: Interfaith Volunteer Caregivers Program, designed to develop interfaith caregiving projects for people of all ages with chronic health conditions. 94.
Interfaith Volunteer Caregivers Association of Estero-San Carlos Park, Estero, FL, $25,000. To replicate Faith in Action: Interfaith Volunteer Caregivers Program, designed to develop interfaith caregiving projects for people of all ages with chronic health conditions. 94.
Interfaith Volunteer Caregivers Coalition of Wicomico County, Salisbury, MD, $25,000. To replicate Faith in Action: Interfaith Volunteer Caregivers Program, designed to develop interfaith caregiving projects for people of all ages with chronic health conditions. 94.
Interfaith Volunteer Caregivers of Upper Pinellas, Dunedin, FL, $25,000. To replicate Faith in Action: Interfaith Volunteer Caregivers Program, designed to develop interfaith caregiving projects for people of all ages with chronic health conditions. 94.
Interfaith Volunteer Caregivers, Southwest, Houston, TX, $25,000. To replicate Faith in Action: Interfaith Volunteer Caregivers Program, designed to develop interfaith caregiving projects for people of all ages with chronic health conditions. 94.
Interfaith Volunteer Caregivers, Wake Area, Raleigh, NC, $25,000. To replicate Faith in Action: Interfaith Volunteer Caregivers Program, designed to develop interfaith caregiving projects for people of all ages with chronic health conditions. 94.
Kingston Hospital, Kingston, NY, $1,048,996. For technical assistance and direction to replicate Faith in Action: Interfaith Volunteer Caregivers Program, designed to develop interfaith caregiving projects for people of all ages with chronic health conditions. 94.
Kresfield Adult Social Daycare Center, Washington, NJ, $188,335. For Phase II of New Jersey Health Services Development Program. 94.
Lakeland Hospice, Fergus Falls, MN, $25,000. To replicate Faith in Action: Interfaith Volunteer Caregivers Program, designed to develop interfaith caregiving projects for people of all ages with chronic health conditions. 94.
Lamoille Elders Networking Services, Johnson, VT, $25,000. To replicate Faith in Action: Interfaith Volunteer Caregivers Program, designed to develop interfaith caregiving projects for people of all ages with chronic health conditions. 94.
Long-Term Care Data Institute, Waltham, MA, $45,295. To develop prevalence-based long-term care financing models. 94.
Macomb Baptist Association, Mount Clemens, MI, $25,000. To replicate Faith in Action: Interfaith Volunteer Caregivers Program, designed to develop interfaith caregiving projects for people of all ages with chronic health conditions. 94.
Metropolitan Jewish Geriatric Center, Brooklyn, NY, $474,038. For Building Health Systems for People with Chronic Illnesses which aims at improving organization, delivery and financing of health services. 94.
Middletown Interfaith Housing, Middletown, PA, $25,000. To replicate Faith in Action: Interfaith Volunteer Caregivers Program, designed to develop interfaith caregiving projects for people of all ages with chronic health conditions. 94.
Monadnock Family Services, Keene, NH, $25,000. To replicate Faith in Action: Interfaith Volunteer Caregivers Program, designed to develop interfaith caregiving projects for people of all ages with chronic health conditions. 94.
Outreach House, Hanover, NH, $25,000. To replicate Faith in Action: Interfaith Volunteer Caregivers Program, designed to develop interfaith caregiving projects for people of all ages with chronic health conditions. 94.
Pacific Home and Community Care, Honolulu, HI, $25,000. To replicate Faith in Action: Interfaith Volunteer Caregivers Program, designed to develop interfaith caregiving projects for people of all ages with chronic health conditions. 94.
Project Word, Fairfax, VA, $25,000. To replicate Faith in Action: Interfaith Volunteer Caregivers Program, designed to develop interfaith caregiving projects for people of all ages with chronic health conditions. 94.
Regional AIDS Interfaith Network (RAIN) of the Southern Piedmont, Charlotte, NC, $25,000. To replicate Faith in Action: Interfaith Volunteer Caregivers Program, designed to develop interfaith caregiving projects for people of all ages with chronic health conditions. 94.
Regional AIDS Interfaith Network (RAIN) of the Guilford Area, Greensboro, NC, $25,000. To replicate Faith in Action: Interfaith Volunteer Caregivers Program, designed to develop interfaith caregiving projects for people of all ages with chronic health conditions. 94.
Round Rock Caregivers, Round Rock, TX, $25,000. To replicate Faith in Action: Interfaith Volunteer Caregivers Program, designed to develop interfaith caregiving projects for people of all ages with chronic health conditions. 94.
Saint Marys Family Respite Center, Philadelphia, PA, $25,000. To replicate Faith in Action: Interfaith Volunteer Caregivers Program, designed to develop interfaith caregiving projects for people of all ages with chronic health conditions. 94.
Shepherd Center, Alexandria, LA, $25,000. To replicate Faith in Action: Interfaith Volunteer Caregivers Program, designed to develop interfaith caregiving projects for people of all ages with chronic health conditions. 94.
Sierra Vista Community United Church of Christ, Sierra Vista, AZ, $25,000. To replicate Faith in Action: Interfaith Volunteer Caregivers Program, designed to develop interfaith caregiving projects for people of all ages with chronic health conditions. 94.
South Carolina Christian Action Council, Columbia, SC, $25,000. To replicate Faith in Action: Interfaith Volunteer Caregivers Program, designed to develop interfaith caregiving projects for people of all ages with chronic health conditions. 94.

Trenton Ecumenical Area Ministry, Trenton, NJ, $25,000. To replicate Faith in Action: Interfaith Volunteer Caregivers Program, designed to develop interfaith caregiving projects for people of all ages with chronic health conditions. 94.
Trinity United Presbyterian Church, Uniontown, PA, $25,000. To replicate Faith in Action: Interfaith Volunteer Caregivers Program, designed to develop interfaith caregiving projects for people of all ages with chronic health conditions. 94.
United Protestant Appeal, Miami, FL, $25,000. To replicate Faith in Action: Interfaith Volunteer Caregivers Program, designed to develop interfaith caregiving projects for people of all ages with chronic health conditions. 94.
United Seniors Health Cooperative, DC, $189,831. For analysis of cash disability allowances for long-term care. 94.
University of Maryland, Center on Aging, College Park, MD, $399,172. For technical assistance and direction for State Initiatives in Long-Term Care, program aimed at reform of long-term care financing and service delivery systems and development of strategies to broaden access to long-term care coverage. 94.
Van Ost Institute for Family Living, Englewood, NJ, $46,775. For research on alcoholism among seniors. 94.
Wake Forest University, Bowman Gray School of Medicine, Winston-Salem, NC, $2,163,743. For technical assistance and direction for Partners in Caregiving: The Dementia Services Program, initiative to promote development and growth of adult day centers to address needs of people with chronic, cognitive disorders. 94.

571
Blanche & Irving Laurie Foundation, Inc.

P.O. Box 53
Roseland 07068-5788 (201) 535-5557
Contact: Gene R. Korf, Trustee

Established in 1983 in NJ.
Donor(s): Irving Laurie.‡
Financial data (yr. ended 09/30/95): Assets, $38,200,300 (M); expenditures, $2,250,638; qualifying distributions, $2,011,537, including $1,811,450 for 69 grants (high: $250,000; low: $100; average: $2,000-$25,000).
Purpose and activities: Support for Jewish social services, secondary schools, and cultural organizations; the arts, particularly for theater; and medical and health centers.
Fields of interest: Theater; Arts/cultural programs; Children & youth, services; Aging, centers & services; Jewish agencies & temples; Aging.
Types of support: Building/renovation, program development.
Limitations: Giving primarily in NJ.
Publications: Informational brochure (including application guidelines).
Application information:
Initial approach: Proposal
Copies of proposal: 6
Deadline(s): None
Officer and Trustees: Adelaide Marcus Zagoren,* Pres.; Gene R. Korf, Ruth Marcus Patt, Albert Rich, Harvey Rich, Charles Sloane.
EIN: 222489725
Grants for Aging:
Daughters of Israel Geriatric Center, West Orange, NJ, $27,100. For general support. 95.

572
Liss Foundation

29 Ridge Rd.
Summit 07901
Contact: Amy C. Liss, Pres.

Established in 1965.
Donor(s): Amy C. Liss, Henry R. Liss.
Financial data (yr. ended 12/31/95): Assets, $412,429 (M); expenditures, $81,899; qualifying distributions, $81,349, including $81,276 for 135 grants (high: $5,000; low: $10; average: $25-$25,000).
Purpose and activities: Preference given to local NJ organizations in which the foundation is personally involved or educational institutions the donors are personally connected to.
Fields of interest: Higher education; Medical school/education; Education; Human services; Aging, centers & services; Jewish federated giving programs; Jewish agencies & temples; Aging.
Types of support: General/operating support, endowment funds, curriculum development, scholarship funds.
Limitations: Applications not accepted. Giving primarily in NY and NJ. No grants to individuals or private foundations.
Application information: Contributes only to pre-selected organizations.
Officers: Amy C. Liss, Pres.; Henry R. Liss, V.P.; Theodore Cohn, Secy.
Number of staff: None.
EIN: 226068425
Grants for Aging:
Daughters of Israel Geriatric Center, West Orange, NJ, $250. 95.

573
Angelo Charles Mazzone Foundation, Inc.

Innovation Plaza
275 Paterson Ave.
Little Falls 07424-1658
Contact: John Mazzone, Trustee

Donor(s): Anthony Mazzone.
Financial data (yr. ended 06/30/95): Assets, $116,821 (M); gifts received, $75,000; expenditures, $61,971; qualifying distributions, $61,795, including $61,795 for 11 grants (high: $20,800; low: $1,000).
Fields of interest: Health care; Food services; Human services; Aging, centers & services; Christian agencies & churches.
Types of support: General/operating support.
Limitations: Giving limited to NJ.
Application information:
Initial approach: Letter
Deadline(s): None
Trustees: Anthony Mazzone, John Mazzone.
EIN: 222259353
Grants for Aging:
Passaic County Nutrition Project, Passaic, NJ, $10,000. For elderly program. 95.
Saint Johns Home for the Elderly, Totowa, NJ, $3,995. 95.

574
The Merck Company Foundation

One Merck Dr.
P.O. Box 100
White House Station 08889-0100
(908) 423-2043
Contact: John R. Taylor, Exec. V.P.

Incorporated in 1957 in NJ.
Donor(s): Merck & Co., Inc.
Foundation type: Company-sponsored
Financial data (yr. ended 12/31/94): Assets, $41,544,538 (M); gifts received, $13,200,000; expenditures, $13,627,928; qualifying distributions, $13,559,328, including $12,137,135 for 316 grants (high: $1,999,948; low: $350; average: $10,000-$50,000) and $1,381,492 for employee matching gifts.
Purpose and activities: Support of education, primarily medical, including the Merck Sharp & Dohme International Fellowships in Clinical Pharmacology; community programs, hospitals, medical, biological, and physical sciences, health agencies, public and civic organizations, and colleges in localities where the company has major operations; and an employee matching gift program for colleges, secondary schools, hospitals, public broadcasting and public libraries.
Fields of interest: Elementary school/education; Secondary school/education; Higher education; Business school/education; Medical school/education; Engineering school/education; Education; Environment; Hospitals (general); Pharmacology; Nursing care; Health care; Eye disease; Heart/circulatory disease; Biomedicine; Health organizations; Medical research; Eye research; Heart/circulatory research; Aging, centers & services; Minorities/immigrants, centers & services; Physical/earth sciences; Chemistry; Engineering & technology; Engineering; Biological sciences; Science; Public policy, research; Minorities; Disabled; Aging; Japan.
Types of support: Equipment, program development, seed money, fellowships, employee matching gifts.
Limitations: Giving primarily in areas of company operations, including NJ, PA, GA, VA, and CA. No support for labor or sectarian groups. No grants to individuals (except for fellowships in clinical pharmacology), or for operating budgets, continuing support, annual campaigns, emergency or endowment funds, deficit financing, land acquisition, travel, conferences, publications, or media productions; no loans.
Publications: Corporate giving report.
Application information: Grants usually made at the initiative of the foundation. Application form not required.
Initial approach: Letter
Copies of proposal: 1
Deadline(s): Aug. 31 for fellowships in clinical pharmacology; no set deadline for other grants

Board meeting date(s): Semiannually and as required
Final notification: 2 months
Officers and Directors:* Raymond V. Gilmartin,* Chair.; Kenneth C. Frazier,* Pres.; John R. Taylor, Exec. V.P.; Shuang Ruy Huang, V.P.; Celia A. Colbert, Secy.; A. John Kearney, Treas.; H. Brewster Atwater, Jr., Sir Derek Birkin, Lawrence A. Bossidy, William G. Bowen, Johnnetta B. Cole, Ph.D., Carolyne K. Davis, Lloyd C. Elam, Charles E. Exley, Jr., William N. Kelley, M.D., Samuel O. Thior, M.D., Dennis Weatherstone.
Number of staff: 3 full-time professional; 3 full-time support.
EIN: 226028476

575
Nabisco Foundation
(also known as The National Biscuit Company Foundation Trust)
c/o Nabisco, Inc.
Seven Campus Dr.
Parsippany 07054 (201) 682-7098
Contact: Henry A. Sandbach, V.P., Public Relations

Incorporated in 1953 in NJ.
Donor(s): Nabisco Brands, Inc.
Foundation type: Company-sponsored
Financial data (yr. ended 12/31/94): Assets, $4,899,553 (M); expenditures, $1,376,544; qualifying distributions, $1,357,719, including $1,338,960 for 86 grants (high: $210,000; low: $1,500; average: $5,000-$50,000).
Purpose and activities: Giving largely for higher education and united funds; support also for education, the aged, handicapped, the homeless, hospitals, youth agencies, and cultural programs, including the performing arts.
Fields of interest: Performing arts; Elementary school/education; Higher education; Adult education—literacy & basic skills; Reading; Education; Hospitals (general); Health care; Health organizations; Food services; Youth, services; Aging, centers & services; Homeless, human services; Federated giving programs; Disabled; Aging; Homeless.
Types of support: Building/renovation, emergency funds, scholarship funds, employee matching gifts, employee-related scholarships.
Limitations: No grants to individuals.
Publications: Occasional report.
Application information: Application form not required.
Copies of proposal: 1
Deadline(s): None
Board meeting date(s): As needed
Final notification: Varies
Administrative Committee: John F. Manfredi, Sr. V.P., Corp. Affairs; Henry A. Sandbach, V.P., Public Relations; Robert K. DeVries.
Trustee: Bankers Trust Co.
EIN: 136042595

576
Theresa and Edward O'Toole Foundation
12 Sullivan St.
Westwood 07675
Contact: Chris Degheri, Trustee

Established in 1971.
Donor(s): Theresa O'Toole.‡
Financial data (yr. ended 06/30/95): Assets, $30,242,862 (M); expenditures, $953,893; qualifying distributions, $812,917, including $734,000 for 161 grants (high: $120,000; low: $500; average: $500-$10,000).
Fields of interest: Higher education; Education; Hospitals (general); Human services; Roman Catholic federated giving programs; Roman Catholic agencies & churches; Native Americans; Aging.
Types of support: General/operating support, continuing support, annual campaigns, capital campaigns, building/renovation, emergency funds, program development, seed money, research, matching funds.
Limitations: Giving primarily in NY, NJ, and FL. No grants to individuals, or for endowment funds, scholarships, or fellowships; no loans.
Application information: Application form not required.
Initial approach: Letter
Copies of proposal: 1
Deadline(s): None
Board meeting date(s): Apr. and Oct.
Final notification: 1 month after board meeting
Trustees: Eskridge V. Culver, Chris Degheri, The Bank of New York.
Number of staff: None.
EIN: 136350175
Grants for Aging:
Cabrini Nursing Home, Dobbs Ferry, NY, $2,000. 95.
Saint Anthony Center for Seniors, NYC, NY, $500. 95.

577
George A. Ohl, Jr. Trust
c/o First Fidelity Bank, N.A., NJ; Philanthropic Services Group
765 Broad St.
Newark 07101 (201) 430-4533

Trust established in 1947 in NJ.
Donor(s): George A. Ohl, Jr.‡
Financial data (yr. ended 12/31/95): Assets, $4,321,243 (M); expenditures, $195,040; qualifying distributions, $160,823, including $157,700 for 29 grants (high: $10,000; low: $1,200; average: $1,000-$20,000).
Purpose and activities: Primary areas of interest include start-up or program support for unique projects that complement the educational system at the secondary school level and promote youth development with emphasis on inner-city youth, and human service activities that provide care for the elderly, the economically disadvantaged and the homeless. Giving also for hospitals, hospital building funds, medical research, and health organizations to improve and expand health care services.
Fields of interest: Arts/cultural programs; Elementary/secondary education; Education; Hospitals (general); Health care; Medical research; Human services; Children & youth, services; Aging, centers & services; Homeless, human services; Aging; Economically disadvantaged; Homeless.
Types of support: Capital campaigns, building/renovation, equipment, program development, seed money, research.
Limitations: Giving limited to NJ. No grants to individuals, or for endowment funds or general operating support; no loans.
Publications: Application guidelines.
Application information: Application form not required.
Initial approach: Proposal
Copies of proposal: 1
Deadline(s): Oct. 31
Board meeting date(s): Mar. and Sept.
Final notification: 1 month after board meets
Trustee: First Fidelity Bank, N.A., NJ.
Number of staff: None.
EIN: 226024900

578
F. Mason Perkins Trust
c/o United Jersey Bank
P.O. Box 547
Hackensack 07602

Established in 1971.
Donor(s): F. Mason Perkins.‡
Financial data (yr. ended 12/31/94): Assets, $2,726,536 (M); expenditures, $238,921; qualifying distributions, $220,140, including $216,830 for 11 grants (high: $40,360; low: $2,000) and $3,200 for 1 grant to an individual.
Purpose and activities: Giving exclusively in Italy for aid to the poor and handicapped, particularly children and the aged, and for the protection of animals; 50 percent of giving to six organizations specified by court order.
Fields of interest: Animal welfare; Speech & hearing centers; Nursing care; Health care; Human services; Children & youth, services; Aging, centers & services; Disabled; Aging; Economically disadvantaged; Italy.
Types of support: Continuing support.
Limitations: Applications not accepted. Giving limited to Italy, with emphasis on Assisi and Rome.
Trustee: United Jersey Bank.
EIN: 226040411

579
Gustavus and Louise Pfeiffer Research Foundation
89 Diamond Spring Rd., C.N. 3050
Denville 07834
Contact: Matthew G. Herold, Secy.

Incorporated in 1942 in NY.
Donor(s): Gustavus A. Pfeiffer,‡ Louise F. Pfeiffer.‡
Financial data (yr. ended 12/31/95): Assets, $19,229,113 (M); expenditures, $1,305,702; qualifying distributions, $1,261,360, including $1,132,108 for 16 grants (high: $500,000; low: $31,749; average: $35,000-$50,000).

Purpose and activities: The improvement of public health through the advancement of medicine and pharmacy; the foundation's primary area of interest is in medical and pharmacological research in the areas of 1) predictive factors in cardiovascular disease; 2) prostate and breast cancer, and ovarian tumors; and 3) gerontological immunology.
Fields of interest: Medical research; Cancer research; Heart/circulatory research; Geriatrics research; Immunology research.
Types of support: Seed money, research.
Limitations: No support for national fundraising organizations or publicly financed projects. No grants to individuals, or for building or endowment funds, scholarships, fellowships, travel, conferences, or general purposes; no loans.
Publications: Biennial report (including application guidelines).
Application information: Only 1 application per organization per year will be considered. Application form not required.
Initial approach: 3 copies of letter of inquiry (not to exceed 2 pages)
Copies of proposal: 3
Deadline(s): Feb. 15 and Aug. 15
Board meeting date(s): 3rd Saturday in Apr. and 3rd Friday in Oct.
Final notification: 1 week after annual board meeting
Officers and Directors:* George R. Pfeiffer,* Pres.; H. Robert Herold II,* V.P., and Treas.; Robert H. Pfeiffer,* V.P.; Matthew G. Herold, Jr.,* Secy.; Kimberly Herold Bakaly, Lise P. Chapman, Anne Herold Keeney, Patricia Herold Nagle, Milton C. Rose.
Number of staff: 1 full-time professional.
EIN: 136086299

580
Puder Foundation
c/o V. Goldfarb
55 Speir Dr.
South Orange 07079
Contact: Robert S. Puder, Pres.
Application address: 184 Bradley Place, Palm Beach, FL 33480

Established in 1951.
Financial data (yr. ended 09/30/94): Assets, $107,560 (M); gifts received, $1; expenditures, $65,832; qualifying distributions, $65,832, including $65,636 for 58 grants (high: $15,275; low: $5).
Fields of interest: Museums; Performing arts centers; Arts/cultural programs; Hospitals (general); Nursing home/convalescent facility; Civil rights, advocacy; Jewish agencies & temples; General charitable giving.
Limitations: Giving primarily in Essex County, NJ, and Palm Beach County, FL. No grants to individuals.
Application information: Application form not required.
Deadline(s): None
Officers: Robert S. Puder, Pres.; Virginia B. Goldfarb, V.P.; Margery N. Puder, V.P.
Trustee: Wendy P. Oren.
EIN: 226041489
Grants for Aging:
Daughters of Israel Geriatric Center, West Orange, NJ, $15,275. 94.

581
Fannie E. Rippel Foundation
180 Mount Airy Rd., Suite 200
Basking Ridge 07920-2021 (908) 766-0404
Contact: Edward W. Probert, Pres.

Incorporated in 1953 in NJ.
Donor(s): Julius S. Rippel.‡
Financial data (yr. ended 04/30/95): Assets, $62,394,411 (M); expenditures, $3,160,886; qualifying distributions, $2,719,910, including $2,010,439 for 13 grants (high: $252,675; low: $25,000; average: $100,000-$200,000).
Purpose and activities: The foundation's activities are legally restricted to aid to hospitals, for treatment and/or research concerning cancer or heart disease and for institutions maintained for the relief and care of aged women.
Fields of interest: Hospitals (general); Cancer; Heart/circulatory disease; Cancer research; Heart/circulatory research; Aging.
Types of support: Building/renovation, equipment, program development, research, matching funds.
Limitations: Giving primarily in the Eastern Seaboard states, particularly NJ and New York, NY. No grants to individuals, or for general purposes, operating budgets, continuing support, annual campaigns, deficit financing, scholarships, fellowships, or building funds, no loans.
Publications: Annual report (including application guidelines).
Application information: Application form not required.
Initial approach: Letter of inquiry
Copies of proposal: 1
Deadline(s): None
Board meeting date(s): Approximately 6 times a year
Final notification: Varies
Officers and Trustees:* S. Jervis Brinton, Jr.,* Chair.; Edward W. Probert,* Pres.; Nancy L. Ryan, Secy.; Janet E. Luther, Treas.; Bruce N. Bensley, G. Frederick Hockenjos, John L. Kidde.
Number of staff: 3 full-time professional; 1 full-time support.
EIN: 221559427

582
The Milton Schamach Foundation, Inc.
810 Belmont Ave.
North Haledon 07508 (201) 423-9494
Contact: Jack Goodman, Secy.-Treas.

Incorporated in 1969 in NJ.
Donor(s): Milton Schamach.‡
Financial data (yr. ended 08/31/95): Assets, $2,863,303 (M); expenditures, $189,799; qualifying distributions, $155,186, including $155,186 for 23 grants (high: $28,425; low: $1,000).
Fields of interest: Hospitals (general); Health care; Cancer; Medical research; Cancer research; Aging, centers & services; Aging.
Types of support: Equipment, research.
Limitations: Giving primarily in NJ. No grants to individuals.
Application information: Application form not required.
Initial approach: Letter
Deadline(s): None
Board meeting date(s): 3 or 4 times a year as required
Final notification: 3 to 4 months
Officers and Trustees:* Gene Schamach,* Pres.; Jack Goodman,* Secy.-Treas.; Nancy Freedman, Andrew E.R. Frommelt, Jr., Alvin Goodman, Jay Rubenstein, Howard Schamach, Rhoda Schamach.
Number of staff: 2
EIN: 237051147
Grants for Aging:
Daughters of Miriam Center for the Aged, Clifton, NJ, $27,000. 94.
Daughters of Miriam Center for the Aged, Clifton, NJ, $22,000. 95.

583
The Arnold A. Schwartz Foundation
c/o Kunzman, Coley, Yospin & Bernstein
15 Mountain Blvd.
Warren 07059-6327 (908) 757-7800
Contact: Edwin D. Kunzman, Pres.

Incorporated in 1953 in NJ.
Donor(s): Arnold A. Schwartz.‡
Financial data (yr. ended 11/30/94): Assets, $4,202,509 (M); expenditures, $234,569; qualifying distributions, $207,726, including $195,150 for 48 grants (high: $20,000; low: $500; average: $1,000-$5,000).
Fields of interest: Visual arts; Performing arts; Child development, education; Elementary school/education; Secondary school/education; Higher education; Libraries/library science; Hospitals (general); Mental health/crisis services; Heart/circulatory disease; AIDS; Heart/circulatory research; AIDS research; Housing/shelter, development; Children & youth, services; Child development, services; Family services; Aging, centers & services; Homeless, human services; Urban/community development; Community development; Voluntarism promotion; Minorities; Disabled; Aging; Homeless; General charitable giving.
Types of support: General/operating support, continuing support, annual campaigns, capital campaigns, building/renovation, program development, scholarship funds, matching funds.
Limitations: Giving primarily in Middlesex, Somerset, and Union counties, NJ. No support for religious purposes. No grants to individuals, or for endowment funds; no loans.
Publications: Occasional report, application guidelines.
Application information: Application form not required.
Initial approach: Letter
Copies of proposal: 2
Deadline(s): Aug. 15
Board meeting date(s): Feb., June, Sept., and Nov.
Final notification: Nov. 30
Officers: Edwin D. Kunzman, Pres.; Louis Harding, V.P.; Steven Kunzman, Secy.-Treas.
Trustees: Victor DiLeo, David Lackland, Robert Shapiro, Kenneth Turnbull.

Number of staff: 1 part-time support.
EIN: 226034152
Grants for Aging:
John F. Kennedy Medical Center Foundation, Adult Medical Day Care Center, Edison, NJ, $5,000. For Alzheimer's patient care. 94.

584
Union Camp Charitable Trust
c/o Union Camp Corp.
1600 Valley Rd.
Wayne 07470 (201) 628-2248
Contact: Phyllis Epp

Trust established in 1951 in NY.
Donor(s): Union Camp Corp.
Foundation type: Company-sponsored
Financial data (yr. ended 12/31/95): Assets, $1,200,870 (M); gifts received, $3,000,000; expenditures, $2,062,812; qualifying distributions, $2,053,787, including $2,052,725 for grants (high: $42,000; low: $50; average: $50-$5,000).
Purpose and activities: Grants largely for community funds, higher and other education, including employee-related scholarships and matching gifts, hospitals and health services, social services, youth and women, civic affairs and public interest, civil rights and law and justice, Jewish giving and Protestant welfare, and cultural programs.
Fields of interest: Media/communications; Museums; Humanities; Historic preservation/historical societies; Arts/cultural programs; Education, association; Education, research; Education, fund raising; Early childhood education; Elementary school/education; Secondary school/education; Higher education; Engineering school/education; Adult education—literacy & basic skills; Reading; Education; Natural resource conservation & protection; Energy; Environment; Hospitals (general); Health care; Substance abuse, services; Health associations; Heart/circulatory disease; Biomedicine; Health organizations; Medical research; Heart/circulatory research; Crime/law enforcement; Food services; Housing/shelter, development; Safety/disasters; Human services; Children & youth, services; Youth, services; Family services; Hospices; Aging, centers & services; Women, centers & services; Community development; Voluntarism promotion; Federated giving programs; Marine science; Computer science; Engineering; Public policy, research; Government/public administration; Public affairs; Jewish agencies & temples; Minorities; Disabled; Aging; Women; Economically disadvantaged; General charitable giving.
Types of support: General/operating support, continuing support, annual campaigns, capital campaigns, building/renovation, equipment, land acquisition, endowment funds, emergency funds, program development, seed money, curriculum development, fellowships, internships, scholarship funds, research, consulting services, employee matching gifts, employee-related scholarships, in-kind gifts, matching funds.
Limitations: Giving primarily in areas of company operations and to national organizations (generally east of the Mason-Dixon line). No grants to individuals (except employee-related scholarships); no loans.
Application information: Application form not required.
Initial approach: Letter to request guidelines
Copies of proposal: 1
Deadline(s): None
Board meeting date(s): Nov.
Final notification: By Feb. 1
Officers and Trustees:* W.C. McClelland, Chair. and C.E.O.; J.M. Reed, Vice Chair. and C.F.O.; J.N. Carter, V.P., Industrial Relations; Morgan Guaranty Trust Co. of New York.
Number of staff: 2 part-time professional.
EIN: 136034666

585
The Edward W. and Stella C. Van Houten Memorial Fund
c/o First Fidelity Bank, N.A., NJ; Philanthropic Svcs. Group
765 Broad St.
Newark 07102 (201) 430-4533
Contact: James S. Hohn, V.P., First Fidelity Bank, N.A., NJ

Established in 1979 in NJ.
Donor(s): Stella C. Van Houten.‡
Financial data (yr. ended 11/30/93): Assets, $14,583,622 (M); expenditures, $1,252,346; qualifying distributions, $1,125,746, including $1,125,731 for 35 grants (high: $134,910; low: $3,859; average: $5,000-$100,000).
Purpose and activities: Interests include: 1) Human service activities in Bergen and Passaic counties in NJ; specific areas of interest include orphaned children, the disabled, and the elderly; 2) Hospitals and health organizations in Bergen and Passaic counties in NJ to improve or expand healthcare services; 3) Higher education - primarily medical and nursing training; and 4) Education and care of children.
Fields of interest: Early childhood education; Child development, education; Medical school/education; Education; Hospitals (general); Nursing care; Health care; Biomedicine; Health organizations; Medical research; Human services; Children & youth, services; Youth, services; Child development, services; Aging, centers & services; Aging.
Types of support: Capital campaigns, building/renovation, equipment, program development, seed money, scholarship funds.
Limitations: Giving primarily in Bergen and Passaic counties, NJ. No grants to individuals, or for general operating support or endowments; no loans.
Publications: Application guidelines.
Application information: Application form not required.
Initial approach: Proposal
Copies of proposal: 1
Deadline(s): Feb. 1, May 1, Aug. 1, and Nov. 1
Board meeting date(s): Mar., June, Sept., and Dec.
Final notification: 1 month after board meets
Trustee: First Fidelity Bank, N.A., NJ.
Number of staff: None.
EIN: 226311438

586
Wallerstein Foundation for Geriatric Life Improvement
c/o Melvin J. Wallerstein
200 Executive Dr., Suite 100
West Orange 07052 (201) 731-2500
Contact: Melvin J. Wallerstein, Pres.

Established in 1956 in NJ.
Donor(s): Julian W. Wallerstein.‡
Financial data (yr. ended 11/30/95): Assets, $10,623,858 (M); expenditures, $531,270; qualifying distributions, $397,326, including $397,326 for 33 grants (high: $128,256; low: $100; average: $500-$30,000).
Purpose and activities: Grants primarily for health, education, and human service organizations.
Fields of interest: Health care; Health organizations; Aging, centers & services; Aging.
Types of support: Program development, seed money.
Limitations: Giving primarily in NJ and NY. No grants to individuals.
Application information: Contributes only to established organizations. Application form not required.
Initial approach: Simple 3-page letter
Copies of proposal: 1
Deadline(s): None
Board meeting date(s): Irregular
Officers and Trustees:* Melvin J. Wallerstein,* Pres.; Rita Wallerstein,* Secy.
Number of staff: 1 part-time professional.
EIN: 223052726
Grants for Aging:
Beth Abraham Foundation, Bronx, NY, $35,000. 95.
Daughters of Israel Geriatric Center, West Orange, NJ, $10,000. 95.
National Council on the Aging, DC, $15,000. 95.

587
Joseph and Yetta Weisberger Fund for the Aged Poor and Needy
c/o Schuhalter, Coughlin & Suozzo
50 Division St., Suite 304
Somerville 08876
Contact: Melvin Eisenberg, Mgr.

Established in 1965 in NJ.
Financial data (yr. ended 03/31/95): Assets, $1,610,157 (M); expenditures, $135,506; qualifying distributions, $72,080, including $61,000 for 23 grants (high: $13,000; low: $1,000).
Purpose and activities: Giving for the benefit of the aged, poor, and needy, primarily through Jewish welfare organizations, social services, and health agencies.
Fields of interest: Health care; Human services; Aging, centers & services; Jewish federated giving programs; Aging.
Limitations: Giving primarily in NJ. No grants to individuals.
Application information:
Deadline(s): None
Officer: Melvin Eisenberg, Mgr.
Trustees: Kenneth Fast, Sheldon Fast, Suzanne Fast, Beverly Schuhalter, Murray Schuhalter.
EIN: 226070831

Grants for Aging:
C. Bierman Home for Aged, Montclair, NJ, $2,000. 94.
Central New Jersey Jewish Home for the Aged, Somerset, NJ, $1,000. 94.
Charles Bierman Home, Montclair, NJ, $2,000. 95.
Daughters of Israel Geriatric Center, West Orange, NJ, $13,000. 94.
Daughters of Israel Geriatric Center, West Orange, NJ, $13,000. For disadvantaged services. 95.
Hebrew Passover Relief, Woodbridge, NJ, $1,000. For poor and elderly matzo program. 95.
Jewish Family Service at Metrowest, Florham Park, NJ, $3,000. For aged and poor counseling programs. 95.
Lighthouse Community Services, Newark, NJ, $2,000. For homeless and needy elderly food program. 95.
Mount Sinai Medical Center of Greater Miami, Miami Beach, FL, $5,000. For elderly care. 94.
Mount Sinai Medical Center of Greater Miami, Miami Beach, FL, $5,000. For elderly indigent care programs. 95.
Newark Beth Israel Medical Center, Newark, NJ, $1,000. For Geriatric Resident program. 95.
Saint Barnabas Burn Foundation, Livingston, NJ, $2,000. For aged care programs. 95.
Saint Vincent de Paul Society, Bethpage, NY, $1,000. For elderly financial aid programs. 95.
YMHA of Fairfield, Fairfield, NJ, $3,500. To transport seniors. 94.

NEW MEXICO

588
The Frost Foundation, Ltd.
314 McKenzie St.
Santa Fe 87501 (505) 986-0208
Contact: Mary Amelia Whited-Howell, Pres.

Incorporated in 1959 in LA.
Donor(s): Virginia C. Frost.‡
Financial data (yr. ended 12/31/93): Assets, $28,193,445 (M); expenditures, $1,300,476; qualifying distributions, $1,056,632, including $914,587 for 58 grants (high: $75,000; low: $1,000; average: $5,000-$15,000).
Purpose and activities: Focus on the following areas: 1) Social service and humanitarian needs - includes, but not limited to, violence in the streets, domestic violence, child abuse, specific public health issues such as alcohol and drug abuse, homelessness, and problems of the elderly; 2) Environment - consideration given to programs in research, education, and action to conserve and protect the environment for the well-being and safety of plants, animals, and human beings; and 3) Education - focus on new, innovative, creative, practical programs to address students' and society's needs today, and which recognize our changing sociological structure and concerns.
Fields of interest: Higher education; Business school/education; Education; Natural resource conservation & protection; Environment; Animal welfare; Health care; Substance abuse, services; Mental health/crisis services; Health associations; AIDS; Health organizations; AIDS research; Food services; Human services; Children & youth, services; Youth, services; Family services; Hospices; Aging, centers & services; Women, centers & services; Minorities/immigrants, centers & services; Homeless, human services; Minorities; Native Americans; Aging; Women; Homeless.
Types of support: Continuing support, capital campaigns, equipment, program development, conferences/seminars, publication, seed money, curriculum development, fellowships, technical assistance, matching funds.
Limitations: No support for animal experimentation. No grants to individuals, or for operating expenses, building funds, endowment funds, or scholarships; no loans.
Publications: Application guidelines, biennial report.
Application information: Application form not required.
Initial approach: Telephone or letter; full proposal at foundation's request
Copies of proposal: 1
Deadline(s): Dec. 1 and June 1
Board meeting date(s): Mar. and Sept.
Final notification: 7 to 10 days
Officers and Directors:* Mary Amelia Whited-Howell,* Pres.; Mitchell R. Woodard, Treas.; John A. LeVan, Member, Exec. Comm.; Ann Rogers Gerber, John W. Loftus, Taylor F. Moore, Lee Wheless, Edwin F. Whited.
Number of staff: 1 full-time professional; 1 part-time professional; 1 full-time support.
EIN: 720520342

589
J. F Maddox Foundation
P.O. Box 2588
Hobbs 88241-2588 (505) 393-6338
Contact: Robert J. Reid, Exec. V.P.

Established in 1963 in NM.
Donor(s): J.F. Maddox,‡ Mabel S. Maddox.‡
Financial data (yr. ended 06/30/95): Assets, $96,966,750 (M); expenditures, $6,099,682; qualifying distributions, $4,692,213, including $4,289,934 for 93 grants (high: $2,215,387; low: $250; average: $500-$62,500), $75,000 for 1 program-related investment and $23,300 for 19 loans to individuals.
Purpose and activities: Giving for higher education, including local student loans, community projects where self-help is evident, activities benefiting the elderly, youth, education, and development programs.
Fields of interest: Higher education; Education; Substance abuse, services; Human services; Youth, services; Aging, centers & services; Aging.
Types of support: Building/renovation, equipment, program development, seed money, program-related investments/loans, matching funds, scholarships—to individuals, student loans—to individuals.
Limitations: Giving primarily in southeast NM and western TX; student loans and scholarships limited to Lea County, NM, residents. No support for private foundations. No grants for operating budgets or endowment funds.
Publications: Application guidelines.
Application information: Application form required for student loans and scholarships.
Initial approach: Letter; telephone for recommended proposal outline
Copies of proposal: 1
Deadline(s): None
Board meeting date(s): As needed
Final notification: Varies
Officers and Directors:* James M. Maddox,* Pres.; Robert J. Reid, Exec. V.P.; Don Maddox,* V.P. and Treas.; Harry H. Lynch.
Number of staff: 3 full-time professional; 2 part-time professional; 3 full-time support; 1 part-time support.
EIN: 756023767
Grants for Aging:
Holiday Hill, Coleman, TX, $38,500. For equipment. 95.

590
McCune Charitable Foundation
(Formerly Marshall & Perrine D. McCune Charitable Foundation)
123 East Marcy St., Suite 201
Santa Fe 87501 (505) 983-8300
Contact: Fran Sowers, Assoc. Dir.
Fax: (505) 983-7887

Established in 1988 in PA.
Donor(s): Perrine Dixon McCune,‡ Marshall L. McCune.‡
Financial data (yr. ended 12/31/94): Assets, $81,981,065 (M); expenditures, $5,236,090; qualifying distributions, $5,075,538, including $4,609,163 for 270 grants (high: $500,000; low: $50; average: $5,000-$50,000).
Purpose and activities: Primary areas of interest include the arts, education, youth, health, and social services.
Fields of interest: Visual arts; Museums; Performing arts; Dance; Theater; Music; History & archaeology; Historic preservation/historical societies; Arts/cultural programs; Early childhood education; Child development, education; Elementary school/education; Secondary school/education; Vocational education; Higher education; Adult/continuing education; Adult education—literacy & basic skills; Libraries/library science; Reading; Education; Natural resource conservation & protection; Environment; Animal welfare; Wildlife preservation & protection; Hospitals (general); Family planning; Medical care, rehabilitation; Health care; Substance abuse, services; Mental health/crisis services; Health associations; Cancer; Heart/circulatory disease; AIDS; Alcoholism; Health organizations; Delinquency prevention/services; Crime/law enforcement; Employment; Agriculture; Food services; Nutrition; Housing/shelter, development; Youth development, services; Youth development, citizenship; Human services; Children & youth, services; Youth, services; Child development, services; Family services; Hospices; Aging, centers & services; Women, centers & services; Minorities/immigrants, centers & services; Homeless, human services; Rural development; Community development; Federated giving programs; Public affairs, citizen participation; Leadership development; Public affairs; Minorities; Native Americans; Disabled; Aging; Women; Gays/lesbians; Economically disadvantaged; Homeless.
Types of support: General/operating support, continuing support, annual campaigns, capital

campaigns, building/renovation, equipment, land acquisition, endowment funds, emergency funds, program development, conferences/seminars, seed money, scholarship funds, technical assistance, matching funds.
Limitations: Giving limited to NM, with emphasis on northern NM. No grants to individuals; no endowments.
Publications: Grants list, informational brochure (including application guidelines).
Application information: Contact foundation for current cycle dates for initial approach and deadlines. Application form required.
Initial approach: Letter of inquiry
Copies of proposal: 2
Deadline(s): Changes annually
Board meeting date(s): Changes annually
Officers: Sarah McCune Losinger, Chair.; Owen M. Lopez, Exec. Dir.; Fran Sowers, Assoc. Dir.
Directors: James McCune Edwards, John R. McCune VI.
Number of staff: 2 full-time professional; 1 full-time support.
EIN: 850375622
Grants for Aging:
Community Outreach Program, Tierra Amarilla, NM, $24,900. For Community Liaison Representative in order to formalize and stabilize community crisis intervention team, mental health and domestic violence intervention and to develop materials for continued outreach efforts to youth, family and elderly. 94.
Ocate Community Center, Ocate, NM, $22,000. For kitchen to enhance services provided to senior citizens and for improvement of facility. 94.
Our Lady of Refuge Church, La Union, NM, $14,000. To continue job program for high school youth including assistance to senior citizens with house and yard work, painting, cleaning, and weeding. 94.
Santa Fe Indian School, Santa Fe, NM, $10,000. For youth-tribal elder mentor program. 94.
Santa Fe, City of, Santa Fe, NM, $20,000. To enhance and expand seniors' activities in Senior Centers. 94.

591
Santa Fe Community Foundation
219 West Manhattan
Santa Fe 87501 (505) 988-9715
Contact: Elizabeth Bremner, Exec. Dir.
Application address: P.O. Box 1827, Sante Fe, NM 87504-1827; FAX: (505) 988-1829

Incorporated in 1981 in NM.
Foundation type: Community
Financial data (yr. ended 12/31/95): Assets, $3,826,140 (M); gifts received, $930,002; expenditures, $765,282, including $330,665 for 92 grants (high: $5,000; low: $300; average: $500-$5,000).
Purpose and activities: Giving in the following areas: 1) Health & Human Services, to address growing concerns of the hungry, homeless, children & youth, physically & mentally ill, aged, substance abusers, and the seriously ill and dying; 2) Environment, to preserve the natural beauty of Santa Fe and northern NM, and to address ecological concerns; also supports the conservation, preservation and restoration of this area; 3) Arts and Humanities, to improve the cultural quality of life, including the performing, visual, literary arts, and the humanities; 4) Education, to support the educational needs of persons in traditional academic settings, in out-of-school programs, and to provide reform and innovation in the schools and new approaches to learning; and 5) Civic Affairs, to support the development and improvement of the community in general, and to foster harmony, leadership, and intercultural understanding.
Fields of interest: Visual arts; Performing arts; Music; Humanities; Arts/cultural programs; Child development, education; Elementary school/education; Education; Natural resource conservation & protection; Environment; Animal welfare; Wildlife preservation & protection; Health care; Mental health/crisis services; Cancer; AIDS; Alcoholism; Health organizations; Cancer research; AIDS research; Domestic violence prevention; Food services; Human services; Children & youth, services; Child development, services; Aging, centers & services; Homeless, human services; Civil rights, immigrants; Civil rights, minorities; Civil rights, disabled; Civil rights, women; Civil rights, aging; Civil rights, gays/lesbians; Race/intergroup relations; Community development; Science; Public affairs; Minorities; Asians/Pacific Islanders; African Americans; Latinos; Native Americans; Disabled; Aging; Women; People with AIDS (PWAs); Gays/lesbians; Immigrants/refugees; Economically disadvantaged; Homeless.
Types of support: Continuing support, annual campaigns, emergency funds, program development, publication, seed money, technical assistance, matching funds.
Limitations: Giving limited to northern NM counties, including Santa Fe, Rio Arriba, Los Alamos, Taos, Mora, and San Miguel. No support for religious or political purposes. No grants for general operating support, capital campaigns, or for endowments.
Publications: Annual report, newsletter, informational brochure, application guidelines.
Application information: Application form not required.
Initial approach: Letter of intent
Copies of proposal: 1
Deadline(s): Summer and winter; call for exact date
Board meeting date(s): Monthly
Officers and Directors:* James Duncan, Sr.,* Chair.; Tish Butler,* Vice-Chair.; Gloria Sawtell,* Vice-Chair.; Shirley Berger,* Secy.; James L. Norris,* Treas.; Elizabeth Bremner, Exec. Dir.; and 22 additional directors.
Staff: M. Carlota Baca, Dir. of Progs.; Ann Wellman, Admin. Coord.
Number of staff: 3 full-time professional.
EIN: 850303044

592
Mary Tresco Foundation for the Aged, Inc.
c/o Western Bank, Trust Dept.
P.O. Box 457
Las Cruces 88004
Application address: Directors, P.O. Box 872, Truth or Consequences, NM 87901; Tel.: (505) 894-7171

Foundation type: Operating
Financial data (yr. ended 12/31/94): Assets, $92,875 (M); expenditures, $7,356; qualifying distributions, $5,947, including $5,887 for 1 grant.
Purpose and activities: Support only for programs that benefit senior citizens in NM.
Fields of interest: Aging, centers & services; Aging.
Limitations: Giving limited to NM. No grants to individuals.
Application information:
Initial approach: Letter
Deadline(s): None
Directors: Kenneth James, C. Alvin Rohne, Jack O. Scott.
Trustee: Western Bank.
EIN: 850241940

NEW YORK

593
Louis and Anne Abrons Foundation, Inc.
c/o First Manhattan Co.
437 Madison Ave.
New York 10017 (212) 756-3376
Contact: Richard Abrons, Pres.

Incorporated in 1950 in NY.
Donor(s): Anne S. Abrons,‡ Louis Abrons.‡
Financial data (yr. ended 12/31/94): Assets, $30,000,000 (M); expenditures, $4,083,000; qualifying distributions, $4,004,300, including $4,004,300 for 186 grants (high: $333,000; low: $500; average: $5,000-$50,000).
Purpose and activities: Giving primarily to social welfare agencies, Jewish charities, major New York, NY institutions, civic improvement programs, education, and environmental and cultural projects.
Fields of interest: Museums; Performing arts; Theater; Arts/cultural programs; Dental school/education; Libraries/library science; Education; Environment; Hospitals (general); Family planning; Legal services; Employment; Human services; Children & youth, services; Youth, services; Family services; Aging, centers & services; Minorities/immigrants, centers & services; Community development; Jewish federated giving programs; Jewish agencies & temples; African Americans; Aging; Economically disadvantaged; Homeless.
Types of support: Continuing support, annual campaigns, building/renovation, program development, seed money, scholarship funds, research, technical assistance, consulting services, program-related investments/loans.

Limitations: Applications not accepted. Giving primarily in the metropolitan New York, NY, area. No grants to individuals.
Application information: Contributes only to pre-selected organizations. Telephone calls not accepted. Unsolicited applications not considered or acknowledged.
Board meeting date(s): Feb., June, and Oct.
Officers and Directors:* Richard Abrons,* Pres.; Herbert L. Abrons,* V.P.; Rita Aranow,* V.P.; Alix Abrons, Anne Abrons, Henry Abrons, John Abrons, Leslie Abrons, Peter Abrons, Judith Aranow, Vicki Feiner.
Number of staff: None.
EIN: 136061329

594
Emma J. Adams Memorial Fund, Inc.
c/o Snow, Becker & Krauss, P.C.
605 Third Ave., 25th Fl.
New York 10158
Contact: Edward R. Finch, Jr., Pres.

Incorporated in 1932 in NY.
Donor(s): Emma J. Adams.‡
Financial data (yr. ended 12/31/94): Assets, $2,685,698 (M); gifts received, $1,060; expenditures, $206,814; qualifying distributions, $94,951, including $18,310 for 13 grants (high: $6,000; low: $100; average: $100-$10,000) and $48,398 for grants to individuals (high: $6,000; low: $100).
Purpose and activities: Giving primarily in the greater New York, NY, area to aid the indigent elderly through a church-sponsored meals program and ecumenical medical care; also limited, non-recurring grants to elderly individuals who are agency-sponsored, medically sponsored, or professionally sponsored.
Fields of interest: Aging, centers & services; Protestant agencies & churches; Aging; Economically disadvantaged.
Types of support: Emergency funds, grants to individuals.
Limitations: Giving primarily in the greater metropolitan New York, NY, area. No grants for operating budgets, annual campaigns, administrative expenses, building funds, special projects, endowments, or scholarships; no loans.
Publications: Application guidelines.
Application information: Application form required.
Initial approach: Letter
Copies of proposal: 1
Deadline(s): None
Board meeting date(s): May 1 and Oct. 1
Final notification: Usually within 60 days
Officer: Edward R. Finch, Jr., Pres.
Directors: Pauline Swayze Finch, Rev. Bruce Forbes, Mary D.F. Haskell, Rev. Elizabeth Jacks, Elizabeth Rowe, Henry Weldon.
Number of staff: 1 part-time professional; 1 part-time support.
EIN: 136116503
Grants for Aging:
Association of the Bar of the City of New York, NYC, NY, $1,000. For Robert B. McKay Community Outreach Law program elderly needy services. 94.
Cathedral Church of Saint John the Divine, NYC, NY, $1,000. For Elderly Seniors program. 94.
Hope House, West Palm Beach, FL, $250. For elderly needy program. 94.
Saint Bartholomews Episcopal Church, NYC, NY, $5,000. For Community Ministry program elderly needy feeding project. 94.
Saint Bartholomews Episcopal Church, NYC, NY, $5,000. For elderly needy program. 94.
Saint Phillip Lutheran Church, Brooklyn, NY, $850. For Silver Circle senior citizen's food program. 94.
Stanley M. Isaacs Neighborhood Center, NYC, NY, $6,000. For elderly needy work program. 94.
Victoria Home for Retired Men and Women, Ossining, NY, $500. 94.
Village Nursing Home, NYC, NY, $1,000. 94.

595
Agnew Foundation of New York
c/o Arthur Rubin, NYU Medical Ctr.
550 First Ave.
New York 10016

Financial data (yr. ended 12/31/94): Assets, $880,412 (M); gifts received, $492; expenditures, $49,193; qualifying distributions, $44,564, including $40,000 for 4 grants (high: $22,500; low: $2,500).
Fields of interest: Higher education; Business school/education; Youth, services; Aging, centers & services.
Types of support: Scholarship funds.
Limitations: Applications not accepted. Giving primarily in NY. No grants to individuals.
Application information: Contributes only to pre-selected organizations.
Trustees: Lester I. Brookner, Nathan Ende, Arthur H. Rubin.
EIN: 136277850

596
Albany's Hospital for Incurables
P.O. Box 3628, Executive Park
Albany 12203-0628 (518) 459-7711
Contact: Arnold Cogswell, Pres.

Established in 1974 in NY.
Foundation type: Operating
Financial data (yr. ended 12/31/95): Assets, $2,206,313 (M); gifts received, $20; expenditures, $867,000; qualifying distributions, $867,000, including $848,253 for 16 grants (high: $500,000; low: $2,500; average: $17,000).
Purpose and activities: Grants to facilitate the development of better health care; support for hospitals and hospital building funds, health services and associations, nursing homes, hospices, community health centers, nutrition and hunger, rehabilitation and AIDS programs, and family and regional health planning groups.
Fields of interest: Hospitals (general); Family planning; Medical care, rehabilitation; Nursing care; Health care; Health associations; AIDS; Health organizations; AIDS research; Food services; Nutrition; Family services; Hospices; Aging, centers & services; Aging.
Types of support: General/operating support, continuing support, capital campaigns, building/renovation, equipment, program development, seed money, matching funds.
Limitations: Giving limited to Albany, Schenectady, Rensselaer, and Saratoga counties, NY. No grants to individuals, or for deficit financing, endowment funds, scholarships, or fellowships.
Publications: Program policy statement, application guidelines, multi-year report.
Application information: Application form required.
Initial approach: Telephone, letter, or proposal
Copies of proposal: 1
Deadline(s): 30 days before board meetings
Board meeting date(s): Jan., Apr., June, and Sept.
Final notification: 5 days after board meets
Officer and Trustees:* Arnold Cogswell,* Pres. and Treas.; Mrs. Lewis Muhlfelder, Mrs. Freeman T. Putney, Jr., Robert H. Randles, M.D., Herbert L. Schultz, Jr., Richard F. Sonneborn.
Number of staff: None.
EIN: 141364443

597
Edith & Jacob G. Albert Foundation, Inc.
c/o Richard G. Albert
100 Old Logging Rd.
Bedford 10506

Established in 1981.
Financial data (yr. ended 11/30/94): Assets, $67,218 (M); expenditures, $34,155; qualifying distributions, $32,425, including $32,425 for 19 grants (high: $15,000; low: $25).
Fields of interest: Arts/cultural programs; Hospitals (general); Health associations; Human services; Aging, centers & services; Jewish federated giving programs; Aging.
Limitations: Applications not accepted. Giving nationally, with some emphasis on FL.
Application information: Contributes only to pre-selected organizations.
Officers: Edith Albert, Pres.; Richard G. Albert, Secy.; Allan Albert, Treas.
EIN: 133075651

598
Joseph Alexander Foundation
400 Madison Ave., Suite 906
New York 10017 (212) 355-3688
Contact: Alfred Mackler, V.P.

Established in 1960 in NY.
Donor(s): Joseph Alexander.‡
Financial data (yr. ended 10/31/95): Assets, $15,018,892 (M); expenditures, $948,790; qualifying distributions, $923,352, including $783,000 for 97 grants (high: $250,000; low: $500).
Purpose and activities: Giving primarily for education, including libraries, law and medical schools, and other higher education; health, especially the medical sciences and research, AIDS programs, the elderly and hospices, cancer care, scientific organizations, and hospitals; museums and other arts groups; and Israel, and Jewish welfare and religious organizations.
Fields of interest: Museums; Arts/cultural programs; Higher education; Law school/education; Medical school/education;

Libraries/library science; Education; Hospitals (general); Health care; Health associations; Cancer; AIDS; Biomedicine; Medical research; Cancer research; AIDS research; Human services; Hospices; Aging, centers & services; Jewish federated giving programs; Chemistry; Engineering & technology; Biological sciences; Science; Jewish agencies & temples; Religion; Aging; Israel.
Types of support: General/operating support, annual campaigns, capital campaigns, building/renovation, equipment, endowment funds, program development, conferences/seminars, curriculum development, scholarship funds, research, exchange programs.
Limitations: Giving primarily in Israel and the continental U.S., with emphasis on New York, NY. No grants to individuals.
Publications: Financial statement.
Application information: Application form not required.
Initial approach: Proposal
Copies of proposal: 1
Deadline(s): Submit proposal preferably in Feb. through Aug.
Board meeting date(s): Jan., Apr., July, and Oct.
Officers and Directors:* Arthur S. Alfert,* Pres.; Alfred Mackler,* V.P.; Robert M. Weintraub,* Secy.; Helen Mackler,* Treas.; Harvey A. Mackler.
EIN: 510175951
Grants for Aging:
Dorot, NYC, NY, $7,500. 95.

599
Altman Foundation
220 East 42nd St., Suite 411
New York 10017 (212) 682-0970
Contact: Karen L. Rosa, V.P. and Exec. Dir.

Incorporated in 1913 in NY.
Donor(s): Benjamin Altman,‡ Col. Michael Friedsam.‡
Financial data (yr. ended 12/31/95): Assets, $163,701,859 (M); expenditures, $8,548,890; qualifying distributions, $7,392,500, including $6,790,500 for 178 grants (high: $400,000; low: $2,500; average: $10,000-$100,000).
Purpose and activities: Support for non-public and independent schools and in particular, programs benefiting talented disadvantaged youth; private voluntary hospitals and health centers to extend medical services to the underserved; artistic and cultural institutions for outreach projects; and social welfare programs providing long-term solutions for the needs of the disadvantaged.
Fields of interest: Arts/cultural programs; Early childhood education; Elementary school/education; Secondary school/education; Education; Hospitals (general); Health care; Mental health/crisis services; AIDS; Health organizations; Employment; Housing/shelter, development; Human services; Youth, services; Family services; Aging, centers & services; Minorities; Aging; Economically disadvantaged.
Types of support: Program development.
Limitations: Giving limited to NY, focusing almost entirely on the boroughs of New York City. No grants to individuals, or for building funds.
Publications: Application guidelines.
Application information: Accepts but does not require NYRAG Common Application Form. Application form not required.
Initial approach: 3- to 5-page letter describing project
Copies of proposal: 1
Deadline(s): None
Board meeting date(s): 6 times a year
Officers and Trustees:* Jane B. O'Connell,* Pres.; Karen Rosa, V.P. and Exec. Dir.; Thomas Burke,* V.P.; Julia V. Shea,* Secy.; John P. Casey, Treas.; Bernard Finkelstein, Maurice A. Selinger, Jr., John W. Townsend IV, Victor D. Ziminsky, Jr.
Number of staff: 3 full-time professional; 3 full-time support.
EIN: 131623879
Grants for Aging:
Cancer Care, NYC, NY, $50,000. To continue to expand Children and Adolescents Outreach Project. 95.
Dorot, NYC, NY, $50,000. To continue support of Volunteer Services program. 95.
Educational Alliance, NYC, NY, $25,000. For Project ORE/ORA for homeless and potentially homeless older adults. 95.
Encore Community Center, NYC, NY, $20,000. For Helping Elderly Achieve Longevity program. 95.
Friends and Relatives of Institutionalized Aged, NYC, NY, $25,000. To continue support for Minority Outreach Project. 95.
Gods Love We Deliver, NYC, NY, $30,000. To continue to expand delivery of meals to homebound people with AIDS. 95.
Home Care Associates Training Institute, Bronx, NY, $70,000. For career upgrading program and for one-time grant for entry-level training. 95.
Jewish Community Council of Greater Coney Island, Brooklyn, NY, $15,000. To continue to support home care and transportation services for frail elderly individuals. 95.
Joint Public Affairs Committee for Older Adults, NYC, NY, $30,000. For Institute for Social Action. Grant made through Jewish Association for Services for the Aged. 95.
Medicare Beneficiaries Defense Fund, NYC, NY, $25,000. For renewed support for educational and telephone hotline services for seniors and people with disabilities. 95.
Nursing Home Community Coalition of New York State, NYC, NY, $20,000. To evaluate subacute nursing home care and educate consumers. 95.
Riverdale Senior Center, Bronx, NY, $20,000. To continue support for health promotion program for seniors. 95.
Senior Employment Service, NYC, NY, $30,000. Toward customer service training center for mature workers. Grant made through Fund for Aging Seniors. 95.
West Side One-Stop for Coordinated Senior Services, NYC, NY, $25,000. For One Stop Senior Support Project to prevent elder abuse. 95.

600
American Chai Trust
c/o Perlman & Perlman
220 Fifth Ave., 7th Fl.
New York 10001
Contact: Clifford Perlman, Trustee
Attn: Grant applications

Established in 1968 in NY.
Financial data (yr. ended 02/28/94): Assets, $1,292,180 (M); expenditures, $69,068; qualifying distributions, $68,112, including $59,014 for 46 grants (high: $2,500; low: $500; average: $500-$5,000).
Purpose and activities: Support for human services, including child and family services, the aged, the handicapped, and aid for the indigent; grants also for health, including AIDS, mental health, alcoholism, drug abuse, and cancer care.
Fields of interest: Arts/cultural programs; Child development, education; Vocational education; Adult education—literacy & basic skills; Reading; Health care; Substance abuse, services; Mental health/crisis services; Cancer; Heart/circulatory disease; AIDS; Alcoholism; Health organizations; Cancer research; Heart/circulatory research; AIDS research; Domestic violence prevention; Food services; Human services; Children & youth, services; Youth, services; Child development, services; Family services; Hospices; Aging, centers & services; Homeless, human services; Community development; Roman Catholic agencies & churches; Disabled; Aging; People with AIDS (PWAs); Gays/lesbians; Economically disadvantaged; Homeless.
Types of support: Program development, seed money, research.
Limitations: Giving primarily in the metropolitan New York, NY, area. No grants to individuals, or for building funds.
Publications: Application guidelines.
Application information: Application form required.
Initial approach: Letter requesting application criteria
Copies of proposal: 6
Deadline(s): None
Board meeting date(s): Quarterly
Trustees: Lis Brewer, Pauline Doynow, Kaye Hirsch, Clifford Perlman, Walter Stern.
Number of staff: None.
EIN: 136130992

601
American Federation for Aging Research, Inc.
(also known as AFAR)
1414 Ave. of the Americas, 18th Fl.
New York 10019 (212) 752-2327
Contact: Stephanie Lederman, Exec. Dir.
FAX: (212) 832-2298

Founded in 1981.
Financial data (yr. ended 12/31/95): Assets, $15,148,317; gifts received, $3,620,815; expenditures, $2,740,307; qualifying distributions, $2,499,274, including $2,356,218 for grants and $143,056 for foundation-administered programs.

Purpose and activities: Support for biomedical research on aging and age-related disorders.
Fields of interest: Geriatrics research; Gerontology.
Types of support: Research.
Application information: Contact federation for application guidelines; Application form required for Faculty Scholars Program.
Deadline(s): Jan. 16; Nov. 15 for Faculty Scholars in Aging Research Program
Officers: Hadley C. Ford, Chair.; Frederick A. Terry, Jr., Vice-Chair. and Secy.; Geoffrey A. Thompson, Vice-Chair. and Treas.; Edward H. Northrop, Vice-Chair.; John P. Blass, M.D., Ph.D., Pres.; Dorothy D. Eweson, V.P.; George Martin, M.D., V.P.
Directors: Horace Andrews, and 19 additional directors.
EIN: 133045282

602
Artists Fellowship, Inc.
c/o Salmagundi Club
47 Fifth Ave.
New York 10003
Contact: Richard Pionk, Trustee

Established in 1925.
Financial data (yr. ended 10/31/95): Assets, $2,343,510 (M); gifts received, $13,270; expenditures, $83,341; qualifying distributions, $71,682, including $67,550 for 30 grants to individuals (high: $8,700; low: $500).
Purpose and activities: Grants for emergency aid to visual artists and their families.
Fields of interest: Visual arts; Aging, centers & services; Disabled; Aging.
Types of support: Grants to individuals.
Limitations: Giving primarily in NY.
Application information: Application form required.
Deadline(s): None
Officers and Trustees:* Marc Mellon, Pres.; Morton Kaish,* V.P.; Robert J. Riedinger, Corresponding Secy.; Joan Brandt, Recording Secy.; John R. McCarthy, Treas.; Anne Auberionois, Kim Borelli, Richard Pionk, Claire Romano, John Ross, Wendy Schrijver, Robert Seyffert, Pamela Singleton, Carl Thompson.
EIN: 136122134

603
An Association Foundation, Inc.
(also known as Association for Relief of the Elderly, Inc.)
c/o Donovan, Leisure, Newton & Irvine
30 Rockefeller Plaza
New York 10112
Contact: Trustees

Incorporated in 1815 in NY by Special Act of Legislation.
Donor(s): Virginia Dodge, Bedell Holmes Harned Trust Fund.
Financial data (yr. ended 12/31/94): Assets, $1,110,807 (M); gifts received, $21,500; expenditures, $79,254; qualifying distributions, $79,254, including $63,375 for 81 grants (high: $20,000; low: $100).
Fields of interest: Arts/cultural programs; Elementary/secondary education; Health care; Aging, centers & services; Christian agencies & churches; Aging.
Limitations: Giving primarily in NY and FL. No grants to individuals.
Application information:
Initial approach: Letter
Deadline(s): None
Officers and Trustees:* Anne F. Cox,* Pres.; Howard E. Cox, Jr.,* V.P.; Barbara Bispham,* Secy.; Edward F. Cox, Mazie Livingston Cox, Mrs. Joseph W. Dorland, Mrs. Gregory Scott Hedberg.
EIN: 132596907
Grants for Aging:
Brigham and Womens Hospital, Boston, MA, $5,000. For aged services. 94.
Dana-Farber Cancer Institute, Boston, MA, $5,000. For aged research. 94.
Family Counseling Service, Westhampton Beach, NY, $1,000. For aged counseling program. 94.
Massachusetts General Hospital, Boston, MA, $2,000. For aged research. 94.

604
Charles J. & Burton S. August Family Foundation
c/o Monro Muffler Brake Inc.
200 Holleder Pkwy.
Rochester 14615-3808 (716) 427-2280
Contact: Charles J. August, Trustee, and Burton S. August, Trustee

Established in 1989 in NY.
Financial data (yr. ended 06/30/95): Assets, $2,312,837 (M); gifts received, $81,187; expenditures, $142,071; qualifying distributions, $127,437, including $125,700 for 47 grants (high: $16,000; low: $200; average: $500-$5,000).
Fields of interest: Higher education; Health care; Domestic violence prevention; Human services; Federated giving programs; Disabled; Aging; People with AIDS (PWAs); Homeless; General charitable giving.
Types of support: General/operating support, annual campaigns, capital campaigns, building/renovation, equipment, emergency funds, program development, scholarship funds.
Limitations: Giving limited to Rochester, NY, and surrounding area. No grants to individuals, or for continuing support.
Application information: Application form not required.
Initial approach: Letter
Deadline(s): May 20 and Nov. 20
Board meeting date(s): June 30 and Dec. 30
Final notification: June 30 and Dec. 30
Trustees: Burton S. August, Charles J. August, Jan Lise August, Jean B. August, Madeleine S. August, Robert W. August, Cortland L. Brovitz, Andrew M. Greenstein.
Number of staff: None.
EIN: 161355601

605
The James E. & Jacob A. Barkey Memorial Fund u/w Jeanne E. Barkey
(Formerly The Jeanne E. & Jacob A. Barkey Memorial Fund)
c/o Citibank, N.A., Tax Dept.
One Court Sq., 22nd Fl.
Long Island City 11120
Contact: M.A. Ingram, Trust Officer, Citibank, N.A.
Application address: c/o Citibank, 153 East 53rd St., 5th Fl., New York, NY 10043

Established in 1970 in NY.
Donor(s): Jeanne E. Barkey.‡
Financial data (yr. ended 12/31/94): Assets, $1,172,835 (M); expenditures, $74,264; qualifying distributions, $52,128, including $51,833 for 5 grants (high: $25,917; low: $1,036).
Fields of interest: Nursing home/convalescent facility; Eye disease; Cancer research; Jewish agencies & temples; Aging.
Types of support: General/operating support.
Limitations: Giving primarily in New York, NY. No grants to individuals.
Application information:
Initial approach: Letter
Deadline(s): Dec. 31
Trustees: Robert M. Arias, Citibank, N.A.
EIN: 136327373
Grants for Aging:
Jewish Home and Hospital for Aged, NYC, NY, $2,592. 94.
Sephardic Home for the Aged, Brooklyn, NY, $11,922. 94.

606
David & Minnie Berk Foundation, Inc.
1101 Stewart Ave.
Garden City 11530
Contact: Ronald Berk, Pres.

Established in 1961 in NY.
Donor(s): Members and friends of the Berk family.
Financial data (yr. ended 10/31/95): Assets, $1,438,997 (M); gifts received, $2,500; expenditures, $58,787; qualifying distributions, $37,193, including $37,193 for 8 grants (high: $7,193; low: $1,000; average: $1,000-$40,000).
Fields of interest: Education; Health care; Health associations; Medical research; Human services; Children & youth, services; Aging, centers & services; Aging; Disabled; Economically disadvantaged.
Types of support: Program development, seed money, research.
Limitations: Giving primarily in the tri-state NY, NJ, and PA, area. No support for major national organizations, except for special programs.
Application information: Application form not required.
Initial approach: Letter
Copies of proposal: 10
Deadline(s): None
Board meeting date(s): Quarterly
Officers and Trustees:* Ronald Berk,* Pres.; Joy Levien,* 1st V.P.; Bruce Ostrow,* 2nd V.P.; Kim Green,* Secy.; Amy Berk Kuhn,* Treas.

Number of staff: None.
EIN: 116038062

607
Rhonie & George F. Berlinger Foundation, Inc.
1120 Park Ave.
New York 10128
Contact: Rhonie H. Berlinger, Pres.

Incorporated in 1958 in NY.
Donor(s): George F. Berlinger,‡ Rhonie H. Berlinger.
Financial data (yr. ended 05/31/94): Assets, $64,214 (M); gifts received, $208,214; expenditures, $151,384; qualifying distributions, $151,397, including $150,332 for 92 grants (high: $75,000; low: $30).
Purpose and activities: Giving primarily to a single-disease association; support also for culture, education, Jewish welfare, and child development.
Fields of interest: Arts/cultural programs; Child development, education; Education; Health associations; Alzheimer's disease; Human services; Child development, services; Jewish federated giving programs.
Limitations: Applications not accepted. Giving primarily in New York, NY. No grants to individuals.
Officers: Rhonie H. Berlinger, Pres.; Nancy K. Stone, Secy.-Treas.
Director: Mary Ellen Klee.
EIN: 136084411
Grants for Aging:
Alzheimers Disease and Related Disorders Association, NYC, NY, $75,000. 94.

608
Bennett & Gertrude Berman Foundation, Inc.
1700 Broadway, 23rd Fl.
New York 10019-5905
Contact: Bennett M. Berman, Pres.

Established about 1964.
Donor(s): Bennett M. Berman.
Financial data (yr. ended 09/30/95): Assets, $1,481,848 (M); expenditures, $68,660; qualifying distributions, $61,810, including $61,810 for 24 grants (high: $14,635; low: $25).
Fields of interest: Arts/cultural programs; Health care; Health associations; Human services; Aging, centers & services; Jewish federated giving programs; Jewish agencies & temples; Aging.
Limitations: Giving primarily in New York, NY, and Palm Beach, FL.
Application information:
Initial approach: Letter
Deadline(s): None
Officers: Bennett M. Berman, Pres.; Gertrude Berman, V.P.
EIN: 136163607
Grants for Aging:
Dorot, NYC, NY, $500. 95.
Jewish Home for the Aged of Palm Beach County, West Palm Beach, FL, $25,000. 94.
Morse Geriatric Center, West Palm Beach, FL, $14,635. 95.
Morse Geriatric Center, West Palm Beach, FL, $3,875. 94.

609
David and Susan Bisgeier Foundation, Inc.
c/o Howard Bisgeier
400 West End Ave.
New York 10024

Financial data (yr. ended 10/31/94): Assets, $1,121,597 (M); gifts received, $645; expenditures, $67,965; qualifying distributions, $66,428, including $66,130 for 16 grants (high: $30,000; low: $50).
Fields of interest: Human services; Aging, centers & services; Jewish federated giving programs; Jewish agencies & temples; Aging.
Limitations: Applications not accepted. Giving primarily in Miami, FL. No grants to individuals.
Application information: Contributes only to pre-selected organizations.
Trustees: Howard Bisgeier.
EIN: 136150131
Grants for Aging:
Alzheimers Association, Boca Raton, FL, $2,025. 94.
Miami Jewish Home and Hospital for the Aged, Miami, FL, $30,000. 94.

610
William and Jane Brachfeld Foundation
1155 Douglas Ave.
Riverdale 10471-3519

Established in 1971.
Financial data (yr. ended 06/30/95): Assets, $1,355,047 (M); expenditures, $79,386; qualifying distributions, $70,961, including $70,750 for 25 grants (high: $25,000; low: $50).
Fields of interest: Higher education; Health associations; Alzheimer's disease; Human services; Child development, services; Aging.
Types of support: General/operating support.
Limitations: Applications not accepted. Giving primarily in New York, NY. No grants to individuals.
Application information: Contributes only to pre-selected organizations.
Officers: William Brachfeld, Pres.; Jane Brachfeld, Secy.
Directors: Jonathan Brachfeld, Kenneth Brachfeld.
EIN: 132688349
Grants for Aging:
Alzheimers Disease and Related Disorders Association, NYC, NY, $20,100. 95.
Alzheimers Disease and Related Disorders Association, NYC, NY, $15,200. 94.
Parker Jewish Geriatric Institute, New Hyde Park, NY, $100. 94.

611
The Brookdale Foundation
126 East 56th St.
New York 10022-3668 (212) 308-7355
Contact: Stephen Schwartz, Pres., or Danylle Rudin, Asst. V.P. and Prog. Officer

Incorporated in 1950 in NY.
Donor(s): Henry L. Schwartz,‡ and his brothers.
Financial data (yr. ended 06/30/95): Assets, $7,836,372 (M); expenditures, $728,843; qualifying distributions, $593,774, including $282,728 for 8 grants (high: $75,000; low: $2,000; average: $3,000-$50,000).
Purpose and activities: Support for gerontological and geriatric research and innovative service programs; giving also for higher education and youth.
Fields of interest: Higher education; Education; Medical research; Human services; Children & youth, services; Aging, centers & services; Jewish agencies & temples; Aging.
Types of support: Program development, conferences/seminars, seed money, research, matching funds.
Limitations: Applications not accepted. No grants to individuals, or for operating budgets, continuing support, or annual campaigns; no loans.
Publications: Program policy statement, newsletter.
Application information: Contributes only to pre-selected organizations.
Board meeting date(s): Monthly
Officers and Directors:* Stephen L. Schwartz,* Pres.; Mary Ann Van Clief,* V.P.; Jeanette Pereira, Secy.-Treas.; Katherine Burns, Stanley Epstein, Arthur Norman Field, Lois Juliber, Roy J. Zuckerberg.
Number of staff: 2 full-time professional; 2 part-time support.
EIN: 136076863
Grants for Aging:
Fund for Aging Services, NYC, NY, $5,000. 95.
National Council on the Aging, DC, $2,000. 95.

612
Brooklyn Home for Aged Men
9701 Shore Rd.
Brooklyn 11209 (718) 745-1638
Contact: Nancy K. Munson, Pres.

Established in 1878 in NY.
Financial data (yr. ended 12/31/94): Assets, $1,005,900 (M); gifts received, $26,352; expenditures, $165,576; qualifying distributions, $150,349, including $86,196 for 9 grants (high: $25,000; low: $1,196).
Purpose and activities: Support for homes for the aged.
Fields of interest: Nursing home/convalescent facility; Aging, centers & services; Aging.
Types of support: Continuing support, building/renovation.
Limitations: Applications not accepted. Giving primarily in Brooklyn, NY. No grants to individuals.
Publications: Informational brochure.
Application information: Contributes only to pre-selected organizations.
Board meeting date(s): Nov. and as needed
Officers and Directors:* Nancy K. Munson,* Pres.; Dorothy C. Beckmann,* V.P.; George C. Schaefer,* Secy.-Treas.; Gary A. Henningsen, Eleanor M. Kaufmann, Annette E. Schaefer, Jean C. Weber.

Number of staff: 1 part-time professional.
EIN: 111630754
Grants for Aging:
Augustana Lutheran Home for the Aged, Brooklyn, NY, $5,000. For building improvements. 94.
Brooklyn United Methodist Church Home, Brooklyn, NY, $25,000. For building improvements. 94.
Concord Nursing Home, Brooklyn, NY, $15,000. For building improvements. 94.
New York Congregational Home for the Aged, Brooklyn, NY, $5,000. For enrichment program. 94.
Norwegian Christian Home and Health Center, Brooklyn, NY, $5,000. 94.
Putnam Berkley Publishing, East Rutherford, NJ, $1,196. For senior educational programs. 94.
Saint John Episcopal Home for the Aged and the Blind, Brooklyn, NY, $5,000. For building improvements. 94.
Swedish Home for the Aged, Staten Island, NY, $20,000. For building improvements. 94.

613
Grandma Brown Foundation, Inc.
Scenic and Watson Aves.
P.O. Box 230
Mexico 13114 (315) 963-7221
Contact: Sandra L. Brown, Trustee

Established in 1961 in NY.
Donor(s): Grandma Brown's Beans, Inc.
Foundation type: Company-sponsored
Financial data (yr. ended 03/31/95): Assets, $125,769 (M); expenditures, $26,632; qualifying distributions, $26,554, including $22,000 for 9 grants (high: $5,000; low: $500) and $3,000 for 3 grants to individuals of $1,000 each.
Purpose and activities: Scholarships are available to local area residents.
Fields of interest: Visual arts; Performing arts; Theater; Arts/cultural programs; Business school/education; Libraries/library science; Hospitals (general); Health care; Health organizations; Medical research; Agriculture; Nutrition; Children & youth, services; Aging, centers & services; Community development; Government/public administration; Aging; Economically disadvantaged; General charitable giving.
Types of support: General/operating support, annual campaigns, building/renovation, equipment, endowment funds, fellowships, scholarship funds, research, scholarships—to individuals, matching funds.
Limitations: Giving primarily in Mexico, NY, and in Oswego and Onondoga counties, NY.
Application information: Application form not required.
Initial approach: Letter or telephone
Copies of proposal: 1
Deadline(s): None
Trustees: Loretta C. Brown, Sandra L. Brown.
EIN: 166052275

614
Louise and Arde Bulova Fund, Inc.
c/o Maurice Silberman, C.P.A.
1120 Ave. of the Americas, Suite 612
New York 10036

Established in 1987 in NY.
Donor(s): Louise B. Guilden.
Financial data (yr. ended 09/30/95): Assets, $1,264,216 (M); gifts received, $497,985; expenditures, $29,747; qualifying distributions, $14,831, including $10,000 for 1 grant.
Fields of interest: Residential/custodial care; Aging.
Types of support: General/operating support.
Limitations: Applications not accepted. Giving primarily in NY. No grants to individuals.
Application information: Contributes only to pre-selected organizations.
Officers and Directors:* Paul B. Guilden,* Pres.; Peter Gale,* Secy.-Treas.; Louise B. Guilden.
EIN: 133470502

615
Byrne Foundation
240 Oneida St.
Syracuse 13202-3373
Contact: James Coughlin

Established in 1960 in NY.
Donor(s): Byrne Dairy, Inc., Sonbyrne Sales, Inc., McMahon's of Central Square, Inc.
Financial data (yr. ended 04/30/95): Assets, $108,994 (M); gifts received, $57,500; expenditures, $44,526; qualifying distributions, $44,526, including $44,050 for 62 grants (high: $5,000; low: $100).
Fields of interest: Higher education; Hospitals (general); Roman Catholic agencies & churches; General charitable giving; Aging.
Types of support: General/operating support.
Limitations: Giving primarily in Syracuse, NY.
Application information: Application form required.
Initial approach: Request pre-grant inquiry form
Deadline(s): None
Officer: C. Vincent Byrne, Mgr.
EIN: 166052248

616
Chase Manhattan Corporation Philanthropy Department
One Chase Manhattan Plaza, 56th Fl.
New York 10081
Contact: Steven W. Gelston, Contribs. Officer, Philanthropy
Additional addresses (outside downstate NY): Lorraine Oglesby, Mgr., Contribs. Comm., Chase BankCard Svcs., 100 West University, 5th Fl., Tempe, AZ 85281; Raquel Castro, Mgr., Contribs. Comm., Chase Natl. Corp. Svcs., 801 S. Grand Ave., 16th Fl., Los Angeles, CA 90017; Susan Murray, 2nd V.P., Mktg., Chase Manhattan Bank/CT, 999 Broad St., 2nd Fl., Bridgeport, CT 06604; David Blank, V.P., Chase Manhattan Bank(USA), 802 Delaware Ave., Wilmington, DE 19801; Peter Arps, V.P., Chase Manhattan Private Bank(FL), NA, 1 Royal Palm Way, Palm Beach, FL 33480; Kristin Zuidema, Mgr., Contribs. Comm., Chase Manhattan Bank/IL, 1420 Kensington Rd., Suite 116, Oakbrook, IL 60521; Susan Miller, Mgr., Contribs. Comm., Chase Manhattan Mortgage Corp., P.O. Box 4025, Monroe, LA 71211-4025; Jacqueline King, Asst. V.P., Chase Manhattan Bank/MD, 10 E. Baltimore St., Baltimore, MD 21202; Barbara Burns, 2nd V.P., Public Affairs, Chase Manhattan-Upstate, 1 Lincoln First Sq., CS5, Rochester, NY 14643; Lora Vesel, Mgr., Contribs. Comm., Chase Manhattan Corp.

Financial data (yr. ended 12/31/94): Total giving, $11,394,309, including $9,787,611 for grants (high: $1,100,000; low: $500), $1,347,866 for 2,110 employee matching gifts and $258,832 for in-kind gifts.
Purpose and activities: "Chase Manhattan is dedicated to working with the communities it serves to enhance the well-being of the people who live in them." The company intends for its philantropic program to be an important part of its overall mission. To further this end, Chase pledges, not only money, but employee talents as well, to its grantees. Chase supports numerous nonprofit groups working in the fields of housing and human services, culture and the arts, and education.
Fields of interest: Visual arts; Museums; Performing arts; Dance; Music; Arts/cultural programs; Secondary school/education; Higher education; Education; Health care; Housing/shelter, development; Human services; Youth, services; Homeless, human services; Human services; International relief; Economic development; Community development; Philanthropy/voluntarism; Federated giving programs; Science; Public affairs; Aging; Economically disadvantaged; Homeless; General charitable giving.
Types of support: General/operating support, continuing support, capital campaigns, program development, scholarship funds, technical assistance, employee volunteer services, employee matching gifts, employee-related scholarships, donated equipment, in-kind gifts, matching funds.
Limitations: Giving primarily in headquarters city and state of NY, and national operating locations in AZ; CA; CT; DE; FL; IL; MD; NJ; TX, and 45 countries where Chase has a business presence. No support for religious, fraternal, or veterans' organizations with limited availability

to the general public, single disease organizations, member organizations of any United Way(s) to which the company already contributes, or for non-501(c)(3) organizations. No grants to individuals, except under the employee scholarship program, or for endowments or medical research.
Publications: Corporate giving report (including application guidelines).
Application information: For information on countries where Chase has a business presence, or for other information, please contact Barbara M. Fitts at (212) 552-7036. Application form required.
Initial approach: Letter or telephone requesting funding guidelines. Organizations based in states in which Chase has a company facility should contact that facility; all others should contact headquarters
Copies of proposal: 1
Deadline(s): None
Corporate Responsibility Committee: Thomas G. Labrecque, Chair.
Number of staff: 6 full-time professional; 2 full-time support.

617
Chenango County Community Trust Fund

c/o NBT Bank, N.A.
52 South Broad St.
Norwich 13815-1646 (607) 337-6193
Contact: Sandra Colton, Trust Administrator, NBT Bank, N.A.

Established in 1966 in NY.
Financial data (yr. ended 08/31/95): Assets, $21,221 (M); expenditures, $355; qualifying distributions, $280.
Purpose and activities: Support for geriatric purposes in Chenango County, NY.
Fields of interest: Aging, centers & services; Aging.
Limitations: Giving limited to Chenango County, NY. No grants to individuals.
Publications: 990-PF.
Application information: No grants paid in fiscal 1995. Application form required.
Initial approach: Letter
Copies of proposal: 1
Deadline(s): None
Trustee: NBT Bank, N.A.
Number of staff: None.
EIN: 237193287

618
Clark Charitable Fund

(Formerly Frank E. Clark Charitable Fund)
c/o Chemical Bank
270 Park Ave.
New York 10017 (212) 270-9094
Contact: J.L. McKechnie, V.P., Chemical Bank

Trust established in 1936 in NY.
Donor(s): Frank E. Clark.‡
Financial data (yr. ended 12/31/94): Assets, $4,797,266 (M); expenditures, $206,258; qualifying distributions, $181,227, including $180,000 for grants.
Fields of interest: Mental health/crisis services; Youth, services; Aging, centers & services; Aging.
Limitations: Giving primarily in the metropolitan New York, NY, area.
Application information: Application form not required.
Initial approach: Proposal
Copies of proposal: 1
Deadline(s): Oct. 31
Board meeting date(s): Dec.
Trustee: Chemical Bank.
EIN: 136049032

619
Robert Sterling Clark Foundation, Inc.

135 East 64th St.
New York 10021 (212) 288-8900
Contact: Margaret C. Ayers, Exec. Dir.
FAX: (212) 288-1033

Incorporated in 1952 in NY.
Donor(s): Robert Sterling Clark.‡
Financial data (yr. ended 10/31/95): Assets, $86,501,244 (M); expenditures, $4,589,656; qualifying distributions, $4,927,714, including $3,606,500 for 111 grants (high: $110,000; low: $2,000; average: $10,000-$100,000).
Purpose and activities: The foundation supports projects that: 1) strengthen the management of cultural institutions in New York City and the greater metropolitan area; 2)support arts advocacy; 3) ensure the effectiveness and accountability of public agencies in New York City and State; and 4) protect reproductive freedom and access to family planning services.
Fields of interest: Visual arts; Museums; Performing arts; Dance; Theater; Music; Arts/cultural programs; Education; Environment; Family planning; Human services; Family services; Aging, centers & services; Reproductive rights; Urban/community development; Community development; Public policy, research; Government/public administration; Public affairs; Aging; Economically disadvantaged; Homeless.
Types of support: Continuing support, program development, research.
Limitations: Giving primarily in NY State in the Public Institutions Program, in New York City in the Cultural Program; giving nationally for reproductive freedom projects. No grants to individuals, or for operating budgets, annual campaigns, seed money, emergency funds, deficit financing, capital or endowment funds, matching gifts, scholarships, fellowships, conferences, or films.
Publications: Annual report (including application guidelines), application guidelines.
Application information: Application form not required.
Initial approach: Proposal
Copies of proposal: 1
Deadline(s): None
Board meeting date(s): Jan., Apr., July, and Oct.
Final notification: 1 to 6 months
Officers and Directors:* Winthrop R. Munyan,* Pres.; Miner D. Crary, Jr.,* Secy.; Richardson Pratt, Jr.,* Treas.; Margaret C. Ayers, Exec. Dir.; Raymond D. Horton, John N. Romans, Virginia Hayes Sibbison, John Hoyt Stookey, Joanna Underwood.
Staff: Darcy Hector, Prog. Officer; Laura Wolff, Prog. Officer.
Number of staff: 3 full-time professional; 1 full-time support.
EIN: 131957792
Grants for Aging:
Low Income Housing Fund, NYC, NY, $40,000. For New York City office to make loans and establish loan pools and funding partnerships with government agencies to finance construction, purchase and rehabilitation of low-income co-ops and other housing for homeless, mentally ill, elderly and HIV positive New Yorkers. 95.

620
The Phyllis and Lee Coffey Foundation, Inc.

460 Park Ave., 22nd Fl.
New York 10022 (212) 751-2660

Established in 1952 in NY.
Donor(s): Lee W. Coffey.‡
Financial data (yr. ended 12/31/94): Assets, $569,740 (M); expenditures, $255,896; qualifying distributions, $252,949, including $250,000 for 2 grants (high: $150,000; low: $100,000).
Fields of interest: Museums (ethnic/folk arts); Aging, centers & services; Jewish agencies & temples.
Types of support: General/operating support, continuing support.
Limitations: Applications not accepted. Giving primarily in New York, NY. No grants to individuals.
Publications: 990-PF.
Application information: Contributes only to pre-selected organizations.
Officers: Hannah H. Schneider, Pres.; Walter I. Nathan, V.P. and Secy.; David Ratner, V.P. and Treas.
EIN: 116014056
Grants for Aging:
Metropolitan Jewish Geriatric Center, Brooklyn, NY, $150,000. 94.

621
The Commonwealth Fund

One East 75th St.
New York 10021-2692 (212) 535-0400
Contact: Adrienne A. Fisher, Dir. of Grants Mgt.
FAX: (212) 606-3500; E-mail: cmwf@cmwf.org; URL: http://www.cmwf.org

Incorporated in 1918 in NY.
Donor(s): Mrs. Stephen V. Harkness,‡ Edward S. Harkness,‡ Mrs. Edward S. Harkness.‡
Financial data (yr. ended 06/30/95): Assets, $404,393,034 (M); gifts received, $750,000; expenditures, $20,784,097; qualifying distributions, $17,147,114, including $9,644,132 for 179 grants (high: $500,000; low: $1,000; average: $10,000-$50,000), $999,903 for 51 grants to individuals, $215,612 for 120 employee matching gifts, $408,438 for foundation-administered programs and $555,000 for 2 program-related investments.
Purpose and activities: The fund carries out its mandate of enhancing the common good by

supporting efforts to help Americans live healthy and productive lives and to assist specific groups with serious and neglected problems. The fund's current four national program areas are improving health care services, bettering the health of minority Americans, advancing the well-being of elderly people, and developing the capacities of children and young people. In all its national programs the fund emphasizes prevention and promoting healthy behavior. In its own community, the fund makes grants toward enhancing the quality of life in New York City. The fund also sponsors Harkness Fellowships, which enable future leaders of the United Kingdom, Australia, and New Zealand to study social issues in the United States. Applicants must be citizens of the United Kingdom, Australia or New Zealand. Requirements and length of fellowship vary depending on the country of origin.
Fields of interest: Health care, insurance; Health organizations; Children & youth, services; Minorities; Aging; Women.
Types of support: Fellowships, research, program development, program-related investments/loans.
Limitations: No grants to individuals for general educational support, or for building or endowment funds, general support, capital funds, construction or renovation of facilities, purchase of equipment, or assistance with operating budgets or deficits of established programs or institutions, scholarships, or matching gifts; no loans (except program-related investments).
Publications: Annual report (including application guidelines), grants list, newsletter.
Application information: Application form not required.
Initial approach: Letter or proposal
Copies of proposal: 3
Deadline(s): None
Board meeting date(s): Apr., July, and Nov.
Final notification: Immediately following board meeting
Officers and Directors:* Charles A. Sanders, M.D.,* Chair.; Karen Davis,* Pres.; John E. Craig, Jr., Exec. V.P. and Treas.; Brian Biles, M.D., Sr. V.P.; Lewis W. Bernard, Frank A. Daniels, Jr., Lawrence S. Huntington, Helene L. Kaplan, Walter E. Massey, Robert M. O'Neil, James R. Tallon, Jr., Blenda J. Wilson.
Staff: Mark Melis, Sr. Prog. Officer, Elderly; Kathryn Taaffe Young, Sr. Prog. Officer, Youth; Adrienne A. Fisher, Dir. of Grants Mgt.
Number of staff: 15 full-time professional; 1 part-time professional; 23 full-time support; 2 part-time support.
EIN: 131635260
Grants for Aging:
Alliance for Aging Research, DC, $198,018. For grant in collaboration with John A. Hartford Foundation and other donors to foster development of cadre of physician-scholars on aging as part of Paul Beeson Physician Faculty Scholars in Aging Research Program. 95.
American Association of Retired Persons, DC, $15,000. For conference on future of Medicare. Grant shared with Andrus Foundation. 95.
American Federation for Aging Research (AFAR), NYC, NY, $1,200,000. For grant in collaboration with John A. Hartford Foundation and other donors to foster development of cadre of physician-scholars on aging as part of Paul Beeson Physician Faculty Scholars in Aging Research Program. 95.
Columbia University, Division of Health Sciences, NYC, NY, $155,000. For study to identify trends in use of screening mammography and in rates of avoidable hospitalizations as indicators of access to primary care for older women and minorities. 95.
Harvard University, Cambridge, MA, $106,025. To survey terminally ill patients and their caregivers about health care and social service issues with goal of developing information to improve care at the end of life. Project co-funded by Nathan Cummings Foundation and conducted at Medical School in Boston. 95.
Harvard University, Cambridge, MA, $55,000. For Phase Two of drafting and testing survey to identify health care and social service issues confronting terminally ill patients and their caregivers. Project co-funded by Nathan Cummings Foundation and conducted at Medical School in Boston. 95.
Health Research, Albany, NY, $344,174. For Phase One of Medicaid Home Care Capitation, demonstration model under development to provide long-term care services on partially capitated basis to Medicaid-eligible elderly people in New York. 95.
Independent Production Fund, NYC, NY, $349,237. For staff training program on eliminating restraints in nursing homes through videos and related materials. Grant made in collaboration with Retirement Research Foundation, Kendal Charitable Funds and Beverly Enterprises. 95.
National Family Caregivers Association, Kensington, MD, $14,000. To develop strategic business plan. 95.
National Opinion Research Center, Chicago, IL, $343,250. To survey terminally ill patients and their caregivers about health care and social service issues with goal of developing information to improve care at the end of life. Project co-funded by Nathan Cummings Foundation. 95.
National Press Foundation, DC, $15,000. For White House Conference on Aging media roundtable. 95.
Sylvan House, Orange, CT, $15,000. For intergenerational greenhouse programs for inner-city residents. 95.
University of California, School of Public Health, Berkeley, CA, $80,600. To analyze recent data from National Survey of Families and Households to obtain comprehensive demographic profile of grandparents rearing grandchildren and to learn more about effects of this arrangement for children and grandparents. 95.
University of Massachusetts, Amherst, MA, $20,000. For educational program for trustees of long-term care institutions. 95.
Urban Institute, DC, $158,691. To administer Picker/Commonwealth Program on Fostering the Independence of Frail Elders including overseeing projects, identifying areas for research and producing issue and methodological papers. 95.
Yale-New Haven Hospital, New Haven, CT, $349,946. To implement program to prevent acute confusion in hospitalized elderly patients. 95.

622
The Community Foundation for the Capital Region, Inc.

Executive Park Dr.
Albany 12203 (518) 446-9638
Contact: Judith Lyons, Exec. Dir.

Incorporated in 1968 in NY.
Foundation type: Community
Financial data (yr. ended 12/31/95): Assets, $6,000,000 (M); gifts received, $1,514,475; expenditures, $445,000, including $362,740 for 125 grants (average: $500-$2,500).
Purpose and activities: Some funds restricted by donor designation; for others, emphasis on giving to otherwise unfinanced projects in the public interest. Primary areas of interest include performing and other arts groups, education, and human services, including programs for the homeless and other disadvantaged groups.
Fields of interest: Performing arts; Dance; Arts/cultural programs; Early childhood education; Child development, education; Adult/continuing education; Adult education—literacy & basic skills; Reading; Education; Natural resource conservation & protection; Energy; Wildlife preservation & protection; Hospitals (general); Medical care, rehabilitation; Health care; Substance abuse, services; Mental health/crisis services; AIDS; Health organizations; AIDS research; Food services; Human services; Children & youth, services; Youth, services; Child development, services; Family services; Aging, centers & services; Homeless, human services; Community development; Voluntarism promotion; Government/public administration; Aging; Economically disadvantaged; Homeless; General charitable giving.
Types of support: Program development, seed money, scholarship funds, technical assistance.
Limitations: Giving primarily in Albany, Renssalaer and Saratoga counties, NY. No support for sectarian religious purposes. No grants to individuals, or for endowment or building funds, operating budgets, deficit financing, consulting services, continuing support, emergency funds, land acquisition, annual campaigns, or fellowships; no loans.
Publications: Annual report, application guidelines, newsletter, informational brochure.
Application information: Application form required.
Initial approach: Letter or telephone inquiry
Copies of proposal: 1
Deadline(s): None
Board meeting date(s): Quarterly
Final notification: Quarterly
Officers and Directors:* Edward R. McEwan,* Pres.; Almeda C. Riley,* 1st V.P.; Helen Desfosses,* 2nd V.P.; Barbara Hoehn,* Secy.; Weston F. Cowles,* Treas.; Judith Lyons, Exec. Dir.; and 21 additional directors.
Number of staff: 3 full-time professional.
EIN: 141505623

623
Compass Foundation, Inc.
c/o Allan Rabinowitz
911 Park Ave.
New York 10021

Financial data (yr. ended 12/31/94): Assets, $86,243 (M); gifts received, $1,068; expenditures, $1,966; qualifying distributions, $1,750, including $1,700 for grants.
Fields of interest: Higher education; Nursing care; Aging, centers & services; Aging.
Limitations: Applications not accepted. Giving on a national basis. No grants to individuals.
Application information: Contributes only to pre-selected organizations.
Officers: David Schaffer, Pres.; Irving Reiter, Secy.; Allan Rabinowitz, Treas.
EIN: 116018258

624
Congel-Pyramid Trust
Four Clinton Sq., Suite 106
Syracuse 13202-1075 (315) 476-0532
Contact: Robert V. Hunter, Trustee

Established in 1986 in NY.
Donor(s): Robert J. Congel, Pyramid Co., and subsidiaries.
Financial data (yr. ended 09/30/95): Assets, $813,408 (M); expenditures, $63,508; qualifying distributions, $60,965, including $60,000 for 4 grants (high: $20,000; low: $10,000).
Fields of interest: Arts/cultural programs; Environmental education; Hospitals (general); Geriatrics; Aging, centers & services.
Limitations: Giving primarily in Syracuse, NY. No grants to individuals.
Application information:
Initial approach: Letter
Deadline(s): None
Trustees: Timothy P. Ahern, Robert J. Congel, Suzanne M. Congel, Robert V. Hunter, Bruce A. Kenan, George J. Schunck.
EIN: 166291475
Grants for Aging:
Loretto Geriatric Corporation, Syracuse, NY, $20,000. 94.
Loretto Geriatric Corporation, Syracuse, NY, $20,000. 95.

625
Peter Cooper Charity Fund
c/o Harry Freed
120-4 Benchley Place, Bldg. 24, Apt. 4L
Bronx 10475

Financial data (yr. ended 08/31/95): Assets, $3,508 (M); gifts received, $986; expenditures, $1,045; qualifying distributions, $1,045, including $1,000 for grants.
Fields of interest: Human services; Aging, centers & services; Aging.
Limitations: Applications not accepted. Giving primarily in NY. No grants to individuals.
Application information: Contributes only to pre-selected organizations.
Officers: Samuel J. Prussak, Pres.; Harry Freed, Secy.-Treas.
EIN: 237202045

626
The Cowles Charitable Trust
630 Fifth Ave., Suite 1612
New York 10111-0144 (212) 765-6262
Contact: Gardner Cowles III, Pres.

Trust established in 1948 in NY.
Donor(s): Gardner Cowles.‡
Financial data (yr. ended 12/31/94): Assets, $16,564,237 (M); expenditures, $1,020,679; qualifying distributions, $747,500, including $747,500 for 130 grants (high: $50,000; low: $500).
Purpose and activities: Grants largely for arts and culture, including museums and the performing arts, education, including early childhood, higher, and secondary, hospitals and AIDS programs, social services, including family planning, and community funds.
Fields of interest: Visual arts; Museums; Performing arts; Dance; Theater; Music; Historic preservation/historical societies; Arts/cultural programs; Education, research; Education, fund raising; Early childhood education; Child development, education; Secondary school/education; Higher education; Medical school/education; Adult/continuing education; Adult education—literacy & basic skills; Libraries/library science; Reading; Education; Natural resource conservation & protection; Environment; Animal welfare; Hospitals (general); Family planning; Health care; Substance abuse, services; Mental health/crisis services; Health associations; Cancer; AIDS; Health organizations; Medical research; Cancer research; AIDS research; Food services; Youth development, services; Human services; Children & youth, services; Youth, services; Child development, services; Family services; Hospices; Aging, centers & services; Women, centers & services; Minorities/immigrants, centers & services; Homeless, human services; Race/intergroup relations; Civil rights; Federated giving programs; Population studies; Leadership development; Minorities; Disabled; Aging; Women; Homeless; General charitable giving.
Types of support: General/operating support, continuing support, annual campaigns, capital campaigns, building/renovation, equipment, endowment funds, emergency funds, program development, professorships, seed money, matching funds.
Limitations: Giving primarily in NY, FL, and on the East Coast. No grants to individuals; no loans.
Publications: Annual report, application guidelines.
Application information: Applications from any organizations submitted more than once every 12 months not considered. Telephone inquiries are not considered. Application form not required.
Initial approach: Proposal or letter
Copies of proposal: 7
Deadline(s): Dec. 1, Mar. 1, June 1, and Sept. 1
Board meeting date(s): Jan., Apr., July, and Oct.
Final notification: Within 2 weeks of board meeting
Officers and Trustees:* Gardner Cowles III,* Pres.; Mary Croft, Secy.-Treas.; Charles Cowles, Jan Cowles, Lois Cowles Harrison, Lois Eleanor Harrison, Kate Cowles Nichols, Virginia Cowles Schroth.
Number of staff: 2 part-time professional.
EIN: 136090295

627
Herbert and Jeanine Coyne Foundation
c/o Loeb & Loeb
345 Park Ave.
New York 10154-0037

Established in 1983 in NY.
Donor(s): Herbert J. Coyne, Jeanine Coyne.
Financial data (yr. ended 12/31/95): Assets, $26,070 (M); gifts received, $50,000; expenditures, $29,555; qualifying distributions, $29,311, including $28,450 for 21 grants (high: $4,500; low: $100).
Fields of interest: Arts education; Museums; Arts/cultural programs; Hospitals (general); Human services; Aging, centers & services; Aging.
Limitations: Applications not accepted. Giving primarily in FL, New York, NY, and MA. No grants to individuals.
Application information: Contributes only to pre-selected organizations.
Officers: Herbert J. Coyne, Pres. and Treas.; Jeanine Coyne, V.P. and Secy.
Director: Robert Pelz.
EIN: 133206423

628
Alan H. Cummings Family Foundation
c/o Bessemer Trust Co., N.A., Tax Dept.
630 Fifth Ave.
New York 10111

Established in 1987 in FL.
Donor(s): Nathan Cummings.‡
Financial data (yr. ended 12/31/93): Assets, $985,136 (M); expenditures, $90,848; qualifying distributions, $77,500, including $77,500 for 15 grants (high: $50,000; low: $100).
Fields of interest: Performing arts; Hospitals (general); Aging, centers & services; Jewish federated giving programs; Jewish agencies & temples; Aging.
Limitations: Giving primarily in West Palm Beach, FL. No grants to individuals.
Application information:
Initial approach: Letter
Deadline(s): None
Officers and Directors:* Ruth Cummings Sorensen,* V.P. and Secy.; Helene C. Gordon,* V.P. and Treas.
EIN: 592635536

629
James H. Cummings Foundation, Inc.
1807 Elmwood Ave., Rm. 112
Buffalo 14207 (716) 874-0040
Contact: William J. McFarland, Exec. Dir.

Incorporated in 1962 in NY.
Donor(s): James H. Cummings.‡

Financial data (yr. ended 05/31/95): Assets, $19,761,189 (M); expenditures, $1,022,911; qualifying distributions, $867,999, including $832,077 for 30 grants (high: $150,000; low: $265).
Purpose and activities: Giving exclusively for charitable purposes in advancing medical science, research, and education in the U.S. and Canada and for charitable work among underprivileged boys and girls and aged and infirm persons in designated areas. Priority is given to medical proposals.
Fields of interest: Medical school/education; Hospitals (general); Biomedicine; Medical research; Human services; Children & youth, services; Youth, services; Aging, centers & services; Aging; Economically disadvantaged; Canada.
Types of support: Capital campaigns, building/renovation, equipment, land acquisition, seed money, research, matching funds.
Limitations: Giving limited to the vicinity of the cities of Buffalo, NY, Hendersonville, NC, and Toronto, Ontario, Canada. No support for national health organizations. No grants to individuals, or for annual campaigns, program support, endowment funds, operating budgets, emergency funds, deficit financing, scholarships, fellowships, publications, conferences, or continuing support; no loans.
Publications: Annual report (including application guidelines).
Application information: Application form not required.
Initial approach: Preliminary letter (not more than 2 pages) or telephone inquiry is encouraged
Copies of proposal: 7
Deadline(s): Feb. 15, May 15, Aug. 15, and Nov.15
Board meeting date(s): Mar., June, Sept., and Dec.
Final notification: 4 to 8 weeks
Officers and Directors:* William G. Gisel,* Pres.; Kenneth M. Alford, M.D.,* V.P.; William J. McFarland, Secy. and Exec. Dir.; Robert J.A. Irwin,* Treas.; John P. Naughton, M.D., Robert S. Scheu, John N. Walsh, Jr.
Number of staff: 1 part-time professional; 1 part-time support.
EIN: 160864200
Grants for Aging:
Baycrest Centre for Geriatric Care, North York, Canada, $35,000. 94.

630
The Charles A. Dana Foundation, Inc.
745 Fifth Ave., Suite 700
New York 10151 (212) 223-4040
Contact: Walter Donway, Prog. Dir. (education), Stephen A. Foster, Pres., Cynthia Read, Dir. (Dana Awards), or Barbara Gill, V.P.

Incorporated in 1950 in CT.
Donor(s): Charles A. Dana,‡ Eleanor Naylor Dana.‡
Financial data (yr. ended 12/31/95): Assets, $248,543,324 (M); expenditures, $17,845,081; qualifying distributions, $16,302,549, including $13,206,783 for grants (high: $1,916,148; low: $200; average: $35,000-$400,000), $175,000 for 5 grants to individuals (high: $50,000; low: $25,000; average: $25,000-$50,000), $14,720 for 13 employee matching gifts and $621,018 for 3 foundation-administered programs.
Purpose and activities: Principal interests in education and health, particularly neuroscience, as well as the Charles A. Dana Awards for Pioneering Achievements in health and education.
Fields of interest: Education; Health care; Aging; People with AIDS (PWAs).
Types of support: General/operating support, research, employee matching gifts, matching funds.
Limitations: No support for professional organizations, or for organizations outside the U.S. No grants to individuals (except for the Charles A. Dana Awards), or for capital or endowment funds, operating budgets, continuing support, annual campaigns, building or emergency funds, deficit financing, publications, equipment, conferences, demonstration projects, or colloquia; no loans.
Publications: Annual report (including application guidelines), newsletter, informational brochure (including application guidelines).
Application information: Applications for the Charles A. Dana Awards by nomination only. Grants require matching support from the organizations involved. Application form not required.
Initial approach: Letter (2 pages)
Copies of proposal: 1
Deadline(s): None
Board meeting date(s): Apr., June, Oct., and Dec.
Final notification: 2 to 3 months
Officers and Directors:* David J. Mahoney,* Chair.; Stephen A. Foster, Pres.; Walter G. Corcoran,* V.P.; Barbara E. Gill, V.P.; Clark M. Whittemore, Jr.,* Secy.-Treas.; Edward C. Andrews, Jr., Wallace L. Cook, Charles A. Dana, Jr., Donald B. Marron, Ann D. McLaughlin, Carlos D. Moseley, L. Guy Palmer II, Edward F. Rover, William L. Safire.
Staff: Barbara D. Best, Dir., Media; Walter Donway, Prog. Dir., Education and Health Grants; Richard A. Maxwell, Dir., Special Events; Cynthia A. Read, Dir., Dana Awards Prog.; James F. O'Sullivan, Prog. Officer, Health.
Number of staff: 12 full-time professional; 14 full-time support.
EIN: 066036761

631
The Davenport-Hatch Foundation, Inc.
c/o Deloitte & Touche, L.L.P.
2200 Chase Sq.
Rochester 14604
Application address: L. Weisenfluh, c/o Fleet Trust Co., 45 East Ave., Rochester, NY 14638

Incorporated in 1952 in NY.
Donor(s): Augustus Hatch.‡
Financial data (yr. ended 05/31/95): Assets, $25,408,464 (M); expenditures, $877,656; qualifying distributions, $798,286, including $741,773 for 66 grants (high: $100,000; low: $1,000; average: $2,000-$10,000).
Fields of interest: Performing arts; Higher education; Nursing care; Health care; Human services; Children & youth, services; Aging, centers & services; Community development; Aging.
Types of support: Continuing support, capital campaigns, building/renovation, equipment, seed money, scholarship funds.
Limitations: Giving primarily in the greater Rochester, NY, area. No grants to individuals.
Application information: Application form not required.
Initial approach: Letter including proposal
Copies of proposal: 1
Deadline(s): None
Board meeting date(s): Approximately the 15th of Apr., June, Sept., and Dec.
Final notification: 3 weeks after board meeting; positive responses only
Officers and Directors:* Austin E. Hildebrandt,* Pres.; Helen H. Heller,* Secy.-Treas.; Robert J. Brinkman, William L. Ely, A. Thomas Hildebrandt, Elizabeth G. Hildebrandt, John W. Ross, David H. Taylor, Douglas F. Taylor, Hart Taylor.
Trustee: Fleet Trust Co.
Number of staff: None.
EIN: 166027105

632
Virginia Evans Devereux Memorial Fund
(also known as Evans Devereux Memorial Fund u/w of Virginia E. Devereux)
120 Delaware Ave.
Buffalo 14202 (716) 845-6000
Contact: Sue S. Gardner, Trustee

Financial data (yr. ended 12/31/95): Assets, $763,737 (M); expenditures, $41,834; qualifying distributions, $31,400, including $31,400 for 15 grants (high: $5,400; low: $500).
Fields of interest: Hospitals (general); Food services; Hospices; Aging, centers & services; Aging.
Types of support: Grants to individuals.
Limitations: Giving primarily in western NY.
Application information:
Initial approach: Letter
Deadline(s): None
Trustees: Carol J. Alaimo, Grace Marie Ange, Sue S. Gardner.
EIN: 223115623

633
The Dime Savings Bank of New York, FSB Corporate Giving Program
589 Fifth Ave., 2nd Fl.
New York 10017 (212) 326-6152
Contact: Lorraine Whiffen, External Affairs Mgr.

Purpose and activities: Dime contributions are used to build partnerships with local community organizations. Dime only considers requests from IRS-certified 501 (c)(3) non-profit organizations whose programs and activities focus primarily on affordable housing, basic education, and community enhancement. Other types of support may be considered on an individual basis.

Fields of interest: Arts/cultural programs; Education; Housing/shelter; Youth development; Aging, centers & services; Human services; Community development.
Types of support: Program development, seed money, scholarship funds, donated equipment, in-kind gifts.
Limitations: Giving primarily in greater NY and NJ metropolitan area.
Application information: Giving handled by Ext. Affairs Dept.
Initial approach: letter of request required before application accepted; send requests to headquarters, attention of Ext. Affairs Dept.
Copies of proposal: 1
Deadline(s): Ongoing
Final notification: Ongoing
Administrators: Franklin L. Wright, Dir.; Lorraine Whiffer, Mgr.

634
Jean and Louis Dreyfus Foundation, Inc.
c/o Decker Hubbard and Welden
30 Rockefeller Plaza
New York 10112 (212) 581-7575
Contact: Thomas J. Hubbard, Secy.

Incorporated about 1978 in NY.
Donor(s): Louis Dreyfus.‡
Financial data (yr. ended 12/31/94): Assets, $14,723,900 (M); expenditures, $1,072,530; qualifying distributions, $961,399, including $892,685 for 70 grants (high: $60,000; low: $1,685; average: $5,000-$20,000).
Purpose and activities: Grants primarily to established institutions of the arts; some support also for health and social services, including youth agencies, women, and the elderly, and education, including literacy.
Fields of interest: Arts/cultural programs; Adult education—literacy & basic skills; Reading; Education; Health care; Health associations; Human services; Children & youth, services; Aging, centers & services; Women, centers & services; Aging; Women.
Types of support: Program development, seed money, matching funds.
Limitations: Giving primarily in the New York, NY, area. No grants to individuals.
Application information: Accepts NYRAG Common Application Form. Application form not required.
Initial approach: Proposal
Copies of proposal: 1
Board meeting date(s): Spring and fall
Officers and Directors:* Nicholas L.D. Firth,* Pres.; Thomas J. Sweeney,* V.P. and Treas.; Katherine V. Firth,* V.P.; Thomas J. Hubbard,* Secy.; Edmee de M. Firth,* Exec. Dir.
Number of staff: 1 part-time professional.
EIN: 132947180

635
The Max and Victoria Dreyfus Foundation, Inc.
50 Main St., Suite 1000
White Plains 10606 (914) 682-2008
Contact: Ms. Lucy Gioia, Office Administrator
Additional address: c/o Mary P. Surrey, V.P., 4722 47th St., N.W., Washington, DC 20016

Incorporated in 1965 in NY.
Donor(s): Victoria Dreyfus,‡ Max Dreyfus.‡
Financial data (yr. ended 12/31/94): Assets, $49,451,122 (M); expenditures, $2,319,510; qualifying distributions, $1,911,777, including $1,497,507 for 258 grants (high: $42,500; low: $1,000; average: $1,000-$10,000).
Purpose and activities: Support for hospitals, medical research, education, health and social services, with emphasis on youth and aid to the aged and handicapped, and cultural programs.
Fields of interest: Arts/cultural programs; Education; Hospitals (general); Health care; Medical research; Human services; Youth, services; Aging, centers & services; Disabled; Aging.
Types of support: Program development, research.
Limitations: No grants to individuals.
Application information:
Initial approach: Letter (not exceeding 3 pages) containing brief description of project
Deadline(s): Mar. 31, July 31, and Nov. 30
Board meeting date(s): Usually in mid-Feb., June, and Oct.
Final notification: 6 weeks after application deadline
Officers and Directors:* David J. Oppenheim,* Chair.; Winifred Riggs Portenoy,* Pres.; Nancy E. Oddo,* V.P.; Norman S. Portenoy,* V.P.; Mary P. Surrey,* Secy.-Treas.
Number of staff: 1 full-time support; 1 part-time support.
EIN: 131687573
Grants for Aging:
Friends in Deed, Green Valley, AZ, $12,500. 94.
Iona Senior Services, DC, $20,500. 94.

636
East New York Savings Bank Corporate Giving Program
350 Park Ave.
New York 10022 (212) 350-2584
Contact: Steve Flax, Community Action Assistance Prog.
Application address: East New York Savings Bank, Community Action Assistance Plan Grants Program, 350 Park Ave., 5th Fl., New York, NY 10022

Established in 1989.
Financial data (yr. ended 12/31/94): Total giving, $300,000, including $285,000 for 101 grants (high: $15,000; low: $500; average: $500-$15,000), $15,000 for 25 employee matching gifts; $7,000,000 for 13 loans.
Fields of interest: Housing/shelter, rehabilitation; Housing/shelter, services; Housing/shelter, repairs; Youth development, association; Economic development; Aging.
Types of support: Continuing support.
Limitations: Giving primarily in areas of company operations.
Application information: The program has a staff that handles only giving. Application form required.
Initial approach: Letter of request to headquarters, or go to local branch office for application form
Copies of proposal: 1
Deadline(s): Apr. 14
Board meeting date(s): Monthly
Final notification: June 15
Number of staff: 1 full-time professional.

637
Samuel & Rae Eckman Charitable Foundation
c/o Baer, Marks & Upham
805 Third Ave.
New York 10022
Contact: Stephen F. Selig, Pres.

Established in 1970 in NY.
Donor(s): Rae Eckman,‡ Samuel Eckman.‡
Financial data (yr. ended 12/31/95): Assets, $2,023,569 (M); expenditures, $154,965; qualifying distributions, $126,400, including $126,400 for 18 grants (high: $25,000; low: $1,000; average: $5,000-$10,000).
Purpose and activities: Support for medical research in the field of cancer and allied diseases, assistance to and support of homes for the aged, and education of indigent or underprivileged children.
Fields of interest: Education; Medical research; Cancer research; AIDS research; Children & youth, services; Aging, centers & services.
Types of support: General/operating support, continuing support, research.
Limitations: Giving primarily in New York, NY.
Publications: Application guidelines.
Application information: Application form not required.
Initial approach: Proposal
Copies of proposal: 1
Deadline(s): None
Board meeting date(s): 3 times annually
Final notification: Positive replies only
Officers and Directors:* Stephen F. Selig,* Pres.; Abraham J. Briloff,* V.P.; William B. Norden,* Secy.-Treas.; Arthur W. Murphy.
Number of staff: None.
EIN: 237051411

638
The Eisner Family Fund
c/o Executive Monetary Mgmt., Inc.
919 Third Ave., 11th Fl.
New York 10022

Established in 1988 in NY.
Donor(s): Michael D. Eisner.
Financial data (yr. ended 12/31/94): Assets, $10,669,101 (M); gifts received, $5,595,000; expenditures, $669,277; qualifying distributions, $635,810, including $635,810 for 145 grants (high: $100,000; low: $50).
Purpose and activities: Support primarily for a Jewish home and hospital for the aged and higher education; giving also to hospitals, health organizations, medical research, museums and other cultural organizations, social services, and public media.
Fields of interest: Media/communications; Museums; Arts/cultural programs; Higher

education; Hospitals (general); Health care; Health associations; Medical research; Human services; Aging, centers & services; Jewish federated giving programs; Aging.
Types of support: Continuing support.
Limitations: Applications not accepted. No grants to individuals.
Application information: Contributes only to pre-selected organizations.
Trustees: Michael D. Eisner, Margot E. Freedman.
Number of staff: None.
EIN: 133486425
Grants for Aging:
Jewish Home and Hospital for Aged, NYC, NY, $100,000. 94.

639
Mark & Helene Eisner Foundation, Inc.
c/o Merwin Lewis
645 Madison Ave.
New York 10022

Established in 1987 in NY.
Donor(s): Helene Rittenberg.
Financial data (yr. ended 08/31/94): Assets, $524,390 (M); expenditures, $26,420; qualifying distributions, $25,965, including $25,000 for 14 grants (high: $5,500; low: $500).
Fields of interest: Music; Education; Aging, centers & services; Jewish agencies & temples; Aging.
Limitations: Applications not accepted. Giving primarily in NY.
Application information: Contributes only to pre-selected organizations.
Officers: Helene Rittenberg, Pres. and Treas.; Mark Eisner, Jr., V.P.; Barbara Lans, V.P.; Deborah Lans, V.P.; Merwin Lewis, Secy.
EIN: 133357583

640
Blanche T. Enders Charitable Trust
c/o Chemical Bank
270 Park Ave., 21st Fl.
New York 10017
Contact: John Boncada

Financial data (yr. ended 12/31/94): Assets, $3,332,006 (M); expenditures, $158,241; qualifying distributions, $123,877, including $120,500 for 27 grants (high: $10,000; low: $2,000).
Purpose and activities: "Grants are restricted to organizations involved with children's education, care of the blind, crippled or aged, and the elimination of cruelty to animals."
Fields of interest: Child development, education; Education; Animal welfare; Children & youth, services; Child development, services; Aging, centers & services; Aging.
Limitations: Giving primarily in New York, NY. No grants to individuals.
Application information: Application form not required.
Initial approach: Letter
Copies of proposal: 1
Deadline(s): Oct.
Board meeting date(s): Nov.
Trustee: Chemical Bank.
EIN: 136164229
Grants for Aging:
Village Center for Care, NYC, NY, $4,000. 94.

641
Faith Home Foundation
Six Flower Hill Ln.
Bayshore 11706
Contact: Mrs. Anna T. Pearson

Incorporated in 1878 in NY.
Financial data (yr. ended 11/30/95): Assets, $3,558,749 (M); gifts received, $750; expenditures, $190,364; qualifying distributions, $150,133, including $130,500 for 32 grants (high: $10,000; low: $1,000).
Purpose and activities: Giving primarily to institutions which provide medical assistance to the elderly in NY.
Fields of interest: Nursing home/convalescent facility; Children & youth, services; Aging, centers & services; Aging.
Limitations: Giving primarily in the metropolitan New York, NY, area, with emphasis on Brooklyn and Staten Island.
Application information:
Initial approach: Letter
Officers and Trustees:* Owen E. Brooks,* Pres.; Gordon M. Brown,* V.P.; William F. deNeergaard,* V.P.; Alexander Pearson,* Secy.; George E. Lawrence,* Treas.; Henry A. Braun, Kenneth S. Heiberg, Allan Larson, George C. Schaefer, Peter M. Syrdahl, William P. Tucker.
EIN: 111776032
Grants for Aging:
Augustana Lutheran Home for the Aged, Brooklyn, NY, $6,500. 94.
Augustana Lutheran Home for the Aged, Brooklyn, NY, $6,000. 95.
Brooklyn United Methodist Church Home, Brooklyn, NY, $6,500. 94.
Danish Home for the Aged, Croton-on-Hudson, NY, $8,000. 95.
Danish Home for the Aged, Croton-on-Hudson, NY, $7,000. 94.
Eger Lutheran Home, Staten Island, NY, $6,500. 94.
Lemberg Home and Geriatrics Institute, Brooklyn, NY, $7,000. 95.
Lemberg Home and Geriatrics Institute, Brooklyn, NY, $7,000. 94.
New York Congregational Home for the Aged, Brooklyn, NY, $7,000. 95.
New York Congregational Home for the Aged, Brooklyn, NY, $6,500. 94.
Saint Johns Episcopal Homes for the Aged and the Blind, Brooklyn, NY, $7,000. 95.
Saint Johns Episcopal Homes for the Aged and the Blind, Brooklyn, NY, $6,500. 94.
Swedish Home for the Aged, Staten Island, NY, $10,000. 95.
Swedish Home for the Aged, Staten Island, NY, $7,000. 94.
Wartburg Lutheran Home for the Aging, Brooklyn, NY, $5,000. 95.

642
Female Charitable Society of Baldwinsville, Inc.
11 Salina St.
Baldwinsville 13027-2510 (315) 635-5666
Contact: Aileen Palmer, Treas.

Established in 1817 in NY; classified as a private operating foundation in 1957.
Foundation type: Operating
Financial data (yr. ended 06/30/94): Assets, $653,472 (M); gifts received, $1,254; expenditures, $26,111; qualifying distributions, $19,807, including $8,034 for 10 grants (high: $5,834; low: $100), $9,773 for grants to individuals and $2,000 for loans to individuals.
Purpose and activities: Interest-free loans to nursing students. Grants and medical equipments to indigent families, and food assistance for elderly and disabled persons (Meals on Wheels). Support also to charitable organizations.
Fields of interest: Health care; Health organizations; Food distribution, meals on wheels; Human services; Family services; Aging, centers & services; Christian agencies & churches; Aging.
Types of support: Emergency funds, grants to individuals, student loans—to individuals.
Limitations: Giving limited to the Baldwinsville, NY, area.
Publications: Informational brochure (including application guidelines).
Application information:
Initial approach: Letter or telephone
Deadline(s): None
Board meeting date(s): Monthly
Officers: Mrs. Gordon Slye, Pres.; Mrs. Robert Bitz, V.P.; Mrs. John Hudson, Secy.; Aileen Palmer, Treas.
EIN: 156019000

643
The Feuerring Foundation
55 Central Park West
New York 10023-6045

Donor(s): Gertrude Feuerring.
Financial data (yr. ended 12/31/94): Assets, $471,097 (M); expenditures, $3,433; qualifying distributions, $500, including $500 for grants.
Fields of interest: Museums; Education; Hospitals (general); Human services; Aging, centers & services; Jewish federated giving programs; Jewish agencies & temples; Religion; Aging; General charitable giving; Israel.
Limitations: Applications not accepted. Giving primarily in New York, NY. No grants to individuals.
Application information: Contributes only to pre-selected organizations.
Officer and Directors:* Gertrude Feuerring,* Pres.; Ralph Feuerring, Eric Sondheimer.
Number of staff: None.
EIN: 136221072

644
The Beth Rosenthal Fisher Foundation, Inc.
c/o Jack Rosenthal
150 East 69th St.
New York 10019

Established in 1990 in NJ.
Donor(s): Jack Rosenthal, Alice Rosenthal.
Financial data (yr. ended 12/31/95): Assets, $8,533 (M); expenditures, $14,504; qualifying distributions, $14,504, including $14,455 for grants.
Fields of interest: Jewish agencies & temples; Aging.
Limitations: Applications not accepted.
Trustees: Harry Fischer, Alice Rosenthal, Jack Rosenthal.
EIN: 223043472

645
Ernst & Elfriede Frank Foundation
85-19 Abingdon Rd.
Kew Gardens 11415

Donor(s): Ernst L. Frank.
Financial data (yr. ended 08/31/94): Assets, $4,851,703 (M); expenditures, $223,220; qualifying distributions, $220,659, including $218,249 for 158 grants (high: $15,000; low: $35).
Fields of interest: Museums; Performing arts; Education; Health care; Human services; Aging.
Limitations: Applications not accepted. Giving primarily in NY. No grants to individuals.
Application information: Contributes only to pre-selected organizations.
Officers: Ernst H. Frank, V.P. and Secy.; Sybil Ann Brennan, V.P.; Eva Maria Tausig, V.P.
EIN: 136106471

646
D. E. French Foundation, Inc.
120 Genesee St., Rm. 503
Auburn 13021
Contact: J. Douglas Pedley, Pres.

Incorporated in 1955 in NY.
Donor(s): Clara M. French,‡ D.E. French.‡
Financial data (yr. ended 12/31/95): Assets, $3,702,207 (M); expenditures, $205,585; qualifying distributions, $196,965, including $180,000 for 71 grants (high: $15,000; low: $100; average: $100-$15,000).
Fields of interest: Dance; Arts/cultural programs; Nursing school/education; Education; Health care; Cancer; Cancer research; Youth, services; Family services; Protestant agencies & churches; Disabled; Aging.
Types of support: General/operating support, continuing support, annual campaigns, capital campaigns, building/renovation, equipment, endowment funds, scholarship funds, matching funds.
Limitations: Giving primarily in the Cayuga County, NY, area.
Application information: Application form not required.
Copies of proposal: 1
Deadline(s): None
Board meeting date(s): Jan., July, and Oct.
Officer and Directors:* J. Douglas Pedley,* Pres.; Frederick J. Atkins, James P. Costello, Walter M. Lowe, Ronald D. West.
Number of staff: 1 part-time support.
EIN: 166052246
Grants for Aging:
Faatz-Crofut Home for the Elderly, Auburn, NY, $10,000. For building fund. 95.
Faatz-Crofut Home for the Elderly, Auburn, NY, $5,000. For building fund. 95.
Mercy Health and Rehabilitation Center Nursing Home Company, Auburn, NY, $10,000. For equipment fund. 95.

647
Jeanne S. Friedman Foundation
c/o Wormser, Kiely, Galef, and Jacobs
711 Third Ave., 19th Fl.
New York 10017

Established in 1984 in NY.
Financial data (yr. ended 12/31/94): Assets, $160,180 (M); gifts received, $20,039; expenditures, $24,959; qualifying distributions, $24,942, including $23,309 for 22 grants (high: $8,000; low: $40).
Fields of interest: Health associations; Aging, centers & services; Aging.
Limitations: Applications not accepted. No grants to individuals.
Application information: Contributes only to pre-selected organizations.
Trustees: Eugene J. Callahan, Douglas E. Friedman, Jeanne S. Friedman, Gwen S. Friedman-McGuire.
EIN: 133230661

648
The Rosamond Gifford Charitable Corporation
731 James St., Rm. 404
Syracuse 13203 (315) 474-2489
Contact: Dean A. Lesinski, Exec. Dir.

Incorporated in 1954 in NY.
Donor(s): Rosamond Gifford.‡
Financial data (yr. ended 12/31/94): Assets, $17,160,049 (M); expenditures, $872,537; qualifying distributions, $781,489, including $670,595 for 24 grants (high: $128,800; low: $400).
Fields of interest: Arts/cultural programs; Higher education; Hospitals (general); Health care; Health organizations; Medical research; Human services; Children & youth, services; Aging, centers & services; Aging.
Types of support: Building/renovation, equipment, emergency funds, program development, conferences/seminars, seed money, research.
Limitations: Giving limited to organizations serving the residents of Syracuse and Onondaga County, NY. No grants to individuals, or for endowment funds, continuing support, deficit financing, land acquisition, special projects, matching gifts, scholarships, or fellowships; no loans.
Publications: Program policy statement, application guidelines, annual report.
Application information: Application form not required.
Initial approach: Letter or telephone
Copies of proposal: 1
Deadline(s): None
Board meeting date(s): Monthly
Final notification: 2 months
Officers and Trustees:* Robert F. Dewey,* Pres.; Roger L. MacDonald,* V.P. and Treas.; John H. Lynch,* Secy.; Dean A. Lesinski, Exec. Dir.; Charles A. Chappell, Jr., Donald M. Mills.
Number of staff: 1 full-time professional; 1 part-time professional; 1 full-time support.
EIN: 150572881

649
The Glickenhaus Foundation
Six East 43rd St.
New York 10017 (212) 953-7867
Contact: Maddy Wehle

Incorporated in 1960 in NY.
Donor(s): Seth M. Glickenhaus.
Financial data (yr. ended 11/30/94): Assets, $1,422,142 (M); gifts received, $161,917; expenditures, $666,222; qualifying distributions, $644,591, including $644,096 for 286 grants (high: $65,000; low: $30).
Purpose and activities: Support for general charitable activities.
Fields of interest: Humanities; Arts/cultural programs; Education, association; Child development, education; Education; Natural resource conservation & protection; Environment; Hospitals (general); Family planning; Health care; Substance abuse, services; Mental health/crisis services; Cancer; AIDS; Biomedicine; Medical research; Cancer research; AIDS research; Delinquency prevention/services; Human services; Children & youth, services; Child development, services; Family services; Aging, centers & services; Arms control; Human rights (international); International affairs; Civil rights; Community development; Minorities; Disabled; Aging; Economically disadvantaged.
Types of support: Endowment funds, emergency funds, research.
Limitations: Giving primarily in the greater metropolitan New York, NY, area, including Westchester County.
Publications: 990-PF.
Application information: Application form not required.
Initial approach: Proposal
Deadline(s): None
Officers: Nancy G. Pier, Pres.; Alfred Feinman, V.P.; James Glickenhaus, V.P.
Number of staff: 1 full-time support.
EIN: 136160941

650
Morris Glickman Foundation, Inc.
12 Moss Run, Box B5
White Plains 10605
Contact: Marvin S. Glickman, Pres.

Donor(s): Marvin S. Glickman.
Financial data (yr. ended 06/30/95): Assets, $516,233 (M); gifts received, $65,906;

expenditures, $53,904; qualifying distributions, $53,754, including $53,230 for grants.
Fields of interest: Health care; Human services; Aging, centers & services; Jewish federated giving programs; Aging.
Limitations: Giving primarily in New York, NY, and CA.
Application information: Application form not required.
Initial approach: Letter
Deadline(s): None
Officers: Marvin S. Glickman, Pres. and Treas.; Linda Levine, V.P.; Nancy Lipton, V.P.; Duanne Singer, V.P.; Alma Glickman, Secy.
EIN: 116015697

651
Horace W. Goldsmith Foundation

375 Park Ave., Suite 1602
New York 10152 (212) 319-8700
Contact: James C. Slaughter, C.E.O.

Incorporated in 1955 in NY.
Donor(s): Horace W. Goldsmith.‡
Financial data (yr. ended 12/31/95): Assets, $491,572,569 (M); expenditures, $21,634,985; qualifying distributions, $20,518,950, including $20,168,590 for 358 grants (high: $600,000; low: $5,000; average: $25,000-$100,000).
Purpose and activities: Support for cultural programs, including the performing arts and museums; Jewish welfare funds and temple support; hospitals and a geriatric center; and education, especially higher education.
Fields of interest: Visual arts; Museums; Performing arts; Dance; Theater; Music; Arts/cultural programs; Education, research; Higher education; Business school/education; Libraries/library science; Education; Natural resource conservation & protection; Hospitals (general); Family planning; Medical care, rehabilitation; Cancer; AIDS; Medical research; Cancer research; AIDS research; Crime/law enforcement; Human services; Aging, centers & services; Homeless, human services; International relief; Jewish federated giving programs; Jewish agencies & temples; Disabled; Aging; Homeless; General charitable giving; Israel.
Types of support: General/operating support, continuing support, capital campaigns, building/renovation, endowment funds, seed money, scholarship funds, matching funds.
Limitations: Applications not accepted. Giving primarily in New York, NY, MA, and AZ. No grants to individuals.
Application information: Foundation depends almost exclusively on internally initiated grants.
Board meeting date(s): 6 times a year
Managing Directors: James C. Slaughter, C.E.O.; Richard L. Menschel, Robert B. Menschel, Thomas Slaughter, William A. Slaughter.
Number of staff: 1 full-time support.
EIN: 136107758
Grants for Aging:
Burden Center for the Aging, NYC, NY, $10,000. 94.
Cancer Care, NYC, NY, $25,000. 94.
University of San Francisco, San Francisco, CA, $25,000. For Senior Net. 94.

652
The Leslie & Roslyn Goldstein Foundation

c/o Nathan Berkman & Co.
29 Broadway, Rm. 2800
New York 10006-3296

Established in 1980.
Donor(s): Leslie Goldstein, Roslyn Goldstein.
Financial data (yr. ended 11/30/94): Assets, $3,149,582 (M); gifts received, $365,875; expenditures, $145,870; qualifying distributions, $124,875, including $124,875 for grants (high: $27,000).
Purpose and activities: Primary areas of interest include education, the elderly, and Jewish organizations, including welfare funds and support for Israel.
Fields of interest: Education; Cancer; Biomedicine; Medical research; Cancer research; Human services; Family services; Aging, centers & services; Jewish federated giving programs; Jewish agencies & temples; Aging; General charitable giving; Israel.
Types of support: Annual campaigns, capital campaigns, building/renovation, program-related investments/loans.
Application information: Application form not required.
Initial approach: Letter
Copies of proposal: 1
Deadline(s): None
Board meeting date(s): Varies
Trustees: Leslie Goldstein, Roslyn Goldstein.
EIN: 061035614

653
Bernard & Barbara Green Charitable Foundation, Inc.

c/o Friedman, Alpren & Green
1700 Broadway, 23rd Fl.
New York 10019

Established in 1986 in NY.
Donor(s): Bernard R. Green.
Financial data (yr. ended 08/31/95): Assets, $149,126 (M); gifts received, $15,000; expenditures, $66,850; qualifying distributions, $66,301, including $66,100 for 7 grants (high: $30,000; low: $1,100).
Fields of interest: Higher education; Aging, centers & services; Jewish federated giving programs; Jewish agencies & temples; Aging.
Types of support: General/operating support, building/renovation.
Limitations: Applications not accepted. Giving primarily in New York, NY, West Palm Beach, FL, and NJ. No grants to individuals.
Application information: Contributes only to pre-selected organizations.
Officers: Bernard R. Green, Pres.; Shirley Dembner, V.P.; Barbara Gordon Green, Secy.; Andrea Green, Treas.
EIN: 133374415
Grants for Aging:
Jewish Home for the Aged of Palm Beach County, West Palm Beach, FL, $10,000. 95.

654
The Green Fund, Inc.

14 East 60th St., Suite 702
New York 10022 (212) 755-2445
Contact: Cynthia Green Colin, Pres.

Incorporated in 1947 in NY.
Donor(s): Evelyn Green Davis,‡ Louis A. Green.‡
Financial data (yr. ended 01/31/95): Assets, $31,115,135 (M); gifts received, $437,600; expenditures, $1,968,073; qualifying distributions, $1,695,825, including $1,543,991 for 213 grants (high: $305,853; low: $20; average: $500-$10,000).
Purpose and activities: Giving primarily for Jewish welfare funds, hospitals within the Jewish Federation network, services to the aged and mentally handicapped, higher and secondary education, the performing arts, social services, and youth agencies.
Fields of interest: Performing arts; Secondary school/education; Higher education; Hospitals (general); Mental health/crisis services; Human services; Youth, services; Aging, centers & services; Jewish federated giving programs; Jewish agencies & temples; Aging.
Limitations: Applications not accepted. Giving primarily in the metropolitan New York, NY, area. No grants to individuals.
Application information: Grants initiated by the fund's members.
Board meeting date(s): Varies
Officers and Directors:* Cynthia Green Colin,* Pres.; S. William Green,* Treas.; Patricia F. Green.
Number of staff: 1 part-time support.
EIN: 136160950
Grants for Aging:
Jewish Association for Services for the Aged, NYC, NY, $10,000. 95.

655
The David J. Greene Foundation, Inc.

599 Lexington Ave., No. 12
New York 10022-6303 (212) 371-4200
Contact: Barbara A. McBride, Secy.

Incorporated in 1966 in NY.
Donor(s): David J. Greene,‡ and members of the Greene family.
Financial data (yr. ended 12/31/94): Assets, $8,240,506 (M); gifts received, $19,180; expenditures, $399,095; qualifying distributions, $385,038, including $382,440 for 148 grants (high: $100,675; low: $50).
Fields of interest: Music; Secondary school/education; Higher education; Education; Environment; Hospitals (general); Eye disease; Eye research; Human services; Children & youth, services; Youth, services; Aging, centers & services; Jewish federated giving programs; Aging.
Types of support: General/operating support.
Limitations: Giving primarily in the metropolitan New York, NY, area. No grants to individuals.
Application information: Application form required.
Copies of proposal: 1
Deadline(s): Dec. 15

Board meeting date(s): Mar., June, Sept., and Dec.
Officers and Directors:* Alan I. Greene,* Pres.; Robert J. Ravitz,* V.P.; Barbara A. McBride,* Secy.; James R. Greene,* Treas.; Michael C. Greene.
Number of staff: None.
EIN: 136209280

656
J. Gurwin Foundation, Inc.
175 Great Neck Rd.
Great Neck 11021
Contact: Joseph Gurwin, Pres.

Incorporated in 1959 in NY.
Donor(s): Joseph Gurwin, Kings Point Industries, Inc.
Financial data (yr. ended 07/31/94): Assets, $14,602,848 (M); expenditures, $993,091; qualifying distributions, $986,377, including $985,555 for 79 grants (high: $233,100; low: $25).
Purpose and activities: Giving primarily for Jewish-affiliated organizations, including welfare funds, temples, educational institutions, geriatric centers and other health facilities, and a holocaust museum.
Fields of interest: Veterans' & war memorials; Elementary/secondary education; University; Medical care, in-patient care; Hospitals (general); Nursing home/convalescent facility; Human services; Aging, centers & services; Jewish federated giving programs; Jewish agencies & temples.
Limitations: Applications not accepted. Giving primarily in NY. No grants to individuals.
Application information: Contributes only to pre-selected organizations.
Officers: Joseph Gurwin, Pres.; Eric Gurwin, V.P.; Rosalind Gurwin, Secy.; Laura Gurwin Glug, Treas.
EIN: 136059258

657
Stella and Charles Guttman Foundation, Inc.
445 Park Ave., 19th Fl.
New York 10022 (212) 371-7082
Contact: Elizabeth Olofson, Exec. Dir.

Incorporated in 1959 in NY.
Donor(s): Charles Guttman,‡ Stella Guttman.‡
Financial data (yr. ended 12/31/94): Assets, $28,206,109 (M); expenditures, $1,601,114; qualifying distributions, $1,259,968, including $1,058,591 for 93 grants (high: $75,000; low: $1,000; average: $5,000-$30,000).
Purpose and activities: Support for organizations providing health, social, educational services; support also for programs that promote the general welfare of the elderly and enhance their quality of life, and for a limited number of charities that conduct activities in the State of Israel, including programs that foster improved relations between Jews and Arabs.
Fields of interest: Early childhood education; Education; Human services; Children & youth, services; Aging, centers & services; Aging; Economically disadvantaged; Israel.
Types of support: General/operating support, continuing support, program development, matching funds.
Limitations: Giving primarily in the metropolitan New York, NY, area. No support for religious organizations for religious purposes, or for public interest litigation or anti-vivisectionist causes. No grants to individuals, or for foreign travel or foreign study.
Publications: Grants list, informational brochure (including application guidelines), multi-year report.
Application information: Application form not required.
Initial approach: Letter
Copies of proposal: 1
Deadline(s): None
Board meeting date(s): As required
Officers and Directors:* Edgar H. Brenner,* Pres.; Peter Herbert,* V.P.; Ernest Rubenstein,* Secy.; Robert S. Gassman,* Treas.; Elizabeth Olofson, Exec. Dir.; Charles S. Brenner, Sonia Rosenberg.
Number of staff: 2 full-time professional.
EIN: 136103039
Grants for Aging:
Dorot, NYC, NY, $10,000. For Homelessness Prevention and Aftercare Program for elders. 94.
Henry Street Settlement, NYC, NY, $15,000. For program of support services for frail, minority elderly residents in Vladeck Houses. 94.
Henry Street Settlement, NYC, NY, $11,000. For youth programs and Good Companions Program for elderly. 94.
United Jewish Appeal-Federation of Jewish Philanthropies, NYC, NY, $25,000. For third payment of grant for NORC Supportive Services Program at Warbasse Houses and Cooperative Village. 94.
United Jewish Appeal-Federation of Jewish Philanthropies, NYC, NY, $15,000. For final payment of grant for transportation services at NORC Supportive Services Program at Warbasse Houses and Cooperative Village. 94.
Volunteers of Legal Service, NYC, NY, $10,000. For Elderly Project providing free civil legal services to low-income seniors in Manhattan. 94.

658
Hagedorn Fund
c/o Chemical Bank
270 Park Ave.
New York 10017 (212) 270-9167
Contact: Robert Rosenthal, V.P., Chemical Bank

Trust established in 1953 in NY.
Donor(s): William Hagedorn.‡
Financial data (yr. ended 12/31/94): Assets, $19,165,017 (M); expenditures, $1,470,944; qualifying distributions, $1,416,951, including $1,309,000 for 83 grants (high: $90,000; low: $1,000; average: $5,000-$15,000).
Purpose and activities: Support for higher and secondary education, hospitals and health agencies, AIDS programs and medical research, the aged, youth agencies, social welfare, community funds, parks and botanical gardens.
Fields of interest: Secondary school/education; Higher education; Botanical gardens; Hospitals (general); Health care; AIDS; Medical research; AIDS research; Housing/shelter, development; Parks/playgrounds; Human services; Children & youth, services; Aging, centers & services; Homeless, human services; Aging; Economically disadvantaged.
Types of support: General/operating support, annual campaigns, capital campaigns, building/renovation.
Limitations: Giving primarily in New York, NY. No grants to individuals, or for continuing support, seed money, emergency funds, deficit financing, endowment funds, matching gifts, scholarships, fellowships, research, special projects, publications, or conferences; no loans.
Application information: Application form not required.
Initial approach: Proposal
Copies of proposal: 1
Deadline(s): Submit proposal preferably in Nov.; deadline Nov. 15
Board meeting date(s): Dec.
Final notification: 1 month
Trustees: W.F. Fischer, Jr., John J. Kindred III, Charles B. Lauren, Chemical Bank.
Number of staff: 5 shared staff
EIN: 136048718

659
The John A. Hartford Foundation, Inc.
55 East 59th St., 23rd Fl.
New York 10022 (212) 832-7788
Contact: Stephen C. Eyre, Exec. Dir.
FAX: (212) 593-4913

Established in 1929; incorporated in 1942 in NY.
Donor(s): John A. Hartford,‡ George L. Hartford.‡
Financial data (yr. ended 12/31/94): Assets, $325,823,480 (M); expenditures, $17,224,546; qualifying distributions, $15,414,366, including $13,112,633 for 76 grants (high: $1,081,250; low: $1,500; average: $50,000-$300,000), $337,365 for employee matching gifts and $317,254 for 2 foundation-administered programs.
Purpose and activities: The foundation provides support through: 1) the Aging and Health Program, to address the unique health needs of the elderly, including long-term care, the use of medication in chronic health problems, increasing the nation's geriatric research and training capability, and improving the integration of financing and care delivery for comprehensive geriatric services; and 2) the Health Care Cost and Quality Program concerned with balancing the quality and cost of medical care. Emphasis is on innovative approaches to health care reform at the community level with a focus on information systems and collective purchasing. Projects are also supported which propose better methods to measure health care provider quality or promise a national impact in reducing inappropriate health care services. The Health Care Financing Program and the John A. and George L. Hartford Fellowship Program were both terminated in 1985; the Hartford Geriatric Faculty Development Award Program was terminated in 1987.

Fields of interest: Health care; Aging, centers & services; Aging.
Types of support: General/operating support, continuing support, program development, conferences/seminars, publication, research, program-related investments/loans, employee matching gifts.
Limitations: Giving primarily on a national basis. No grants to individuals, or for annual or capital campaigns, seed money, emergency or endowment funds, or deficit financing.
Publications: Annual report, program policy statement, application guidelines.
Application information: No new grants to individuals will be awarded. Application form not required.
Initial approach: Letter or proposal
Copies of proposal: 1
Deadline(s): No set deadline, but initial inquiry should be made at least 6 months before funding is required
Board meeting date(s): Mar., June, Sept., and Dec.
Final notification: 6 weeks
Officers and Trustees:* James D. Farley,* Chair.; Charles E. Murphy, Jr.,* Vice-Chair.; Norman H. Volk,* Vice-Chair.; Robert H. Mulreany,* Secy.; Stephen C. Eyre, Treas. and Exec. Dir.; Samuel R. Gische, Finance Dir. and Cont.; Michael D. Dingman, Alexander M. Laughlin, Nuala Pell, Thomas A. Reynolds, Jr., Kathryn D. Wriston.
Staff: Donna I. Regenstreif, Sr. Prog. Officer; Laura A. Robbins, Prog. Officer; Richard S. Sharpe, Prog. Dir.
Number of staff: 6 full-time professional; 6 full-time support.
EIN: 131667057
Grants for Aging:
American Federation for Aging Research (AFAR), NYC, NY, $1,481,439. For continued support for Medical Student Geriatric Scholars Program to develop geriatric scholars with research opportunities and career development. 95.
Baylor College of Medicine, Houston, TX, $100,000. For planning grant to organize and coordinate practicums for non-physician professionals in care of elderly as part of Geriatric Interdisciplinary Team Training (GITT) Initiative. 95.
Dartmouth Medical School, Hanover, NH, $2,000,000. For program, in coordination with John D. and Catherine T. MacArthur Foundation, to improve treatment of depression in elderly patients. 95.
Harvard University, Cambridge, MA, $100,000. For planning grant to organize and coordinate practicums for non-physician professionals in care of elderly as part of Geriatric Interdisciplinary Team Training (GITT) Initiative at Medical School in Boston. 95.
Henry Ford Health System, Troy, MI, $100,000. For planning grant to organize and coordinate practicums for non-physician professionals in care of elderly as part of Geriatric Interdisciplinary Team Training (GITT) Initiative. 95.
Johns Hopkins Bayview Medical Center, Baltimore, MD, $770,803. For Phase II of Hospital Outcomes Program for the Elderly (HOPE) to establish Johns Hopkins Home Hospital, testing safety and efficacy of hospital care at home for older patients. 95.
Kaiser Foundation Hospitals, Pasadena, CA, $100,000. For planning grant to organize and coordinate practicums for non-physician professionals in care of elderly as part of Geriatric Interdisciplinary Team Training (GITT) Initiative. 95.
Mount Sinai School of Medicine, NYC, NY, $100,000. For planning grant to organize and coordinate practicums for non-physician professionals in care of elderly as part of Geriatric Interdisciplinary Team Training (GITT) Initiative. 95.
New York University, NYC, NY, $1,549,981. For Resource Center to organize and coordinate practicums for non-physician professionals in care of elderly and to assist in evaluation and dissemination of new models as part of Geriatric Interdisciplinary Team Training (GITT) Initiative. 95.
New York University, NYC, NY, $750,397. To improve hospital care for elders through dissemination of effective inpatient nursing models. 95.
On Lok Senior Health Services, San Francisco, CA, $100,000. For planning grant to organize and coordinate practicums for non-physician professionals in care of elderly as part of Geriatric Interdisciplinary Team Training (GITT) Initiative. 95.
Rush-Presbyterian-Saint Lukes Medical Center, Chicago, IL, $100,000. For planning grant to organize and coordinate practicums for non-physician professionals in care of elderly as part of Geriatric Interdisciplinary Team Training (GITT) Initiative. 95.
University Hospitals of Cleveland, Cleveland, OH, $100,000. For planning grant to organize and coordinate practicums for non-physician professionals in care of elderly as part of Geriatric Interdisciplinary Team Training (GITT) Initiative. 95.
University of Colorado, Denver, CO, $100,000. For planning grant to organize and coordinate practicums for non-physician professionals in care of elderly as part of Geriatric Interdisciplinary Team Training (GITT) Initiative. 95.
University of Minnesota, Minneapolis, MN, $100,000. For planning grant to organize and coordinate practicums for non-physician professionals in care of elderly as part of Geriatric Interdisciplinary Team Training (GITT) Initiative. 95.
University of North Carolina, Chapel Hill, NC, $100,000. For planning grant to organize and coordinate practicums for non-physician professionals in care of elderly as part of Geriatric Interdisciplinary Team Training (GITT) Initiative. 95.
University of Pennsylvania, Philadelphia, PA, $100,000. For planning grant to organize and coordinate practicums for non-physician professionals in care of elderly as part of Geriatric Interdisciplinary Team Training (GITT) Initiative. 95.
University of South Florida Foundation, Tampa, FL, $100,000. For planning grant to organize and coordinate practicums for non-physician professionals in care of elderly as part of Geriatric Interdisciplinary Team Training (GITT) Initiative. 95.

660
The Hearthstone Foundation

(Formerly Rochester Friendly Home Foundation, Inc.)
3156 East Ave.
Rochester 14618
Contact: Denise Hubler, Dir.

Established in 1992 in NY.
Financial data (yr. ended 12/31/95): Assets, $8,941,912 (M); expenditures, $691,006; qualifying distributions, $578,160, including $549,088 for 2 grants (high: $545,088; low: $4,000).
Purpose and activities: "The mission of the foundation is to develop resources and distribute grants to enhance the quality of our aging population. The foundation shall promote and support programs, research, education, and services that benefit the elderly in Monroe County."
Fields of interest: Aging, centers & services; Aging.
Types of support: Building/renovation, land acquisition, program development, conferences/seminars, research.
Limitations: Applications not accepted. Giving limited to Monroe County, NY. No grants to individuals.
Application information: Contributes only to pre-selected organizations.
Officers and Directors:* Jane S. Hatch,* Chair.; Crofts K. Gorsline,* Vice-Chair.; Marion M. Morse,* Secy.; Bruce B. Bates,* Treas.; Thomas J. Hargrave, John Henderson, Patrick D. Martin, Ellen G. Neisner, Robert W. Warren, Marie G. Whitbeck.
Number of staff: 1 part-time professional; 1 part-time support.
EIN: 223174636
Grants for Aging:
Alzheimers Disease and Related Disorders Association, Rochester, NY, $4,000. For emergency respite program. 95.
Rochester Friendly Home, Rochester, NY, $545,088. For housing development program. 95.

661
The Harry B. Helmsley Foundation, Inc.

230 Park Ave., 17th Fl.
New York 10169

Incorporated in 1954 in NY.
Donor(s): Harry B. Helmsley.
Financial data (yr. ended 05/31/95): Assets, $26,214,005 (M); expenditures, $181,350; qualifying distributions, $155,350, including $154,600 for 8 grants (high: $75,000; low: $100).
Fields of interest: Health care; Health associations; Alzheimer's disease research.
Limitations: Applications not accepted. Giving primarily in NY.
Application information: Contributes only to pre-selected organizations.
Officers and Directors:* Harry B. Helmsley,* Pres.; Leona M. Helmsley,* V.P.; David Panzirer.
EIN: 136123336
Grants for Aging:

Alzheimers Disease and Related Disorders Association, NYC, NY, $100,000. 94.
Alzheimers Disease and Related Disorders Association, NYC, NY, $75,000. 95.

662
Emy & Emil Herzfeld Foundation, Inc.

420 Lexington Ave., Suite 1745
New York 10170
Contact: William P. Holm, Esq., Secy.

Established in 1952 in NY.
Financial data (yr. ended 12/31/94): Assets, $1,367,599 (M); expenditures, $101,386; qualifying distributions, $77,271, including $76,500 for 61 grants (high: $10,000; low: $500).
Fields of interest: Food services; Human services; Youth, services; Aging, centers & services; Homeless, human services; Aging; Homeless.
Limitations: Giving primarily in the metropolitan New York, NY, area. No grants to individuals.
Application information:
Initial approach: Proposal
Deadline(s): None
Officer and Directors:* William P. Holm,* Secy.; Countess Emilie de Rohan-Chandor, Esther R. Dyer, Jane H. Rowen, Joseph R. Rowen, Gary B. Schreiner, Alice E. Schwartz.
EIN: 136161598

663
Holland Lodge Foundation, Inc.

71 West 23rd St.
New York 10010-4102 (212) 675-0323

Established in 1929 in NY.
Financial data (yr. ended 09/30/95): Assets, $1,509,398 (M); gifts received, $420; expenditures, $87,474; qualifying distributions, $65,969, including $19,500 for 20 grants (high: $1,000; low: $500) and $27,000 for 3 grants to individuals (high: $12,000; low: $6,000).
Purpose and activities: Support limited to assisting the elderly or the young.
Fields of interest: Human services; Children & youth, services; Aging, centers & services; Christian agencies & churches; Aging.
Types of support: General/operating support, grants to individuals.
Limitations: Giving primarily in New York, NY.
Application information:
Initial approach: Proposal
Deadline(s): None
Officers: Henry C.B. Lindh, Pres.; Jonathan K. Bitting, Treas.
Directors: Charles E. Baskett, Hans H.A. Bielenstein, Robert C. Hubbard, Daniel E. Peterson, Robert W. Redsch, Stephen W. Spencer, Byan K. Stevens, Edgar P.E. White.
Number of staff: 1 full-time support.
EIN: 136126132

664
Helen Thomas Howland Testamentary Trust Foundation

c/o The Chase Manhattan Bank, N.A.
P.O. Box 1412
Rochester 14603-1412
Application address: c/o Chase Manhattan Bank, N.A., attn.: Sue Smith, Box 700, Binghamton, NY 13902

Established in 1991 in NY.
Financial data (yr. ended 06/30/95): Assets, $1,381,667 (M); expenditures, $77,205; qualifying distributions, $63,645, including $59,480 for 11 grants (high: $24,000; low: $480).
Fields of interest: Environment; Animal welfare; Health care; Children & youth, services; Aging, centers & services; Federated giving programs; Aging.
Types of support: Capital campaigns, program development.
Limitations: Giving primarily in NY. No support for churches or organizations for religious purposes. No grants to individuals.
Application information: Application form required.
Initial approach: Write for guidelines
Deadline(s): None
Trustee: The Chase Manhattan Bank, N.A.
EIN: 166353030
Grants for Aging:
Tompkins County Senior Citizens Council, Ithaca, NY, $1,200. 95.

665
Stewart W. & Willma C. Hoyt Foundation, Inc.

105-107 Court St., Suite 400
Binghamton 13901 (607) 722-6706
Contact: Judith C. Peckham, Exec. Dir.

Established in 1993 in NY as successor to Stewart W. & Willma C. Hoyt Foundation, which was established in 1970.
Donor(s): Willma C. Hoyt.‡
Financial data (yr. ended 12/31/95): Assets, $16,173,294 (M); gifts received, $19,630; expenditures, $626,226; qualifying distributions, $519,393, including $408,320 for 30 grants (high: $47,500; low: $1,922).
Purpose and activities: Primary areas of interest include the arts and humanities, education, health, and social and human services, with preference for capital campaigns, special projects, and seed money.
Fields of interest: Humanities; Arts/cultural programs; Child development, education; Higher education; Education; Health care; Substance abuse, services; AIDS; Alcoholism; Health organizations; Human services; Children & youth, services; Aging, centers & services; Disabled.
Types of support: Continuing support, capital campaigns, building/renovation, equipment, emergency funds, program development, seed money, scholarship funds, technical assistance, consulting services, program-related investments/loans, matching funds.
Limitations: Giving limited to Broome County, NY. No support for religious purposes. No grants to individuals, or for annual campaigns of local chapters of national organizations, deficit financing, general endowments, research, or publications.
Publications: Annual report, application guidelines.
Application information: No grants considered at Jan., May, and Sept. meetings. Application form required.
Initial approach: Telephone or letter
Copies of proposal: 1
Deadline(s): 1st of the month prior to board meeting dates
Board meeting date(s): Bimonthly, beginning in Jan.; no grants awarded in Jan., May, and Sept.
Final notification: 1 to 3 days following board meetings
Officers and Directors:* John F. Russell,* Chair.; John M. Keeler,* Vice-Chair.; William H. Rincker,* Secy.-Treas.; Fannie R. Linder, Albert Mamary, Jacqueline Visser, Priscilla H. Young.
Trustee: The Chase Manhattan Bank, N.A.
Number of staff: 1 full-time professional; 1 part-time support.
EIN: 223209342

666
Fannie C. Hyde Testamentary Trust

c/o Chemung Canal Trust
203 Main St.
Owego 13827
Contact: Robin A. Allen, Trust Officer, Chemung Canal Trust

Established in 1963 in NY.
Donor(s): Fannie C. Hyde.‡
Financial data (yr. ended 04/30/95): Assets, $1,341,225 (M); expenditures, $66,155; qualifying distributions, $45,800, including $45,800 for 15 grants (high: $15,000; low: $350; average: $300-$7,500).
Purpose and activities: Giving only to benefit residents of the Village of Owego, NY.
Fields of interest: Arts/cultural programs; Child development, education; Libraries/library science; Natural resource conservation & protection; Health care; Recreation; Human services; Youth, services; Child development, services; Aging, centers & services; Community development; Aging.
Types of support: General/operating support, equipment, program development, scholarship funds.
Limitations: Giving limited to the village of Owego, NY.
Publications: Annual report.
Application information: Application form not required.
Initial approach: Letter
Copies of proposal: 1
Deadline(s): None
Board meeting date(s): Quarterly
Trustee: Chemung Canal Trust Co.
EIN: 156020596

667
J.L.M. Benevolent Fund
c/o Kelley, Drye & Warren
101 Park Ave.
New York 10178-0002 (212) 808-7933
Contact: Michael S. Insel, Trustee

Established around 1947 in NY.
Donor(s): Francois Monohan.‡
Financial data (yr. ended 10/31/95): Assets, $8,854 (M); gifts received, $8,177; expenditures, $9,339; qualifying distributions, $9,261, including $3,000 for 4 grants (high: $1,500; low: $500) and $4,341 for 1 grant to an individual.
Fields of interest: Education; Aging, centers & services; Aging; France.
Types of support: Grants to individuals.
Limitations: Giving primarily in France and the northeastern U.S.
Application information:
Initial approach: Letter
Deadline(s): None
Trustees: John J. Costello, Michael S. Insel, Winthrop R. Munyan.
EIN: 136272298

668
The Jedra Charitable Foundation, Inc.
110-11 Queens Blvd., Apt. 20B
Forest Hills 11375 (718) 263-4956
Contact: David Shechet, Pres.

Established in 1964 in NY.
Donor(s): David Shechet.
Financial data (yr. ended 06/30/95): Assets, $596,719 (M); gifts received, $30,004; expenditures, $37,229; qualifying distributions, $37,229, including $36,674 for 51 grants (high: $10,610; low: $22).
Fields of interest: Arts/cultural programs; Education, fund raising; Elementary/secondary education; Early childhood education; Higher education; Medical school/education; Education; Hospitals (general); Medical care, rehabilitation; Health care; Mental health/crisis services; Eye disease; Health organizations; Medical research; Eye research; Human services; Aging, centers & services; Jewish federated giving programs; Jewish agencies & temples; Religion; Aging; Israel.
Types of support: General/operating support, annual campaigns, capital campaigns, building/renovation, emergency funds.
Limitations: Giving primarily in New York, NY, FL, and Israel.
Application information: Application form not required.
Deadline(s): None
Officers: David Shechet, Pres.; Arthur Shechet, V.P.; Jean Shechet, Secy.
Number of staff: None.
EIN: 136163612
Grants for Aging:
Gurwin Jewish Geriatric Center of Long Island, Commack, NY, $400. 94.

669
Daisy Marquis Jones Foundation
500 Granite Bldg.
130 East Main St.
Rochester 14604-1689 (716) 263-3331
Contact: Roger L. Gardner, Pres.

Established in 1968 in NY.
Donor(s): Daisy Marquis Jones.‡
Financial data (yr. ended 12/31/95): Assets, $27,850,000 (M); expenditures, $1,360,127; qualifying distributions, $1,288,127, including $1,258,127 for 82 grants (high: $100,000; low: $750; average: $5,000-$25,000) and $30,000 for 1 program-related investment.
Purpose and activities: Grants primarily to stablize and support families in the city of Rochester; support also for services for senior citizens, women and youth, with special emphasis on the disadvantaged and toward improving the administration of justice. Special attention to preventive programs.
Fields of interest: Early childhood education; Education; Health care; Legal services; Human services; Children & youth, services; Aging, centers & services; Women, centers & services; Community development; Public affairs; Aging; Women; Economically disadvantaged.
Types of support: General/operating support, capital campaigns, building/renovation, equipment, land acquisition, emergency funds, program development, publication, seed money, technical assistance, matching funds.
Limitations: Giving limited to Monroe and Yates counties, NY. No support for the arts, religious purposes, private schools, or local chapters of national health-related organizations. No grants to individuals, or for endowment funds, research, continuing support, scholarships, fellowships, annual campaigns, or deficit financing; no loans.
Publications: Annual report (including application guidelines), application guidelines.
Application information: Application form required.
Initial approach: Letter
Copies of proposal: 1
Deadline(s): None
Board meeting date(s): Monthly (except summer)
Final notification: 2 to 3 months
Officers and Trustees:* Leo M. Lyons,* Chair.; Donald W. Whitney,* Vice-Chair.; Roger L. Gardner,* Pres.; Pearl W. Rubin, Marine Midland Bank, N.A.
Number of staff: 1 full-time professional; 1 part-time support.
EIN: 237000227
Grants for Aging:
Saint Johns Home Foundation, Rochester, NY, $25,000. For expansion of Home Care Center. 95.

670
Joy Family Foundation
107-111 Goundry St.
North Tonawanda 14120 (716) 692-6665
Contact: Mrs. Marsha J. Sullivan, Exec. Dir.

Established in 1989 in NY.
Donor(s): Paul W. Joy, H. Joan Joy.
Financial data (yr. ended 12/31/93): Assets, $4,100,426 (M); gifts received, $181,311; expenditures, $234,506; qualifying distributions, $213,519, including $197,636 for 27 grants (high: $25,600; low: $100; average: $1,000-$15,000).
Fields of interest: Child development, education; Adult education—literacy & basic skills; Reading; Education; Hospitals (general); Substance abuse, services; AIDS; Alcoholism; AIDS research; Housing/shelter, development; Human services; Children & youth, services; Youth, services; Child development, services; Family services; Aging, centers & services; Women, centers & services; Roman Catholic agencies & churches; Aging; Women; Economically disadvantaged.
Types of support: General/operating support, building/renovation, program development, consulting services, grants to individuals.
Limitations: Giving primarily in the City of Buffalo and Genesse, Erie, and Niagara counties, NY.
Application information: Application form required.
Initial approach: Letter requesting application form
Copies of proposal: 1
Deadline(s): None
Board meeting date(s): Quarterly
Trustees: H. Joan Joy, Paul W. Joy, Stephen T. Joy, John D. Reinhold, Paula Joy Reinhold, Marsha Joy Sullivan, Michael F. Sullivan.
Number of staff: 1 part-time support.
EIN: 166335211

671
Julia R. and Estelle L. Foundation, Inc.
3600 Marine Midland Ctr.
Buffalo 14203 (716) 856-9491
Contact: Richard L. Wolf, V.P.

Incorporated in 1941 in NY.
Donor(s): Peter C. Cornell Trust, R. John Oishei.‡
Financial data (yr. ended 12/31/94): Assets, $44,581,557 (M); gifts received, $916,170; expenditures, $3,244,061; qualifying distributions, $3,056,704, including $3,040,717 for 140 grants (high: $461,381; low: $250; average: $5,000-$100,000).
Purpose and activities: Emphasis on hospitals and medical research, higher and secondary education, and social services, including programs for the aged and youth; some support for health agencies and cultural programs.
Fields of interest: Arts/cultural programs; Secondary school/education; Higher education; Hospitals (general); Health care; Medical research; Human services; Children & youth, services; Youth, services; Aging, centers & services; Disabled; Aging.
Types of support: General/operating support, building/renovation, research.
Limitations: Giving primarily in Buffalo, NY. Generally, no grants to individuals.
Application information: Application form not required.
Deadline(s): None
Officers and Directors:* Rupert Warren,* Pres.; Richard L. Wolf,* V.P. and Secy.-Treas.; Carl E. Larson,* V.P.

Members: Patricia O. Colby, Albert R. Mugel, Julian R. Oishei, Allan R. Wiegley.
Number of staff: None.
EIN: 160874319

672
Rita J. and Stanley H. Kaplan Foundation, Inc.

866 United Nations Plaza, Suite 306
New York 10017 (212) 688-1047
Contact: Rita J. Kaplan, Dir.
FAX: (212) 688-6907

Incorporated in 1984 in NY.
Donor(s): Stanley H. Kaplan, Rita J. Kaplan.
Financial data (yr. ended 12/31/95): Assets, $20,076,756 (M); expenditures, $1,850,650; qualifying distributions, $1,446,745, including $1,337,960 for grants (high: $150,000; low: $100; average: $100-$150,000).
Purpose and activities: Support for cultural programs, including music, arts, theater, performing arts, and museums; libraries; medical research and education, including mental illness, AIDS and cancer research, and hospital building funds; social and family services, including programs for the homeless, for children, and for women; Jewish giving; and organizations promoting human rights.
Fields of interest: Visual arts; Museums; Performing arts; Dance; Theater; Music; Humanities; Arts/cultural programs; Education, association; Education, research; Education, fund raising; Elementary/secondary education; Early childhood education; Child development, education; Elementary school/education; Higher education; Medical school/education; Theological school/education; Libraries/library science; Education; Hospitals (general); Health care; Mental health/crisis services; Cancer; AIDS; Biomedicine; Medical research; Cancer research; AIDS research; Gun control; Domestic violence prevention; Recreation; Youth development, services; Human services; Children & youth, services; Youth, services; Child development, services; Family services; Aging, centers & services; Women, centers & services; Homeless, human services; International affairs, goodwill promotion; Human rights (international); Race/intergroup relations; Roman Catholic federated giving programs; Jewish federated giving programs; Leadership development; Jewish agencies & temples; Religion; Disabled; Aging; Women; Gays/lesbians; Economically disadvantaged; Homeless; General charitable giving; Israel.
Types of support: General/operating support, continuing support, annual campaigns, capital campaigns, building/renovation, equipment, endowment funds, program development, professorships, seed money, fellowships, internships, research, in-kind gifts.
Limitations: Applications not accepted. Giving primarily in NY; some giving also in Boston, MA, and Israel. No grants to individuals.
Application information: Contributes only to pre-selected organizations.
Officers and Directors:* Stanley H. Kaplan,* Pres.; Nancy Kaplan Belsky, V.P.; Susan Beth Kaplan, V.P.; Rita J. Kaplan,* Secy.
Number of staff: 1 full-time professional; 1 part-time support.
EIN: 133221298

673
The Iris J. & Saul B. Katz Foundation, Inc.

111 Great Neck Rd., Suite 408
Great Neck 11021-5476
Contact: Saul B. Katz, Pres.

Established in 1982.
Donor(s): Saul B. Katz.
Financial data (yr. ended 12/31/94): Assets, $867,767 (M); gifts received, $50,250; expenditures, $92,546; qualifying distributions, $88,785, including $88,785 for 19 grants (high: $25,700; low: $10).
Fields of interest: Higher education; Hospitals (general); Human services; Aging, centers & services; Jewish federated giving programs; Jewish agencies & temples; Aging; General charitable giving.
Limitations: Giving primarily in NY. No grants to individuals.
Application information: Application form not required.
Initial approach: Letter
Deadline(s): None
Officers and Directors:* Saul B. Katz,* Pres.; David M. Katz, Secy.-Treas.; Iris J. Katz.
EIN: 112626656
Grants for Aging:
Parker Jewish Geriatric Institute, New Hyde Park, NY, $1,000. 94.

674
Henry Kaufmann Foundation

1585 Broadway
New York 10036 (212) 969-3229
Contact: Jeffrey A. Horwitz, Secy.

Incorporated in 1928 in NY.
Donor(s): Henry Kaufmann.‡
Financial data (yr. ended 12/31/94): Assets, $1,857,365 (M); expenditures, $1,003,302; qualifying distributions, $961,298, including $940,000 for 21 grants (high: $425,000; low: $1,000; average: $5,000-$100,000).
Purpose and activities: Capital grants principally for geriatric care facilities, arts and educational institutions, Jewish giving and welfare funds, and camping and community centers.
Fields of interest: Arts/cultural programs; Education; Health care; Health organizations; Recreation; Human services; Aging, centers & services; Jewish federated giving programs; Jewish agencies & temples; Aging.
Types of support: Capital campaigns, building/renovation, equipment, land acquisition, professorships.
Limitations: Giving primarily in the metropolitan New York, NY, and Pittsburgh, PA, areas. No grants to individuals, or for endowment funds, operating budgets, scholarships, fellowships, or matching gifts; no loans.
Publications: 990-PF, financial statement, application guidelines.
Application information: Application form not required.
Initial approach: Written proposal
Copies of proposal: 2
Deadline(s): Submit written proposal preferably 1 or 2 months before board meeting dates; no set deadline
Board meeting date(s): May and Nov.
Final notification: After board meetings (positive replies only)
Officers and Directors:* Philip J. Hirsch,* Pres.; Leonard N. Block,* V.P.; Jeffrey A. Horwitz, Secy.; William T. Golden,* Treas.; Jerome Goldsmith, Exec. Dir.; Charles Looker, Frederick P. Rose, John M. Wolf, Sr., Arnold Levine.
Number of staff: None.
EIN: 136034179

675
Walter H. D. Killough Trust

c/o Marine Midland Bank, N.A.
250 Park Ave., 4th Fl.
New York 10177 (212) 503-2768
Contact: Deborah S. Metrick, Trust Officer, Marine Midland Bank, N.A.

Trust established in 1929 in NY.
Donor(s): Walter H.D. Killough.‡
Financial data (yr. ended 07/31/95): Assets, $2,851,247 (M); expenditures, $136,403; qualifying distributions, $91,132, including $81,795 for 22 grants (high: $21,283; low: $1,000).
Purpose and activities: Specific grants to designated educational and humane organizations; discretionary grants restricted primarily to hospitals and homes for the aged; scholarship funds.
Fields of interest: Hospitals (general); Aging, centers & services; Aging.
Types of support: General/operating support, continuing support, building/renovation, equipment, emergency funds, program development, scholarship funds, research.
Limitations: Giving primarily in NJ and NY. No grants to individuals.
Application information: Application form not required.
Initial approach: Proposal
Copies of proposal: 1
Deadline(s): Oct. 15
Board meeting date(s): Nov. 30
Final notification: Jan. 15
Trustees: Norman S. Fink, Rt. Rev. Robert C. Witcher, Marine Midland Bank, N.A.
Number of staff: None.
EIN: 136063894
Grants for Aging:
Parker Jewish Geriatric Institute, New Hyde Park, NY, $1,000. 94.
Saint Josephs Home for the Elderly, $1,000. 94.
Village Nursing Home, NYC, NY, $1,000. 94.

676
Kinney Memorial Foundation

c/o The Bank of New York, Tax Dept.
One Wall St., 28th Fl.
New York 10286 (212) 495-1205
Contact: Andrew Roman, V.P., The Bank of New York

Established in 1991 in NY.
Financial data (yr. ended 12/31/94): Assets, $3,050,040 (M); expenditures, $296,920; qualifying distributions, $266,124, including

$262,217 for 101 grants (high: $53,382; low: $100).
Fields of interest: Elementary/secondary education; Higher education; Hospitals (general); Aging, centers & services; Christian agencies & churches.
Types of support: General/operating support.
Limitations: Giving primarily in NY, NJ, and PA. No grants to individuals.
Application information:
Initial approach: Letter
Deadline(s): None
Trustees: Edward Holloway, Jr., Col. George R. Kinney, Jr., The Bank of New York.
EIN: 136968427

677
Kvistad Foundation
Route 1, Box 381A
West Hurley 12491 (914) 331-2450
Contact: Gina Van Hentenryck

Established in 1988.
Donor(s): Garry Kvistad, Diane Kvistad, Woodstock Percussion, Inc.
Foundation type: Operating
Financial data (yr. ended 12/31/95): Assets, $264,338 (M); gifts received, $102,250; expenditures, $96,997; qualifying distributions, $96,997, including $95,853 for 96 grants (high: $8,764; low: $35).
Purpose and activities: Support primarily to organizations which provide food and shelter for the poor, including the elderly and children, and to arts organizations and libraries.
Fields of interest: Arts/cultural programs; Libraries/library science; Education; Food services; Human services; Children & youth, services; Aging, centers & services; Aging; Economically disadvantaged.
Limitations: Giving primarily in Ulster County, NY. No grants to individuals.
Application information: Application form not required.
Deadline(s): None
Officers: Diane Herrick Kvistad, Pres.; Garry Kvistad, Secy.
EIN: 141702791
Grants for Aging:
New York Foundation for Senior Citizens, NYC, NY, $500. 95.
Ulster County Office of Aging, Kingston, NY, $2,000. For meals program. 95.

678
The Morris P. Leibovitz Foundation
c/o Feldman Radin and Co., P.C.
805 Third Ave., 21st Fl.
New York 10022

Established in 1988 in NY.
Donor(s): Morris P. Leibovitz.‡
Financial data (yr. ended 12/31/94): Assets, $2,437,173 (M); expenditures, $236,448; qualifying distributions, $185,500, including $125,000 for 3 grants (high: $85,000; low: $15,000).
Fields of interest: Health associations; Human services; Aging, centers & services; Jewish federated giving programs; Jewish agencies & temples; Disabled; Aging.
Limitations: Applications not accepted. Giving primarily in NY. No grants to individuals.
Application information: Contributes only to pre-selected organizations.
Trustees: Brian Leibovitz, Al Marston, Carole Ann McLeod.
EIN: 133442686

679
Louis Levin Foundation
c/o A. Zell
392 Central Park West, Apt. 1217
New York 10025
Contact: Joan Rose, Trustee

Established in 1967.
Financial data (yr. ended 12/31/93): Assets, $1,210,684 (M); expenditures, $69,594; qualifying distributions, $36,436, including $36,436 for 40 grants (high: $5,000; low: $50).
Purpose and activities: Support for synagogues, the aged, orphanages, medical research, and medical colleges.
Fields of interest: Medical school/education; Medical research; Children & youth, services; Aging, centers & services; Jewish agencies & temples; Aging.
Limitations: Giving primarily in NY. No grants to individuals.
Application information: Application form not required.
Initial approach: Proposal
Deadline(s): None
Trustees: David Rose, Joan Rose, Saul Rose.
EIN: 226076671

680
Lindenbaum Family Charitable Trust
c/o Belle and Samuel H. Lindenbaum
575 Madison Ave.
New York 10022

Established in 1989 in NY.
Financial data (yr. ended 09/30/94): Assets, $827,104 (M); expenditures, $91,138; qualifying distributions, $83,690, including $82,250 for 26 grants (high: $32,100; low: $50).
Fields of interest: Museums; Arts/cultural programs; Secondary school/education; Education; Aging, centers & services.
Limitations: Applications not accepted. Giving primarily in New York, NY. No grants to individuals.
Application information: Contributes only to pre-selected organizations.
Trustees: Belle Lindenbaum, Samuel Lindenbaum.
EIN: 136929327

681
Fay J. Lindner Foundation
1161 Meadowbrook Rd.
North Merrick 11566
Contact: Robert M. Goldberg, Pres.

Established in 1966.
Donor(s): Fay J. Lindner.‡
Financial data (yr. ended 08/31/95): Assets, $22,516,452 (M); expenditures, $1,033,814; qualifying distributions, $1,012,136, including $973,643 for 78 grants (high: $66,000; low: $575).
Purpose and activities: Giving primarily for hospitals, child welfare, the elderly, and social services; grants also to a university and Jewish organizations, including a welfare fund.
Fields of interest: Performing arts; Hospitals (general); Health care; Health associations; Human services; Children & youth, services; Hospices; Aging, centers & services; Jewish agencies & temples; Aging.
Types of support: Building/renovation, program development, seed money, fellowships, program-related investments/loans.
Limitations: Applications not accepted. Giving primarily in Long Island, NY. No grants to individuals.
Application information: Contributes only to pre-selected organizations.
Officers and Directors:* Robert M. Goldberg,* Pres.; Robin Goldberg,* Secy.; Herman Scheffer,* Secy.; David Goldberg.
EIN: 116043320
Grants for Aging:
Gurwin Jewish Geriatric Center of Long Island, Commack, NY, $65,000. 94.
Gurwin Jewish Geriatric Center of Long Island, Commack, NY, $50,000. 95.
Parker Jewish Geriatric Institute, New Hyde Park, NY, $50,000. 95.

682
The Kenneth & Evelyn Lipper Foundation
c/o Lipper & Co., Inc.
101 Park Ave., 6th Fl.
New York 10178 (212) 883-6333
Contact: Kenneth Lipper, Trustee

Established about 1982 in NY.
Donor(s): Gruss Petroleum Corp., Evmar Oil Corp.
Financial data (yr. ended 08/31/94): Assets, $9,709,022 (M); gifts received, $9,462,971; expenditures, $2,308,418; qualifying distributions, $2,266,674, including $2,247,382 for 138 grants (high: $1,000,000; low: $200; average: $1,000-$10,000).
Purpose and activities: Giving primarily for education and arts, giving also for nursing homes and Jewish welfare funds.
Fields of interest: Arts/cultural programs; Elementary/secondary education; University; Nursing home/convalescent facility; Human services; Children & youth, services; Jewish federated giving programs; Jewish agencies & temples.
Limitations: Giving primarily in New York, NY.
Application information: Application form not required.
Deadline(s): None
Trustees: Evelyn Gruss Lipper, Kenneth Lipper.
EIN: 133188873

683
Gerda Lissner Foundation, Inc.
135 East 55th St., 8th Fl.
New York 10022
Contact: Betty Smith, Pres.

Established in 1994 in NY.
Donor(s): Gerda Lissner.‡
Financial data (yr. ended 12/31/94): Assets, $9,495,221 (M); gifts received, $9,811,204; expenditures, $266,566; qualifying distributions, $262,059, including $100 for 1 grant.
Fields of interest: Alzheimer's disease; Medical research.
Limitations: Giving primarily in New York, NY.
Application information: Application form not required.
Deadline(s): None
Officers: Betty Smith, Pres.; Lynn Barnett, V.P.
Directors: Edmund Badgley, Angelene Rasmussen.
EIN: 133566516

684
Marquis George MacDonald Foundation, Inc.
c/o Chase Manhattan Bank, N.A.
1345 Ave. of the Americas, 48th Fl.
New York 10105
Contact: Donna M. Bowers, Administrator

Incorporated in 1951 in NY.
Donor(s): Marquis George MacDonald.‡
Financial data (yr. ended 12/31/95): Assets, $6,592,933 (M); expenditures, $328,670; qualifying distributions, $324,631, including $296,724 for 140 grants (high: $20,000; low: $500).
Purpose and activities: Giving for the arts, environment, higher and secondary education, church support, religious associations, hospitals, health, cancer and AIDS research, welfare funds, and organizations providing benefit to the community and serving the public interest.
Fields of interest: Media/communications; Visual arts; Museums; Performing arts; Dance; Theater; Music; Arts/cultural programs; Secondary school/education; Higher education; Natural resource conservation & protection; Environment; Animal welfare; Hospitals (general); Health care; Health associations; Cancer; AIDS; Alcoholism; Cancer research; AIDS research; Food services; Human services; Aging, centers & services; Women, centers & services; Arms control; Community development; Roman Catholic agencies & churches; Jewish agencies & temples; Religion; Disabled; Aging; Women.
Types of support: Continuing support, program development, scholarship funds.
Limitations: Applications not accepted. No grants to individuals, or for matching gifts; no loans.
Application information: Contributes only to pre-selected organizations; unsolicited proposals not considered.
Board meeting date(s): May 7, Aug. 6, and Dec. 10
Officers and Directors:* Catherine MacDonald,* Pres.; Kevin McDonald,* V.P.; John L. McDonald, Jr.,* V.P. and Treas.; Elizabeth McDonald,* Secy.; Helen McDonald, Joseph MacDonald.
Number of staff: 1 part-time professional.
EIN: 131957181

685
Mary W. MacKinnon Fund
c/o Wilber National Bank, Trust Dept.
245 Main St.
Oneonta 13820-2502 (607) 432-1700

Established in 1968 in NY.
Donor(s): Mary W. MacKinnon.‡
Financial data (yr. ended 12/31/94): Assets, $1,312,019 (M); expenditures, $70,462; qualifying distributions, $66,782, including $64,755 for grants to individuals.
Purpose and activities: To provide medical, hospital, rehabilitation, and nursing home care for local aged and indigent individuals.
Fields of interest: Aging, centers & services; Aging; Economically disadvantaged.
Types of support: Grants to individuals.
Limitations: Giving limited to Sidney, NY, residents.
Application information:
Initial approach: Application must be submitted through doctor or hospital
Deadline(s): None
Trustees: Rev. Irving Ballert, Jr., Roma Haag, Theodore Wilklow.
EIN: 237234921

686
The Anna D. Mahan Foundation
800 Mony Tower I
Syracuse 13202-2721 (315) 474-6448
Contact: John J. Costello, Secy.

Established in 1984 in NY.
Financial data (yr. ended 06/30/95): Assets, $846,546 (M); expenditures, $59,249; qualifying distributions, $52,000, including $52,000 for 1 grant.
Purpose and activities: Support limited to the care and treatment of elderly and infirm persons in central NY.
Fields of interest: Aging, centers & services; Aging.
Types of support: General/operating support, capital campaigns, program development, technical assistance, matching funds.
Limitations: Giving limited to the central NY area. No grants to individuals.
Publications: Informational brochure (including application guidelines).
Application information: Application form not required.
Initial approach: Letter
Copies of proposal: 3
Deadline(s): None
Board meeting date(s): As needed
Officers and Directors:* Charlotte G. Holstein, Chair.; John J. Costello, Secy.; Msgr. Charles J. Fahey.
Number of staff: None.
EIN: 222695315

687
Marble Fund, Inc.
c/o Rosenberg Selsman and Co.
655 Third Ave., Suite 1610
New York 10017
Contact: Marion H. Levy, Pres.

Established in 1952 in NY.
Donor(s): M. William Levy,‡ Marion H. Levy, Caryn L. Magid, William Guy Levy.
Financial data (yr. ended 12/31/95): Assets, $2,237,847 (M); expenditures, $143,525; qualifying distributions, $138,109, including $137,322 for 95 grants (high: $15,000; low: $20).
Fields of interest: Performing arts; Theater; Education, fund raising; Secondary school/education; Education; Environment; Wildlife preservation & protection; Health care; Health organizations; Medical research; Aging, centers & services; Peace; Rural development; Community development; Biological sciences; Anthropology & sociology; Aging; General charitable giving; Africa.
Types of support: General/operating support, annual campaigns, capital campaigns, building/renovation, seed money, research, technical assistance.
Limitations: Giving primarily in NY. No grants to individuals.
Application information:
Initial approach: Letter
Deadline(s): None
Officers and Director:* Marion H. Levy,* Pres.; William Guy Levy, V.P.; Caryn L. Magid, V.P.
Number of staff: None.
EIN: 136084387

688
J. M. McDonald Foundation, Inc.
48 West Court St.
P.O. Box 470
Cortland 13045 (607) 756-9283
Contact: Reed L. McJunkin, Secy.

Incorporated in 1952 in NE.
Donor(s): James M. McDonald, Sr.‡
Financial data (yr. ended 12/31/94): Assets, $12,842,277 (M); expenditures, $770,636; qualifying distributions, $670,000, including $670,000 for grants (average: $3,500-$50,000).
Purpose and activities: Grants for the aged, orphans, and children who are sick, infirm, blind, or crippled; support for youth and child care in an effort to combat juvenile delinquency and to aid underprivileged, mentally or physically handicapped children; other interests include health and hospitals and education, especially higher education. Prefers funding capital projects.
Fields of interest: Higher education; Education; Hospitals (general); Health care; Crime/law enforcement; Human services; Children & youth, services; Youth, services; Aging, centers & services; Disabled; Aging.
Types of support: General/operating support, continuing support, annual campaigns, capital campaigns, building/renovation, equipment.
Limitations: Giving limited to the U.S., with emphasis on the Northeast. No grants to individuals, or for seminars, workshops,

endowment funds, scholarships, fellowships, travel, exhibits, or conferences; no loans.
Publications: Application guidelines.
Application information: Application form not required.
Initial approach: Letter, proposal, or telephone
Copies of proposal: 1
Deadline(s): Apr. 15 and Sept. 15
Board meeting date(s): May and Oct.
Final notification: May 30 or Oct. 30 for positive responses
Officers and Trustees:* Eleanor F. McJunkin,* Pres.; Donald R. McJunkin,* V.P.; Reed L. McJunkin,* Secy.; Donald C. Berry, Jr.,* Treas.
Number of staff: 1 part-time support.
EIN: 471431059

689
Dextra Baldwin McGonagle Foundation, Inc.
P.O. Box 58, Main Post Office
Purchase 10577
Contact: Maury L. Spanier, Chair.

Incorporated in 1967 in NY.
Donor(s): Dextra Baldwin McGonagle.‡
Financial data (yr. ended 12/31/95): Assets, $8,670,969 (M); expenditures, $576,917; qualifying distributions, $488,415, including $488,415 for 74 grants (high: $126,500; low: $25; average: $25-$130,000).
Purpose and activities: Primary areas of interest include hospitals, the medical sciences, and medical research, including cancer research; grants also for higher and medical education, social service agencies, and cultural programs.
Fields of interest: Arts/cultural programs; Higher education; Medical school/education; Hospitals (general); Health care; Cancer; Biomedicine; Medical research; Cancer research; Human services; Biological sciences; Aging.
Types of support: Annual campaigns, building/renovation, equipment, endowment funds, seed money, research.
Limitations: Giving primarily in NY and CA. No grants to individuals, or for matching gifts.
Application information: Application form not required.
Copies of proposal: 1
Deadline(s): None
Board meeting date(s): As required
Officers and Directors:* Maury L. Spanier,* Chair.; David B. Spanier,* Pres.; Helen G. Spanier,* V.P. and Secy.-Treas.
Number of staff: 1 part-time support.
EIN: 136219236

690
Merrill Lynch & Co. Inc.
World Financial Center, South Tower
World Headquarters
New York 10080-6106 (212) 236-4319
Contact: Westina L. Matthews, V.P., Philanthropic Prog.
For Special Events: Linda Federici, V.P., Special Events, at above address

Established in 1950 in NY.
Financial data (yr. ended 12/31/95): Total giving, $8,209,910, including $8,209,910 for grants.
Purpose and activities: Merrill Lynch and its subsidiaries support: education, health and hospitals, the environment, culture and the arts, civic affairs, and human services. In addition to direct cash grants, the company underwrites cultural events, and awards grants on behalf of employee volunteers through the Employee Community Involvement Program.
Fields of interest: Museums; Dance; Theater; Music; Historic preservation/historical societies; Arts/cultural programs; Higher education; Business school/education; Libraries/library science; Education; Natural resource conservation & protection; Energy; Hospitals (general); Health care; Substance abuse, services; Health organizations; Housing/shelter, development; Human services; Youth, services; Family services; Aging, centers & services; Women, centers & services; Minorities/immigrants, centers & services; Homeless, human services; Business & industry; Community development; Voluntarism promotion; Government/public administration; Public affairs; Minorities; Economically disadvantaged; Homeless.
Types of support: General/operating support, continuing support, capital campaigns, building/renovation, endowment funds, scholarship funds, employee volunteer services, employee matching gifts, employee-related scholarships, donated equipment.
Limitations: Giving primarily in the main headquarters area of the greater New York, NY area, and in other cities where the company has offices. No support for fraternal, social, or athletic organizations, nor to political parties, groups, or candidates. No grants to individuals, or for operating support of government agencies, or to reduce an operating deficit or liquidate a debt.
Publications: Corporate giving report (including application guidelines).
Application information: Company has a staff that only handles contributions. Application form not required.
Initial approach: Letter (3 page maximum) to headquarters; organizations outside the greater New York area should send requests to nearest branch office
Copies of proposal: 1
Deadline(s): No deadlines; decisions are made continuously
Board meeting date(s): Quarterly
Final notification: Within 60 days
Administrators: John A. Fitzgerald, Pres., Merrill Lynch and Co. Fdn., Inc.; Westina L. Matthews, V.P., Philanthropic Progs. and Secy. of the Fdn.
Number of staff: 5 full-time professional; 1 part-time professional; 4 full-time support.

691
Stanley W. Metcalf Foundation, Inc.
120 Genesee St., Rm. 503
Auburn 13021
Contact: J. Douglas Pedley, Pres.

Established in 1962.
Donor(s): Stanley W. Metcalf.‡
Financial data (yr. ended 12/31/95): Assets, $6,483,316 (M); expenditures, $402,176; qualifying distributions, $385,435, including $346,500 for 67 grants (high: $25,000; low: $1,000; average: $500-$50,000).
Purpose and activities: Emphasis on youth organizations and church support; grants also for hospitals, welfare, and education.
Fields of interest: Nursing school/education; Education; Hospitals (general); Human services; Youth, services; Protestant agencies & churches; Disabled; Aging.
Types of support: General/operating support, continuing support, annual campaigns, capital campaigns, building/renovation, endowment funds, emergency funds, scholarship funds, matching funds.
Limitations: Giving primarily in Cayuga County, NY.
Application information: Application form not required.
Initial approach: Letter
Copies of proposal: 1
Deadline(s): None
Board meeting date(s): Jan., July, and Oct.
Officers and Directors:* J. Douglas Pedley,* Pres.; Caryl W. Adams, Secy.; Herbert T. Anderson, James P. Costello, Walter M. Lowe, Marjorie S. Pedley, Ronald D. West.
Number of staff: None.
EIN: 156017859
Grants for Aging:
Faatz-Crofut Home for the Elderly, Auburn, NY, $25,000. 95.
Mercy Health and Rehabilitation Center Nursing Home Company, Auburn, NY, $10,000. 95.

692
Metzger-Price Fund, Inc.
230 Park Ave., Suite 2300
New York 10169 (212) 867-9500
Contact: Isaac A. Saufer, Secy.-Treas.

Trust established in 1970 in NY.
Donor(s): Estelle Metzger,‡ Leonard Metzger.‡
Financial data (yr. ended 06/30/95): Assets, $618,550 (M); gifts received, $170,257; expenditures, $200,124; qualifying distributions, $196,017, including $183,000 for 98 grants (high: $4,500; low: $1,000; average: $1,000-$3,000).
Purpose and activities: Giving for aid to the handicapped and health services; support also for child welfare and social service agencies, recreation, and the elderly.
Fields of interest: Education; Health care; AIDS; AIDS research; Food services; Recreation; Human services; Children & youth, services; Youth, services; Family services; Aging, centers & services; Women, centers & services; Homeless, human services; Community development; Public affairs; Minorities; Disabled; Aging; Women; Economically disadvantaged; Homeless.
Types of support: General/operating support, continuing support, program development.
Limitations: Giving primarily in New York, NY. No grants to individuals, or for capital campaigns or building funds; no multiple grants in single calendar year to same organization.
Publications: Financial statement.
Application information: Application form not required.
Initial approach: Letter
Copies of proposal: 1

Deadline(s): Submit proposal preferably 1 month before board meetings
Board meeting date(s): Jan., Apr., July, and Oct.
Final notification: Only if decision is affirmative
Officers and Directors:* Ronald B. Sobel,* Pres.; Don Robert Johnson,* V.P.; Isaac A. Saufer,* Secy.-Treas.
Number of staff: None.
EIN: 237072764
Grants for Aging:
Jewish Home and Hospital for Aged, NYC, NY, $3,000. 94.
Jewish Home and Hospital for Aged, NYC, NY, $3,000. 95.

693
The Midgard Foundation

Two World Trade Ctr., 39th Fl.
New York 10048
Contact: Phillip C. Broughton, Pres.

Established in 1975 in NY.
Donor(s): Richard W. Weatherhead.‡
Financial data (yr. ended 12/31/93): Assets, $2,247,562 (M); expenditures, $181,661; qualifying distributions, $174,573, including $168,625 for 17 grants (high: $112,500; low: $100).
Fields of interest: Visual arts; Performing arts; Historic preservation/historical societies; Arts/cultural programs; Higher education; Civil rights, women; Civil rights, aging; Civil rights, gays/lesbians; Protestant agencies & churches; Asians/Pacific Islanders; Aging; Women; Gays/lesbians; Asia; Japan.
Types of support: Continuing support, capital campaigns, program development, conferences/seminars, publication, seed money, fellowships, scholarship funds, exchange programs, matching funds.
Limitations: Giving primarily in the eastern U.S. No grants to individuals.
Application information: Application form not required.
Initial approach: Letter
Copies of proposal: 1
Deadline(s): None
Officer and Directors:* Phillip C. Broughton,* Pres. and Treas.; Phillip C. Broughton, Jr., V.P.; C. Hardiman, Secy.
Number of staff: None.
EIN: 136206619

694
The Llewellyn Miller Fund of the American Society of Journalists and Authors Charitable Trust

1501 Broadway, Suite 302
New York 10036 (212) 997-0947
Contact: Murray Teigh Bloom, Chair.

Established in 1972 in NY; became operational in 1982.
Donor(s): New York Times Foundation, Reader's Digest Foundation, Newhouse Foundation.
Financial data (yr. ended 08/31/95): Assets, $118,550 (M); gifts received, $10,243; expenditures, $9,296; qualifying distributions, $8,000, including $8,000 for grants to individuals (high: $2,500).
Purpose and activities: Relief assistance to needy, established, professional freelance writers who are 60 years of age or older or disabled who are in financial need or caught up in an "extraordinary professional crisis."
Fields of interest: Journalism & publishing; Language & linguistics; Literature; Aging, centers & services; Disabled; Aging.
Types of support: Continuing support, grants to individuals.
Publications: Informational brochure, application guidelines.
Application information:
Initial approach: Letter
Deadline(s): None
Trustees: Murray Teigh Bloom, Chair.; Paul W. Bradley, Sey Chassler, Arlene Eisenberg, Glen Evans, Lewis Burke Frumkes, Joan Rattner Heilman, Terry Morris, Ray Robinson, Al Silverman.
Number of staff: 1 part-time support.
EIN: 136625578

695
The Ambrose Monell Foundation

c/o Fulton, Duncombe & Rowe
One Rockefeller Plaza, Suite 301
New York 10020-2002 (212) 586-0700
Contact: George Rowe, Jr., Pres.

Incorporated in 1952 in NY.
Donor(s): Maude Monell Vetlesen.‡
Financial data (yr. ended 12/31/94): Assets, $174,585,567 (M); expenditures, $8,810,953; qualifying distributions, $8,573,998, including $8,441,000 for 94 grants (high: $750,000; low: $1,000; average: $5,000-$100,000).
Purpose and activities: For the "improvement of the physical, mental, and moral condition of humanity throughout the world." Giving largely for hospitals and health services, scientific research, museums, performing arts, and other cultural activities, and higher and secondary education; support also for social services, research in political science, mental health, and aid to the handicapped.
Fields of interest: Secondary school/education; Higher education; Education; Animal welfare; Hospitals (general); Health care; Mental health/crisis services; AIDS; Alcoholism; Health organizations; Medical research; AIDS research; Human services; Aging, centers & services; Physical/earth sciences; Political science; Public policy, research; Disabled; Aging.
Types of support: General/operating support, continuing support, building/renovation, endowment funds, scholarship funds, research.
Limitations: No grants to individuals.
Application information: Proposal not exceeding 10 pages. Application form not required.
Initial approach: Proposal
Copies of proposal: 1
Deadline(s): Dec. 1
Board meeting date(s): Dec.
Officers and Directors:* George Rowe, Jr.,* Pres. and Treas.; Joseph T.C. Hart, Secy.; Eugene P. Grisanti, Henry G. Walter, Jr.
Number of staff: None.
EIN: 131982683
Grants for Aging:
Alzheimers Disease and Related Disorders Association, Chicago, IL, $150,000. For general support. 94.
American Federation for Aging Research (AFAR), NYC, NY, $100,000. For general support. 94.

696
J. P. Morgan Charitable Trust

(Formerly Morgan Guaranty Trust Company of New York Charitable Trust)
60 Wall St., 46th Fl.
New York 10260-0060 (212) 648-9673
Contact: Marilyn Montay, V.P., J.P. Morgan & Co. Incorporated

Trust established in 1961 in NY.
Donor(s): J.P. Morgan & Co. Incorporated.
Foundation type: Company-sponsored
Financial data (yr. ended 12/31/95): Assets, $35,360,638 (M); gifts received, $5,000,000; expenditures, $11,417,673; qualifying distributions, $11,225,750, including $7,564,517 for 440 grants (high: $325,000; low: $5,000; average: $5,000-$50,000) and $3,661,233 for 11,719 employee matching gifts.
Purpose and activities: Emphasis is on helping to find solutions to social problems and needs through support of competent agencies in fields of health, social services, culture, education, the environment, and international affairs. Special attention to job training, youth programs, international relief, housing, economic development, and advocacy and citizen involvement programs in New York City. Matches employee gifts to educational programs, cultural institutions, hospitals and health care agencies, human services and local development organizations, and environmental and international organizations.
Fields of interest: Performing arts; Arts/cultural programs; Elementary school/education; Higher education; Libraries/library science; Education; Environment; Hospitals (general); Health care; AIDS; Health organizations; AIDS research; Housing/shelter, development; Human services; Children & youth, services; Aging, centers & services; Minorities/immigrants, centers & services; International relief; International affairs; Economic development; Community development; Minorities; Eastern Europe; South Africa; Latin America; Asia.
Types of support: General/operating support, annual campaigns, capital campaigns, building/renovation, equipment, endowment funds, program development, seed money, technical assistance, employee matching gifts, matching funds.
Limitations: Giving limited to New York, NY, except for international affairs. No support for organizations working with chemical dependency, specific disabilities or diseases (except AIDS), or churches for non-secular purposes. No grants to individuals, or for scholarly research, scholarships, fellowships, or conferences; no loans.
Publications: Corporate giving report (including application guidelines).
Application information: Accepts New York Common Application form. Application form required.
Initial approach: Letter
Copies of proposal: 1

Deadline(s): Sept. 15
Board meeting date(s): Every 6 weeks
Final notification: 3 months
Advisory Committee: Roberto G. Mendoza, Jr., Michael E. Patterson, Hildy J. Simmons.
Trustee: J.P. Morgan & Co. Incorporated.
Number of staff: 7 full-time professional; 4 full-time support.
EIN: 136037931
Grants for Aging:
Coalition of Institutionalized Aged and Disabled, Bronx, NY, $10,000. For general support. 94.
Friends and Relatives of Institutionalized Aged, NYC, NY, $15,000. For general support. 94.
Medicare Beneficiaries Defense Fund, NYC, NY, $10,000. For general support. 94.
Mid-Bronx Senior Citizens Council, Bronx, NY, $15,000. For general support. 94.
Rivington House Health Care Facility, NYC, NY, $25,000. For start-up support. 94.
United Seniors Health Cooperative, DC, $20,000. For second payment for Benefits Outreach and Screening Software program. 94.

697
Morgan Stanley Group Corporate Giving Program
1251 Ave. of the Americas, 31st Fl.
New York 10020 (212) 703-6610
Contact: Patricia Schaefer, V.P. and Fdn. Officer

Purpose and activities: Each year, Morgan Stanley supports a wide variety of civic and cultural organizations, hospitals, social service agencies and educational institutions. The company does this as a way of demonstrating its commitment to the communities in which it operates. While corporate grants have increased steadily over the years, the firm has expanded its philanthropic mission to include more than the distribution of grant dollars. The company is also establishing productive partnerships with national and local organizations testing new ideas in education, employment training, health care and social services. These organizations are uniquely placed to understand and address the specific challenges facing urban communities. They are also a vital channel through which Morgan Stanley can participate in its communities.
Fields of interest: Arts/cultural programs; Education; Hospitals (general); AIDS; AIDS research; Employment; Food services; Housing/shelter, development; Human services; Aging, centers & services; Minorities/immigrants, centers & services; Community development.
Types of support: Fellowships, internships, scholarship funds, employee volunteer services, loaned talent, use of facilities.
Limitations: Giving primarily in New York, NY, Chicago, IL, and Los Angeles, CA. No support for United Way member agencies. No grants to individuals.
Application information:
Initial approach: Letter to headquarters requesting application guidelines
Copies of proposal: 1
Final notification: 3 to 6 months

698
Henry and Lucy Moses Fund, Inc.
c/o Moses and Singer
1301 Ave. of the Americas
New York 10019 (212) 554-7800
Contact: Henry Schneider, Esq., Pres.

Incorporated in 1942 in NY.
Donor(s): Henry L. Moses,‡ Lucy G. Moses.‡
Financial data (yr. ended 12/31/94): Assets, $1,725,389 (M); gifts received, $2,170,000; expenditures, $2,298,620; qualifying distributions, $2,277,394, including $2,273,100 for 100 grants (high: $500,000; low: $500; average: $10,000-$25,000).
Purpose and activities: Support for hospitals, including building funds, and rehabilitation and medical schools; Jewish and other welfare funds; higher and legal education and educational programs for minorities; social service agencies, including those for youth, child welfare, minorities, the aged, and the handicapped; arts and cultural programs, including dance; environmental concerns, including Central Park in New York City; and AIDS programs.
Fields of interest: Performing arts; Dance; Music; Arts/cultural programs; Higher education; Law school/education; Medical school/education; Environment; Hospitals (general); Medical care, rehabilitation; AIDS; AIDS research; Human services; Children & youth, services; Youth, services; Aging, centers & services; Minorities/immigrants, centers & services; Jewish federated giving programs; Minorities; Disabled; Aging; Israel.
Types of support: General/operating support, continuing support, annual campaigns, capital campaigns, building/renovation, endowment funds, professorships, fellowships, scholarship funds, research, matching funds.
Limitations: Giving primarily in the metropolitan New York, NY, area. No grants to individuals; no loans.
Application information: Support generally limited to previous grant recipients. Application form not required.
Initial approach: Letter
Copies of proposal: 1
Deadline(s): None
Board meeting date(s): Usually in Feb., May, Aug., and Oct.
Officers and Directors:* Henry Schneider,* Pres. and Treas.; Alfred W. Bressler,* V.P.; Joseph Fishman,* V.P.; Irving Sitnick,* Secy.
Number of staff: None.
EIN: 136092967
Grants for Aging:
Hebrew Home for the Aged at Riverdale, Bronx, NY, $10,000. 94.
Jewish Association for Services for the Aged, NYC, NY, $20,000. 94.
Jewish Home and Hospital for Aged, NYC, NY, $10,000. 94.

699
Mount Moriah Benevolent Fund, Inc.
c/o Skender Selman
112 Whitehill Ave.
Jamestown 14701-7928

Financial data (yr. ended 12/31/95): Assets, $4,671 (M); expenditures, $188; qualifying distributions, $175, including $150 for 2 grants (high: $100; low: $50) and $25 for grants to individuals.
Fields of interest: Aging, centers & services; Aging; Economically disadvantaged.
Types of support: Grants to individuals.
Limitations: Giving primarily in NY.
Officers: Jerome Erickson, Pres.; John Sundeen, V.P.; Murry Marsh, Jr., Secy.; Skender Selman, Treas.
EIN: 166030457

700
The Neisloss Family Foundation, Inc.
1787-6 Veterans Hwy.
Islandia 11722-1595 (516) 234-1600
Contact: Stanley Neisloss, Pres.

Established in 1991 in NY.
Donor(s): Stanley Neisloss.
Financial data (yr. ended 07/31/95): Assets, $1,165,063 (M); gifts received, $100,000; expenditures, $43,335; qualifying distributions, $38,600, including $38,425 for 20 grants (high: $23,300; low: $100).
Fields of interest: Hospitals (general); Health associations; AIDS; Human services; Aging, centers & services; Jewish federated giving programs; Aging.
Limitations: Giving primarily in New York, NY. No grants to individuals.
Application information: Application form not required.
Deadline(s): None
Officers: Stanley Neisloss, Pres. and Treas.; Irma Neisloss, V.P. and Secy.
Director: Martin Mones.
EIN: 113086865

701
The New York Community Trust
Two Park Ave., 24th Fl.
New York 10016-9385 (212) 686-0010
Contact: Lorie A. Slutsky, Dir.
FAX: (212) 532-8528

Established in 1924 in NY by resolution and declaration of trust.
Foundation type: Community
Financial data (yr. ended 12/31/95): Assets, $1,206,806,603 (M); gifts received, $168,494,797; expenditures, $112,807,977, including $107,795,883 for 3,100 grants (high: $3,310,708; low: $100; average: $5,000-$35,000).
Purpose and activities: A grantmaking community foundation. Priority given to applications for projects having particular significance for the New York City area. Loan guarantee program improves access to commercial lending. Program areas of major interest are 1) Children, youth and families - includes issues of hunger and homelessness, social services, substance abuse, and youth development; 2) Community development and the environment - includes civic affairs, conservation, economic development, housing, neighborhood revitalization, and technical assistance; 3) Education, arts and the humanities

- includes arts and culture, education, and human justice; and 4) Health and people with special needs - includes health services and policy, biomedical research, AIDS, visual handicaps, children and youth with disabilities, the elderly, and mental health and retardation.
Fields of interest: Arts/cultural programs; Child development, education; Education, public education; Environment; Health care; Substance abuse, services; Mental health/crisis services; Cancer; AIDS; Health organizations; Domestic violence prevention; Legal services; Employment; Food services; Housing/shelter, development; Human services; Children & youth, services; Family services; Aging, centers & services; Women, centers & services; Homeless, human services; Civil rights, immigrants; Civil rights, minorities; Civil rights, disabled; Civil rights, women; Civil rights, aging; Civil rights, gays/lesbians; Reproductive rights; Community development; Government/public administration.
Types of support: Program development, publication, seed money, fellowships, scholarship funds, research, technical assistance, consulting services, program-related investments/loans, employee matching gifts.
Limitations: Giving limited to the metropolitan New York, NY, area. No support for religious purposes. No grants to individuals, or for deficit financing, emergency funds, building campaigns, endowment funds, or general operating support.
Publications: Annual report, informational brochure (including application guidelines), newsletter, occasional report, financial statement.
Application information: Accepts NYRAG Common Application Form. Application form required.
Initial approach: Proposal with cover letter
Copies of proposal: 1
Deadline(s): None
Board meeting date(s): Feb., Apr., June, July, Oct., and Dec.
Final notification: Up to 25 weeks
Officers and Distribution Committee:* William M. Evarts, Jr.,* Chair.; Lorie A. Slutsky,* Pres. and Dir.; Karen Metcalf, V.P., Finance and Administration and Treas.; Joyce M. Bove, V.P., Progs. and Projects; Jane L. Wilton, Secy. and General Counsel; Kathryn Conroy, Cont.; Arthur G. Altschul, Bruce L. Ballard, M.D., Charlotte M. Fischman, Barry H. Garfinkel, Robert M. Kaufman, Anne Sidamon-Eristoff, Donald M. Stewart, Carroll L. Wainwright, Jr., Lulu C. Wang.
Trustees: The Bank of New York, Bankers Trust Co., Bessemer Trust Co., N.A., Brown Brothers, Harriman Trust Co., Chase, Citibank, N.A., Fiduciary Trust Co. International, IBJ Schroder Bank & Trust Co., Marine Midland Bank, N.A., Morgan Guaranty Trust Co. of New York, National Westminster Bank USA, Newberger and Berman Trust Co., Republic National Bank of New York, Rockefeller Trust Co., U.S. Trust Co. of New York.
Staff: Anita Nager, Sr. Prog. Officer, Community Devel. & Environment; Luiz Velez, Sr. Prog. Officer, Children, Youth & Families; Patricia White, Sr. Prog. Officer, Children, Youth & Families; Taryn Higashi, Prog. Officer, Education, Arts & Humanities; Len McNally, Prog. Dir., Health/People with Special Needs; Jane Stern, Prog. Dir., Education, Arts & Humanities; Jacqueline Elias, Prog. Assoc.
Number of staff: 20 full-time professional; 2 part-time professional; 16 full-time support; 1 part-time support.
EIN: 133062214
Grants for Aging:
A Very Special Place, Staten Island, NY, $10,000. To integrate developmentally disabled elders in mainstream Staten Island senior centers. 95.
American Society on Aging, San Francisco, CA, $10,000. For continued support for leadership development of New York City minority professionals in field of aging. 95.
Betances Health Unit, NYC, NY, $50,000. For physician House Call program for elderly residents and homebound persons with AIDS on Lower East Side. 95.
Bronx AIDS Services, Bronx, NY, $15,000. To expand food distribution program for poor persons with AIDS. 95.
Brooklyn Bar Association Volunteer Lawyers Project, Brooklyn, NY, $30,000. To expand pro bono legal assistance to low-income elderly. 95.
Burden Center for the Aging, NYC, NY, $25,000. To serve isolated gay and lesbian elders. 95.
Cancer Care, NYC, NY, $480,000. For financial support program for indigent cancer patients. 95.
Casita Maria, Bronx, NY, $30,000. To serve isolated Spanish-speaking elderly residents of East Harlem. 95.
Coalition of Institutionalized Aged and Disabled, Bronx, NY, $30,000. To teach peer training in advocacy to residents of nursing and adult homes. 95.
Coler Memorial Hospital, NYC, NY, $100,000. To expand physical rehabilitation services for patients preparing to re-enter community life. 95.
Dorot, NYC, NY, $30,000. For program to prevent falls among homebound elderly. 95.
Friends and Relatives of Institutionalized Aged, NYC, NY, $35,000. To involve more Latinos in family councils in nursing homes. 95.
Greater Chinatown Community Association, NYC, NY, $15,000. To serve isolated Chinese elders on lower East Side. 95.
Harlem Hospital Center, NYC, NY, $42,000. To continue and to document program that helps grandparents caring for their drug-exposed grandchildren. 95.
Hunter College of the City University of New York, Brookdale Center on Aging, NYC, NY, $45,000. To serve isolated African-American elders in Harlem. 95.
Medicare Beneficiaries Defense Fund, NYC, NY, $30,000. To help elderly people receive medicare benefits and advocate for improved medicare policies. 95.
Mid-Bronx Senior Citizens Council, Bronx, NY, $25,000. To promote economic development initiatives. 95.
Morningside Retirement and Health Services, NYC, NY, $40,000. For supportive services. 95.
Mount Sinai Hospital and Medical Center, NYC, NY, $35,000. For intergenerational program that provides housing for elderly people and day care for children. 95.
New York City Department for the Aging, NYC, NY, $30,000. For program to assist grandparents raising their grandchildren. 95.
New York Legal Assistance Group, NYC, NY, $20,000. To expand pro bono legal assistance to low-income elderly. 95.
Pregones Touring Puerto Rican Theater Collection, NYC, NY, $10,000. For bilingual, cultural programs for children, youth and seniors. 95.
Spanish Speaking Elderly Council of Brooklyn, Brooklyn, NY, $45,000. To serve isolated Latino elders caring for their grandchildren. 95.
Sunnyside Home Care Project, Long Island City, NY, $32,000. To continue program that integrates home care clients into senior senters. 95.
United Jewish Appeal-Federation of Jewish Philanthropies, NYC, NY, $50,000. For nursing services to elderly residents of naturally occurring retirement community in Brooklyn. 95.
Visiting Nurse Service of New York, NYC, NY, $32,000. For support program for children of women with AIDS served by home care agency. 95.
West Side Federation for Senior Housing, NYC, NY, $30,000. To assess and respond to impact of entitlement cutbacks on tenants. 95.
YM-YWHA of the Bronx, Graenum Berger Bronx Jewish Federated Service Center, Bronx, NY, $15,000. For emergency feeding program for poor, Jewish elderly residents. 95.

702
New York Foundation

350 Fifth Ave., No. 2901
New York 10118 (212) 594-8009
Contact: Madeline Lee, Exec. Dir.

Incorporated in 1909 in NY.
Donor(s): Louis A. Heinsheimer,‡ Alfred M. Heinsheimer,‡ Lionel J. Salomon.‡
Financial data (yr. ended 12/31/95): Assets, $61,997,010 (M); expenditures, $4,142,016; qualifying distributions, $3,040,934, including $3,040,934 for 111 grants (high: $40,000; low: $1,600; average: $5,000-$35,000).
Purpose and activities: Support for projects designed to improve the quality of life for disadvantaged, handicapped, and minority populations, with extra emphasis on youth and the elderly, especially projects that involve community organizing and advocacy.
Fields of interest: Housing/shelter, development; Youth development, services; Human services; Youth, services; Aging, centers & services; Minorities/immigrants, centers & services; Homeless, human services; Civil rights, immigrants; Civil rights, minorities; Civil rights, disabled; Civil rights, women; Civil rights, aging; Civil rights, gays/lesbians; Race/intergroup relations; Reproductive rights; Community development; Minorities; African Americans; Latinos; Disabled; Aging; People with AIDS (PWAs); Immigrants/refugees; Economically disadvantaged; Homeless.
Types of support: General/operating support, continuing support, program development, seed money, technical assistance, program-related investments/loans.
Limitations: Giving limited to local programs in the New York, NY, metropolitan area. No support for the arts, medical research, or films. No grants to individuals, or to capital campaigns, renovations, emergency funds,

deficit financing, building or endowment funds, equipment, scholarships, fellowships, land acquisition, research, conferences, publications, or demonstration projects.
Publications: Annual report (including application guidelines).
Application information: Accepts NYRAG Common Application Form. Application form not required.
Initial approach: Letter outlining project and budget needs
Copies of proposal: 1
Deadline(s): Nov. 1, Mar. 1, and July 1
Board meeting date(s): Feb., June, and Oct.
Final notification: 3 to 6 months
Officers and Trustees:* Stephen D. Heyman,* Chair.; R. Harcourt Dodds,* Vice-Chair.; Margaret Fung,* Secy.; Edgar Wachenheim III,* Treas.; Madeline Lee, Exec. Dir.; Susan Bellinger, Emilio Bermiss, Angela Diaz, M.D., Rose Dobrof, A. Carleton Dukess, Angelo Falcon, Madeline Einhorn Glick, David R. Jones, William M. Kelly, Thomas J. Kline, Elba Montalvo, Brian P. Mooney, Malcolm B. Smith, Arthur Zankel.
Staff: Vicente Martinez, Prog. Officer; Maria Mottola, Prog. Officer.
Number of staff: 4 full-time professional; 4 full-time support.
EIN: 135626345
Grants for Aging:
Asian-American Task Force on Aging, NYC, NY, $30,000. For coalition of agencies serving and advocating for Asian-American elderly. 94.
Bronx Regional Interagency Council on Aging, Bronx, NY, $37,000. To hire staff to help increase membership and enhance clearinghouse function and advocacy abilities. 94.
Casita Maria, Bronx, NY, $30,000. For Homebound Visitors Program, neighbor-to neighbor network providing outreach to homebound elderly in East Harlem. 94.
Council of Senior Centers and Services of New York City, NYC, NY, $36,540. For continued support for Training Unit Coordinator providing technical assistance and training to senior citizens centers. 94.
Friends and Relatives of Institutionalized Aged, NYC, NY, $40,000. For general support. 94.
Institute for the Puerto Rican/Hispanic Elderly, NYC, NY, $30,000. For consortium with RAICES and VISIONES, providing minority and visually-impaired elderly with enrollment information on Supplemental Security Income. 94.
Joint Public Affairs Committee for Older Adults, NYC, NY, $35,000. For Queens community organizer. 94.
Korean Community Services of Metropolitan New York, Woodside, NY, $33,000. For home care service program for Korean homebound elderly in northern Queens. 94.
Latino Gerontological Center, NYC, NY, $35,000. For general support. 94.
New York State Conference for the Aging, Albany, NY, $35,000. For general support. 94.
New York Statewide Senior Action Council, Albany, NY, $43,218. For advocacy campaign to unite elderly and youth groups in coordinated effort to dispel intergenerational competition for government resources. 94.

703
Ethel & Alexander Nichoson Foundation

18 West Carver St.
Huntington 11743
Contact: Arthur Goldstein, Trustee

Established in 1970.
Financial data (yr. ended 05/31/95): Assets, $1,540,122 (M); expenditures, $101,619; qualifying distributions, $84,360, including $84,360 for grants (high: $7,500).
Fields of interest: Human services; Children & youth, services; Family services; Aging, centers & services; Jewish federated giving programs; Jewish agencies & temples; Aging.
Limitations: Giving primarily in the metropolitan New York, NY, area, including Long Island. No grants to individuals.
Application information: Application form not required.
Deadline(s): None.
Trustee: Arthur Goldstein.
EIN: 116101005

704
The William F. Nicklin Charitable Foundation

33 Grand Ave.
Newburgh 12550-1932
Contact: William F. Nicklin, Trustee

Financial data (yr. ended 11/30/95): Assets, $38,882 (M); expenditures, $28,178; qualifying distributions, $27,163, including $27,163 for 6 grants (high: $15,413; low: $250).
Fields of interest: Education; Hospitals (general); Youth, services; Aging.
Types of support: Grants to individuals.
Limitations: Giving primarily in the Hudson Valley, NY, area.
Application information:
Initial approach: Proposal
Deadline(s): None
Trustee: William F. Nicklin.
EIN: 222454314

705
Northern Chautauqua Community Foundation, Inc.

212 Lake Shore Dr. West
Dunkirk 14048 (716) 366-4892
Contact: David J. Doino, Exec. Dir.

Incorporated in 1986 in NY.
Foundation type: Community
Financial data (yr. ended 12/31/95): Assets, $4,481,790 (M); gifts received, $539,324; expenditures, $307,348, including $197,649 for 36 grants (high: $10,000; low: $500; average: $500-$10,000), $50,500 for grants to individuals (average: $70-$2,000) and $50,000 for 1 loan.
Purpose and activities: Primary areas of interest include education, libraries, family services, community funds, cultural programs, and other general charitable activities.
Fields of interest: Arts/cultural programs; Higher education; Adult education—literacy & basic skills; Libraries/library science; Reading; Education; Environment; Hospitals (general); Substance abuse, services; Recreation; Family services; Hospices; Aging, centers & services; Community development; Voluntarism promotion; Federated giving programs; Aging; General charitable giving.
Types of support: General/operating support, continuing support, endowment funds, program development, scholarship funds, scholarships—to individuals, matching funds.
Limitations: Giving limited to northern Chautauqua County, NY. No support for religious organizations. No grants to individuals (except for designated scholarship funds), or for capital campaigns, general operating budgets, publication of books, conferences, or annual fundraising campaigns.
Publications: Annual report (including application guidelines), application guidelines.
Application information: Application form required.
Initial approach: Letter or telephone
Copies of proposal: 1
Deadline(s): 15 days prior to grants committee meetings
Board meeting date(s): Quarterly
Final notification: 10 days following board meeting
Officers and Directors:* Rocco R. Doino,* Pres.; Thomas Reed,* V.P.; Susan Marsh,* Secy.; Andrew W. Dorn, Jr.,* Treas.; David J. Doino, Exec. Dir.; Richard Anson, James F. Carpenter, Maxine Cole, Donald Eno, D.V.M., Richard S. Johnson, James H. Minton, Jr., Horace Pantano, Jeffrey G. Passafaro, Bruce H. Rittenburg III, Gerald Rocque, George B. Weaver, Jr., Thomas K. Webb, Jr., Susan Wells, H.K. Williams III.
Number of staff: 1 full-time professional; 1 part-time professional; 1 part-time support.
EIN: 161271663

706
Northern New York Community Foundation, Inc.

(Formerly Watertown Foundation, Inc.)
120 Washington St.
Watertown 13601 (315) 782-7110
Contact: Alex C. Velto, Exec. Dir.

Incorporated in 1929 in NY.
Foundation type: Community
Financial data (yr. ended 12/31/95): Assets, $12,150,398 (M); gifts received, $658,313; expenditures, $829,587, including $437,883 for 41 grants (high: $40,000; low: $250) and $207,000 for 152 grants to individuals (high: $3,000; low: $200).
Purpose and activities: To promote charitable, educational, cultural, recreational, and health programs through grants to community organizations and agencies, and through a student scholarship program in Jefferson and Lewis counties, NY.
Fields of interest: Historic preservation/historical societies; Arts/cultural programs; Education, fund raising; Child development, education; Adult/continuing education; Libraries/library science; Education; Environment; Hospitals (general); Nursing care; Health care; Substance abuse, services; AIDS; Health organizations; Food services; Housing/shelter, development; Recreation;

Human services; Children & youth, services; Youth, services; Child development, services; Family services; Hospices; Aging, centers & services; Homeless, human services; Community development; Federated giving programs; Government/public administration; Disabled; Aging; Economically disadvantaged; Homeless; General charitable giving.
Types of support: Annual campaigns, capital campaigns, building/renovation, equipment, land acquisition, program development, conferences/seminars, publication, seed money, scholarship funds, technical assistance, scholarships—to individuals, matching funds.
Limitations: Giving limited to organizations and individuals in Jefferson and Lewis counties, NY. No grants for endowment funds or deficit financing.
Publications: Annual report, newsletter.
Application information: Application form not required.
Initial approach: Letter
Copies of proposal: 1
Deadline(s): Feb. 1, May 1, Aug. 1, and Nov. 1
Board meeting date(s): Mar., June, Sept., and Dec.
Final notification: 1 to 2 months
Officers and Directors:* Lee T. Hirschey,* Pres.; Donna D. Macsuga,* V.P.; Grace A. Wright,* Secy.-Treas.; Alex C. Velto, Exec. Dir.; Janet J. George, James R. Kanik, Jane N. Lormore, Tony Morgia, James L. O'Donnell, Mark S. Purcell, Richard E. Smith, Jan K. Turcotte, Anderson Wise.
Number of staff: 1 full-time professional; 1 full-time support; 1 part-time support.
EIN: 156020989

707
The Ogilvy Foundation
309 West 49th St.
New York 10019
Contact: Nancy Nolan

Established in 1984 in NY.
Donor(s): The Ogilvy Group, Inc.
Foundation type: Company-sponsored
Financial data (yr. ended 06/30/95): Assets, $1,136,818 (M); expenditures, $81,711; qualifying distributions, $81,711, including $80,000 for 5 grants (high: $20,000; low: $15,000).
Purpose and activities: Giving primarily for wildlife conservation; support also for an outdoor educational and recreational program, the aged, and medical research.
Fields of interest: Adult/continuing education; Education; Natural resource conservation & protection; Wildlife preservation & protection; Medical research; Aging, centers & services.
Types of support: General/operating support, continuing support, research.
Limitations: Applications not accepted. Giving on a national and international basis. No grants to individuals.
Officers and Directors:* Graham Phillips,* Pres.; John Elliott, Jr.,* V.P.; William E. Phillips,* V.P.; Edward Harrigan,* Treas.; David Ogilvy.
EIN: 133230406

708
Open Society Fund
888 Seventh Ave., 33rd Fl.
New York 10106 (212) 757-2323
Contact: Steve Gutmann

Established about 1981 in NY.
Donor(s): George Soros, Tivadar Charitable Lead Trust.
Financial data (yr. ended 12/31/94): Assets, $5,415,088 (M); gifts received, $7,524,009; expenditures, $8,265,068; qualifying distributions, $8,073,470, including $3,351,834 for grants (low: $431; average: $20,000-$500,000), $692,935 for 209 grants to individuals and $450,477 for foundation-administered programs.
Purpose and activities: Support for independent institutions in the countries of Central and Eastern Europe, the former Soviet Union, and South Africa during the period of transition from repression to openness. Through its local foundations, its aim is to help build the infrastructures and institutions of an open society and to support a variety of educational, cultural, and economic restructuring activities. Support also for major regional programs in English language teaching and training, health education, library support and development, management training, media, medical training and equipment donation, publishing, student exchange and scholarships, contemporary art, student advising, and education reform.
Fields of interest: Media/communications; Journalism & publishing; Arts/cultural programs; Higher education; Libraries/library science; Education; Environment; Health care; Substance abuse, services; Biomedicine; Health organizations; Medical research; Aging, centers & services; Human rights (international); International affairs; International studies; Minorities; Aging; Europe; Eastern Europe; Soviet Union (Former); South Africa.
Types of support: General/operating support, continuing support, seed money, fellowships, scholarship funds, research.
Limitations: Giving primarily in Central and Eastern Europe, the former Soviet Union, and South Africa. No loans for individuals.
Publications: Newsletter, informational brochure.
Application information: Applicants will be solicited through contacts with educational institutions.
Initial approach: Telephone or letter to request application
Deadline(s): None
Officers and Directors:* George Soros,* Pres.; Gary Gladstein,* V.P. and Secy.; Susan Weber Soros,* V.P. and Treas.; Aryeh Neier, William D. Zabel.
EIN: 133095822

709
The Ostberg Foundation, Inc.
225 Park Ave. South
New York 10003
Contact: Isabelle Liebman

Established in 1980 in NY.
Donor(s): Henry D. Ostberg.
Financial data (yr. ended 11/30/94): Assets, $627,079 (M); gifts received, $36,580; expenditures, $197,459; qualifying distributions, $187,977, including $123,603 for 15 grants (high: $70,934; low: $50) and $64,374 for 42 grants to individuals (high: $4,436; low: $200).
Fields of interest: Aging, centers & services; Disabled; Aging; Economically disadvantaged; Homeless; Haiti.
Types of support: General/operating support, grants to individuals.
Limitations: Applications not accepted. Giving on an international basis.
Application information:
Board meeting date(s): Quarterly
Officers and Director:* Henry D. Ostberg,* Pres.; Neal Ostberg, V.P.; Sydelle Ostberg, Secy.
Number of staff: None.
EIN: 132963335

710
The Parodneck Foundation for Self-Help, Housing & Community Development, Inc.
(Formerly The Consumer-Farmer Foundation, Inc.)
121 Ave. of the Americas, Suite 501
New York 10013 (212) 431-9700
Contact: Harold DeRienzo, Pres.
FAX: (212) 431-9783

Established in 1970 in NY.
Donor(s): Meyer Parodneck.‡
Financial data (yr. ended 12/31/95): Assets, $30,430,414 (M); gifts received, $93,950; expenditures, $629,450, including $4,258,197 for program-related investments.
Purpose and activities: Support for low-income housing, planning, and community development with emphasis on assistance to senior citizens, including grants and loans to at-risk senior citizen homeowners to make necessary repairs.
Fields of interest: Housing/shelter, development; Housing/shelter, aging; Housing/shelter, repairs; Urban/community development; Community development, real estate; Community development; Aging.
Types of support: Building/renovation, seed money, technical assistance, program-related investments/loans, grants to individuals.
Limitations: Giving limited to New York, NY.
Publications: Annual report, 990-PF, application guidelines, newsletter, financial statement.
Application information: Application form required.
Initial approach: Letter
Deadline(s): None
Board meeting date(s): Quarterly
Officer and Directors:* Irma Rodriquez,* Chair.; Harold DeRienzo,* Pres.; Karolyn Gould,* Secy.; Dr. Harold Wattel,* Treas.; Eugenia M. Flatow,* Asst. Treas.; Mark B. Anderson, Susan Hyman, Jerome Liblit, Luis Sierra, Ozenith Tate.
Staff: Rebecca Dib, Housing Specialist; Glenn Duncan, Senior Citizen Prog. Mgr.; Amanda Ortiz, Bookkeeper; Rosina Crawford, Receptionist; Rey Rodriguez, Bronx Community Forum Coord.
Number of staff: 4 full-time professional; 2 part-time professional; 1 full-time support.
EIN: 112229635

711
Moses L. Parshelsky Foundation
26 Court St., Rm. 904
Brooklyn 11242 (718) 875-8883
Contact: Tony B. Berk, Trustee

Trust established in 1949 in NY.
Donor(s): Moses L. Parshelsky.‡
Financial data (yr. ended 12/31/95): Assets, $6,235,277 (M); expenditures, $284,070; qualifying distributions, $234,850, including $234,850 for 49 grants (high: $30,000; low: $100; average: $100-$30,000).
Purpose and activities: Emphasis on the aged, the handicapped, and hospitals; support also for higher and secondary education, temple support and religious activities, youth agencies, mental health, and Jewish welfare funds.
Fields of interest: Dance; Arts/cultural programs; Secondary school/education; Higher education; Hospitals (general); Mental health/crisis services; Cancer; Cancer research; Human services; Youth, services; Aging, centers & services; Jewish federated giving programs; Jewish agencies & temples; Disabled; Aging.
Limitations: Giving primarily in Brooklyn and Queens, NY. No grants to individuals, or for building or endowment funds, or operating budgets.
Application information: Application form not required.
Initial approach: Letter
Copies of proposal: 1
Deadline(s): May 31
Board meeting date(s): Monthly
Trustees: Tony B. Berk, Josephine B. Krinsky, Robert D. Krinsky.
Number of staff: 1 part-time professional.
EIN: 111848260
Grants for Aging:
Cancer Care, NYC, NY, $4,000. 94.
Metropolitan Jewish Geriatric Center, Brooklyn, NY, $27,500. For unkeep and improvement. 94.

712
Pfizer Inc Corporate Philanthropy Program
c/o Pfizer Inc
235 East 42nd St.
New York 10017-5755 (212) 573-5936
Contact: Grants Administrator, Corporate Philanthropy Dept.

Financial data (yr. ended 12/31/94): Total giving, $2,483,800, including $2,483,800 for 132 grants (high: $200,000; low: $1,000).
Purpose and activities: The broad objectives of Pfizer's corporate philanthropy program are to improve educational, health, cultural, social, and other community services in areas of company facilities; to make grants to educational and research institutions, academic departments, and programs which involve significant mutual, intellectual, or scientific interests; and to support selected national organizations and institutions whose programs address social problems of interest to Pfizer. Support for nonprofit organizations whose programs are of interest to the company as a whole or to the company's particular divisions, such as pharmaceuticals, chemicals, agriculture, materials science, consumer and hospital products. Programs in which Pfizer employees are active volunteers receive special consideration; Pfizer encourages individual employee support of health care and social service organizations through the United Way. Part of the contributions program focuses on encouraging studies, analyses, and discussions of policy issues; Pfizer seeks to recognize academic and other institutions engaged in research, writing, and publishing on policy issues. Additional support for organizations engaged in international activities, focusing on projects that enrich the development process worldwide and that directly relate to international public policy concerns; also support for organizations and institutions overseas through Pfizer International. The company often responds to emergencies and natural disasters with donations of medicine and/or equipment; this assistance is generally coordinated through established international relief agencies.
Fields of interest: Arts/cultural programs; Education, research; Education, fund raising; Elementary/secondary education; Higher education; Business school/education; Adult/continuing education; Adult education—literacy & basic skills; Libraries/library science; Education; Natural resource conservation & protection; Environment; Hospitals (general); Medical care, rehabilitation; Health care; Substance abuse, services; Cancer; Heart/circulatory disease; AIDS; Health organizations; Cancer research; Heart/circulatory research; AIDS research; Human services; Children & youth, services; Child development, services; Aging, centers & services; Minorities/immigrants, centers & services; Homeless, human services; International relief; International affairs; Business & industry; Community development; Science, formal/general education; Mathematics; Biological sciences; Political science; International studies; Government/public administration; Public affairs; Minorities; Disabled; Aging; Economically disadvantaged; Homeless; General charitable giving.
Types of support: General/operating support, continuing support, annual campaigns, capital campaigns, building/renovation, program development, conferences/seminars, professorships, publication, seed money, fellowships, research, technical assistance, employee volunteer services, use of facilities, employee matching gifts, donated equipment, donated products, in-kind gifts.
Limitations: Giving primarily in areas of company operations; support also for national organizations. No support for organizations that discriminate on the basis of race, creed, religion, gender, or nationality, religious organizations, fraternal, labor, or veterans' organizations unless they are engaged in a significant program benefiting the entire community, political parties or candidates, partisan political organizations, anti-business organizations, organizations related to the business interests of Pfizer Inc; generally no support for organizations receiving support from the United Way. No grants to individuals, or for courtesy advertising, or unsolicited fundraising events. Pfizer's corporate contributions program does not support conferences and symposia, disease-specific organizations, or research. Proposals or this nature pertaining to Pfizer's products or research should be directed to the appropriate operating group; no loans; usually no general, unrestricted contributions.
Publications: Corporate giving report (including application guidelines), grants list, corporate report.
Application information: Organizations serving regional interests in Pfizer communities are handled by local facility management; organizations whose programs complement Pfizer's business areas are handled by headquarters staff under the auspices of the division whose interests relate to the program; contributions to organizations with a broad-based, corporate-wide focus are handled by the Corporate Contributions Committee, which is comprised of Pfizer employees who meet regularly to review proposals; international contributions are handled by management in that country. Application form not required.
Initial approach: 3- to 5-page proposal or letter to headquarters or nearest company facility. No videos or audiocassettes
Copies of proposal: 1
Deadline(s): None
Board meeting date(s): Every 1 to 3 months
Final notification: Within 90 days
Number of staff: 3 full-time professional; 4 full-time support.

713
The Louis and Harold Price Foundation, Inc.
450 Park Ave., Suite 1102
New York 10022 (212) 753-0240
Contact: Harold Price, Chair., Gloria W. Appel, Pres., or Rosemary L. Guidone, Exec. V.P.
Additional tel.: (212) 752-9335

Incorporated in 1951 in NY.
Donor(s): Louis Price,‡ Harold Price.
Financial data (yr. ended 12/31/95): Assets, $68,550,160 (M); expenditures, $3,006,881; qualifying distributions, $2,586,212, including $2,470,008 for 182 grants.
Purpose and activities: Support for a business institute, Jewish welfare funds, hospitals, community funds, and higher education, including scholarship funds; grants also for youth agencies, camps for children, temple support, medical research, the arts, and services for the handicapped, including the blind.
Fields of interest: Theater; Arts/cultural programs; Education, fund raising; Elementary/secondary education; Child development, education; Higher education; Medical school/education; Adult/continuing education; Adult education—literacy & basic skills; Libraries/library science; Reading; Education; Animal welfare; Wildlife preservation & protection; Hospitals (general); Medical care, rehabilitation; Health care; Mental health/crisis services; Health associations; Cancer; Heart/circulatory disease; Skin disorders; AIDS; Biomedicine; Health organizations; Medical research; Cancer research; Heart/circulatory research; Skin research; AIDS research; Crime/law enforcement; Food services; Camps;

Recreation; Human services; Children & youth, services; Youth, services; Child development, services; Family services; Aging, centers & services; Minorities/immigrants, centers & services; Homeless, human services; Federated giving programs; Jewish federated giving programs; Roman Catholic agencies & churches; Jewish agencies & temples; Religion; Minorities; Disabled; Aging; Economically disadvantaged; Homeless; Israel.
Types of support: General/operating support, continuing support, annual campaigns, endowment funds, program development, scholarship funds, research.
Limitations: Giving primarily in the metropolitan New York, NY, area and Los Angeles, CA; support for Israel. No grants to individuals, or for building funds.
Application information: Application form not required.
Initial approach: Letter
Copies of proposal: 1
Deadline(s): None
Board meeting date(s): Feb., May, and as required
Final notification: 1 to 3 months
Officers and Trustees:* Harold Price,* Chair. and Treas.; Gloria W. Appel,* Pres.; Rosemary L. Guidone,* Exec. V.P.; Pauline Price,* V.P. and Secy.; George Asch, David Gerstein, Linda Vitti Herbst.
Number of staff: 1 full-time professional.
EIN: 136121358
Grants for Aging:
Jewish Homes for the Aging of Greater Los Angeles, Reseda, CA, $25,000. 94.

714
Ramapo Trust
126 East 56th St.
New York 10022 (212) 308-7355
Contact: Nora O'Brien by telephone, or Stephen L. Schwartz, Trustee, by mail

Trust established in 1973 in NY.
Donor(s): Henry L. Schwartz,‡ Montebello Trust.
Financial data (yr. ended 06/30/95): Assets, $38,928,832 (M); expenditures, $8,131,702; qualifying distributions, $7,951,789, including $7,424,858 for 68 grants (high: $4,739,500; low: $329; average: $7,500-$55,000).
Purpose and activities: Giving for gerontological and geriatric research and innovative services; support also for health, higher and other education.
Fields of interest: Higher education; Health care; Health organizations; Medical research; Aging, centers & services; Aging.
Types of support: Emergency funds, program development, conferences/seminars, seed money, research, matching funds.
Limitations: No grants to individuals, or for capital or building campaigns, operating budgets, continuing support, annual campaigns, or deficit financing; no loans.
Publications: Newsletter, application guidelines.
Application information: Application form not required.
Initial approach: Letter of intent
Deadline(s): None
Board meeting date(s): Monthly
Trustees: Arthur Norman Field, Karen Schwartz Hart, Andrew M. Schreier, William Schreier, Stephen L. Schwartz, Rebecca Shaffer, Mary Ann Van Clief.
Number of staff: 1 full-time professional; 1 part-time professional; 2 part-time support.
EIN: 136594279
Grants for Aging:
American Association of Retired Persons Foundation, DC, $100,000. 95.
Medicare Beneficiaries Defense Fund, NYC, NY, $25,695. 95.
National Institute on Aging, Bethesda, MD, $20,000. 95.

715
Republic New York Corporate Giving Program
452 Fifth Ave.
New York 10018 (212) 525-6597
Contact: J. Phillip Burgess, 1st V.P.

Purpose and activities: Main areas of interest are arts, education, Jewish welfare, health and human services and urban development. Support also for performing arts, cultural institutes, economic development, business and minority education, and private colleges. Provides employee matching gifts for higher education, advertising and public relations, general operation expenses, and donations of in-kind goods and services.
Fields of interest: Performing arts; Arts/cultural programs; Higher education; Business school/education; Adult/continuing education; Education; Substance abuse, services; AIDS; AIDS research; Food services; Human services; Children & youth, services; Family services; Aging, centers & services; Minorities/immigrants, centers & services; Homeless, human services; International affairs; Urban/community development; Community development; Jewish federated giving programs; Minorities; Disabled; Aging; Economically disadvantaged; Homeless.
Types of support: General/operating support, capital campaigns, program development, in-kind gifts.
Limitations: Giving primarily in the metropolitan New York, NY, area. No support for political organizations.
Application information:
Initial approach: Letter describing program
Deadline(s): None
Final notification: 2 to 3 weeks required for full review and decision

716
Rhodebeck Charitable Trust
245 Park Ave., 40th Fl.
New York 10167-0034
Contact: Huyler C. Held, Trustee

Established in 1987 in AZ.
Donor(s): Mildred T. Rhodebeck.‡
Financial data (yr. ended 04/30/95): Assets, $20,247,410 (M); expenditures, $1,402,225; qualifying distributions, $1,242,100, including $1,241,305 for 26 grants (high: $250,000; low: $1,500).
Purpose and activities: "To alleviate the plight of disadvantaged people in the New York metropolitan area, including homeless, hungry, elderly, children, and sick by making grants to publicly supported tax-exempt organizations concerned with one or more of these objectives."
Fields of interest: Mental health/crisis services; Legal services; Food services; Human services; Children & youth, services; Family services; Aging, centers & services; Homeless, human services; Federated giving programs; Aging; Economically disadvantaged; Homeless.
Types of support: Endowment funds, program development, seed money, matching funds.
Limitations: Giving limited to the metropolitan New York, NY, area. No grants to individuals.
Application information: Unsolicited applications are discouraged.
Trustee: Huyler C. Held.
Number of staff: 1 part-time support.
EIN: 133413293

717
The William and Mary Rosenwald Foundation
122 East 42nd St., 24th Fl.
New York 10168-0001

Established in 1984 in NY.
Donor(s): Nina Rosenwald.
Financial data (yr. ended 04/30/95): Assets, $72,185 (M); expenditures, $4,209; qualifying distributions, $3,125, including $2,075 for grants.
Fields of interest: Arts/cultural programs; Medical research; Aging, centers & services; Jewish agencies & temples; Aging.
Limitations: Applications not accepted. Giving primarily in the metropolitan New York, NY, area. No grants to individuals.
Application information: Contributes only to pre-selected organizations.
Officers and Directors:* Nina Rosenwald,* Pres.; Alice R. Sigelman,* V.P.; Elizabeth R. Varet,* V.P.; David P. Steinmann, Secy.-Treas.
EIN: 133179190

718
Arthur Ross Foundation, Inc.
20 East 74th St., 4-C
New York 10021 (212) 737-7311
Contact: Arthur Ross, Pres.

Incorporated in 1955 in NY.
Donor(s): Arthur Ross.
Financial data (yr. ended 12/31/95): Assets, $8,187,231 (M); gifts received, $1,905,813; expenditures, $2,052,992; qualifying distributions, $1,929,407, including $1,885,055 for 134 grants (high: $149,750; low: $1,000; average: $1,000-$100,000).
Purpose and activities: Giving for higher education and cultural institutions, especially museums and parks; support also for environmental organizations and historic preservation.
Fields of interest: Museums; Historic preservation/historical societies; Arts/cultural programs; Higher education; Medical

school/education; Environment; Disabled; Aging; Homeless.
Types of support: Continuing support, capital campaigns, endowment funds, conferences/seminars, scholarship funds, matching funds.
Limitations: Applications not accepted. Giving primarily in NY.
Application information: Contributes only to pre-selected organizations.
Officers and Directors:* Arthur Ross,* Pres. and Treas.; Clifford A. Ross,* Exec. V.P.; Janet C. Ross,* V.P.; George J. Gillespie III,* Secy.; Tom A. Bernstein, John H. Dobkin, William T. Golden, Ralph M. Sussman, Paul E. Taylor, Jr., Hon. William J. Vanden Heuvel, Edgar Wachenheim III.
Number of staff: 2
EIN: 136121436

719
The Fan Fox and Leslie R. Samuels Foundation, Inc.

630 Fifth Ave., Suite 2255
New York 10111-0002 (212) 315-2940
Contact: Eva Burt, Prog. Asst.
FAX: (212) 765-3319

Incorporated in 1959 in UT; reincorporated in 1981 in NY.
Donor(s): Leslie R. Samuels,‡ Fan Fox Samuels.‡
Financial data (yr. ended 07/31/95): Assets, $138,505,000 (M); expenditures, $5,964,000; qualifying distributions, $4,811,867, including $4,811,867 for 148 grants (high: $500,000; low: $400; average: $5,000-$200,000).
Purpose and activities: Grants for the performing arts and hospitals and health care, especially programs for the young and elderly; and a small budget for arts-in-education.
Fields of interest: Arts education; Performing arts; Opera; Dance; Theater; Music; Hospitals (general); Health care; Health organizations; Hospices; Aging, centers & services; Aging.
Types of support: General/operating support, program development, seed money, program-related investments/loans, matching funds.
Limitations: Giving limited to New York, NY. No support for social service or education. No grants to individuals, or for scholarships, fellowships, or film or video projects.
Publications: Biennial report (including application guidelines).
Application information: Application form not required.
Initial approach: Letter of inquiry not exceeding 3 typed pages
Copies of proposal: 1
Deadline(s): Sept. 1, Dec. 1, Mar. 1, and June 1
Board meeting date(s): Oct., Jan., Apr., July, and as necessary
Final notification: 3 months
Officers and Directors:* Marvin A. Kaufman,* Pres.; Joseph C. Mitchell,* V.P. and Treas.; Carlos D. Moseley,* V.P.; Morton J. Bernstein, Mary Jane Koven, M.D., Robert Marx.
Staff: Mo Katz, Health Prog. Advisor; Alexandra Francis, Prog. Assoc.; Eva M. Burt, Prog. Asst.
Number of staff: 2 full-time professional; 1 part-time professional; 2 full-time support.
EIN: 133124818

Grants for Aging:
Cobble Hill Nursing Home, Brooklyn, NY, $65,000. For study of nursing assistants' conception of care and actual provisions of care and to raise professionalism of caregivers of persons with dementia. 95.
Frances Schervier Home and Hospital, Riverdale, NY, $25,000. To establish long term care ethics network in New York City. 95.
Hospital for Joint Diseases Orthopedic Institute, NYC, NY, $50,000. For Geriatric Falls Program to better treat older people who have fallen, to work in community and teach people how to prevent falls. 95.
Jewish Home and Hospital for Aged, NYC, NY, $75,000. To complete, furnish and equip Therapeutic Arts and Recreation Center. 95.
Jewish Home and Hospital for Aged, NYC, NY, $34,800. To enhance communication ability of Alzheimer patients. 95.
Morningside House, Bronx, NY, $25,000. For research project, Stability of Preferences for Treatment in Nursing Home Population. 95.
New York Hospital-Cornell Medical Center, NYC, NY, $95,000. For study of treatment of high blood pressure in elderly using home blood pressure readings. 95.
New York University, NYC, NY, $77,400. To develop and test clinical guidelines for determining decisionmaking capacity in elderly. 95.
Nursing Home Community Coalition of New York State, NYC, NY, $15,000. To study costs and quality in nursing home care in New York City. 95.
Saint Vincents Hospital and Medical Center of New York, NYC, NY, $108,000. To evaluate interdisciplinary acute care geriatric service. 95.
Saint Vincents Hospital and Medical Center of New York, NYC, NY, $15,000. For planning and development of interdisciplinary acute care geriatric service. 95.

720
The Carole & Alvin Schragis Foundation, Inc.

c/o Doral Hotel and Resorts
122 East 42nd St., Suite 1601
New York 10168-1694

Established in 1988 in NY.
Donor(s): Alvin Schragis, Carole Schragis.
Financial data (yr. ended 12/31/94): Assets, $4 (M); gifts received, $20,080; expenditures, $24,819; qualifying distributions, $24,819, including $19,236 for 42 grants (high: $3,750; low: $20).
Fields of interest: Higher education; Aging, centers & services; Community development; Jewish agencies & temples; Aging.
Limitations: Applications not accepted. Giving primarily in NY. No grants to individuals.
Application information: Contributes only to pre-selected organizations.
Officers and Directors:* Carole Schragis,* Pres.; Alvin Schragis, V.P.; Steven Schragis,* Secy.; Cathy Heller, Gary Schragis.
EIN: 133505306

721
Samuel & Bertha Schwartz Foundation, Inc.

501 Fleet Bank Bldg.
Auburn 13021 (315) 253-6205
Contact: Margaret A. Schwartz, Pres.
Application address: P.O. Box 693, Auburn, NY 13021

Established in 1951.
Donor(s): Herman H. Schwartz.‡
Financial data (yr. ended 12/31/94): Assets, $2,123,054 (M); expenditures, $126,623; qualifying distributions, $101,560, including $101,560 for 35 grants (high: $25,000; low: $100).
Purpose and activities: Giving primarily for Jewish welfare and temple support and higher education; support also for social and human services, including programs for youth and the aged.
Fields of interest: Higher education; Human services; Children & youth, services; Aging, centers & services; Jewish federated giving programs; Jewish agencies & temples; Aging.
Types of support: Annual campaigns, building/renovation, equipment, scholarship funds.
Limitations: Giving primarily in Auburn, Rochester and New York, NY, Palm Beach and Miami, FL, and Boston, MA. No grants to individuals.
Application information:
Initial approach: Letter
Deadline(s): None
Officers and Trustees:* Margaret A. Schwartz,* Pres.; Vincent M. Klein,* Secy.; Lois Ellenoff, Bradley W. Schwartz.
Number of staff: 1 part-time support.
EIN: 156017667

722
Edith M. Schweckendieck Trusts

c/o Citibank, N.A.
One Court Sq., 22nd Fl.
Long Island City 11120
Contact: Michael Festa, Sr. Trust Officer, Citibank, N.A.
Application address: PBG Trusts, 153 East 53rd St., 25th Fl., New York, NY 10043; Tel.: (212) 715-0100

Trust established in 1922 in NY; second trust established in 1936 in NY.
Donor(s): Edith M. Schweckendieck.‡
Financial data (yr. ended 12/31/94): Assets, $2,725,397 (M); expenditures, $126,174; qualifying distributions, $89,885, including $89,840 for 19 grants (high: $6,530; low: $2,680).
Purpose and activities: Grants to charitable institutions to provide assistance for care and maintenance of the aged and feeble; care, maintenance, and education of crippled children; and prevention and relief of cancer.
Fields of interest: Cancer; Cancer research; Children & youth, services; Aging, centers & services; Disabled; Aging.
Types of support: General/operating support, building/renovation, endowment funds.

Limitations: Giving limited to NY. No grants to individuals.
Application information:
Initial approach: Letter
Deadline(s): Dec. 31
Board meeting date(s): Oct.
Trustee: Citibank, N.A.
EIN: 136055135

723
Marty and Dorothy Silverman Foundation
150 East 58th St., 21st Fl.
New York 10155
Contact: Lorin Silverman, Secy.-Treas.

Established in 1986.
Donor(s): Marty Silverman.
Financial data (yr. ended 07/31/94): Assets, $164,179,495 (M); gifts received, $3,203,815; expenditures, $7,202,064; qualifying distributions, $7,500,650, including $7,000,650 for 63 grants (high: $4,075,000; average: $10,000-$50,000) and $500,000 for 1 program-related investment.
Purpose and activities: Support for programs that address the special needs of indigent senior citizens, including nursing homes and hospitals. Grants may also be made to educational and cultural organizations, and health and welfare agencies.
Fields of interest: Arts/cultural programs; Education, association, Hospitals (general), Health associations; Human services; Aging, centers & services; Aging.
Types of support: Program-related investments/loans.
Limitations: Applications not accepted. Giving primarily in NY. No grants to individuals.
Application information: Contributes only to pre-selected organizations.
Officers and Directors:* Marty Silverman,* Pres.; Carol Goldsmith,* V.P.; Joan Noritz,* V.P.; Lorin Silverman,* Secy.-Treas.
EIN: 222777449
Grants for Aging:
Bedford Park Multi-Service Center for Senior Citizens, Bronx, NY, $35,000. 94.
Burden Center for the Aging, NYC, NY, $25,000. 94.
Caring Community, NYC, NY, $20,000. 94.
Citymeals-on-Wheels, NYC, NY, $300,000. 94.
Council of Senior Centers and Services of New York City, NYC, NY, $40,000. 94.
Hunter College of the City University of New York, Brookdale Center on Aging, NYC, NY, $50,000. 94.
Isaac H. Tuttle Fund, NYC, NY, $10,000. 94.
Metropolitan Jewish Geriatric Center, Brooklyn, NY, $30,000. 94.
Montefiore Medical Center, Division of Geriatrics, Bronx, NY, $12,700. 94.
New York Statewide Senior Action Council, Albany, NY, $10,000. 94.
Parker Jewish Geriatric Institute Foundation, New Hyde Park, NY, $30,000. 94.
Project Ezra, NYC, NY, $25,000. 94.
Selfhelp Community Services, NYC, NY, $47,500. 94.
United Jewish Appeal-Federation of Jewish Philanthropies, Fund for Programs for the Aging, NYC, NY, $4,075,000. 94.
United Neighbors of East Midtown, NYC, NY, $12,500. 94.
West Side One-Stop for Coordinated Senior Services, NYC, NY, $21,000. 94.

724
The Skadden Fellowship Foundation, Inc.
(Formerly Skadden, Arps, Slate, Meagher & Flom Fellowship Foundation)
919 Third Ave.
New York 10022 (212) 735-2956
Contact: Susan Butler Plum

Established in 1988 in NY.
Donor(s): Skadden, Arps, Slate, Meagher & Flom.
Foundation type: Company-sponsored
Financial data (yr. ended 12/31/94): Assets, $4,165,468 (M); gifts received, $1,239,427; expenditures, $2,192,656; qualifying distributions, $2,192,656, including $2,017,363 for grants to individuals of $32,500 each.
Purpose and activities: Awards fellowships to graduating law students and outgoing judicial clerks who want to work in the public interest for organizations that provide civil legal services to the poor, including the homeless, the elderly, the disabled, and those deprived of their civil or human rights. Grants are made to the public interest organizations chosen by the fellows.
Fields of interest: Education; AIDS; Employment; Housing/shelter, development; Human services; Youth, services; Aging, centers & services; Homeless, human services; Civil rights; Community development; Minorities; Native Americans; Gays/lesbians; Economically disadvantaged; Homeless.
Types of support: Fellowships.
Publications: Multi-year report, application guidelines, informational brochure.
Application information: Applicants must secure a potential position with a sponsoring public interest organization before applying for a fellowship. Application form required.
Copies of proposal: 1
Deadline(s): Oct. 10
Board meeting date(s): Mid-Dec.
Final notification: Dec. 9
Officers and Directors:* Joseph Flom,* Chair.; Peter Mullen, Pres.; Michael Connery, V.P.; Barry H. Garfinkel, V.P.; Earle Yaffa, Secy.-Treas.; Archibald Cox, Marian Wright Edelman, Rev. Theodore Hesburgh, Edward Levi, Kurt Schmoke, Sargent Shriver.
Number of staff: 1 full-time professional; 1 part-time support.
EIN: 133455231

725
Louis Skalny Foundation Trust
c/o Marine Midland Bank, N.A.
One Marine Midland Ctr., 17th Fl.
Buffalo 14240

Established in 1970 in NY.
Financial data (yr. ended 12/31/94): Assets, $1,216,608 (M); expenditures, $122,447; qualifying distributions, $110,299, including $108,830 for 45 grants (high: $78,080; low: $2,000).
Fields of interest: Higher education; Nursing home/convalescent facility; General charitable giving.
Limitations: Applications not accepted. Giving primarily in Rochester, NY. No grants to individuals.
Application information: Contributes only to pre-selected organizations.
Trustee: Marine Midland Bank, N.A.
EIN: 166119085
Grants for Aging:
Saint Johns Home Foundation, Rochester, NY, $25,000. 94.

726
The Jo Sokolski Foundation
1133 Broadway
New York 10010

Established in 1987 in NY.
Donor(s): Josephine Sokolski.
Financial data (yr. ended 11/30/95): Assets, $65,687 (M); gifts received, $700; expenditures, $59,603; qualifying distributions, $59,603, including $59,603 for grants.
Fields of interest: Performing arts, education; Arts/cultural programs; Food services; Aging, centers & services.
Types of support: General/operating support.
Limitations: Applications not accepted. Giving primarily in New York, NY. No grants to individuals.
Application information: Contributes only to pre-selected organizations.
Officer and Directors:* Josephine Sokolski,* Pres.; Edith Klein, Jon Sokolski.
EIN: 133446225
Grants for Aging:
Citymeals-on-Wheels, NYC, NY, $8,800. 95.
YM-YWHA, 92nd Street, NYC, NY, $15,000. For senior adult program. 95.

727
The Thanks Be To Grandmother Winifred Foundation
P.O. Box 1449
Wainscott 11975-1449 (516) 725-0323

Established in 1991 in NY; funded in 1992.
Financial data (yr. ended 06/30/95): Assets, $456 (M); gifts received, $131,115; expenditures, $132,447; qualifying distributions, $132,447, including $102,935 for 34 grants to individuals (high: $5,000; low: $750; average: $500-$5,000).
Purpose and activities: "Encourages, through individual grants, the creativity of women 54 years of age and older to develop and implement projects, programs or policies that empower and enrich one or more aspects of the cultural, economic, educational, ethnic, mental, physical, professional, racial, sexual, social, and spiritual well-being of women."
Fields of interest: Aging; Women.
Types of support: Grants to individuals.
Limitations: Giving limited to U.S. citizens. No support for projects involving children or adolescents in any way.

Publications: Annual report, informational brochure (including application guidelines), application guidelines.
Application information: Applicant must be a woman who has experienced her 54th birthday; budget may not exceed $5,000; women holding public or elective office are not eligible.
Initial approach: Write for guidelines
Copies of proposal: 8
Deadline(s): Postmarked Mar. 21 and Sept. 21
Board meeting date(s): Apr. and Oct.
Final notification: After May 1 and Oct. 31
Officer and Trustee:* Deborah Ann Light,* Pres.
Number of staff: 1 part-time support.
EIN: 116404146

728
Annie Rensselaer Tinker Memorial Fund
369 Lexington Ave., 7th Fl.
New York 10017 (212) 983-9300
Contact: Nancy Houghton, Trustee

Established in 1924 in NY.
Donor(s): Annie Rensselaer Tinker.‡
Foundation type: Operating
Financial data (yr. ended 11/30/95): Assets, $2,150,597 (M); gifts received, $8,340; expenditures, $118,085; qualifying distributions, $93,605, including $1,500 for 3 grants (high: $1,000; low: $250) and $48,222 for 21 grants to individuals (high: $5,400; low: $700).
Purpose and activities: Support primarily for retired people who are physically, mentally or emotionally capable of living independently, but are in need of financial assistance.
Fields of interest: Human services; Aging, centers & services; Aging.
Types of support: Grants to individuals.
Limitations: Giving primarily in the greater metropolitan New York, NY, area.
Application information: Application form required.
Initial approach: Letter
Deadline(s): None
Officers and Trustees:* R. Dyke Benjamin,* Pres.; Mary Rogers,* V.P. and Secy.; Frederic Howard,* Treas.; Sue Chandler, Meg Dooley, George P. Engbert, Jr., Nancy Houghton, Phyliss Ross Schless, Carolyn Smith.
Number of staff: 1 part-time professional.
EIN: 136405671

729
Tioga County Senior Citizens Foundation
c/o Chemung Canal Trust Co.
P.O. Box 1522
Elmira 14902
Contact: Dean Fowler, Treas.
Application address: 348 Front St., Owego, NY 13827; Tel.: (607) 687-3083

Financial data (yr. ended 09/30/95): Assets, $892,536 (M); expenditures, $47,009; qualifying distributions, $36,000, including $36,000 for grants.
Purpose and activities: Support only to senior citizen related programs in Tioga County, NY.
Fields of interest: Performing arts; Libraries/library science; Human services; Aging.
Limitations: Giving limited to Tioga County, NY.
Application information: Request application form. Application form required.
Deadline(s): June 1
Officers: J. Dickson Edson, Pres.; Sheldon Guile, V.P.; Pauline Oliver, Secy.; Dean Fowler, Treas.
EIN: 150543615

730
The Alan & Peggy Tishman Foundation, Inc.
55 East 59th St.
New York 10022
Contact: Alan V. Tishman, Pres.

Incorporated in 1956 in NY; name changed in 1988.
Donor(s): Alan V. Tishman.
Financial data (yr. ended 11/30/95): Assets, $1,077,374 (M); expenditures, $81,557; qualifying distributions, $73,834, including $72,164 for 110 grants (high: $3,000; low: $100).
Purpose and activities: Primary areas of interest include aged, family services, hospital, and Jewish giving.
Fields of interest: Visual arts; Performing arts; Arts/cultural programs; Higher education; Adult/continuing education; Education; Hospitals (general); Health care; Health associations; Human services; Children & youth, services; Family services; Aging, centers & services; International economic development; Foreign policy; Jewish federated giving programs; Biological sciences; Science; Christian agencies & churches; Jewish agencies & temples; Disabled; Aging; General charitable giving.
Types of support: Annual campaigns, capital campaigns, building/renovation.
Limitations: Applications not accepted. Giving primarily in NY. No grants to individuals.
Application information: Contributes only to pre-selected organizations.
Officers: Alan V. Tishman, Pres.; Peggy Tishman, V.P.
Number of staff: None.
EIN: 136099395

731
George W. Tower Foundation
130 East Main St.
Waterville 13480-1108
Contact: Richard S. Woodman, Treas.
Application address: P.O. Box 26, Waterville, NY 13480; Tel.: (315) 841-8021

Financial data (yr. ended 12/31/93): Assets, $204,100 (M); expenditures, $8,829; qualifying distributions, $8,829.
Fields of interest: Hospitals (general); Aging, centers & services; Federated giving programs; Aging.
Limitations: Giving limited to the Waterville, NY, area.
Application information:
Initial approach: Letter
Deadline(s): None
Officers: Gail H. Gale, Pres.; Richard S. Woodman, Treas.
EIN: 150543664

732
Utica Foundation, Inc.
270 Genesee St.
Utica 13502 (315) 735-8212
Contact: Gordon M. Hayes, Jr., Exec. Dir.

Incorporated in 1952 in NY.
Foundation type: Community
Financial data (yr. ended 12/31/94): Assets, $23,242,768 (L); gifts received, $4,869,090; expenditures, $959,817, including $597,227 for grants.
Purpose and activities: Primary areas of interest include the aged and youth; support also for social and health services, scholarship programs of institutions for aid to local students, and cultural programs.
Fields of interest: Arts/cultural programs; Higher education; Libraries/library science; Education; Environment; Hospitals (general); Health care; Housing/shelter, development; Human services; Youth, services; Family services; Aging, centers & services; Disabled; Aging; Economically disadvantaged.
Types of support: Capital campaigns, building/renovation, equipment, seed money, scholarship funds, matching funds.
Limitations: Giving limited to Oneida and Herkimer counties, NY. No support for religious purposes. No grants to individuals, or for endowment funds, deficit financing, or operating budgets; no loans.
Publications: Annual report, application guidelines, newsletter.
Application information: Application form required.
Initial approach: Letter
Copies of proposal: 8
Board meeting date(s): May, and as required (3 to 4 times a year)
Final notification: 2 to 3 months
Officers and Directors:* Dwight E. Vicks, Jr.,* Pres.; Judith B. Gorman,* V.P.; Mrs. Thomas G. Hineline,* V.P.; William L. Schrauth, V.P.; Arthur H. Turner,* V.P.; Susan M. Blatt, M.D.,* Secy.; James E. Raymonda,* Treas.; Rev. P. Arthur Brindisi, Lauren E. Bull, Harold T. Clark, Jr., Vincent R. Corrou, Jr., Mary K. Griffith, Joseph H. Hobika, Sr., James S. Kernan, Jr., John L. Knower, David L. Mathis, Harold J. Moore, Burrel Samuels, Tom Sinnott.
Trustee Banks: Fleet Bank, N.A., Marine Midland Bank, N.A.
Number of staff: 2 full-time professional; 2 full-time support.
EIN: 156016932
Grants for Aging:
Presbyterian Home for Central New York, New Hartford, NY, $75,000. To construct residential health care facility. 94.

733
Veatch Program of the Unitarian Universalist Congregation at Shelter Rock

48 Shelter Rock Rd.
Manhasset 11030 (516) 627-6576
Contact: Marjorie Fine, Exec. Dir.
FAX: (516) 627-6596

Established in 1959 in NY.
Donor(s): Caroline Veatch.‡
Financial data (yr. ended 06/30/95): , including $9,400,000 for 191 grants (high: $1,000,000; low: $15,000).
Purpose and activities: Support for organizations and institutions whose purposes are to strengthen the democratic process and promote justice, equity, and compassion in human relations. The program strives to address broad social, economic, and political problems in the United States with particular emphasis on efforts to promote progressive changes in the way in which public and private institutions relate to disadvantaged sectors of the population. Grantmaking is aimed at encouraging institutions to be more responsive to the needs of the poor and disenfranchised, rather than at providing direct services to individuals who are neglected or underserved. The program intends to support activities that address the causes of social problems, rather than those that treat their symptoms.
Fields of interest: Environment; Family planning; AIDS; AIDS research; Employment; Youth development, services; Human services; Aging, centers & services; Civil rights; Community development; Leadership development; Public affairs; Protestant agencies & churches; Religion; Aging.
Limitations: No support for governmental institutions, historic preservation, cultural activities, or media programs. No grants to individuals, or to non-denominational organizations for capital projects, endowments, annual contribution drives, direct services, publications, meetings and conferences, scholarship funds, or scientific or academic research.
Publications: Annual report, informational brochure (including application guidelines).
Application information: Accepts NYRAG and NNG Common Application Forms. The Veatch Program funds the Unitarian Universalist Funding Program of Boston, MA. Organizations may not receive funding from both programs during the same 12-month period. Additionally, organizations with a current grant from the Unitarian Universalist Fund for a Just Society, the Fund for Unitarian Universalism, or the Fund for Unitarian Social Responsibility are ineligible.
Initial approach: Proposal 5 to 15 pages
Deadline(s): None
Final notification: Within 120 days
Officers and Governors: Robert Adams, Chair.; Ruth Reeves, Vice-Chair.; Marjorie Fine, Exec. Dir.; Judith Albert, Paul Drezner, Jean Judd, Judith Rymer, Chester Thompson, Linda Welles.
EIN: 111855655

734
The Vidda Foundation

c/o Carter, Rupp & Roberts
Ten East 40th St., Suite 3808
New York 10016 (212) 696-4050
Contact: Gerald E. Rupp, Mgr.

Established in 1979 in NY.
Donor(s): Ursula Corning.
Financial data (yr. ended 05/31/95): Assets, $909,511 (M); gifts received, $403,884; expenditures, $1,079,142; qualifying distributions, $1,029,020, including $944,339 for 32 grants (high: $150,000; low: $1,000; average: $500-$500,000).
Purpose and activities: Giving primarily to higher education and educational projects, cultural programs, including fine arts and museums, an educational film-making company, church music funds, animal welfare, the environment and conservation, hospitals, and social services, including child welfare and the elderly.
Fields of interest: Visual arts; Museums; Performing arts; Dance; Theater; Music; Arts/cultural programs; Higher education; Education; Natural resource conservation & protection; Environment; Animal welfare; Wildlife preservation & protection; Hospitals (general); Human services; Children & youth, services; Aging, centers & services; Community development; Protestant agencies & churches; Roman Catholic agencies & churches; Aging; Economically disadvantaged.
Types of support: General/operating support, building/renovation, endowment funds, program development, research.
Limitations: Giving primarily in NY. No grants to individuals.
Application information: Application form not required.
Initial approach: Letter or proposal
Copies of proposal: 1
Deadline(s): None
Board meeting date(s): Nov. and May
Final notification: Approximately 2 months
Officer and Trustees:* Gerald E. Rupp,* Mgr.; John A. Downey, M.D., Helen C. Evarts, Ian Fraser, Christophe Velay.
Number of staff: 2 part-time support.
EIN: 132981105
Grants for Aging:
Search and Care, NYC, NY, $10,000. 94.

735
Vinmont Foundation, Inc.

888 East 19th St.
Brooklyn 11230 (718) 377-0178
Contact: William R. Nye, Pres.

Incorporated in 1947 in NY.
Donor(s): Lily H. Weinberg,‡ Robert C. Weinberg,‡ Ruth Weinberg.‡
Financial data (yr. ended 12/31/95): Assets, $1,319,406 (M); expenditures, $160,568; qualifying distributions, $156,632, including $155,550 for 66 grants (high: $10,000; low: $850).
Purpose and activities: Giving primarily for national African-American development organizations and for social service agencies, urban planning, and restoration in metropolitan New York City.
Fields of interest: Historic preservation/historical societies; Human services; Minorities/immigrants, centers & services; Civil rights, disabled; Civil rights, aging; Urban/community development; Community development; Public affairs; Minorities; African Americans; Disabled; Aging; Immigrants/refugees; Economically disadvantaged.
Types of support: General/operating support, continuing support, annual campaigns, emergency funds, seed money.
Limitations: Giving primarily in the New York, NY, metropolitan area; support for national African-American agencies. No grants to individuals, or for capital or endowment funds, research, special projects, publications, conferences, scholarships, fellowships, or matching gifts; no loans.
Publications: Program policy statement.
Application information: Rarely funds unsolicited proposals. Application form not required.
Initial approach: Letter
Copies of proposal: 1
Deadline(s): None
Board meeting date(s): Feb. and Oct.
Final notification: 6 months
Officers and Directors:* William R. Nye,* Pres.; Carolyn L. Whittle,* V.P.; Paul S. Byard,* Secy.; Bruce L. Bozeman, L. Franklyn Lowenstein.
Number of staff: None.
EIN: 131577203
Grants for Aging:
WISE Individualized Senior Experience, White Plains, NY, $7,500. 95.

736
The Laura B. Vogler Foundation, Inc.

P.O. Box 610508
Bayside 11361-0508 (718) 423-3000
Contact: D. Donald D'Amato, Pres.

Incorporated in 1959 in NY.
Donor(s): Laura B. Vogler,‡ John J. Vogler.‡
Financial data (yr. ended 10/31/95): Assets, $4,378,213 (M); expenditures, $230,016; qualifying distributions, $195,647, including $143,800 for 59 grants (high: $5,000; low: $1,000; average: $1,000-$5,000).
Purpose and activities: "Awards one-time non-renewable grants for new programs in the areas of health, youth, child welfare, the disadvantaged, the elderly, and other related services."
Fields of interest: Education; Health care; Health associations; Human services; Children & youth, services; Aging, centers & services; Aging.
Types of support: Emergency funds, program development, seed money, scholarship funds, research.
Limitations: Giving limited to New York City and Long Island. No grants to individuals, or for building or endowment funds, annual fundraising campaigns, or matching gifts; no loans.
Publications: Annual report (including application guidelines).

Application information: Accepts NYRAG Common Application Form. Application form required.
Initial approach: Letter
Copies of proposal: 1
Deadline(s): Jan. 1, Apr. 1, July 1, and Oct. 1
Board meeting date(s): Jan., Apr., July, and Oct.
Final notification: 2 to 3 months
Officers and Trustees:* D. Donald D'Amato,* Pres. and C.E.O.; Lawrence L. D'Amato,* Secy.-Treas.; Max L. Kupferberg, I. Jerry Lasurdo, Rev. Stephen S. Schwander, Robert T. Waldbauer, Karen M. Yost.
Number of staff: 2 part-time professional; 1 part-time support.
EIN: 116022241
Grants for Aging:
Community Programs Center of Long Island, Deer Park, NY, $2,500. For elder care program. 95.

737
Walter & Lorenz Foundation, Inc.
866 United Nations Plaza, Rm. 471
New York 10017
Contact: Otto L. Walter, Pres.

Established in 1954 in NY.
Donor(s): Anton Lorenz.‡
Financial data (yr. ended 12/31/94): Assets, $563,633 (M); expenditures, $110,388; qualifying distributions, $81,184, including $58,212 for 42 grants (high: $11,100; low: $50).
Purpose and activities: Primary areas of interest include education, hunger, the disadvantaged, and Germany.
Fields of interest: Museums; Arts/cultural programs; Secondary school/education; Higher education; Law school/education; Adult/continuing education; Education; Food services; Human services; Aging, centers & services; International affairs, goodwill promotion; Foreign policy; Race/intergroup relations; Public policy, research; Aging; Economically disadvantaged; Germany.
Types of support: General/operating support, debt reduction, professorships, matching funds.
Limitations: Applications not accepted. Giving primarily in NY. No grants to individuals.
Publications: Annual report (including application guidelines).
Application information: Application funds are severely limited.
Officers and Directors:* Otto L. Walter,* Pres. and Treas.; Frances Doonen Walter,* V.P.; Frank G. Helman,* Secy.
Number of staff: 1 full-time professional; 1 part-time support.
EIN: 131625529
Grants for Aging:
Gods Love We Deliver, NYC, NY, $900. 94.
Selfhelp Community Services, NYC, NY, $250. 94.

738
Washington County Home for Aged Women, Inc.
c/o Glens Falls National Bank
250 Glen St., P.O. Box 307
Glens Falls 12801-9989
Application address: Alvin E. Dunnem, One Washington St., Cambridge, NY 12816; Tel.: (518) 677-3130

Donor(s): J. Sheldon Trust.
Financial data (yr. ended 09/30/95): Assets, $598,168 (M); gifts received, $6,498; expenditures, $34,835; qualifying distributions, $29,238, including $22,865 for grants.
Fields of interest: Libraries (public); Hospitals (general); Aging, centers & services; Foundations (private grantmaking); Christian agencies & churches; Aging; Economically disadvantaged.
Types of support: Equipment.
Limitations: Giving limited to Washington County, NY.
Application information:
Deadline(s): July 1
Officer and Directors:* Charles R. Clark,* Pres.; James A. Catalfimo, Clyde Cook, Lawrence E. Corbett, Jr., Daniel Hayes, Robert I. Rozell.
EIN: 141372655

739
Sanford I. Weill Charitable Foundation, Inc.
388 Greenwich St.
New York 10013 (212) 891-8888
Contact: Sanford I. Weill, Pres.

Donor(s): Sanford I. Weill.
Financial data (yr. ended 12/31/94): Assets, $5,975,599 (M); gifts received, $2,270,625; expenditures, $356,565; qualifying distributions, $341,470, including $341,425 for 29 grants (high: $100,000; low: $100).
Fields of interest: Arts/cultural programs; Education; Hospitals (general); Human services; Aging, centers & services; Jewish agencies & temples; Aging.
Limitations: Giving primarily in the metropolitan New York, NY, area.
Application information: Application form required.
Initial approach: Proposal
Deadline(s): None
Officers: Sanford I. Weill, Pres.; Kenneth J. Bialkin, Mgr.; Joan H. Weill, Mgr.
EIN: 136223609
Grants for Aging:
Hebrew Home for the Aged at Riverdale, Bronx, NY, $100,000. 94.

740
The Margaret L. Wendt Foundation
40 Fountain Plaza, Suite 277
Buffalo 14202-2220 (716) 855-2146
Contact: Robert J. Kresse, Secy.

Trust established in 1956 in NY.
Donor(s): Margaret L. Wendt.‡
Financial data (yr. ended 01/31/95): Assets, $56,786,491 (M); expenditures, $2,562,737; qualifying distributions, $4,639,819, including $1,928,377 for 100 grants (high: $125,000; low: $750; average: $5,000-$50,000) and $2,505,396 for 2 program-related investments.
Purpose and activities: Emphasis on education, the arts, and social services; support also for churches and religious organizations, health associations, public interest organizations, and youth agencies.
Fields of interest: Visual arts; Museums; Performing arts; Theater; History & archaeology; Historic preservation/historical societies; Arts/cultural programs; Education, fund raising; Early childhood education; Higher education; Libraries/library science; Education; Natural resource conservation & protection; Hospitals (general); Substance abuse, services; Mental health/crisis services; Health associations; Cancer; AIDS; Alcoholism; Biomedicine; Medical research; Cancer research; AIDS research; Legal services; Crime/law enforcement; Human services; Children & youth, services; Youth, services; Hospices; Aging, centers & services; Minorities/immigrants, centers & services; Human rights (international); Community development; Federated giving programs; Political science; Government/public administration; Public affairs; Religion; Minorities; Disabled; Aging; Economically disadvantaged.
Types of support: Program-related investments/loans.
Limitations: Giving primarily in Buffalo and western NY. No grants to individuals, or for scholarships.
Publications: Application guidelines.
Application information: Application form not required.
Initial approach: Letter or application form
Copies of proposal: 4
Deadline(s): 1 month prior to board meeting
Board meeting date(s): Quarterly; no fixed dates
Final notification: Usually 4 to 6 months
Officers and Trustees:* Ralph W. Loew,* Chair.; Robert J. Kresse,* Secy.; Thomas D. Lunt.
Number of staff: 1 part-time support.
EIN: 166030037

741
The Western New York Foundation
Main Seneca Bldg., Suite 1402
237 Main St.
Buffalo 14203 (716) 847-6440
Contact: Welles V. Moot, Jr., Pres.

Incorporated in 1951 in NY as the Wildroot Foundation; present name adopted in 1958.
Donor(s): Welles V. Moot.‡
Financial data (yr. ended 07/31/95): Assets, $6,361,936 (M); expenditures, $312,910; qualifying distributions, $260,460, including $199,657 for 19 grants (high: $25,000; low: $42; average: $2,500-$75,000) and $55,000 for 1 loan.
Purpose and activities: Grants to nonprofit institutions, with emphasis on capital needs, seed funds for new projects, or expanding services. Support primarily for the fine and performing arts, youth agencies, the natural sciences, and social service agencies; some support also for health services and libraries and other educational institutions.

Fields of interest: Visual arts; Museums; Performing arts; Dance; Theater; Music; Arts/cultural programs; Education, fund raising; Child development, education; Secondary school/education; Business school/education; Adult/continuing education; Adult education—literacy & basic skills; Libraries/library science; Reading; Education; Animal welfare; Medical care, rehabilitation; Health care; Substance abuse, services; Mental health/crisis services; Health associations; AIDS; Alcoholism; Health organizations; AIDS research; Legal services; Crime/law enforcement; Housing/shelter, development; Human services; Children & youth, services; Youth, services; Child development, services; Family services; Hospices; Aging, centers & services; Women, centers & services; Minorities/immigrants, centers & services; Human rights (international); Community development; Engineering & technology; Science; Minorities; Disabled; Aging; Women.
Types of support: Capital campaigns, building/renovation, equipment, land acquisition, endowment funds, emergency funds, program development, conferences/seminars, publication, seed money, technical assistance, program-related investments/loans, matching funds.
Limitations: Giving limited to the 8th Judicial District of NY (Erie, Niagara, Genesee, Wyoming, Allegany, Cattaraugus, and Chautauqua counties). No support for hospitals or religious organizations. No grants to individuals, or for scholarships, fellowships, or generally for operating budgets or deficit financing.
Publications: Annual report.
Application information: Application form required.
Initial approach: Letter (not more than 1 1/2 pages) from unpaid officer of applicant organization, not staff member
Copies of proposal: 2
Deadline(s): None
Board meeting date(s): 3 or 4 times a year
Final notification: 8 to 12 weeks
Officers and Trustees:* Welles V. Moot, Jr.,* Pres.; Cecily M. Johnson,* V.P.; John R. Moot,* Secy.; Richard E. Moot,* Treas.; Trudy A. Mollenberg, Andrew R. Moot, John N. Walsh III.
Number of staff: 1 full-time professional; 1 part-time support.
EIN: 160845962

742
Fred & Floy Willmott Foundation
c/o Marine Midland Bank, N.A.
One Marine Midland Ctr.
Buffalo 14240

Established in 1984 in NY.
Financial data (yr. ended 12/31/94): Assets, $5,006,233 (M); expenditures, $381,964; qualifying distributions, $308,406, including $302,858 for 67 grants (high: $25,000; low: $500).
Purpose and activities: Giving primarily for Methodist churches and other religious organizations; support also for aging, education, including higher education, and social services.
Fields of interest: Higher education; Education; Human services; Christian agencies & churches; Protestant agencies & churches; Aging.
Limitations: Giving primarily in Monroe County, NY. No grants to individuals.
Application information: Application form required.
Initial approach: Letter requesting application
Deadline(s): None
Final notification: 60 days or more
Trustees: Rev. John D. Cooke, Marine Midland Bank, N.A.
EIN: 222587484

743
Judy and Fred Wilpon Family Foundation, Inc.
111 Great Neck Rd., Suite 408
Great Neck 11021-5476
Contact: Fred Wilpon, Pres.

Established in 1982.
Donor(s): Fred Wilpon.
Financial data (yr. ended 12/31/94): Assets, $493,068 (M); gifts received, $63,000; expenditures, $59,810; qualifying distributions, $57,700, including $57,700 for 8 grants (high: $30,000; low: $200).
Fields of interest: Nursing home/convalescent facility; Recreation; Jewish federated giving programs.
Types of support: General/operating support.
Limitations: Giving primarily in the greater metropolitan New York, NY, area, including Long Island.
Application information: Application form not required.
Initial approach: Letter
Deadline(s): None
Officer and Directors:* Fred Wilpon,* Pres.; Robin Wilpon Wachtler, Secy.-Treas.; Jeffrey Wilpon, Judith Wilpon.
EIN: 112626618
Grants for Aging:
Parker Jewish Geriatric Institute, New Hyde Park, NY, $20,000. 94.

744
Jessie C. Wilson Memorial Trust Fund
20 Bliss St.
Westfield 14787
Contact: David Gross, Trustee
Application address: 11 Holt St., Westfield, NY 14787

Established in 1983 in NY.
Foundation type: Operating
Financial data (yr. ended 12/31/94): Assets, $37,760 (M); gifts received, $1,040; expenditures, $1,756; qualifying distributions, $1,567, including $1,567 for grants.
Fields of interest: Education; Aging, centers & services; Rural development; Community development; Federated giving programs; Christian agencies & churches; Aging.
Limitations: Giving primarily in the Westfield NY, area. No grants to individuals.
Application information: Application form not required.
Initial approach: Letter
Deadline(s): None
Board meeting date(s): Feb.
Trustees: David Gross, David McCabe, Priscilla Nixon, David Wilson, Janice D. Wilson, Jodi Wilson.
Number of staff: 4
EIN: 166253879

745
Yaron Foundation, Inc.
201 East 37th St., Lobby Suite
New York 10016-3142
Contact: Norman Horowitz, Exec. Dir.

Established in 1984.
Donor(s): Isaac Steven Herschkopf, Moses Z. Berman, Debrah Lee Charatan, Leon Miller, Howard Miller, Harry Stern, Martin L. Markowitz, Ivan Kaufman, Robert Mitzman.
Financial data (yr. ended 12/31/94): Assets, $631,276 (M); gifts received, $34,116; expenditures, $84,510; qualifying distributions, $84,421, including $82,656 for 64 grants (high: $10,000; low: $2; average: $2-$15,050).
Fields of interest: Film/video; Museums; Theater; Music; Arts/cultural programs; Education, research; Education, fund raising; Higher education; Medical school/education; Adult/continuing education; Adult education—literacy & basic skills; Libraries/library science; Reading; Education; Natural resource conservation & protection; Environment; Wildlife preservation & protection; Hospitals (general); Health care; Health associations; Biomedicine; Health organizations; Medical research; Human services; Youth, services; Hospices; Aging, centers & services; Women, centers & services; Minorities/immigrants, centers & services; Peace; Human rights (international); Jewish federated giving programs; Psychology/behavioral science; Jewish agencies & temples; Minorities; Disabled; Aging; Women; General charitable giving; Israel.
Types of support: Annual campaigns, building/renovation, equipment, emergency funds, curriculum development, research.
Limitations: Giving primarily in New York, NY.
Application information: Academic qualifications required for individual applicants; proposal required for research grants. Application form not required.
Copies of proposal: 1
Deadline(s): None
Board meeting date(s): Monthly
Final notification: 2 months
Officers: Isaac Steven Herschkopf, Pres.; and six additional board members.
Number of staff: 1 full-time professional; 1 part-time support.
EIN: 133209791

746
The Zausner Foundation, Inc.
c/o Martin Zausner
923 Fifth Ave.
New York 10021-2649

Financial data (yr. ended 12/31/95): Assets, $274,423 (M); expenditures, $9,833; qualifying

distributions, $8,662, including $7,870 for 31 grants (high: $600; low: $40).
Fields of interest: Health care; Health organizations; Aging, centers & services; Aging; General charitable giving.
Limitations: Applications not accepted. Giving primarily in New York, NY. No grants to individuals.
Application information: Contributes only to pre-selected organizations.
Officers: Martin Zausner, Pres. and Treas.; Adrienne B. Zausner, V.P. and Secy.
Director: Judith S. Borten.
EIN: 136089201

NORTH CAROLINA

747
Harry Borns Trust
c/o First Union National Bank
CMG-1161
Charlotte 28288-1161

Financial data (yr. ended 03/31/95): Assets, $502,893 (M); expenditures, $28,619; qualifying distributions, $22,468, including $21,811 for grants.
Fields of interest: Aging, centers & services; Aging.
Limitations: Applications not accepted.
Application information: Contributes only to pre-selected organizations.
Trustee: First Union National Bank.
EIN: 596131334

748
The Community Foundation of Henderson County, Inc.
Fourth Ave. and Main St.
P.O. Box 1108
Hendersonville 28793 (704) 697-6224
Contact: Priscilla Cantrell, Exec. Dir., or Crystal Reese, Office Administrator
FAX: (704) 696-4026

Incorporated in 1982 in NC.
Foundation type: Community
Financial data (yr. ended 06/30/95): Assets, $10,133,325 (M); gifts received, $1,259,188; expenditures, $689,823, including $419,441 for 78 grants (high: $76,634; low: $50; average: $50-$5,000) and $51,200 for 50 grants to individuals (high: $2,000; low: $250).
Purpose and activities: To maintain and improve the quality of life in the community and to make a difference in the fight against homelessness, caring for children and the elderly, and providing educational services; awards to individuals include scholarships, medical assistance, and aid to women in need.
Fields of interest: Arts/cultural programs; Child development, education; Education; Human services; Child development, services; Aging, centers & services; Homeless, human services; Community development; Aging; Homeless; General charitable giving.
Types of support: Equipment, emergency funds, program development, publication, seed money, curriculum development, scholarship funds, scholarships—to individuals, matching funds.
Limitations: Giving limited to the Henderson County, NC, area. No grants for endowment funds or capital campaigns; no loans.
Publications: Annual report, newsletter, application guidelines, 990-PF, informational brochure.
Application information: Application form required.
Initial approach: Letter or telephone
Copies of proposal: 2
Deadline(s): Mar. 1, June 1, Sept. 1, and Dec. 1
Board meeting date(s): Monthly
Officers and Directors:* R.E. Harmon,* Pres.; Theron Mullinax, Jr., V.P., Development; R. Charles Waters,* V.P., Distrib.; Edna Lutz, Secy.; F. Lee Thomas, Treas.; Priscilla Cantrell, Exec. Dir.; Betsy Armstrong-Price, Rebecca Boswell, Warren Carlson, Glenavin Cason, Eugenia Dowdeswell, Steve Greene, Steve Johnson, James Marshall, Jeff Miller, Richard Porter, Robert Sanford, William Stokes, Jr., Grace Vineyard.
Staff: Kathryn McConnell, Prog. Officer; Crystal Reese, Administrator.
Number of staff: 2 full-time professional; 1 full-time support.
EIN: 561330792

749
The Katherine H. Daveler and David R. Hayworth Foundation
c/o Wachovia Bank & Trust Co., N.A.
P.O. Box 3099
Winston-Salem 27150-1022
Contact: David Hayworth, Pres.
Application address: 800 Rockford Rd., High Point, NC 27260; Tel.: (919) 889-4439

Established in 1986.
Financial data (yr. ended 12/31/94): Assets, $2,983,274 (M); expenditures, $167,757; qualifying distributions, $158,563, including $156,750 for grants.
Fields of interest: Children & youth, services; Family services; Aging, centers & services; Federated giving programs; Protestant agencies & churches; Aging.
Limitations: Giving limited to NC, with emphasis on High Point.
Application information: Application form not required.
Deadline(s): None
Officers and Directors:* David R. Hayworth,* Pres. and Treas.; Charles E. Hayworth,* V.P. and Secy.; Margaret Dalton.
Trustee: Wachovia Bank of North Carolina, N.A.
EIN: 581705607

750
Champion McDowell Davis Charitable Foundation
P.O. Box 1268
Wilmington 28402 (910) 763-4748
Contact: Cyrus D. Hogue, Jr., Secy.

Established in 1963 in NC.
Donor(s): Champion McDowell Davis.‡
Financial data (yr. ended 12/31/94): Assets, $10,707,679 (M); expenditures, $607,980; qualifying distributions, $527,424, including $526,682 for 3 grants (high: $467,700; low: $1,000).
Purpose and activities: Giving primarily for a health center; support for other health services and care for the elderly; limited to capital projects.
Fields of interest: Health care; Aging, centers & services; Aging.
Types of support: Capital campaigns, building/renovation.
Limitations: Giving primarily in Wilmington, NC. No grants to individuals.
Application information: Funds fully committed through 1997. Application form not required.
Initial approach: Letter
Copies of proposal: 1
Deadline(s): 2 weeks before meetings
Board meeting date(s): Bimonthly meetings on 2nd Wednesday commencing in Feb.
Officers and Trustees:* Robey T. Sinclair, Jr., M.D.,* Chair.; Cyrus D. Hogue, Jr.,* Secy.; Raymond H. Holland, Jr.,* Treas.; Emsley A. Laney, John R. Murchison II, Peter B. Ruffin.
Number of staff: 1 part-time support.
EIN: 566055716

751
The First Union Foundation
Two First Union
Charlotte 28288-0143
Contact: Judith N. Allison, Dir., Corp. Contribs.
Additional local bank addresses: Fin. Div., Box 1329, Greenville, SC 29602; Box 740074, Atlanta, GA 30374; Box 44250-FL004, Jacksonville, FL 32231-4250; 150 Fourth Ave. N., Nashville, TN 37219; Box 13327, Roanoke, VA 24040 for VA, MD, and DC

Established in 1987 in NC.
Donor(s): First Union National Bank of Virginia.
Foundation type: Company-sponsored
Financial data (yr. ended 12/31/94): Assets, $9,484,000 (M); gifts received, $15,950,000; expenditures, $6,568,125; qualifying distributions, $6,571,125, including $6,249,156 for 1,708 grants (high: $790,738; low: $25; average: $100-$20,000) and $318,969 for employee matching gifts.
Purpose and activities: Support for higher education and special programs for public elementary and secondary schools; arts funds or councils; community improvement; family and social services, minorities, and the handicapped. Special consideration for children and youth and the disadvantaged to help them become productive and self-sufficient. Types of support include capital grants, made only when there is a community-wide fundraising campaign that includes the entire business community. Grants are made for one year only unless a multi-year pledge is made.
Fields of interest: Visual arts; Museums; Performing arts; Dance; Music; Education, fund raising; Early childhood education; Child development, education; Elementary school/education; Secondary school/education; Higher education; Business school/education; Adult/continuing education; Adult education—literacy & basic skills;

Libraries/library science; Reading; Education; Natural resource conservation & protection; Environment; Hospitals (general); Medical care, rehabilitation; Health care; Substance abuse, services; Mental health/crisis services; Heart/circulatory disease; Alcoholism; Health organizations; Heart/circulatory research; Youth development, citizenship; Human services; Children & youth, services; Youth, services; Child development, services; Family services; Hospices; Aging, centers & services; Minorities/immigrants, centers & services; Homeless, human services; Urban/community development; Community development; Voluntarism promotion; Federated giving programs; Government/public administration; Public affairs, citizen participation; Minorities; Disabled; Aging; Economically disadvantaged; Homeless.
Types of support: General/operating support, capital campaigns, building/renovation, endowment funds, program development, seed money, scholarship funds, employee matching gifts.
Limitations: Giving limited to Washington, DC, FL, GA, MD, NC, SC, TN, and VA. No support for religious, veterans', or fraternal organizations, retirement homes, pre-college level private schools except through employee matching gifts, or organizations supported through the United Way, except for approved capital campaigns.
Publications: Informational brochure (including application guidelines), application guidelines.
Application information: Application form not required.
Initial approach: Proposal to the nearest First Union National Bank
Copies of proposal: 1
Deadline(s): None
Directors: Judith N. Allison, Dir., Corp. Contribs.; Robert Atwood, Marion A. Cowell, Jr., Edward E. Crutchfield, Jr., Malcolm E. Everett, John R. Georgius, Don Johnson, Burt Melton, Alvin Sale.
Trustee: First Union National Bank of North Carolina.
EIN: 566288589

752

The Thad W. Garner, Mildred B. Garner, and Kathryn W. Garner Foundation, Inc.

2104 Nisbet Court
Winston-Salem 27106

Incorporated in 1991 in NC; funded in 1992.
Donor(s): Thad W. Garner.
Financial data (yr. ended 12/31/94): Assets, $43,097 (M); gifts received, $10,000; expenditures, $5,500; qualifying distributions, $5,500, including $5,400 for 2 grants (high: $3,500; low: $1,900).
Fields of interest: Business school/education; Alzheimer's disease.
Types of support: Scholarship funds.
Limitations: Applications not accepted. Giving limited to Winston-Salem, NC.
Application information: Contributes only to pre-selected organizations.
Officers and Directors:* Thad W. Garner,* Pres.; Kathryn W. Garner,* V.P. and Secy.-Treas.; Mildred B. Garner,* V.P.; Patricia R. Guy, Earline Heath King.
EIN: 561748418

753

The Adelaide Gurganus Jackson Foundation

5219 Trent Woods Dr.
New Bern 28562
Contact: Ann J. Johnson, Pres.

Established in 1987 in NC.
Donor(s): Rudolph Hoyt Jackson.‡
Foundation type: Operating
Financial data (yr. ended 06/30/94): Assets, $154,538 (M); expenditures, $15,218; qualifying distributions, $14,000, including $10,881 for 4 grants (high: $6,206; low: $50) and $3,120 for 3 grants to individuals (high: $1,636; low: $164).
Fields of interest: Aging, centers & services; Aging.
Limitations: Giving primarily in Craven County, NC.
Application information:
Initial approach: Letter
Deadline(s): None
Officers: Ann J. Johnson, Pres.; Leann Johnson, Secy.; Lester W. Johnson, Jr., Treas.
Directors: Pam Fillinger, Lucille Stewart.
EIN: 561570654

754

The Melvin R. Lane Charitable Trust

c/o Wachovia Bank of North Carolina, N.A.
P.O. Box 3099
Winston-Salem 27150-7131 (910) 732-6090
Contact: Nola Miller, Trust Officer, Wachovia Bank of North Carolina, N.A.

Established in 1989 in NC.
Donor(s): Melvin R. Lane.‡
Financial data (yr. ended 06/30/94): Assets, $4,712,144 (M); gifts received, $233; expenditures, $224,047; qualifying distributions, $187,269, including $166,700 for 17 grants (high: $25,000; low: $3,000).
Fields of interest: Health care; Human services; Aging, centers & services; Religious federated giving programs; Christian agencies & churches; Aging.
Limitations: Giving limited to Henderson and Buncombe counties, NC. No support for arts and humanities. No grants to individuals; no loans.
Application information: Application form required.
Copies of proposal: 6
Deadline(s): Jan. 15 and July 15
Board meeting date(s): July and Oct.
Trustees: Evelyn Lane Fozzard, Wachovia Bank of North Carolina, N.A.
Advisory Committee: Peter Allen Fozzard, Miriam Kussrow, Carolyn McCall, Scott Pierson.
EIN: 581854812

755

North Carolina Community Foundation

333 Fayetteville St. Mall, Suite 1410
Raleigh 27601 (919) 828-4387
Contact: Elizabeth C. Fentress, Exec. Dir.
FAX: (919) 828-5495; Western Regional Office address: 317 West Main St., Sylva, NC 28779; Tel.: (704) 586-4616; FAX: (704) 586-4757

Established in 1985 in NC.
Foundation type: Community
Financial data (yr. ended 03/31/95): Assets, $9,063,957 (M); gifts received, $2,187,365; expenditures, $771,424, including $366,978 for grants (average: $50-$40,000).
Purpose and activities: Primary areas of interest include higher and other education, conservation, community funds, and other general charitable activities.
Fields of interest: Museums; Performing arts; Historic preservation/historical societies; Higher education; Adult education—literacy & basic skills; Reading; Education; Natural resource conservation & protection; Environment; Health care; Substance abuse, services; Health organizations; Youth, services; Hospices; Aging, centers & services; Women, centers & services; Homeless, human services; Federated giving programs; Christian agencies & churches; Aging; Women; Homeless; General charitable giving.
Types of support: Endowment funds, program development, conferences/seminars, technical assistance, consulting services.
Limitations: Applications not accepted. Giving primarily in NC.
Publications: Annual report, informational brochure, newsletter.
Application information:
Board meeting date(s): June and Dec.
Officers and Directors:* Lewis R. Holding,* Pres.; Charles W. Gaddy,* V.P.; Victor E. Bell, Jr.,* 2nd V.P.; William J. Cathecart,* Secy.; John A. Williams, Jr.,* Treas.; Elizabeth C. Fentress, Exec. Dir.; Waverly F. Akins, John A. Allison IV, R. Marks Arnold, and 20 additional directors.
Staff: Esther S. Hall, Prog. Coord.
Number of staff: 4 full-time professional; 2 part-time professional.
EIN: 581661700

756

Kate B. Reynolds Charitable Trust

128 Reynolda Village
Winston-Salem 27106-5123 (910) 723-1456
Contact: E. Ray Cope, Exec Dir., or John H. Frank, Dir., Health Care Division

Established in 1947 in NC.
Donor(s): Kate B. Reynolds.‡
Financial data (yr. ended 08/31/95): Assets, $359,580,556 (M); expenditures, $17,826,270; qualifying distributions, $16,946,446, including $16,549,922 for 221 grants (high: $669,225; low: $4,000; average: $20,000-$200,000).
Purpose and activities: Seventy-five percent of net income is to be distributed for the health care of those in need statewide, to increase the availability of health services to underserved groups and to support other programs that have merit and are related to the goal of the division.

Twenty-five percent is for the benefit of poor and needy residents of Winston-Salem and Forsyth County to support organizations that provide for basic needs (food, clothing, shelter, and health care), to fund efforts that seek to reduce reliance upon support services or that promote maximum levels of functioning for those with chronic problems, and to support other programs that have merit and are related to the goal of the division.
Fields of interest: Early childhood education; Child development, education; Nursing school/education; Education; Hospitals (general); Medical care, rehabilitation; Nursing care; Health care; Substance abuse, services; Mental health/crisis services; Health associations; Cancer; AIDS; Alcoholism; Health organizations; Domestic violence prevention; Food services; Nutrition; Housing/shelter, development; Human services; Children & youth, services; Child development, services; Family services; Hospices; Aging, centers & services; Homeless, human services; Rural development; Disabled; Aging; Economically disadvantaged; Homeless.
Types of support: General/operating support, continuing support, annual campaigns, capital campaigns, building/renovation, equipment, program development, seed money, matching funds.
Limitations: Giving limited to NC; social welfare grants limited to Winston-Salem and Forsyth County; health care giving, statewide. No grants to individuals, or for endowment funds or medical research; grants on a highly selective basis for construction of facilities or purchase of equipment.
Publications: Annual report (including application guidelines), application guidelines, informational brochure.
Application information: Applicant should contact the trust staff to discuss the proposal prior to submitting a written application. Application form required.
Initial approach: Telephone to inquire about guidelines and to request an application
Copies of proposal: 1
Deadline(s): 1st business day of Jan., May, and Aug. for Poor and Needy Division; Mar. 15 and Sept. 15 for Health Care Division, or the 1st business day thereafter if the deadline falls on a weekend or holiday
Board meeting date(s): Poor and Needy Division Advisory Board meets in Sept., Feb., and June; Health Care Division Advisory Board meets in Nov. and May
Final notification: Within 2 weeks after advisory board meeting
Officer: E. Ray Cope, Exec. Dir.
Trustee: Wachovia Bank of North Carolina, N.A.
Staff: John H. Frank, Dir., Health Care Div.; Markita A. Moore, Prog. Officer; Sara C. Smith, Prog. Officer.
Number of staff: 4 full-time professional; 2 full-time support.
EIN: 566036515
Grants for Aging:
Alamance County Council on Elderly Services and Support, Burlington, NC, $13,430. For vehicle to deliver meals to home-bound patients. 95.
Ashe Services for Aging, Jefferson, NC, $300,000. Toward construction of new facility from which home and community-based services to elderly and disabled will be provided. 95.
Campbell University, Buies Creek, NC, $96,075. For clinical pharmacist/faculty position at Dorothea Dix Hospital providing services for elderly psychiatric patients. 95.
Chatham County Council on Aging, Pittsboro, NC, $50,000. To construct space for expanded and better coordinated services for elderly. 95.
Clay County Health Department, Hayesville, NC, $75,000. For start-up support of Medicaid Community Alternatives Programs to provide case-managed services for low-income, frail elderly and disabled individuals as part of Kate B. Reynolds Aging at Home Program, Round two. 95.
Cross Roads Rest and Retirement Center, Asheboro, NC, $50,000. For construction for adult day care and day health services to residents with Alzheimer's Disease. 95.
District Memorial Hospital of Southwestern North Carolina, Andrews, NC, $69,795. For start-up support of Medicaid Community Alternatives Programs to provide case-managed services for low-income, frail elderly and disabled individuals as part of Kate B. Reynolds Aging at Home Program, Round two. 95.
Duke University Medical Center, Durham, NC, $135,009. For operating support for management of Round Two of Aging at Home Program. 95.
Gates County Department of Social Services, Gatesville, NC, $75,000. For start-up support of Medicaid Community Alternatives Programs to provide case-managed services for low-income, frail elderly and disabled individuals as part of Kate B. Reynolds Aging at Home Program, Round two. 95.
Greene County Department of Social Services, Snow Hill, NC, $74,116. For start-up support of Medicaid Community Alternatives Programs to provide case-managed services for low-income, frail elderly and disabled individuals as part of Kate B. Reynolds Aging at Home Program, Round two. 95.
Hyde County Department of Social Services, Swan Quarter, NC, $75,000. For start-up support of Medicaid Community Alternatives Programs to provide case-managed services for low-income, frail elderly and disabled individuals as part of Kate B. Reynolds Aging at Home Program, Round two. 95.
Lenoir Memorial Hospital, Kinston, NC, $71,999. For start-up support of Medicaid Community Alternatives Programs to provide case-managed services for low-income, frail elderly and disabled individuals as part of Kate B. Reynolds Aging at Home Program, Round two. 95.
Life Enrichment Center of Cleveland County, Shelby, NC, $90,000. For construction and equipment toward expansion of adult day care/day health services for disabled and frail elderly. 95.
Living Independently Through Volunteers for the Elderly of Cleveland County, Shelby, NC, $314,358. For start-up operating support to serve frail elderly and disabled who are not eligible for Medicaid and cannot afford to pay for skilled care. 95.
Martin County Department of Social Services, Williamston, NC, $74,991. For start-up support of Medicaid Community Alternatives Programs to provide case-managed services for low-income, frail elderly and disabled individuals as part of Kate B. Reynolds Aging at Home Program, Round two. 95.
Mountain Geri-Care Center, Asheville, NC, $50,000. For renovation and equipment to expand day care and day health care services for older and impaired adults. 95.
Piedmont Residential Development Center, Concord, NC, $34,217. For renovation and equipment for day program to meet specialized needs of adults with severe mental and physical disabilities. 95.
Richmond Memorial Hospital, Rockingham, NC, $75,000. For start-up support of Medicaid Community Alternatives Programs to provide case-managed services for low-income, frail elderly and disabled individuals as part of Kate B. Reynolds Aging at Home Program, Round two. 95.
Shepherds Staff, Belhaven, NC, $10,000. For direct client assistance with medication expenses to meet emergency needs of low-income, elderly and handicapped individuals. 95.
Vance County Department of Social Services, Henderson, NC, $66,565. For start-up support of Medicaid Community Alternatives Programs to provide case-managed services for low-income, frail elderly and disabled individuals as part of Kate B. Reynolds Aging at Home Program, Round two. 95.
Warren County Department of Social Services, Warrenton, NC, $75,000. For start-up support of Medicaid Community Alternatives Programs to provide case-managed services for low-income, frail elderly and disabled individuals as part of Kate B. Reynolds Aging at Home Program, Round two. 95.
Washington County Department of Social Services, Plymouth, NC, $69,566. For start-up support of Medicaid Community Alternatives Programs to provide case-managed services for low-income, frail elderly and disabled individuals as part of Kate B. Reynolds Aging at Home Program, Round two. 95.
Wayne Memorial Hospital, Goldsboro, NC, $67,119. For start-up support of Medicaid Community Alternatives Programs to provide case-managed services for low-income, frail elderly and disabled individuals as part of Kate B. Reynolds Aging at Home Program, Round two. 95.

757
The Mary Lynn Richardson Fund

P.O. Box 20124
Greensboro 27420 (910) 274-5471
Contact: Managing Trustee

Trust established in 1940 in NC.
Donor(s): Mary Lynn Richardson.‡
Financial data (yr. ended 12/31/94): Assets, $5,155,750 (M); expenditures, $216,898; qualifying distributions, $167,254, including $136,184 for 30 grants (high: $15,000; low: $500) and $14,875 for 6 grants to individuals.
Purpose and activities: Grants to organizations which aid the needy and to foreign Presbyterian causes.
Fields of interest: Human services; Children & youth, services; Family services; Aging, centers

& services; Christian agencies & churches; Protestant agencies & churches; Aging; Economically disadvantaged.
Types of support: General/operating support, seed money.
Limitations: Giving limited to Guilford County, NC, for domestic programs; giving also on an international basis. No grants to individuals, or for building funds, research programs, or matching gifts; no loans.
Application information: No new grants to individuals will be awarded. Application form not required.
Initial approach: Proposal
Copies of proposal: 1
Deadline(s): Submit proposal preferably between Jan. and Mar.; deadline Apr. 1 and Oct. 1
Board meeting date(s): Late spring and fall
Trustees: Eric R. Calhoun, Betsy Boney Mead, William Y. Preyer, Jr., Lisa B. Prochnow, Adele Richardson Ray.
Number of staff: 1 shared staff
EIN: 066025946

758
The Schechter Foundation, Inc.
P.O. Box 614
Kinston 28502-0614 (919) 527-8011
Contact: Sol Schechter, Pres.

Established in 1982.
Financial data (yr. ended 12/31/92): Assets, $1,353,185 (M); gifts received, $115,000; expenditures, $62,691; qualifying distributions, $62,691, including $62,633 for 118 grants (high: $10,175; low: $10).
Fields of interest: Higher education; Aging, centers & services; Jewish agencies & temples; Aging; General charitable giving.
Limitations: Giving primarily in NC.
Application information: Application form not required.
Initial approach: Letter of proposal
Deadline(s): None
Officers: Sol Schechter, Pres. and Treas.; Arnold M. Schechter, V.P.; Pearl F. Schechter, Secy.
EIN: 561318527

759
The Thomas Foundation
c/o Wachovia Bank of North Carolina, N.A.
P.O. Box 3099
Winston-Salem 27150-1022
Contact: Douglas M. Harrison, Secy.
Application address: c/o Thomas Built Buses, Inc., P.O. Box 2450, High Point, NC 27261; Tel.: (910) 889-4781

Established in 1976 in NC.
Donor(s): Thomas Built Buses, Inc.
Foundation type: Company-sponsored
Financial data (yr. ended 12/31/93): Assets, $350,720 (M); expenditures, $35,625; qualifying distributions, $30,825, including $30,000 for 12 grants (high: $6,000; low: $1,000).
Fields of interest: Higher education; Nursing care; Alcoholism; Youth, services; Aging, centers & services; Religion; Aging.
Limitations: Giving primarily in High Point, NC. No grants to individuals.
Application information:
Initial approach: Letter
Deadline(s): None
Officers and Trustees:* P.A. Thomas,* Chair. and Pres.; James E. Thomas,* Vice-Chair. and V.P.; Douglas M. Harrison,* Secy.; John W. Thomas III,* Treas.; L.T. Gayle, R.A. Price, Albert L. Thomas, B.L. Thomas, John W. Thomas, Jr.
EIN: 510189803

760
Triangle Community Foundation
100 Park Offices, Suite 209
P.O. Box 12834
Research Triangle Park 27709 (919) 549-9840
Contact: Polly Guthrie, Prog. Officer

Incorporated in 1983 in NC.
Foundation type: Community
Financial data (yr. ended 06/30/95): Assets, $22,797,671 (M); gifts received, $12,816,018; expenditures, $1,660,763, including $1,148,378 for 25 grants (high: $15,000; average: $500-$20,000) and $154,000 for 20 grants to individuals (high: $4,400).
Fields of interest: Visual arts; Museums; Performing arts; Dance; Theater; Music; Humanities; Historic preservation/historical societies; Arts/cultural programs; Early childhood education; Child development, education; Elementary school/education; Vocational education; Higher education; Adult/continuing education; Adult education—literacy & basic skills; Libraries/library science; Reading; Education; Natural resource conservation & protection; Energy; Environment; Animal welfare; Wildlife preservation & protection; Family planning; Medical care, rehabilitation; Health care; Substance abuse, services; Mental health/crisis services; AIDS; Alcoholism; Health organizations; Delinquency prevention/services; Legal services; Crime/law enforcement; Food services; Housing/shelter, development; Recreation; Youth development, services; Human services; Children & youth, services; Child development, services; Family services; Hospices; Aging, centers & services; Women, centers & services; Minorities/immigrants, centers & services; Homeless, human services; Peace; Race/intergroup relations; Urban/community development; Rural development; Community development; Voluntarism promotion; Government/public administration; Leadership development; Public affairs; Minorities; Native Americans; Disabled; Aging; Women; Gays/lesbians; Economically disadvantaged; Homeless; General charitable giving.
Types of support: Continuing support, emergency funds, program development, seed money, scholarship funds, technical assistance, program-related investments/loans, employee-related scholarships, scholarships—to individuals.
Limitations: Giving limited to Durham, Orange, and Wake counties, NC. No grants for annual campaigns or operating budgets.
Publications: Annual report (including application guidelines), newsletter, application guidelines, financial statement, grants list.
Application information: Application form required.
Initial approach: Narrative and application form
Copies of proposal: 6
Deadline(s): Feb. 1 and Aug. 1
Board meeting date(s): Feb., May, Aug., and Nov.
Final notification: June 1 and Dec. 1
Officers and Directors:* Mary L. Hill,* Pres.; Beth Head, C.O.O.; R. Peyton Woodson III,* V.P.; Charles Neely,* Secy.; Bert Collins, Treas.; Stephen D. Corman,* Finance Chair.; Carol W. Bilbro,* Distribs. Chair.; Shannon St. John, Exec. Dir.; and 16 additional directors.
Staff: Polly Guthrie, Prog. Officer; Fred Stang, Development Officer.
Number of staff: 4 full-time professional; 1 part-time professional; 1 full-time support; 1 part-time support.
EIN: 561380796

761
John H. Wellons Foundation, Inc.
(Formerly Wellons Foundation, Inc.)
P.O. Box 1254
Dunn 28335 (910) 892-0436
Contact: John H. Wellons, Sr., Pres.

Established in 1950 in NC.
Financial data (yr. ended 12/31/94): Assets, $2,669,654 (M); gifts received, $98,361; expenditures, $526,876; qualifying distributions, $469,752, including $36,259 for 19 grants (high: $5,011; low: $10), $343,453 for 1 foundation-administered program and $90,040 for loans to individuals.
Purpose and activities: Awards student loans to local area residents and provides housing for the elderly and/or handicapped.
Fields of interest: Housing/shelter, development; Aging, centers & services; Disabled; Aging.
Types of support: General/operating support, student loans—to individuals.
Limitations: Giving limited to the Dunn, NC, area.
Application information: Student loans limited to students of local area high schools and universities. Application form required.
Deadline(s): None
Officers and Directors:* John H. Wellons, Sr.,* Pres.; John H. Wellons, Jr.,* V.P.; Llewellyn Jernigan, Secy.; Sylvia W. Craft, Gene T. Jernigan, Donald McCoy.
EIN: 566061476

762
The Winston-Salem Foundation
310 West Fourth St., Suite 229
Winston-Salem 27101-2889 (910) 725-2382
Contact: Henry M. Carter, Jr., Pres.

Established in 1919 in NC by declaration of trust.
Foundation type: Community
Financial data (yr. ended 12/31/95): Assets, $97,783,601 (M); gifts received, $12,086,154; expenditures, $7,241,838, including $5,981,274 for grants (high: $288,887; low: $25; average: $1,000-$25,000), $164,000 for

121 grants to individuals, $20,000 for 1 loan to an organization and $79,000 for 40 loans to individuals.
Purpose and activities: Student aid primarily to bona fide residents of Forsyth County, NC; support also for nonprofit organizations of all types, especially educational, social service and health programs, the arts, and civic affairs.
Fields of interest: Arts/cultural programs; Education; Health care; Substance abuse, services; Health organizations; Human services; Youth, services; Aging, centers & services; Community development; Government/public administration; Aging.
Types of support: General/operating support, continuing support, endowment funds, emergency funds, program development, seed money, fellowships, scholarship funds, technical assistance, program-related investments/loans, employee matching gifts, scholarships—to individuals, matching funds, student loans—to individuals.
Limitations: Giving primarily in the greater Forsyth County, NC, area; some support for northwest NC. No grants for annual campaigns, land acquisition, publications, or conferences.
Publications: Annual report, application guidelines, newsletter, grants list, informational brochure (including application guidelines).
Application information: Application form required for student aid or student loans only and includes $20 application fee.
Initial approach: Telephone
Copies of proposal: 1
Deadline(s): Jan. 1, Apr. 1, July 1, and Oct. 1
Board meeting date(s): Mar., June, Sept., and Dec.
Final notification: 1 month
Officer: Henry M. Carter, Jr., Pres.
Foundation Committee: Roberta W. Irwin, Chair.; Willard W. Bass, Jr., Graham F. Bennett, Richard P. Budd, Richard N. Davis, Victor I. Flow, Jr., Richard Janeway, M.D., John G. Medlin, Jr., Joseph F. Neely, Elizabeth L. Quick, Ann Ring, Robert C. Vaughn, Jr.
Trustees: Branch Banking & Trust Co., Central Carolina Bank & Trust Co., First Citizens Bank & Trust Co., First Union National Bank of North Carolina, NationsBank of North Carolina, N.A., Wachovia Bank of North Carolina, N.A., Salem Trust Bank.
Number of staff: 8 full-time professional; 1 part-time professional; 5 full-time support.
EIN: 566037615
Grants for Aging:
Alzheimers Disease and Related Disorders Association, Piedmont Triad North Carolina Chapter, Winston-Salem, NC, $35,000. For salary for director of development. 95.
Shepherds Center of Kernersville, Kernersville, NC, $20,000. For position of administrative assistant. 95.

763
World of Clothing Foundation
P.O. Box 2360
Hendersonville 28793
Contact: Robert D. Williams, Pres.
Application address: 135 Sugarloaf Rd., Hendersonville, NC 28793; Tel.: (704) 693-1507

Established in 1988 in NC.
Donor(s): Robert D. Williams.
Financial data (yr. ended 09/30/93): Assets, $20,815 (M); gifts received, $10,650; expenditures, $98,481; qualifying distributions, $98,481, including $82,950 for 1 grant and $11,803 for 3 grants to individuals (high: $11,167; low: $222).
Fields of interest: Nursing school/education; Aging; Economically disadvantaged.
Types of support: Scholarship funds, grants to individuals.
Limitations: Giving primarily in Hendersonville, NC.
Application information:
Initial approach: Letter, with references
Deadline(s): None
Officers and Directors:* Robert D. Williams,* Pres.; Gary Jones, Secy.-Treas.; Mickey Marvin.
EIN: 581648745

NORTH DAKOTA

764
Myra Foundation
P.O. Box 13536
Grand Forks 58208-3536 (701) 772-8111
Contact: Alan B. Warcup, Pres.

Incorporated in 1941 in ND.
Donor(s): John E. Myra.‡
Financial data (yr. ended 12/31/93): Assets, $2,724,057 (M); expenditures, $282,156; qualifying distributions, $217,082, including $207,782 for grants.
Fields of interest: Arts/cultural programs; Secondary school/education; Higher education; Health care; Health organizations; Human services; Youth, services; Aging, centers & services; Government/public administration; Aging.
Types of support: Building/renovation, equipment, scholarship funds.
Limitations: Giving limited to Grand Forks County, ND. No grants to individuals, or for endowment funds, research, or matching gifts; no loans.
Publications: Informational brochure (including application guidelines).
Application information: Application form required.
Initial approach: Letter
Copies of proposal: 1
Deadline(s): None
Board meeting date(s): Quarterly
Officers: Alan B. Warcup, Pres.; Donna J. Gillig, V.P.; Robert F. Hansen, Secy.-Treas.
EIN: 450215088

765
North Dakota Community Foundation
P.O. Box 387
Bismarck 58502-0387 (701) 222-8349
Contact: Kevin J. Dvorak, Pres.

Established in 1977 in ND.
Foundation type: Community
Financial data (yr. ended 12/31/95): Assets, $6,239,603 (L); gifts received, $1,017,097; expenditures, $617,137, including $444,685 for 263 grants (high: $16,000; low: $50; average: $1,000).
Purpose and activities: Unrestricted funds largely for aid to the elderly and disadvantaged; support also for health services, including mental health, youth agencies, parks and recreation, and arts and cultural programs in ND.
Fields of interest: Arts/cultural programs; Health care; Mental health/crisis services; Recreation; Human services; Youth, services; Aging, centers & services; Community development; Aging; Economically disadvantaged.
Types of support: General/operating support, continuing support, annual campaigns, building/renovation, equipment, program development, conferences/seminars, publication, seed money, scholarship funds, research, scholarships—to individuals, matching funds.
Limitations: Giving primarily in ND. No support for sectarian purposes; low priority given to national or out-of-state organizations, hospitals, organizations with substantial and professional fundraising programs, or organizations that raise money through gambling activities. No grants to individuals (except for scholarships), or for emergency or endowment funds, deficit financing, or land acquisition; no loans.
Publications: Annual report, newsletter, informational brochure, application guidelines.
Application information: Application form not required.
Initial approach: Letter
Copies of proposal: 1
Deadline(s): Aug. 31
Board meeting date(s): Annually in 2nd quarter of year
Officers and Directors:* Vernon Wagner,* Chair.; Kevin J. Dvorak,* Pres.; Donald Schmid,* Secy.-Treas.; George Cox, Irma Dulmage, David M. Gipp, Cornelius Grant, Ray Hoffman, Frank P. Keogh, William Kretschmar, Agnes Palanuk, Marlys Prince, Jacque Schauer, Rita Staloch.
Number of staff: 2 full-time professional; 1 full-time support.
EIN: 450336015

766
Alex Stern Family Foundation
Bill Stern Bldg., Suite 205
609 1/2 First Ave. North
Fargo 58102
Contact: E.G. Preston, Dir.

Established in 1964 in ND.
Donor(s): William Stern,‡ Sam Stern,‡ Edward A. Stern.‡
Financial data (yr. ended 12/31/93): Assets, $8,367,666 (M); expenditures, $437,625; qualifying distributions, $420,891, including $367,610 for 46 grants (high: $62,500; low: $800; average: $6,417).
Purpose and activities: Primary areas of interest include the arts, child welfare, the elderly, alcohol abuse programs, and community funds. Support also for family and social services, including legal services, and welfare for the homeless and disabled; community organizations; higher, business, minority, and

other education; and hospices and cancer research.
Fields of interest: Museums; Performing arts; Dance; Theater; Historic preservation/historical societies; Arts/cultural programs; Elementary/secondary education; Child development, education; Elementary school/education; Higher education; Hospitals (general); Substance abuse, services; Cancer; Alcoholism; Cancer research; Legal services; Housing/shelter, development; Human services; Children & youth, services; Child development, services; Family services; Hospices; Aging, centers & services; Homeless, human services; Biological sciences; Religion; Minorities; Native Americans; Disabled; Aging; Economically disadvantaged; Homeless; General charitable giving.
Types of support: General/operating support, continuing support, annual campaigns, building/renovation, equipment, emergency funds, program development, scholarship funds, research, matching funds.
Limitations: Giving limited to the Fargo, ND, and Moorhead, MN, areas. No grants to individuals, or for endowment funds; no loans.
Publications: Application guidelines, annual report.
Application information: Application form required.
Initial approach: Letter requesting application and guidelines
Copies of proposal: 4
Deadline(s): Apr. 30 for June consideration and Sept. 30 for Nov. consideration
Board meeting date(s): Varies
Final notification: Within a few months
Officer and Trustees:* E.G. Preston,* Dir.; J.L. McCormick, S. Stroud.
Number of staff: 1 part-time professional.
EIN: 456013981

OHIO

767
The Abington Foundation
c/o Foundation Mgmt. Svcs., Inc.
1422 Euclid Ave., Suite 627
Cleveland 44115-1901 (216) 621-2901
Contact: Janet E. Narten, Consultant

Established in 1983 in OH.
Donor(s): David Knight Ford,‡ Elizabeth Brooks Ford.‡
Financial data (yr. ended 12/31/95): Assets, $24,853,848 (M); gifts received, $177,893; expenditures, $1,077,252; qualifying distributions, $952,246, including $903,020 for 38 grants (high: $100,000; low: $500).
Purpose and activities: Giving primarily for educational programs, geriatrics, healthcare, social services, and the arts and cultural programs in northeast OH.
Fields of interest: Arts/cultural programs; Education; Health care; Human services; Aging.
Types of support: Annual campaigns, capital campaigns, equipment, emergency funds, program development, seed money, matching funds.
Limitations: Giving primarily in Cleveland, OH. No grants to individuals.
Publications: Annual report, application guidelines.
Application information: Application form required.
Copies of proposal: 6
Deadline(s): 6 weeks prior to meetings
Board meeting date(s): Jan., Apr., July, and Oct.
Officers and Trustees:* Amasa B. Ford, M.D.,* Pres.; Allen H. Ford,* V.P. and Treas.; David Kingsley Ford,* V.P.; Oliver M. Ford,* V.P.
Number of staff: None.
EIN: 341404854
Grants for Aging:
Benjamin Rose Institute, Cleveland, OH, $100,000. For Margaret Wagner House program Care Giver Resource Center capital campaign. 95.
Benjamin Rose Institute, Cleveland, OH, $100,000. For Margaret Wagner House Care Giver Resource Center capital campaign. 95.
Long-Term Care Ombudsman, Cleveland, OH, $9,000. 95.

768
Akron Community Foundation
Society Bldg., Suite 830
159 South Main St.
Akron 44308-1318 (330) 376-8522
Contact: Jody Bacon, Exec. Dir.
FAX: (330) 376-0202

Incorporated in 1955 in OH.
Foundation type: Community
Financial data (yr. ended 03/31/96): Assets, $42,792,570 (M); gifts received, $5,307,078; expenditures, $1,652,658, including $1,132,455 for 245 grants (high: $137,680; low: $35; average: $100-$136,300).
Purpose and activities: To promote charitable, benevolent, educational, recreational, health, esthetic, cultural, and public welfare activities; to support a program of research leading to the improvement of the health, education, and general well-being of all citizens of the Akron area; to give toward the support of experimental and demonstration programs, through established or new agencies; to test the validity of research findings in various fields of community planning directed toward the efficient and adequate coordination of public and private services organized to meet human needs.
Fields of interest: Arts/cultural programs; Education; Health care; Health associations; Recreation; Human services; Children & youth, services; Community development; African Americans; Disabled; Aging; Women; People with AIDS (PWAs); Gays/lesbians; Immigrants/refugees; Economically disadvantaged; Homeless.
Types of support: Program development, seed money, scholarship funds, research, matching funds.
Limitations: Giving primarily in Akron, Summit, and Medina counties, OH. No grants to individuals, or for endowment funds, capital campaigns, or fellowships; no loans.
Publications: Annual report (including application guidelines), application guidelines, newsletter.
Application information: No more than 1 grant to an organization in a 12-month period. Application form not required.
Initial approach: Letter or telephone requesting application guidelines
Copies of proposal: 20
Deadline(s): Jan. 2, Apr. 1, July 1, and Oct. 1
Board meeting date(s): Generally Feb., May, Aug., and Nov.
Final notification: 6 weeks
Officers and Trustees:* Edward S. Gaffney,* Chair.; Ernest J. Novack, Jr.,* Vice-Chair.; R. Briggs, Secy.; D. Wilson, Treas.; Jody Bacon, Exec. Dir.; Lolita K. Adair, Ronald C. Allan, John C. Curry, John Dotson, Ernest Estep, Donald R. Fair, Stanley Gault, Stuart Giller, J. Harvey Graves, Richard L. Hardgrove, Willard Holland, Kathryn M. Hunter, Clifford Isroff, Mary Ann Jackson, Mary Myers, Janise B. Parry, Judith Read, Edwin Schrank, Sandra Smith, Robert Stefanko, Gale R. Urda, James R. Williams.
Trustee Banks: Bank One Akron, N.A., First National Bank of Ohio, Key Trust Co. of Ohio, N.A., National City Bank.
Number of staff: 2 full-time professional; 2 part-time professional; 2 full-time support.
EIN: 341087615
Grants for Aging:
Arlington Housing Options Plus Elderly Services (HOPES), Akron, OH, $15,000. For Arlington Shared Elderly Living Facility. 95.
Mobile Meals Foundation, Akron, OH, $10,000. For computer system network. 95.

769
The Ruth H. Beecher Charitable Trust
c/o National City Bank, Akron
P.O. Box 450
Youngstown 44501 (330) 742-4254
Contact: James H. Sisek, Sr. V.P. and Sr. Trust Officer, National City Bank, Akron

Established in 1986 in OH.
Financial data (yr. ended 09/30/95): Assets, $1,680,071 (M); expenditures, $76,687; qualifying distributions, $66,152, including $65,500 for 37 grants (high: $6,000; low: $1,000; average: $1,000-$5,000).
Purpose and activities: Giving primarily for the arts, including a symphony society, the performing arts, theater, fine arts, and museums; support also for civic affairs, a historical society, the elderly, child development, family planning, Jewish organizations, and other general charitable giving.
Fields of interest: Visual arts; Museums; Performing arts; Theater; Historic preservation/historical societies; Arts/cultural programs; Child development, education; Child development, services; Aging, centers & services; Government/public administration; Aging; General charitable giving.
Types of support: Capital campaigns, building/renovation, equipment, land acquisition, program development.
Limitations: Giving primarily in Youngstown, OH.
Application information: Application form not required.
Initial approach: Letter and proposal
Copies of proposal: 4
Deadline(s): None

Board meeting date(s): Mar., June, and Oct.
Trustees: John Weed Powers, National City Bank, Northeast.
EIN: 346861417
Grants for Aging:
Blackburn Home for Aged People, Poland, OH, $3,500. 95.
Park Vista Retirement Community, Youngstown, OH, $2,500. For Life Care fund. 95.

770
Britton Fund

c/o Advisory Svcs., Inc.
1422 Euclid Ave., 1010 Hanna Bldg.
Cleveland 44115-2078 (216) 363-6489
Contact: Nick Valentino, Treas.

Incorporated in 1952 in OH.
Donor(s): Gertrude H. Britton,‡ Charles S. Britton II,‡ Brigham Britton.‡
Financial data (yr. ended 12/31/95): Assets, $20,131,983 (M); gifts received, $419,697; expenditures, $850,827; qualifying distributions, $791,008, including $780,750 for 52 grants (high: $187,250; low: $100; average: $2,000-$5,000).
Fields of interest: Education, research; Secondary school/education; Higher education; Hospitals (general); Family planning; Health care; Medical research; Alzheimer's disease research; Food services; Human services; Children & youth, services; Women, centers & services; Disabled; Women.
Types of support: General/operating support, continuing support, annual campaigns, endowment funds, emergency funds, scholarship funds, research.
Limitations: Giving primarily in OH. No grants to individuals.
Publications: Annual report.
Application information: Funds substantially committed. Application form not required.
Initial approach: Letter
Copies of proposal: 1
Deadline(s): Prior to board meetings
Board meeting date(s): May and Nov.
Officers and Trustees:* Lynda R. Britton,* Pres.; Terence B. Britton,* V.P.; Timothy C. Britton,* V.P.; Julie R. Hamilton, Secy.; Nick Valentino, Treas.
Number of staff: None.
EIN: 346513616

771
Eva L. and Joseph M. Bruening Foundation

1422 Euclid Ave., Suite 627
Cleveland 44115 (216) 621-2632
Contact: Janet E. Narten, Exec. Dir.

Established in 1988 in OH.
Donor(s): Joseph M. Bruening,‡ Eva L. Bruening.‡
Financial data (yr. ended 12/31/95): Assets, $48,075,076 (M); expenditures, $2,187,365; qualifying distributions, $1,664,400, including $1,664,400 for 72 grants (high: $100,000; low: $2,000; average: $5,000-$100,000).
Purpose and activities: The foundation's current focus areas are health, education and social services with an emphasis on care for the elderly, disabled, and disadvantaged.
Fields of interest: Education, fund raising; Early childhood education; Higher education; Education; Domestic violence prevention; Human services; Children & youth, services; Youth, services; Aging, centers & services; Roman Catholic agencies & churches; Minorities; Disabled; Aging; Women; People with AIDS (PWAs); Economically disadvantaged; Homeless.
Types of support: Capital campaigns, building/renovation, equipment, emergency funds, program development, seed money, matching funds.
Limitations: Giving limited to the greater Cleveland, OH, area. No grants to individuals, or for endowment funds, general operating budgets, research, publications, or symposiums and seminars.
Publications: Informational brochure, annual report (including application guidelines).
Application information: The foundation does not respond to mass mailings or annual campaign appeals. Application form not required.
Initial approach: Proposal
Copies of proposal: 1
Deadline(s): Mar. 1, July 1, and Nov. 1
Board meeting date(s): Apr., Aug., and Dec.
Final notification: Within several weeks of board meeting
Distribution Committee: Anne B. Blaine, Marilyn A. Cunin, John A. Fauret, E. Lorrie Robertson.
Trustee: Key Trust Co. of Ohio, N.A.
Number of staff: None.
EIN: 341584378
Grants for Aging:
Altenheim, Strongsville, OH, $15,000. For start-up of Adult Day Care Center. 94.
Eliza Bryant Center, Cleveland, OH, $36,000. To develop Coordinated Volunteer Program. 94.
Fairhill Institute for the Elderly, Cleveland, OH, $10,000. For start-up support of Intergenerational Resource Center. 94.
Golden Age Centers of Greater Cleveland, Cleveland, OH, $15,000. For general support. 94.
Judson Retirement Community, Cleveland Heights, OH, $50,000. For capital campaign. 94.
Saint Augustine Manor, Cleveland, OH, $100,000. For relocation of Nursing Care Manor. 94.

772
The Greater Cincinnati Foundation

425 Walnut St., Suite 1110
Cincinnati 45202-3915 (513) 241-2880
Contact: Ruth A. Cronenberg, Prog. Dir.

Established in 1963 in OH by bank resolution and declaration of trust.
Foundation type: Community
Financial data (yr. ended 12/31/95): Assets, $160,024,485 (M); gifts received, $19,168,229; expenditures, $11,452,790, including $10,330,995 for grants (high: $90,000; low: $400).
Purpose and activities: Grants for a broad range of both new and existing activities in general categories of arts and culture, community progress, environmental needs, education, health, and social and human services, including youth agencies.
Fields of interest: Arts/cultural programs; Early childhood education; Education; Environment; Health care; Housing/shelter, home owners; Human services; Youth, services; Community development; Voluntarism promotion; African Americans; Disabled; Aging; Economically disadvantaged; Homeless.
Types of support: Capital campaigns, building/renovation, equipment, emergency funds, program development, seed money, technical assistance, program-related investments/loans, matching funds.
Limitations: Giving limited to the greater Cincinnati, OH, area. No support for sectarian religious purposes. No grants to individuals, or for operating budgets, annual campaigns, deficit financing, scholarships, fellowships, internships, exchange programs, or scholarly research.
Publications: Annual report (including application guidelines), newsletter, informational brochure (including application guidelines), application guidelines.
Application information: Application form required.
Initial approach: Letter or telephone, followed by interview with foundation staff and volunteers
Copies of proposal: 15
Deadline(s): 90 days prior to board meetings
Board meeting date(s): Feb., May, Aug., and Dec.
Final notification: Immediately following board meetings
Officers: Karen D. Hoeb, C.E.O. and Pres.; Lawrence D. Graziani, V.P., Operations.
Governing Board: Herbert R. Brown, Chair.; Dwight Hibbard, Vice-Chair.; Richard J. Ruebel, Legal Counsel; Frank Bloom, Cynthia Booth, William R. Burleigh, Frank W. Cianciolo, M.D., Elizabeth D. Goldsmith, Louise A. Head, John T. Lawrence III, Joseph A. Pichler, Paul G. Sittenfeld, Merri Gaither Smith, John A. Stith, Robert I. Westheimer.
Trustee Banks: Bank One Ohio Trust Co., N.A., Fifth Third Bank, Huntington National Bank, Key Corp., The Lebanon Citizens National Bank, The North Side Bank & Trust Co., PNC Bank, N.A., The Provident Bank, Star Bank, N.A.
Staff: Ruth A. Cronenberg, Prog. Dir.; Amy L. Bick, Advancement Dir.; Tracy J. Loesing, Financial Svcs. Dir.; Michael A. Cheney, Financial Services. Dir.
Number of staff: 6 full-time professional; 5 full-time support.
EIN: 310669700
Grants for Aging:
Council on Aging of the Cincinnati Area, Cincinnati, OH, $50,000. For WMKV, educational radio station for seniors. 94.
Dearborn Adult Center, Lawrenceburg, IN, $15,000. 94.

773
The Cincinnati Foundation for the Aged

2100 Central Trust Tower
Five West 4th St.
Cincinnati 45202
Contact: Ruth Avram, Secy.

Established in 1891 in OH.
Donor(s): Oscar Cohrs,‡ Otto Luedeking.‡
Financial data (yr. ended 03/31/95): Assets, $11,002,993 (M); gifts received, $78,899; expenditures, $319,368; qualifying distributions, $303,196, including $297,761 for 7 grants (high: $137,640; low: $1,440).
Purpose and activities: "The sole purpose of the foundation is to assist indigent persons in the greater Cincinnati, OH, area to gain admission to nonprofit nursing homes."
Fields of interest: Aging, centers & services; Aging.
Limitations: Giving limited to the greater Cincinnati, OH, area.
Application information: Disbursements limited to the foundation's single mission described in "Purpose & activities"; funding requests for studies or any other activity not eligible for consideration. Application form required.
Deadline(s): None
Board meeting date(s): Mar., June, Sept., and Dec.
Officers: William Dock Meyer, Pres.; Robert Porter, Jr., 1st V.P.; Gene Weber, 2nd V.P.; Ruth Avram, Secy.; Donald Hathaway, Treas.
Trustees: Bernice Gartrell, Guido Gores, Jack Greer, Richard Hoeffinghoff, Jon Hoffheimer, Philip Walters.
Number of staff: 1 full-time support.
EIN: 310536971
Grants for Aging:
Bayley Place, Cincinnati, OH, $20,638. 95.
Bayley Place, Cincinnati, OH, $19,000. 94.
Carmel Manor, Fort Thomas, KY, $137,640. 95.
Carmel Manor, Fort Thomas, KY, $126,079. 94.
Cottingham Retirement Center, Cincinnati, OH, $53,106. 95.
Cottingham Retirement Center, Cincinnati, OH, $19,225. 94.
Lakeside Place, Highland Heights, KY, $375. 94.
New England Club, Cincinnati, OH, $1,125. 94.
Ohio Presbyterian Homes, LLanfair Terrace, Cincinnati, OH, $35,282. 94.
Saint Charles Nursing Home, Covington, KY, $3,803. 94.
Saint Theresa Home for the Aged, Cincinnati, OH, $8,385. 94.
Saint Theresa Home for the Aged, Cincinnati, OH, $4,000. 95.
West Park Retirement Community, Cincinnati, OH, $90,200. 94.
West Park Retirement Community, Cincinnati, OH, $56,100. 95.

774
The Cleveland Foundation

1422 Euclid Ave., Suite 1400
Cleveland 44115-2001 (216) 861-3810
Contact: Steven A. Minter, Exec. Dir.
FAX: (216) 861-1729; TTY: (216) 861-3806

Established in 1914 in OH by bank resolution and declaration of trust.
Foundation type: Community
Financial data (yr. ended 12/31/94): Assets, $733,950,639 (M); gifts received, $33,782,492; expenditures, $38,294,569, including $30,723,125 for 1,047 grants (high: $1,500,000; low: $36), $561,045 for 24 foundation-administered programs and $3,250,000 for 4 program-related investments.
Purpose and activities: The pioneer community foundation which has served as a model for most community foundations in the U.S.; grants are made to private tax-exempt and governmental agencies and programs serving the greater Cleveland area in the fields of civic and cultural affairs, education and economic development, and health and social services. Current priorities are in economic development, neighborhood development, downtown revitalization, lakefront enhancement, programs dealing with the young, the aged and special constituencies, health care for the medically indigent and for underserved populations, and the professional performing and visual arts. Grants are given mainly as seed money for innovative projects or to developing institutions or services addressing unmet needs in the community. Very limited support for capital purposes for highly selective construction or equipment projects which serve the program priorities listed above. Special initiatives include neighborhoods, education (public school improvement), and persistent poverty.
Fields of interest: Visual arts; Performing arts; Arts/cultural programs; Elementary school/education; Secondary school/education; Higher education; Medical school/education; Health care; AIDS; Health organizations; Medical research; AIDS research; Housing/shelter, development; Human services; Youth, services; Aging, centers & services; Urban/community development; Community development; Economics; Government/public administration; Aging.
Types of support: Program development, seed money, scholarship funds, research, technical assistance, consulting services, program-related investments/loans, matching funds.
Limitations: Giving limited to the greater Cleveland, OH, area, with primary emphasis on Cleveland, Cuyahoga, Lake, and Geauga counties, unless specified by donor. No support for sectarian or religious activities, community services such as fire and police protection, and library and welfare services. No grants to individuals, or for endowment funds, operating costs, debt reduction, fundraising campaigns, publications, films and audiovisual materials (unless they are an integral part of a program already being supported), memberships, travel for bands, sports teams, classes and similar groups; capital support for planning, construction, renovation, or purchase of buildings, equipment and materials, land acquisition, or renovation of public space unless there is strong evidence that the program is of priority to the foundation.
Publications: Annual report (including application guidelines), newsletter, occasional report, application guidelines, financial statement, informational brochure.
Application information: Application form not required.
Initial approach: Letter
Copies of proposal: 2
Deadline(s): Mar. 31, June 30, Sept. 15, and Dec. 31
Board meeting date(s): Distribution committee meets in Mar., June, Sept., and Dec.
Final notification: 1 month
Officers: Roberta W. Allport, Secy.; J.T. Mullen, C.F.O.; Steven A. Minter, Exec. Dir.; Susan N. Lajoie, Assoc. Dir.
Distribution Committee: Charles A. Ratner, Chair.; Jerry V. Jarrett, Vice-Chair.; Rev. Elmo A. Bean, James E. Bennett, James M. Delaney, Doris A. Evans, M.D., Adrienne Lash Jones, Catherine Monroe Lewis, James V. Patton, Alfred M. Rankin, Jr., Jerry Sue Thorton.
Trustees: Bank One, Cleveland, N.A., First National Bank of Ohio, Huntington National Bank, National City Bank, Key Trust Co. of Ohio, N.A.
Staff: Susan N. Lajoie, Assoc. Dir.; Goldie K. Alvis, Sr. Prog. Officer, Social Services; Robert E. Eckardt, Sr. Prog. Officer, Health; Jay Talbot, Sr. Prog. Officer, Civic Affairs and Econ. Devel.; Carol Kleiner Willen, Sr. Prog. Officer, Education; Kathleen A. Cereny, Prog. Officer, Cultural Affairs; Barbara M. Deerhake, Prog. Officer, The L. Dale Dorney Fund; Pamela L. George, Prog. Assoc., Civic Affairs and Econ. Devel.; Terri Kovach, Prog. Assoc., Health and Human Services.
Number of staff: 25 full-time professional; 2 part-time professional; 17 full-time support.
EIN: 340714588
Grants for Aging:
A. M. McGregor Home, Cleveland, OH, $36,750. For general support. 95.
Alzheimers Disease and Related Disorders Association, Cleveland, OH, $30,000. For improvement of Helpline services. 95.
Alzheimers Disease and Related Disorders Association, Cleveland, OH, $25,000. For start-up support of new office in Mentor. 95.
Alzheimers Respite Care Society of Hancock County, Findlay, OH, $17,935. For marketing consultant assistance for promotional plan and social worker to assess needs of clients and families. 95.
American Red Cross, Greater Cleveland Chapter, Cleveland, OH, $134,000. For programs for elderly. 95.
American Society on Aging, San Francisco, CA, $35,000. For Cleveland participants in New Ventures in Leadership program. 95.
Benjamin Rose Institute, Cleveland, OH, $40,000. For feasibility study of intensive home care program for frail elderly in collaboration with University Hospitals of Cleveland. 95.
Benjamin Rose Institute, Cleveland, OH, $36,750. For general support. 95.
Case Western Reserve University, Cleveland, OH, $133,000. For start-up support for training center in geriatric oral health. 95.
Cleveland Neighborhood Health Services, Cleveland, OH, $52,000. For improved services to elderly patients with chronic conditions. 95.
Cleveland Senior Council, Cleveland, OH, $15,000. To diversify user base in private sector. 95.

Cleveland Society for the Blind, Cleveland, OH, $135,000. For Share the Vision program for visually impaired older adults. 95.
Retired Senior Volunteer Program (RSVP) of Cleveland, Cleveland, OH, $49,150. For implementation of strategic plan. 95.
Visiting Nurse Association of Cleveland, Cleveland, OH, $40,000. For geriatric and pediatric nurse-based care at University Settlement. 95.

775
Clinton County Foundation

224 North Mulberry St.
Wilmington 45177 (513) 382-5700
Contact: Campbell Graf, Exec. Secy.
Application address: P.O. Box 831, Wilmington, OH 45177

Established in 1972 in OH.
Foundation type: Community
Financial data (yr. ended 12/31/93): Assets, $189,950 (M); gifts received, $100,693; expenditures, $39,864, including $34,806 for 21 grants (high: $9,372; low: $14; average: $14-$9,372) and $1,100 for 3 grants to individuals (high: $500; low: $100; average: $100-$500).
Fields of interest: Performing arts; Theater; Historic preservation/historical societies; Arts/cultural programs; Education, association; Nursing school/education; Education; Domestic violence prevention; Youth development, services; Human services; Youth, services; Rural development; Community development; Voluntarism promotion; Federated giving programs; Government/public administration; Leadership development; Public affairs; Disabled; Aging; Economically disadvantaged; General charitable giving.
Types of support: General/operating support, endowment funds, program development, seed money, scholarship funds, scholarships—to individuals.
Limitations: Giving limited to Clinton County, OH.
Publications: Informational brochure, annual report.
Application information: Application form not required.
Initial approach: Letter
Copies of proposal: 5
Deadline(s): Jan. 31
Board meeting date(s): Monthly
Final notification: Mar. or Apr.
Officers and Trustees:* Karen Buckley,* Pres.; Mike Cottle,* V.P.; Campbell Graf,* Exec. Secy.; Sarah Barker,* Treas.; Raymond L. Baver, John Filkins, Marque Jones, Bruce Miller, C. Kent Vandervort, C. Ted Vandervort, E. Jonathan Walt, Charles Watts, Mark Williams.
Number of staff: None.
EIN: 311140087

776
John F. and Doris E. Ernsthausen Charitable Foundation

c/o Key Trust Co. of Ohio, N.A.
127 Public Sq., 16th Fl.
Cleveland 44114-1306
Contact: Cornelius J. Ruffing, Mgr.
Application address: Citizens Bank Bldg., Norwalk, OH 44857

Trust established in 1956 in OH.
Donor(s): John F. Ernsthausen, Doris E. Ernsthausen.
Financial data (yr. ended 06/30/95): Assets, $6,764,917 (M); expenditures, $326,885; qualifying distributions, $300,943, including $295,500 for 13 grants (high: $55,000; low: $5,000).
Purpose and activities: Giving for a Methodist church, care of the aged, higher and secondary education, and a community fund.
Fields of interest: Secondary school/education; Higher education; Aging, centers & services; Federated giving programs; Christian agencies & churches; Aging.
Limitations: Giving primarily in OH. No loans or program-related investments.
Application information: Application form not required.
Deadline(s): None
Officer: Cornelius J. Ruffing, Mgr.
Trustee: Key Trust Co. of Ohio, N.A.
EIN: 346501908

777
Fairfield County Foundation

P.O. Box 2450
Lancaster 43130 (614) 653-8251
Contact: Diane W. Eversole, Exec. Dir.

Established in 1989 in OH.
Donor(s): Alma S. Busby,‡ Nannie B. Martens,‡ Charles H. Drinkle,‡ Hubert Amstutz, Elsie Cox-Smith, E. Trevor Jones,‡ Edgar A. Work, William Queen, Cyrus Fulton,‡ Bess Floyd,‡ Ed Sands,‡ Phil Floyd.‡
Foundation type: Community
Financial data (yr. ended 12/31/93): Assets, $3,858,750 (M); expenditures, $192,901, including $192,901 for grants.
Fields of interest: Hospitals (general); Health care; Substance abuse, services; Health associations; Health organizations; Food services; Recreation; Human services; Children & youth, services; Aging, centers & services; Disabled; Aging; Economically disadvantaged; Homeless; General charitable giving.
Types of support: Continuing support, building/renovation, seed money, scholarship funds, matching funds.
Limitations: Giving limited to Fairfield County, OH. No grants to individuals.
Publications: Annual report, application guidelines, informational brochure.
Application information: Contact foundation for application form. Application form required.
Copies of proposal: 3
Deadline(s): Dec., Mar., June, and Sept.
Board meeting date(s): 4th Thursday in Feb., Apr., June, Sept. and Nov.
Officers: Robert E. Johnston, Chair.; Nancy J. Frick, Exec. Dir.
Number of staff: 1 part-time support.
EIN: 341623983

778
John D. Finnegan Foundation

c/o Mahoning National Bank of Youngstown, Trust Dept.
P.O. Box 479
Youngstown 44501 (330) 742-7000
Contact: Patrick A. Sebastiano, Secy.

Trust established in 1957 in OH.
Donor(s): John D. Finnegan.‡
Financial data (yr. ended 12/31/95): Assets, $4,513,064 (M); expenditures, $161,479; qualifying distributions, $146,966, including $139,150 for 11 grants (high: $75,000; low: $1,000; average: $1,000-$75,000).
Purpose and activities: Giving for care of the aged; support also for Roman Catholic religious and welfare associations and for higher education.
Fields of interest: Higher education; Human services; Aging, centers & services; Roman Catholic federated giving programs; Roman Catholic agencies & churches; Aging.
Types of support: Capital campaigns, building/renovation, equipment.
Limitations: Giving primarily in Youngstown, OH. No grants to individuals, or for operating budgets, scholarships, fellowships, or matching gifts; no loans.
Application information:
Initial approach: Letter or proposal
Copies of proposal: 1
Deadline(s): Submit proposal preferably from Jan. through Mar.
Board meeting date(s): May, Sept., and Nov.
Final notification: Mar.
Officers and Directors:* John M. Newman,* Chair.; W.W. Bresnahan,* Vice-Chair.; Patrick A. Sebastiano,* Secy.; William J. Mullen, Gregory L. Ridler.
Trustee: Mahoning National Bank of Youngstown.
Number of staff: None.
EIN: 346516439
Grants for Aging:
Assumption Nursing Home, Youngstown, OH, $75,000. For enlargement and relocation. 95.
Park Vista Retirement Community, Youngstown, OH, $10,000. For center fund. 95.

779
The S. N. Ford and Ada Ford Fund

c/o Key Trust Co. of Ohio, N.A.
P.O. Box 849
Mansfield 44901 (419) 525-7668
Contact: Tracey Williamson, Trust Officer, Key Trust Co. of Ohio, N.A.

Trust established in 1947 in OH.
Donor(s): Ada Ford, M.D.‡
Financial data (yr. ended 12/31/95): Assets, $8,618,905 (M); gifts received, $1,573,672; expenditures, $390,951; qualifying distributions, $317,288, including $32,000 for 10 grants (high: $7,000; low: $1,000) and $285,288 for 583 grants to individuals.

Purpose and activities: Assistance to the aged and the sick, and scholarships for the youth of Richland County.
Fields of interest: Education; Health care, reproductive health; Aging; Economically disadvantaged.
Types of support: Building/renovation, grants to individuals, scholarships—to individuals.
Limitations: Giving primarily in Richland County, OH. No grants for endowment funds, or for operating budgets, special projects, general support, research, or matching gifts; no loans.
Publications: Annual report.
Application information: Application form required.
Initial approach: Telephone
Deadline(s): None
Board meeting date(s): Monthly
Final notification: 2 months
Distribution Committee: Ralph H. LeMunyon, Pres.; Burton Preston, V.P.; Stephen B. Bogner, Secy.; W. Thomas Ross, David L. Upham, John W. Welsh.
Trustee: Key Trust Co. of Ohio, N.A.
EIN: 340842282

780
Thomas B. Fordham Foundation
P.O. Box 1805
Dayton 45401 (513) 228-2411
Contact: Chester E. Finn, Pres.

Established in 1959 in OH.
Donor(s): Thelma Fordham Pruett.‡
Financial data (yr. ended 12/31/95): Assets, $1,746,764 (M); expenditures, $103,928; qualifying distributions, $95,552, including $82,350 for 21 grants (high: $25,000; low: $500).
Fields of interest: Education, fund raising; Higher education; Aging, centers & services; Urban/community development; Aging; General charitable giving.
Types of support: Continuing support, seed money, fellowships.
Limitations: Giving primarily in Dayton, OH. No grants to individuals.
Application information: Application form not required.
Initial approach: Letter
Deadline(s): None
Board meeting date(s): Varies
Officers and Trustees:* Chester E. Finn,* Pres. and Treas.; Belinda A. Burns, V.P.; Thomas A. Holton,* Secy.; Chester E. Finn, Jr.
Number of staff: None.
EIN: 316032844
Grants for Aging:
Wright State University, School of Medicine, Office of Geriatric Medicine and Gerontology, Department of Community Health, Dayton, OH, $25,000. 95.

781
The GAR Foundation
50 South Main St.
P.O. Box 1500
Akron 44309 (330) 376-5300
Contact: Robert W. Briggs, Exec. Dir.

Trust established in 1967 in OH.
Donor(s): Ruth C. Roush,‡ Galen Roush.‡
Financial data (yr. ended 12/31/94): Assets, $169,328,592 (M); expenditures, $9,576,057; qualifying distributions, $9,381,832, including $8,684,676 for 160 grants (high: $1,000,000; low: $552; average: $10,000-$50,000).
Purpose and activities: Grants to higher and secondary educational institutions, and for the arts, hospitals, and civic and social service agencies, including youth activities.
Fields of interest: Arts/cultural programs; Secondary school/education; Higher education; Education; Hospitals (general); Domestic violence prevention; Human services; Youth, services; Economics; African Americans; Disabled; Aging; Economically disadvantaged; Homeless.
Types of support: General/operating support, capital campaigns, building/renovation, equipment, endowment funds, program development, seed money, scholarship funds, research, matching funds.
Limitations: Giving primarily in the Akron-Summit County area and secondarily in northeastern OH. No support for medical research or private non-operating foundations. No grants to individuals, or for fundraising campaigns or general operating expenses of the donee not directly related to its exempt purpose.
Publications: Application guidelines.
Application information: Application form required.
Initial approach: Request application form
Copies of proposal: 1
Deadline(s): Feb. 1, May 1, Aug. 1, and Nov. 1
Board meeting date(s): Feb., May, Aug., and Nov.
Final notification: 2 to 3 weeks after meeting
Officer and Trustees:* Robert W. Briggs,* Exec. Dir.; National City Bank.
Distribution Committee: Richard A. Chenoweth, Joseph Clapp, John L. Tormey, S.R. Werner, Douglas A. Wilson.
Number of staff: 1 full-time professional; 4 part-time professional.
EIN: 346577710
Grants for Aging:
Interfaith Volunteer Caregivers Program of the Akron Area, Akron, OH, $14,500. For services to elderly persons in African-American community in Akron. 94.
Mobile Meals Foundation, Akron, OH, $75,000. Toward permanent endowment for operations. 94.
Ohio Presbyterian Retirement Services, Rockynol Retirement Community, Akron, OH, $35,000. For Life Care Endowment Fund. 94.
Senior Workers Action Program, Akron, OH, $20,000. For operating support for Cherry Creek Acres. 94.

782
Della B. Gardner Trust
c/o Bank One Ohio Trust Co., N.A.
235 West Schrock Rd.
Westerville 43081
Contact: Martha Puffenberger, Trust Officer, Bank One Ohio Trust Co., N.A.
Application address: c/o Bank One Ohio Trust Co., N.A., Two South Main St., Middletown, OH, 45042; Tel.: (513) 425-8430

Financial data (yr. ended 12/31/95): Assets, $307,422 (M); expenditures, $17,416; qualifying distributions, $13,680, including $13,500 for 5 grants (high: $6,500; low: $500).
Fields of interest: Hospitals (general); Aging, centers & services; Aging.
Limitations: Giving limited to Middletown, OH. No grants to individuals.
Application information:
Initial approach: Letter
Deadline(s): None
Trustee: Bank One Ohio Trust Co., N.A.
EIN: 316020705

783
Virginia Gay Fund
c/o National City Bank, Columbus
155 East Broad St.
Columbus 43251
Contact: Trustees

Established in 1914.
Financial data (yr. ended 12/31/95): Assets, $1,923,084 (M); gifts received, $120; expenditures, $93,294; qualifying distributions, $72,655, including $2,000 for 1 grant and $65,837 for 23 grants to individuals (high: $5,544; low: $319).
Purpose and activities: Primarily provides relief assistance to retired, elderly female school teachers.
Fields of interest: Aging, centers & services; Women, centers & services; Aging; Women; Economically disadvantaged.
Types of support: Grants to individuals.
Limitations: Giving limited to OH.
Application information: Application form required.
Initial approach: Contact board for application
Deadline(s): None
Board meeting date(s): Apr. and Nov.
Officers and Trustees:* L.D. Shuter,* Pres.; Marjorie Ater,* V.P.; Joseph Endry,* Exec. Dir.; Maryellen Meredith, Orin E. Morris, George D. Norris.
Number of staff: 1 part-time professional.
EIN: 314379588

784
Grace A. Gossens Testamentary Trust
One SeaGate, 24th Fl.
P.O. Box 10032
Toledo 43604
Contact: Alice J. Servais, Trustee
Application address: 416 West Wayne St., Maumee, OH 43537; Tel.: (419) 893-8603

Financial data (yr. ended 09/30/95): Assets, $368,584 (M); expenditures, $9,980; qualifying distributions, $9,980, including $4,500 for 2 grants to individuals (high: $2,500; low: $2,000).
Purpose and activities: Support only to needy elderly women residing in the Maumee, OH, area.
Fields of interest: Aging, centers & services; Women, centers & services; Aging; Women.
Types of support: Grants to individuals.
Limitations: Giving limited to the Maumee, OH, area.
Application information:
Initial approach: Letter

Deadline(s): None
Trustees: Richard R. Dardenne, Alice J. Servais, Donald J. Servais.
EIN: 346526725

785
H & H Foundation

c/o Rea & Assocs., Inc.
2301 Baton Rouge Ave.
Lima 45805
Contact: Leo J. Hawk, Pres.

Established in 1989 in OH.
Donor(s): Henry J. Hawk, Jr., Beverly Ann Hawk, Leo Hawk, Arlene F. Hawk.
Financial data (yr. ended 12/31/94): Assets, $456,016 (M); gifts received, $106,052; expenditures, $123,310; qualifying distributions, $120,500, including $120,500 for 15 grants (high: $32,500; low: $1,250).
Fields of interest: Arts, multipurpose centers/programs; Television; Elementary/secondary education; Human services; Aging, centers & services; Roman Catholic agencies & churches.
Types of support: General/operating support.
Limitations: Giving primarily in OH. No grants to individuals.
Application information:
Deadline(s): None
Officers: Henry J. Hawk, Jr., Chair.; Leo Hawk, Pres.; Arlene F. Hawk, V.P.; Beverly Ann Hawk, V.P.
EIN: 341625352
Grants for Aging:
Senior Citizens Services, $5,000. 94.

786
Robert E. Hillier Family Charitable Trust

1365 Sharon-Copley Rd.
P.O. Box 70
Sharon Center 44274 (330) 239-2711
Contact: Robert C. Bolon, Exec. Dir.

Established in 1974 in OH.
Donor(s): Pleadis Hillier,‡ Colon C. Hillier,‡ Ruth E. Hillier.‡
Financial data (yr. ended 11/30/94): Assets, $7,631,402 (M); gifts received, $84,448; expenditures, $572,195; qualifying distributions, $468,153, including $415,975 for 29 grants (high: $155,000; low: $200; average: $500-$10,000).
Fields of interest: Higher education; Education; Hospitals (general); Health associations; Human services; Aging, centers & services; Christian agencies & churches; Aging.
Types of support: General/operating support, annual campaigns, program development, scholarship funds.
Limitations: Giving primarily in Medina and Summit counties, OH. No grants to individuals.
Application information: Application form not required.
Initial approach: Letter
Deadline(s): Early in the year
Officer and Trustees:* Robert C. Bolon,* Exec. Dir.; Henry L. Metzger, John C. Swartz.
Number of staff: None.
EIN: 237425779

787
The Herbert W. Hoover Foundation

220 Market Ave. South
United Bank Plaza, Suite 40
Canton 44702
Contact: Herbert W. Hoover, Jr., Chair.

Established in 1989 in OH.
Donor(s): The Hoover Foundation.
Financial data (yr. ended 12/31/95): Assets, $15,066,085 (M); expenditures, $739,874; qualifying distributions, $689,443, including $583,084 for 41 grants (high: $50,000; low: $1,000).
Fields of interest: Visual arts; Performing arts; Humanities; Arts/cultural programs; Education, research; Child development, education; Elementary school/education; Secondary school/education; Higher education; Education; Natural resource conservation & protection; Environment; Wildlife preservation & protection; Hospitals (general); Health care; Mental health/crisis services; Health associations; Heart/circulatory disease; Biomedicine; Medical research; Heart/circulatory research; Recreation; Human services; Children & youth, services; Child development, services; Family services; Aging, centers & services; Women, centers & services; Community development; Marine science; Government/public administration; Disabled; Aging; Women.
Types of support: General/operating support, annual campaigns, capital campaigns, building/renovation, equipment, program development, publication, seed money, scholarship funds, research.
Limitations: Giving primarily in Stark County, OH. No grants to individuals, or for continuing support.
Publications: Application guidelines.
Application information:
Initial approach: Letter
Copies of proposal: 6
Deadline(s): None
Officer and Trustees:* Herbert W. Hoover, Jr.,* Chair.; Ruth H. Basner, Elizabeth Hoover Chase, Robert S. O'Brien, Blair C. Woodside, Jr., Key Trust Co. of Ohio, N.A.
Number of staff: 1 full-time professional; 1 part-time support.
EIN: 346905388

788
John F. Hynes and John D. Finnegan Foundation

(also known as Hynes Finnegan Foundation)
c/o Mahoning National Bank of Youngstown
23 Federal Plaza, P.O. Box 479
Youngstown 44501 (330) 742-7000
Contact: Patrick A. Sebastiano, Sr. V.P., Mahoning National Bank of Youngstown

Financial data (yr. ended 12/31/95): Assets, $362,885 (M); expenditures, $15,998; qualifying distributions, $13,296, including $11,000 for 3 grants (high: $5,000; low: $1,000).
Fields of interest: Youth development, services; Youth, services; Aging, centers & services; Leadership development; Aging.
Limitations: Giving primarily in Youngstown, OH. No grants to individuals.
Application information:
Initial approach: Proposal
Deadline(s): None
Officers and Members:* John M. Newman,* Chair.; William W. Bresnahan,* Vice-Chair.; William J. Mullen, Gregory L. Ridler, Patrick A. Sebastiano.
Trustee: Mahoning National Bank of Youngstown.
EIN: 346554850

789
William H. Kilcawley Fund

c/o National City Bank
P.O. Box 450
Youngstown 44501-0450 (330) 744-9000
Contact: James H. Sisek

Established in 1946.
Financial data (yr. ended 12/31/95): Assets, $2,653,743 (M); expenditures, $112,306; qualifying distributions, $100,759, including $100,500 for 6 grants (high: $50,000; low: $2,000; average: $1,500-$25,000).
Purpose and activities: Giving primarily for higher and other education, Christian churches, community funds, performing and other arts, including museums, and health and social services, including youth and child development, programs for the aged and the homeless, and alcohol abuse programs.
Fields of interest: Museums; Performing arts; Arts/cultural programs; Child development, education; Higher education; Medical school/education; Education; Health care; Health associations; Alcoholism; Children & youth, services; Child development, services; Aging, centers & services; Homeless, human services; Community development; Federated giving programs; Christian agencies & churches; Protestant agencies & churches; Roman Catholic agencies & churches; Aging; Homeless.
Types of support: General/operating support, annual campaigns, capital campaigns, building/renovation, equipment.
Limitations: Giving primarily in Youngstown, OH. No grants to individuals.
Application information: Application form not required.
Initial approach: Letter or proposal
Copies of proposal: 1
Deadline(s): None
Appointing Committee: Anne K. Christman, Herbert H. Pridham.
Trustee: National City Bank.
Number of staff: None.
EIN: 346515643

790
Lake County Foundation

c/o Bank One
30 South Park Place
Painesville 44077 (216) 352-5920

Foundation type: Community

Financial data (yr. ended 12/31/95): Assets, $88,246 (M); expenditures, $8,062, including $5,050 for 9 grants (high: $1,000; low: $300).
Fields of interest: Food services; Human services; Aging, centers & services; Aging; Economically disadvantaged.
Types of support: Grants to individuals.
Limitations: Giving limited to Lake County, OH.
Application information: Application form not required.
Deadline(s): None
Board meeting date(s): June and Dec.
Officers: Arthur Sidley, Pres.; John J. Hurley, Jr., Secy.; George Milbourn, Treas.
Number of staff: None.
EIN: 346536532

791
Loeb Foundation
c/o Lebanon Citizens National Bank
P.O. Box 59
Lebanon 45036-0059 (513) 932-1414
Contact: B.H. Wright, Jr., Trustee

Established in 1992 in OH.
Donor(s): Justus H. Loeb.‡
Financial data (yr. ended 09/30/95): Assets, $5,993,328 (M); expenditures, $252,843; qualifying distributions, $246,569, including $235,689 for 16 grants (high: $43,361; low: $1,185), $1,680 for 2 grants to individuals (high: $1,480; low: $200) and $4,600 for 1 loan to an individual.
Purpose and activities: Giving primarily for fire and police protection.
Fields of interest: Government/public administration; Aging.
Types of support: Equipment, grants to individuals.
Limitations: Giving limited to Warren County, OH.
Application information: Application form not required.
Initial approach: Letter
Copies of proposal: 3
Deadline(s): Aug. 15
Board meeting date(s): Early Sept.
Final notification: Late Sept.
Trustees: Michael E. Foley, Bernard H. Wright, Jr., The Lebanon Citizens National Bank.
Number of staff: None.
EIN: 316225986

792
Middletown Community Foundation
United Way Bldg.
29 City Centre Plaza
Middletown 45042 (513) 424-7369
Contact: Norman M. Hayes, Exec. Dir.

Incorporated in 1976 in OH.
Foundation type: Community
Financial data (yr. ended 12/31/95): Assets, $8,440,275 (M); gifts received, $1,040,174; expenditures, $639,373, including $308,394 for 97 grants (high: $50,000; low: $500; average: $500-$50,000) and $220,000 for 210 grants to individuals (high: $2,600; low: $250; average: $250-$2,600).
Purpose and activities: Primary areas of interest include higher and other education, the arts, youth, and social services.
Fields of interest: Performing arts; Arts/cultural programs; Elementary/secondary education; Early childhood education; Elementary school/education; Higher education; Libraries/library science; Education; Hospitals (general); Health care; Youth development, services; Youth development, citizenship; Human services; Youth, services; Family services; Homeless, human services; Community development; Public affairs, citizen participation; Leadership development; Religion; Aging; Homeless.
Types of support: Building/renovation, equipment, endowment funds, emergency funds, program development, seed money, scholarship funds, consulting services, scholarships—to individuals, matching funds.
Limitations: Giving limited to the greater Middletown, OH, area. No support for religious organizations other than religious schools. No grants to individuals (except for scholarships).
Publications: Annual report, newsletter, application guidelines, informational brochure.
Application information: Application form not required.
Initial approach: Proposal
Copies of proposal: 1
Deadline(s): Mar. 1, June 1, Sept. 1, and Dec. 1
Board meeting date(s): Quarterly
Final notification: Apr. 30, July 30, Oct. 30, and Dec. 30
Officers and Trustees:* Thomas Blake,* Pres.; Frank Chapman,* V.P.; Donna Switzer,* Secy.; B.K. Parnell,* Treas.; Norman M. Hayes, Exec. Dir.; Joseph Baker, Jacqueline Banks, Bill Barnes, Charles Barton, John Bilich, Wilson Breiel, Sanford Casper, Wilbur Cohen, Adam Cristo, David Daugherty, Michael Governanti, David Harrison, Michael Miller, Ronald Olsen, William Parnell, Michael J. Sanders, Gene Snow, Aimee Snyder, Janet Thatcher, James Waxweiler, Thomas Wortley.
Number of staff: 1 full-time professional.
EIN: 310898380

793
The Monarch Machine Tool Company Foundation
615 North Oak St.
Sidney 45365

Trust established in 1952 in OH.
Donor(s): Monarch Machine Tool Co.
Foundation type: Company-sponsored
Financial data (yr. ended 12/31/94): Assets, $2,704,859 (M); gifts received, $115,508; expenditures, $189,182; qualifying distributions, $171,403, including $167,550 for 40 grants (high: $25,000; low: $100).
Fields of interest: Higher education; Hospitals (general); Human services; Salvation Army; YM/YWCAs & YM/YWHAs; Children & youth, services; Aging, centers & services; Federated giving programs; Aging.
Types of support: General/operating support, building/renovation.
Limitations: Applications not accepted. Giving primarily in OH, with some emphasis on Sidney. No grants to individuals.
Application information: Contributes only to pre-selected organizations.
Officers: R.J. Siewert, Pres.; R.B. Riethman, Secy.-Treas.
Trustees: J.A. Dunlap, N.V. Gushing.
EIN: 346556088

794
The Harry C. Moores Foundation
3010 Hayden Rd.
Columbus 43235 (614) 764-8999
Contact: David L. Fenner, Trustee

Trust established in 1961 in OH.
Donor(s): Harry C. Moores.‡
Financial data (yr. ended 09/30/94): Assets, $25,033,367 (M); expenditures, $1,325,550; qualifying distributions, $1,278,635, including $1,275,500 for 79 grants (high: $75,000; low: $2,000; average: $1,000-$20,000).
Purpose and activities: Grants largely for rehabilitation of the handicapped, Protestant church support, hospitals, higher education, cultural programs, and social service agencies concerned with the aged, child welfare, and the retarded.
Fields of interest: Arts/cultural programs; Higher education; Hospitals (general); Health care; Health organizations; Human services; Children & youth, services; Aging, centers & services; Protestant agencies & churches; Disabled; Aging.
Types of support: General/operating support, annual campaigns, capital campaigns, seed money, scholarship funds.
Limitations: Giving primarily in the Columbus, OH, area. No support for private foundations. No grants to individuals, or for endowment funds or matching gifts; no loans.
Application information: Application form not required.
Initial approach: Proposal in letter form
Copies of proposal: 1
Deadline(s): Submit proposal between Oct. and July; deadline Aug. 1
Board meeting date(s): Apr. or May and Aug. or Sept.
Final notification: By Oct. 15 (if affirmative)
Trustees: Neil B. Distelhorst, David L. Fenner, William C. Jones, William H. Leighner.
Number of staff: None.
EIN: 316035344
Grants for Aging:
Alzheimers Disease and Related Disorders Association, Columbus, OH, $10,000. 94.
Elder Focus, Columbus, OH, $10,000. 94.

795
Nationwide Insurance Enterprise Foundation
(Formerly Nationwide Insurance Foundation)
One Nationwide Plaza
Columbus 43215-2220 (614) 249-5095
Contact: Stephen A. Rish, Pres.

Incorporated in 1959 in OH.
Donor(s): Nationwide Mutual Insurance Co., and affiliates.
Foundation type: Company-sponsored
Financial data (yr. ended 12/31/94): Assets, $36,430,357 (M); gifts received, $12,838,390;

expenditures, $12,294,646; qualifying distributions, $12,219,839, including $8,480,280 for 318 grants (high: $500,000; average: $1,000-$30,000) and $3,620,355 for employee matching gifts.
Purpose and activities: Giving primarily for human services agencies; support also for cultural programs, community funds, and higher education, including employee matching gifts.
Fields of interest: Performing arts; Arts/cultural programs; Education, association; Higher education; Business school/education; Health care; Health organizations; Human services; Youth, services; Family services; Aging, centers & services; Minorities/immigrants, centers & services; Federated giving programs; Minorities; Disabled; Aging; Economically disadvantaged.
Types of support: General/operating support, continuing support, annual campaigns, capital campaigns, emergency funds, program development, seed money, employee matching gifts, matching funds.
Limitations: Giving primarily in OH, particularly Columbus, and other communities where the company maintains offices. No support for public elementary and secondary schools, or fraternal or veterans' organizations. No grants to individuals, or for building funds; no loans.
Publications: Informational brochure (including application guidelines).
Application information: The foundation has a specific format for requests for funding, which is listed in the Guidelines for Grant Consideration brochure. Application form not required.
Initial approach: Letter
Copies of proposal: 1
Deadline(s): Sept. 1
Board meeting date(s): Feb., May, Aug., and Nov.
Final notification: Feb.
Officers and Trustees:* D. Richard McFerson,* Chair. and C.E.O.; Stephen A. Rish, Pres.; Gordon E. McCutchan, Exec. V.P., General Counsel; Robert A. Oakley, Exec. V.P. and C.F.O.; Robert J. Woodward, Jr., Exec. V.P.; Dennis W. Click, V.P. and Secy.; Mark Thresher, V.P. and Treas.; Harry A. Schermer, V.P.; Charles L. Fuellgraf, Jr., Henry S. Holloway, David O. Miller, James F. Patterson, Arden L. Shisler.
Number of staff: 1 part-time professional; 1 full-time support.
EIN: 316022301
Grants for Aging:
Alzheimers Disease and Related Disorders Association, Columbus, OH, $17,000. 94.
Lifecare Alliance, Columbus, OH, $30,000. 94.
Westminster-Thurber Community, Columbus, OH, $20,000. 94.
Wexner Heritage House, Columbus, OH, $20,000. 94.

796
Nordson Corporate Giving Program

28601 Clemens Rd.
Westlake 44145 (216) 892-1580
Contact: Constance T. Haqq, Exec. Dir., Nordson Corp. Fdn.

Established in 1950 in OH.
Financial data (yr. ended 10/31/94): Total giving, $693,186, including $505,863 for grants and $187,323 for employee matching gifts.
Purpose and activities: The corporation sets aside 5 percent of its pre-tax domestic profit for use in those communities where it has major facilities. "Contributions are made directly by the corporation to meet its obligations and commitments to these communities."
Fields of interest: Visual arts; Museums; Performing arts; Dance; Theater; Music; Humanities; Arts/cultural programs; Early childhood education; Child development, education; Elementary school/education; Vocational education; Higher education; Adult/continuing education; Adult education—literacy & basic skills; Reading; Education; Medical care, rehabilitation; Mental health/crisis services; Food services; Housing/shelter, development; Human services; Children & youth, services; Child development, services; Family services; Aging, centers & services; Women, centers & services; Minorities/immigrants, centers & services; Homeless, human services; Race/intergroup relations; Urban/community development; Business & industry; Community development; Engineering & technology; Science; Government/public administration; Public affairs; Minorities; Disabled; Aging; Women; Economically disadvantaged; Homeless.
Types of support: General/operating support, annual campaigns, capital campaigns, building/renovation, emergency funds, technical assistance, employee volunteer services, loaned talent, use of facilities, employee matching gifts, donated equipment, donated products, matching funds.
Limitations: Giving limited to Lorain County in northeastern OH, and the greater metro-Atlanta, GA, area. No support for non-education, non-human welfare, non-civic, or non-arts/culture organizations.
Publications: Corporate report, corporate giving report, informational brochure (including application guidelines), grants list.
Application information: Contributions are handled by Corp. Contribs. Dept.; application procedures are the same as those of the foundation. Application form not required.
Initial approach: Letter to headquarters
Copies of proposal: 1
Deadline(s): Dec. 1, Apr. 1, July 1, and Oct. 1
Board meeting date(s): Jan., May, Aug., and Nov.
Final notification: Within 1 month of trustee meeting
Administrators: Constance T. Haqq, Exec. Dir., Nordson Corp. Foun.; Karen M. Sayre, Prog. Off., Northern Ohio; Nancy J. Scott, Mgr., Community Rels., Lorain County; Carolyn Gibson, Community Affairs Liaison, Atlanta.
Number of staff: 3 full-time professional; 1 part-time professional.

797
The Nordson Corporation Foundation

28601 Clemens Rd.
Westlake 44145-1148 (216) 892-1580
Contact: Constance T. Haqq, Exec. Dir.
Additional tel.: (216) 988-9411

Established in 1988 in OH.
Donor(s): Nordson Corp.
Foundation type: Company-sponsored
Financial data (yr. ended 10/31/94): Assets, $5,000,000 (M); expenditures, $1,754,442; qualifying distributions, $1,754,442, including $1,567,119 for 155 grants (high: $250,000; low: $350; average: $550-$25,000) and $187,323 for employee matching gifts.
Purpose and activities: To provide a source of stable funding for community programs and projects in the areas of education, human welfare, civics, and art and culture. Educational support is generally limited to improving elementary and secondary public schools and certain programs for public and private higher education. The foundation is willing to consider a number of funding areas, including urban affairs, volunteerism, public policy, and literacy.
Fields of interest: Visual arts; Performing arts; Humanities; Education, association; Education, research; Education, fund raising; Early childhood education; Elementary school/education; Secondary school/education; Higher education; Business school/education; Adult/continuing education; Adult education—literacy & basic skills; Reading; Environment; Health care; Mental health/crisis services; Alcoholism; Health organizations; Employment; Food services; Youth development, services; Youth development, citizenship; Human services; Youth, services; Aging, centers & services; Minorities/immigrants, centers & services; Homeless, human services; International affairs; Race/intergroup relations; Community development; Voluntarism promotion; Federated giving programs; Mathematics; Public policy, research; Government/public administration; Public affairs, citizen participation; Leadership development; Public affairs; Minorities; African Americans; Latinos; Disabled; Aging; Women; Economically disadvantaged; Homeless.
Types of support: General/operating support, continuing support, annual campaigns, capital campaigns, building/renovation, equipment, emergency funds, seed money, employee matching gifts, in-kind gifts, matching funds.
Limitations: Giving limited to the northern OH, Atlanta, GA, and Monterey Peninsula, CA areas.
Publications: Annual report (including application guidelines), grants list, corporate giving report.
Application information: Application form not required.
Initial approach: Letter or proposal
Copies of proposal: 2
Deadline(s): Feb., May, Aug., and Nov.
Board meeting date(s): 4 times yearly, once each calendar quarter
Final notification: Within 1 month after meeting
Officer: Constance T. Haqq, Exec. Dir.
Trustees: Edward P. Campbell, John E. Jackson, William P. Madar, Thomas L. Moorhead.
Staff: Karen M. Sayre, Prog. Officer; Carolyn L. Gibson, Mgr., Community Affairs, Atlanta; Nancy J. Scott, Mgr. Community Relations, Lorain County.
Number of staff: 4 full-time professional; 1 part-time professional; 1 part-time support.
EIN: 341596194
Grants for Aging:
Catholic Social Service Bureau, Elyria, OH, $15,000. For Senior Link Program. 94.

Elyria United Methodist Home, Elyria, OH, $40,000. For capital campaign for Elyria Senior Center. 94.

798
Oglebay Norton Foundation

P.O. Box 6508
Cleveland 44101-1508 (216) 861-2852
Contact: Kenneth R. Fair, Secy.

Trust established in 1952 in OH; incorporated in 1959.
Donor(s): Oglebay Norton Co.
Foundation type: Company-sponsored
Financial data (yr. ended 12/31/95): Assets, $40,361 (M); gifts received, $141,945; expenditures, $116,679; qualifying distributions, $116,215, including $116,215 for 46 grants (high: $45,000; low: $25; average: $25-$45,000).
Fields of interest: Arts, multipurpose centers/programs; Visual arts; Museums; Performing arts; Education, association; Education; Health care; Human services; Aging, centers & services; Community development; Engineering & technology; Science; Public affairs; Aging.
Types of support: General/operating support, continuing support, annual campaigns, capital campaigns, endowment funds, employee matching gifts.
Limitations: Giving primarily in Cleveland, OH. No grants to individuals, or for seed money, deficit financing, equipment and materials, land acquisition, matching or challenge grants, scholarships, fellowships, publications, or conferences; no loans.
Application information: Application form not required.
Initial approach: Proposal
Copies of proposal: 1
Deadline(s): Sept.
Board meeting date(s): Nov.
Final notification: Within 3 months
Officers and Trustees:* R. Thomas Green, Jr.,* Pres.; Richard J. Kessler, V.P. and Treas.; Kenneth R. Fair, Secy.; Brent D. Baird, Malvin E. Bank, William G. Bares, A.C. Bersticker, John J. Dwyer, R.D. Ketchum, H.S. Richey, Renold D. Thompson, J.D. Weil.
Number of staff: 2 part-time support.
EIN: 346513722

799
Omnicare Foundation

2800 Chemed Ctr.
255 East Fifth St.
Cincinnati 45202-4728 (513) 762-6967
Contact: Cheryl D. Hodges, Secy.

Established in 1993 in OH.
Donor(s): Omnicare, Inc.
Foundation type: Company-sponsored
Financial data (yr. ended 12/31/95): Assets, $390,415 (M); expenditures, $29,222; qualifying distributions, $29,222, including $24,500 for 6 grants (high: $6,000; low: $500).
Purpose and activities: "Preference is given to organizations that benefit the geriatric population."
Fields of interest: Higher education; Pharmacology; Health care; Health organizations; Aging, centers & services; Aging.
Application information:
Initial approach: Letter
Deadline(s): None
Officers and Trustees:* Joel F. Gemunder,* Pres.; Herbert A. Langsam,* V.P.; Cheryl D. Hodges,* Secy.; Jeffrey A. Glancy, Treas.; Kenneth W. Chesterman, Patrick E. Keefe, Janice M. Rice.
EIN: 311389112

800
The Reinberger Foundation

27600 Chagrin Blvd.
Cleveland 44122 (216) 292-2790
Contact: Robert N. Reinberger, Co-Dir.

Established in 1968 in OH.
Donor(s): Clarence T. Reinberger,‡ Louise F. Reinberger.‡
Financial data (yr. ended 12/31/94): Assets, $56,350,366 (M); expenditures, $3,410,075; qualifying distributions, $3,021,591, including $2,841,285 for 64 grants (high: $166,667; low: $1,000; average: $20,000-$100,000).
Purpose and activities: Support for the arts, social welfare, Protestant churches, higher education, and medical research.
Fields of interest: Media/communications; Visual arts; Museums; Performing arts; Dance; Theater; Music; Historic preservation/historical societies; Arts/cultural programs; Education, research; Education, fund raising; Environment; Wildlife preservation & protection; Hospitals (general); Health care; Cancer; Biomedicine; Health organizations; Medical research; Cancer research; Youth, services; Family services; Aging, centers & services; Community development; Aging.
Types of support: General/operating support, continuing support, annual campaigns, capital campaigns, building/renovation, equipment, endowment funds, debt reduction, program development, publication, scholarship funds, research, matching funds.
Limitations: Giving primarily in the Cleveland and Columbus, OH, areas. No grants to individuals, or for seed money, emergency funds, land acquisition, demonstration projects, or conferences; no loans.
Publications: 990-PF, grants list, informational brochure (including application guidelines).
Application information: Application form not required.
Initial approach: Proposal
Copies of proposal: 1
Deadline(s): None
Board meeting date(s): Feb., May, Aug., and Nov.
Final notification: 6 months
Officer: Richard H. Oman, Secy.
Directors: Sara R. Dyer, Karen R. Hooser, Robert N. Reinberger, William C. Reinberger.
Trustee: Key Trust Co. of Ohio, N.A.
Number of staff: 2 full-time professional.
EIN: 346574879

801
Reliance Electric Company Charitable, Scientific and Educational Trust

6065 Parkland Blvd.
Cleveland 44124-8020 (216) 266-5826
Contact: Edward R. Towns, Secy.

Trust established in 1974 in OH.
Donor(s): Reliance Electric Co.
Foundation type: Company-sponsored
Financial data (yr. ended 12/31/95): Assets, $8,757 (M); gifts received, $660,000; expenditures, $701,114; qualifying distributions, $699,207, including $697,270 for 473 grants (high: $141,000; low: $20; average: $500-$5,000).
Purpose and activities: Emphasis on community funds, higher education, hospitals, cultural programs, and social services; also funds an employee matching gift program.
Fields of interest: Arts/cultural programs; Higher education; Engineering school/education; Education; Hospitals (general); Health care; Human services; Family services; Federated giving programs; Engineering; Aging; Economically disadvantaged; Homeless.
Types of support: Continuing support, annual campaigns, capital campaigns, employee matching gifts.
Limitations: Giving primarily in Cleveland, OH, and other areas of major company facilities. No support for national health organizations. No grants to individuals, or for dinners or special events.
Publications: Program policy statement.
Application information: Application form not required.
Initial approach: Proposal
Copies of proposal: 1
Deadline(s): None
Board meeting date(s): Quarterly
Final notification: Immediately following board meetings
Officer: Edward R. Towns, Secy.
Trustees: E.S. Dalton, D.P. Sheffler, P.J. Tsiuitse, Key Trust Co. of Ohio, N.A.
Number of staff: None.
EIN: 346505329
Grants for Aging:
Eliza Bryant Center, Cleveland, OH, $1,000. 95.
Judson Retirement Community, Cleveland Heights, OH, $2,000. 95.

802
The Helen Steiner Rice Foundation

221 East Fourth St., Suite 2100, Atrium 2
P.O. Box 0236
Cincinnati 45201-0236 (513) 451-9241
Contact: Andrea Cornett, Grant Coord.

Established in 1980 in OH.
Donor(s): Helen Steiner Rice.‡
Financial data (yr. ended 06/30/95): Assets, $8,253,224 (M); gifts received, $592; expenditures, $549,191; qualifying distributions, $342,388, including $305,300 for 49 grants (high: $35,000; low: $800; average: $5,000-$10,000).
Purpose and activities: Emphasis on the elderly, the homeless, health services, and the issue of

hunger; support also for family services, youth and child welfare, women, and adult and early childhood education; preference for meeting immediate needs.
Fields of interest: Early childhood education; Child development, education; Adult/continuing education; Adult education—literacy & basic skills; Reading; Medical care, rehabilitation; Health care; Delinquency prevention/services; Food services; Human services; Children & youth, services; Youth, services; Child development, services; Family services; Aging, centers & services; Women, centers & services; Homeless, human services; Voluntarism promotion; Christian agencies & churches; Minorities; Disabled; Aging; Women; Economically disadvantaged; Homeless.
Types of support: General/operating support, continuing support, emergency funds, program development, seed money, consulting services.
Limitations: Giving limited to the greater Cincinnati area and Lorain, OH. No grants to individuals, or for capital campaigns or building funds.
Publications: Annual report (including application guidelines), application guidelines, informational brochure, program policy statement.
Application information: Application form required.
Initial approach: Letter
Copies of proposal: 5
Deadline(s): July 1
Board meeting date(s): As required
Final notification: Nov.
Trustees: Willis D. Gradison, Jr., Eugene P. Ruehlmann, Donald E. Weston.
Number of staff: 1 full-time professional; 1 part-time support.
EIN: 310978383
Grants for Aging:
Center for the Visually Impaired, Elyria, OH, $16,000. For disadvantaged elderly and preschool walk-in clinic program. 95.
Council on Aging of the Cincinnati Area, Cincinnati, OH, $10,000. For senior radio station start-up. 95.
Radio Reading Services of Greater Cincinnati, Cincinnati, OH, $8,000. For Personal Reader program for the elderly. 94.
Radio Reading Services of Greater Cincinnati, Cincinnati, OH, $8,000. For Personal Reader senior citizens' program. 95.
Resident Home for the Mentally Retarded, Cincinnati, OH, $15,000. For In-Home Attendant Care program. 94.
Saint Claire Retirement Community, Cincinnati, OH, $10,000. For long-term care for AIDS patients. 94.
Wesley Hall, Cincinnati, OH, $35,000. For disadvantaged elderly community services program. 95.

803
Richland County Foundation
(Formerly The Richland County Foundation of Mansfield, Ohio)
24 West Third St., Suite 100
Mansfield 44902-1209 (419) 525-3020
Contact: Pamela H. Siegenthaler, Pres.
FAX: (419) 525-1590

Incorporated in 1945 in OH.
Foundation type: Community
Financial data (yr. ended 12/31/95): Assets, $30,799,160 (M); gifts received, $1,214,344; expenditures, $1,610,525, including $1,133,835 for 132 grants (high: $342,870; low: $100) and $179,447 for grants to individuals.
Purpose and activities: To improve the quality of life in Richland County through organized philanthropy; to provide leadership and act as catalyst in identifying and addressing evolving community needs, and to distribute grants for charitable purposes in the areas of health, economic development, basic human needs, education, cultural activities, environment, and community services.
Fields of interest: Historic preservation/historical societies; Arts/cultural programs; Early childhood education; Child development, education; Elementary school/education; Secondary school/education; Vocational education; Higher education; Adult/continuing education; Adult education—literacy & basic skills; Libraries/library science; Reading; Education; Hospitals (general); Health care; Substance abuse, services; Mental health/crisis services; Health organizations; Human services; Children & youth, services; Youth, services; Child development, services; Aging, centers & services; Women, centers & services; Minorities/immigrants, centers & services; Race/intergroup relations; Community development; Government/public administration; Minorities; Disabled; Aging; Women; Economically disadvantaged; General charitable giving.
Types of support: General/operating support, capital campaigns, building/renovation, equipment, endowment funds, emergency funds, program development, publication, seed money, scholarship funds, technical assistance, program-related investments/loans, grants to individuals, scholarships—to individuals, matching funds.
Limitations: Giving primarily in Richland County, OH. No support for sectarian religious purposes. No grants for annual campaigns, fellowships, highly technical or specialized research, operating or maintenance funds, or travel.
Publications: Annual report (including application guidelines), application guidelines, newsletter, informational brochure.
Application information: Application form required for college scholarships. Applications available after Jan. 1. Application form required.
Initial approach: Telephone or appointment
Copies of proposal: 1
Deadline(s): 1st Friday of Jan., May, July, Sept., and Nov.
Board meeting date(s): 3rd Monday of Feb., Apr., June, Aug., Oct., and Dec. Annual Meeting in May
Final notification: At least 8 weeks
Officers and Trustees:* Jeffery S. Gorman,* Chair.; Wray C. Smith, D.D.,* Vice-Chair.; Pamela H. Siegenthaler, Pres.; Inge S. Vucelic, Ph.D.,* Secy.; W. Thomas Ross,* Treas.; Ivy Amos, Pete Bailey, Donald N. Beddard, M.D., Rex E. Collins, Otis M. Cummins III, Richard S. Cummins, Katherine N. Fernyak, Bill Goldman, William J. Hartnett, Edith B. Humphrey, Robert L. Lee, Sarah S. Lichtenstein, James D. Miller, Elizabeth H. Prestel, Burton Preston, John D. Robinson, Allen M. Sanford, John H. Siegenthaler, Richard G. Taylor, Fred J. Wiecher, M.D.
Trustee Banks: Bank One, Mansfield, N.A., Key Trust Co. of Ohio, N.A., National City Bank, Cleveland, Richland Bank, Mansfield.
Staff: Amy L. Marinelli, Prog. Officer.
Number of staff: 2 full-time professional; 1 part-time professional; 1 full-time support.
EIN: 340872883

804
Richman Brothers Foundation
P.O. Box 657
Chagrin Falls 44022
Contact: Richard R. Moore, Pres.

Incorporated in 1932 in OH.
Donor(s): Nathan G. Richman,‡ Charles L. Richman,‡ Henry C. Richman.‡
Financial data (yr. ended 12/31/95): Assets, $2,128,107 (M); expenditures, $129,156; qualifying distributions, $98,691, including $44,000 for 22 grants (high: $10,000; low: $500) and $54,360 for 163 grants to individuals (high: $650; low: $170).
Purpose and activities: Giving principally for health care and to agencies providing support to children and the aged; also provides relief assistance to pensioners of Richman Brothers Co. or their widows.
Fields of interest: Higher education; Human services; Youth, services; Aging, centers & services; Federated giving programs; Aging.
Types of support: Building/renovation, program development, grants to individuals, matching funds.
Limitations: Giving primarily in OH, with emphasis on Cleveland.
Application information: Application form not required.
Initial approach: Proposal
Deadline(s): Nov. 25
Board meeting date(s): Nov.
Officers and Trustees:* Richard R. Moore,* Pres.; Ernest J. Marvar,* V.P.; Frank Hribar, Secy.; Raymond J. Novack, Treas.; Frank Harding.
EIN: 346504927
Grants for Aging:
Eliza Bryant Center, Cleveland, OH, $2,000. 95.
Golden Age Centers of Greater Cleveland, Cleveland, OH, $3,000. 95.
Senior Citizen Resources, Cleveland, OH, $1,000. 95.
Slovene Home for the Aged, Cleveland, OH, $2,000. 95.

805
The Samuel Rosenthal Foundation
Halle Bldg., Suite 310
1228 Euclid Ave.
Cleveland 44115 (216) 523-8125
Contact: Charlotte R. Kramer, Trustee
Application address: c/o Foundation Mgmt. Svcs., Inc., 1422 Euclid Ave., Suite 627, Cleveland, OH 44115-1901

Trust established in 1959 in OH.

Financial data (yr. ended 12/31/95): Assets, $9,082,023 (M); expenditures, $1,897,607; qualifying distributions, $1,852,432, including $1,801,350 for 65 grants (high: $450,296; low: $100).
Purpose and activities: Giving primarily for traditional education, the health and well-being of children and the elderly, Cleveland-based human services and cultural institutions, and the basic roots of Jewish heritage.
Fields of interest: Museums; Performing arts; Theater; Arts/cultural programs; Health care, infants; Health care; Food services; Human services; Children & youth, services; Aging, centers & services; Jewish federated giving programs; Jewish agencies & temples; Disabled; Aging; Economically disadvantaged.
Types of support: General/operating support, continuing support, capital campaigns, building/renovation, equipment, endowment funds, program development, seed money.
Limitations: Giving primarily in Cleveland, OH. No grants to individuals.
Publications: Informational brochure (including application guidelines).
Application information: Application form not required.
Initial approach: Letter
Copies of proposal: 6
Deadline(s): Jan. 1, May 1, and Oct. 1
Board meeting date(s): 3 times a year
Final notification: After meeting
Trustees: Cynthia R. Boardman, Jane R. Horvitz, Charlotte R. Kramer, Mark R. Kramer, Leighton A. Rosenthal.
Number of staff: None.
EIN: 346558832
Grants for Aging:
Menorah Park Center for Aging, Beachwood, OH, $20,000. For building campaign. 94.

806
Ruth G. & Sam H. Sampliner Foundation

c/o Hans Loeser & Parks
3300 BP America Bldg.
Cleveland 44114
Contact: Sidney Nudelman, Trustee

Donor(s): Sam H. Sampliner.
Financial data (yr. ended 12/31/95): Assets, $1,304,560 (M); expenditures, $32,592; qualifying distributions, $26,019, including $25,000 for 1 grant.
Purpose and activities: Giving primarily to an institute for the elderly.
Fields of interest: Music; Aging, centers & services; Aging; General charitable giving.
Limitations: Giving primarily in Cleveland, OH. No grants to individuals.
Application information: Application form not required.
Initial approach: Letter
Deadline(s): None
Trustees: P.E. Leon, Jr., Sidney Nudelman, Bud Slessinger.
EIN: 346520228

807
Albert G. and Olive H. Schlink Foundation

401 Citizens National Bank Bldg.
Norwalk 44857
Contact: Robert A. Wiedemann, Pres.

Established in 1966 in OH.
Donor(s): Albert G. Schlink,‡ Olive H. Schlink.‡
Financial data (yr. ended 12/31/95): Assets, $10,499,632 (M); expenditures, $640,407; qualifying distributions, $604,283, including $555,693 for 21 grants (high: $100,000; low: $1,947).
Purpose and activities: Grants to organizations providing aid to the indigent, aged, including health agencies and hospitals; support also for the blind.
Fields of interest: Museums; Education, fund raising; Medical school/education; Education; Hospitals (general); Nursing care; Health care; Medical research; Human services; Hospices; Aging, centers & services; Engineering & technology; Biological sciences; Science; Disabled; Aging; Economically disadvantaged.
Types of support: General/operating support, continuing support, capital campaigns, building/renovation, equipment, endowment funds, program development, scholarship funds, research.
Limitations: Giving primarily in OH. No grants to individuals.
Application information: Application form not required.
Initial approach: Letter
Copies of proposal: 1
Deadline(s): None
Board meeting date(s): Monthly
Final notification: Dec.
Officers and Trustees:* Robert A. Wiedemann,* Pres. and Secy.; Curtis J. Koch,* V.P.; John D. Allton,* Treas.; Thomas D. Huff, Dorothy E. Wiedemann.
Number of staff: None.
EIN: 346574722
Grants for Aging:
Saint Francis Home, Tiffin, OH, $30,000. 95.
Saint Francis Home, Tiffin, OH, $26,550. 94.

808
Jacob G. Schmidlapp Trust No. 1 and No. 2

(Formerly Jacob G. Schmidlapp Trust No. 1)
c/o Fifth Third Bank
Fifth Third Ctr., ML 1090C7; Foundation Office
Cincinnati 45263 (513) 579-6034
Contact: Lawra J. Baumann, Fdn. Officer

Trust established in 1927 in OH.
Donor(s): Jacob G. Schmidlapp.‡
Financial data (yr. ended 09/30/95): Assets, $44,377,761 (M); expenditures, $2,034,534; qualifying distributions, $1,876,717, including $1,757,777 for 72 grants (high: $100,000; low: $3,000; average: $10,000-$50,000).
Purpose and activities: Grants for the relief of sickness, suffering, and distress, and for care of young children or the helpless and afflicted; support also for education including child care training.
Fields of interest: Child development, education; Education; Hospitals (general); Health care; Health organizations; Food services; Housing/shelter, development; Human services; Children & youth, services; Youth, services; Child development, services; Aging, centers & services; Homeless, human services; Minorities; Aging; Homeless.
Types of support: Capital campaigns, building/renovation, equipment, land acquisition, endowment funds, seed money, scholarship funds, technical assistance.
Limitations: Giving primarily in the greater Cincinnati, OH, area. No support for religious purposes. No grants to individuals, or for annual campaigns, deficit financing, general support, fellowships, operating budgets, or continuing support; no loans.
Publications: Annual report (including application guidelines).
Application information: Application form not required.
Initial approach: Letter
Copies of proposal: 1
Deadline(s): Feb. 1, May 1, Aug. 1, and Nov. 1
Board meeting date(s): Mar., June, Sept., and Dec.
Final notification: Middle of months in which board meets
Trustee: Fifth Third Bank.
Number of staff: 1 full-time professional; 1 full-time support.
EIN: 316019680
Grants for Aging:
Episcopal Retirement Home, Cincinnati, OH, $50,000. For capital campaign. 95.

809
Jasper H. Sheadle Trust

c/o Key Trust Co. of Ohio, N.A.
127 Public Sq., 16th Fl.
Cleveland 44114-1306 (216) 689-5829

Trust established in 1917 in OH.
Donor(s): Jasper H. Sheadle.‡
Financial data (yr. ended 12/31/95): Assets, $3,124,386 (M); expenditures, $311,957; qualifying distributions, $295,264, including $295,060 for 63 grants to individuals (high: $7,900; low: $600).
Purpose and activities: To provide pensions for elderly American-born women or couples (62 and over) only, who are residing in Cuyahoga or Mahoning counties, OH.
Fields of interest: Aging, centers & services; Aging.
Types of support: Grants to individuals.
Limitations: Giving limited to Cuyahoga and Mahoning counties, OH.
Application information: Applicants usually nominated by outside organizations.
Initial approach: Letter by sponsor
Board meeting date(s): Varies
Officers: Hon. John J. Donnelly, Mgr.; Bishop J. Clark Grew, Mgr.; Frank I. Harding III, Mgr.
Trustee: Key Trust Co. of Ohio, N.A.
Number of staff: 1 part-time professional.
EIN: 346506457

810
The Sisler McFawn Foundation

(Formerly Lois Sisler McFawn Trust No. 2)
3925 Embassy Pkwy.
Akron 44333-1799 (330) 374-2628
Contact: Charlotte M. Stanley, Grants Mgr.
FAX: (330) 374-2333

Trust established in 1959 in OH.
Donor(s): Lois Sisler McFawn.‡
Financial data (yr. ended 12/31/95): Assets, $15,010,235 (M); expenditures, $666,218; qualifying distributions, $532,440, including $520,790 for 71 grants (high: $50,000; low: $280; average: $500-$60,000).
Fields of interest: Education; Health care; Health associations; Human services; Children & youth, services; Aging, centers & services; Disabled; Aging.
Types of support: General/operating support, continuing support, annual campaigns, capital campaigns, building/renovation, equipment, endowment funds, program development, seed money, curriculum development, scholarship funds, matching funds.
Limitations: Giving primarily in Summit County, OH. No grants to individuals; no loans.
Publications: Application guidelines, grants list.
Application information: Application form not required.
Initial approach: Proposal
Copies of proposal: 1
Deadline(s): 30 days prior to board meeting
Board meeting date(s): 1st week of May, Sept., and Dec.
Distribution Committee: Patricia A. Kemph, Chair.; Michael J. Connor, Howard L. Flood, Jon V. Heider, John L. Macso, Justin T. Rogers, Jr.
Trustee: Key Trust Co. of Ohio, N.A.
Staff: Charlotte M. Stanley, Grants Mgr.
Number of staff: 1 part-time professional.
EIN: 346508111
Grants for Aging:
Senior Workers Action Program, Akron, OH, $5,000. 95.

811
The Stark County Foundation

The Saxton House
331 Market Ave. South
Canton 44702-2107 (330) 454-3426
Contact: James A. Bower, Exec. Dir.
FAX: (330) 454-5855

Established in 1963 in OH by resolution and declaration of trust.
Foundation type: Community
Financial data (yr. ended 12/31/94): Assets, $51,754,294 (M); gifts received, $2,818,353; expenditures, $3,030,272, including $2,126,492 for 177 grants (high: $213,551; low: $150; average: $2,500-$20,000), $72,924 for 134 grants to individuals and $131,650 for 118 loans to individuals.
Purpose and activities: To maintain the sound health and general welfare of the citizens through support for civic improvement programs and educational institutions. Primary areas of interest include the arts, education, community development, health and wellness, youth, and social services.
Fields of interest: Visual arts; Performing arts; Historic preservation/historical societies; Arts/cultural programs; Early childhood education; Child development, education; Elementary school/education; Higher education; Business school/education; Law school/education; Education; Natural resource conservation & protection; Environment; Health care; Substance abuse, services; AIDS; AIDS research; Crime/law enforcement; Food services; Housing/shelter, development; Recreation; Youth development, services; Human services; Children & youth, services; Child development, services; Family services; Aging, centers & services; Minorities/immigrants, centers & services; Homeless, human services; Urban/community development; Community development; Government/public administration; Leadership development; Minorities; Disabled; Aging; Homeless.
Types of support: General/operating support, capital campaigns, building/renovation, equipment, land acquisition, emergency funds, program development, seed money, scholarship funds, research, technical assistance, consulting services, program-related investments/loans, scholarships—to individuals, matching funds, student loans—to individuals.
Limitations: Giving limited to Stark County, OH. No grants for endowment funds, operating budgets, continuing support, annual campaigns, publications, or deficit financing; no grants or loans to individuals (except to college students who are permanent residents of Stark County).
Publications: Biennial report (including application guidelines), program policy statement, application guidelines, financial statement, grants list, newsletter, 990-PF.
Application information: Application form not required.
Initial approach: Letter or proposal
Copies of proposal: 10
Deadline(s): Mar. 1 for student aid; none for other grants
Board meeting date(s): 8 to 10 times per year
Final notification: 60 to 90 days
Officers: Patricia C. Quick, Financial Officer; James A. Bower, Exec. Dir.
Distribution Committee: William L. Luntz, Chair.; William H. Belden, Jr., Paul R. Bishop, Theodore V. Boyd, Paralee W. Compton, Lynne S. Dragomier, Randolph L. Snow.
Trustee Banks: Bank One Ohio Trust Co., N.A., First National Bank in Massillon, Key Trust Co. of Ohio, N.A., National City Bank, Northeast, United National Bank.
Staff: Cynthia M. Lazor, Prog. Officer.
Number of staff: 3 full-time professional; 1 full-time support; 1 part-time support.
EIN: 340943665
Grants for Aging:
Saint Joseph Hospice, Louisville, OH, $10,000. For classroom and furnishings in assisted living/elderly. 94.

812
The Stocker Foundation

209 Sixth St., Suite 25
Lorain 44052 (216) 246-5719
Contact: Jane Norton, Exec. Dir.

Incorporated in 1979 in OH.
Donor(s): Beth K. Stocker.
Financial data (yr. ended 09/30/95): Assets, $14,007,704 (M); gifts received, $500,000; expenditures, $699,976; qualifying distributions, $640,435, including $568,054 for 122 grants (high: $17,000; low: $25; average: $2,000-$15,000).
Purpose and activities: Emphasis on short-term youth development programs; social service agencies offering solutions to specific problems, such as literacy, hunger, and homelessness; education (including early childhood, elementary, secondary, and higher education); aid to the disabled; self-help programs; theater and the performing arts, and other cultural programs; women's issues and the strengthening of families.
Fields of interest: Arts/cultural programs; Early childhood education; Elementary school/education; Secondary school/education; Adult education—literacy & basic skills; Family planning; Mental health/crisis services; Domestic violence prevention; Housing/shelter; Youth development, services; Human services; Family services; Hospices; Aging, centers & services; Women, centers & services; Homeless, human services; Reproductive rights; Voluntarism promotion; Psychology/behavioral science; Public affairs, citizen participation; Leadership development; Disabled; Economically disadvantaged.
Types of support: General/operating support, building/renovation, equipment, endowment funds, emergency funds, program development, publication, seed money, curriculum development, technical assistance, matching funds.
Limitations: Giving primarily in Lorain County, OH, southern AZ (Cochise, Pima, and Santa Cruz counties), and Bexar County, TX. No support for religious organizations for religious purposes, governmental services, or public school services required by law. No grants to individuals, or for annual campaigns, deficit financing, multi-year proposals except under special circumstances, or fundraising; no loans.
Publications: Application guidelines, informational brochure (including application guidelines), grants list.
Application information: Faxed proposals not accepted. Application form not required.
Initial approach: Telephone or letter
Copies of proposal: 5
Deadline(s): Jan. 15, May 15, and Sept. 1
Board meeting date(s): Mid-winter, summer, and fall
Final notification: 8 to 10 weeks after deadline
Officers and Trustees:* Beth K. Stocker, Pres.; Jane Norton,* Secy.-Treas. and Exec. Dir.; Mary Ann Dobras, Wendy Dobras, Benjamin P. Norton, Anne Woodling, Nancy Elizabeth Woodling.
Corporate Trustee: Key Trust Co. of Ohio, N.A.
Number of staff: 1 full-time professional; 1 part-time support.
EIN: 341293603

813
Tipp City Foundation

c/o Star Bank, N.A., Cincinnati
910 West Main St.
Troy 45373
Contact: Richard Fraas, Trust Officer, Star Bank, N.A.
Application address: 730 Hathaway Terr., Tipp City, OH 45371

Established in 1943 in OH.
Financial data (yr. ended 12/31/95): Assets, $1,493,587 (M); gifts received, $2,650; expenditures, $86,891; qualifying distributions, $76,674, including $75,819 for 20 grants (high: $9,038; low: $250).
Purpose and activities: Support for city schools, including library, art, and computer programs, community services, including civic groups, aid for the handicapped, the hungry, and recreation.
Fields of interest: Libraries/library science; Education; Human services; Federated giving programs; Disabled; Aging.
Limitations: Giving limited to Tipp City, OH.
Application information: Application form not required.
Initial approach: Letter
Deadline(s): None
Board meeting date(s): As needed
Trustee: Star Bank, N.A.
Number of staff: None.
EIN: 316018697

814
Toledo Community Foundation, Inc.

608 Madison Ave., Suite 1540
Toledo 43604-1151 (419) 241-5049
Contact: Pam Howell-Beach, Dir.
FAX: (419) 242-5549

Established in 1924 in OH by trust agreement; reactivated in 1973.
Foundation type: Community
Financial data (yr. ended 12/31/94): Assets, $38,900,000 (M); gifts received, $7,300,000; expenditures, $2,750,343, including $2,500,000 for grants.
Purpose and activities: Support for projects which promise to affect a broad segment of the citizens of northwestern OH or which tend to help those living in an area not being adequately served by local community resources. Areas of interest include social services and youth programs, arts and culture, education, natural resources, government and urban affairs, and physical and mental health.
Fields of interest: Arts/cultural programs; Child development, education; Education; Natural resource conservation & protection; Health care; Mental health/crisis services; Health organizations; Human services; Children & youth, services; Youth, services; Child development, services; Aging, centers & services; Homeless, human services; Community development; Government/public administration; Public affairs; Aging; Homeless.
Types of support: Program development, seed money, matching funds.
Limitations: Giving primarily in northwestern OH, with emphasis on the greater Toledo area. No grants to individuals, or for annual campaigns, operating budgets, or endowment funds.
Publications: Annual report (including application guidelines), informational brochure, application guidelines, newsletter.
Application information: Application form not required.
Initial approach: Telephone followed by proposal
Copies of proposal: 1
Deadline(s): Mar. 1, June 1, Sept. 1, and Dec. 1
Board meeting date(s): Jan., Apr., July, and Oct.
Final notification: 2 months
Officers and Trustees:* Joel A. Levine,* Pres.; Elizabeth Brady,* V.P.; Stephen Stranahan,* Secy.; Donald Saunders,* Treas.; Ronald C. Boller, Ardath Danford, Hon. Charles Doneghy, Nancy Fairhurst, Scott Libbe, Julie Taylor, John R. Wanick, David K. Welles, Jr.
Staff: Pamela Howell-Beach, Dir.; Mary Sobecki, Sr. Prog. Officer; Bridget Brell Holt, Prog. Officer; Bridgett Stonerock, Donor Relations Coord.
Number of staff: 3 full-time professional; 1 part-time professional; 1 full-time support; 1 part-time support.
EIN: 237284004

815
The Waddell Ladies Home Association

1101 East Barks Rd.
P.O. Box 358
Marion 43302-0358 (614) 389-3677
Contact: William E. Payette, Secy.-Treas.

Established in 1901 in OH.
Donor(s): Benjamin Waddell.‡
Financial data (yr. ended 05/31/95): Assets, $2,062,960 (M); expenditures, $103,670; qualifying distributions, $96,330, including $90,282 for 3 grants (high: $47,148; low: $1,505).
Purpose and activities: Giving primarily for social services, with emphasis on programs for senior citizens, including transportation and meals.
Fields of interest: Human services; Aging, centers & services; Aging.
Types of support: General/operating support, continuing support, building/renovation, equipment, emergency funds, program development.
Limitations: Giving primarily in Marion County, OH. No grants to individuals.
Publications: Annual report.
Application information: Application form required.
Initial approach: Letter
Board meeting date(s): 2nd or 3rd Tuesday quarterly
Officers: James P. Waddell, Pres.; William Dunn, V.P.; William Payette, Secy.-Treas.
Trustee: Betty Dendinger.
Number of staff: None.
EIN: 314386851
Grants for Aging:
Marion Senior Citizens, Marion, OH, $41,629. For transportation program. 95.
Marion Senior Citizens, Marion, OH, $39,972. For transportation. 94.
Marion Senior Citizens, Marion, OH, $10,000. For building fund. 94.
Marion Senior Citizens, Marion, OH, $4,500. 94.
Marion Senior Citizens, Marion, OH, $1,505. For Reassurance program. 95.
Marion Senior Citizens, Marion, OH, $530. For reassurance program. 94.
Mobile Meals of Marion, Marion, OH, $47,128. 95.
Mobile Meals of Marion, Marion, OH, $10,000. 94.

816
Bill & Edith Walter Foundation

6711 Elmers Court
Worthington 43085

Donor(s): William Walter Trust, Edith Walter Trust.
Financial data (yr. ended 12/31/94): Assets, $422,556 (M); expenditures, $45,843; qualifying distributions, $45,843, including $36,000 for 4 grants (high: $15,000; low: $5,000).
Fields of interest: Environment; Human services; Aging, centers & services; Protestant agencies & churches.
Limitations: Applications not accepted. Giving primarily in Columbus, OH. No grants to individuals.
Application information: Contributes only to pre-selected organizations.
Officers and Trustees:* James E. Lane,* Pres.; Fredrick L. Fisher,* Secy.-Treas.; Betty B. Lane.
EIN: 311102570

817
Virginia Wright Mothers Guild, Inc.

c/o M. Courtwright
426 East Clinton St.
Columbus 43202-2741

Financial data (yr. ended 06/30/95): Assets, $69,887 (M); gifts received, $2,164; expenditures, $14,256; qualifying distributions, $12,050, including $12,050 for 11 grants to individuals (high: $1,225; low: $400).
Fields of interest: Aging, centers & services; Aging.
Types of support: Grants to individuals.
Limitations: Applications not accepted. Giving limited to female residents of the Columbus, OH, area.
Officers: Florence Sanders, Pres.; Majorie Courtwright, Treas.
EIN: 316034381

818
The Wuliger Foundation, Inc.

28601 Chagrin Blvd., Suite 410
Woodmere 44122 (216) 999-8922
Contact: Timothy F. Wuliger, Dir.

Incorporated in 1956 in OH.
Donor(s): Ernest M. Wuliger.‡
Financial data (yr. ended 12/31/94): Assets, $9,838,462 (M); expenditures, $115,915; qualifying distributions, $3,550, including $3,550 for 4 grants (high: $1,050; low: $500; average: $1,000-$10,000).

Purpose and activities: Giving for Jewish welfare funds; support also for education, hospitals, Jewish community organizations, and social services.
Fields of interest: Education; Hospitals (general); Health care; Health organizations; Crime/violence prevention; Human services; Children & youth, services; Aging, centers & services; Community development; Aging; Economically disadvantaged.
Types of support: General/operating support, annual campaigns, capital campaigns, building/renovation.
Limitations: Giving primarily in OH. No grants to individuals.
Publications: 990-PF.
Application information: Application form not required.
Initial approach: Written proposal
Copies of proposal: 3
Deadline(s): None
Board meeting date(s): As necessary
Final notification: Within 2 months if possible
Officers and Directors:* E. Jeffrey Wuliger,* Pres.; Gregory Wuliger,* V.P.; Timothy F. Wuliger,* Secy.-Treas.
Number of staff: None.
EIN: 346527281

OKLAHOMA

819
Irvin E. and Sharna Frank Trust

Nine East Fourth St., Suite 702
Tulsa 74103

Established in 1992 in OK.
Donor(s): Irvin E. Frank, Sharna Frank.
Financial data (yr. ended 04/30/95): Assets, $101,428 (M); gifts received, $150,000; expenditures, $343,781; qualifying distributions, $341,691, including $341,691 for 22 grants (high: $167,125; low: $150).
Fields of interest: Human services; Aging, centers & services; Jewish federated giving programs.
Limitations: Applications not accepted. Giving on a national basis with emphasis on OK. No grants to individuals.
Application information: Contributes only to pre-selected organizations.
Trustees: Irvin E. Frank, Donald H. Newman, Coleman L. Robison.
EIN: 731412060
Grants for Aging:
Tulsa Jewish Community Retirement and Health Care Center, Tulsa, OK, $100,000. 95.

OREGON

820
Leslie G. Ehmann Trust

c/o U.S. National Bank of Oregon, Trust Group
P.O. Box 3168
Portland 97208-3168 (503) 275-5718
Contact: C. Gordon Childs, Trustee

Established in 1985 in OR.
Donor(s): Leslie G. Ehmann.‡
Financial data (yr. ended 06/30/95): Assets, $1,534,497 (M); expenditures, $99,212; qualifying distributions, $68,583, including $64,500 for 6 grants (high: $16,000; low: $8,000).
Purpose and activities: "To aid the elderly or the needy by the use and enjoyment of pets."
Fields of interest: Animal welfare; Aging, centers & services; Disabled; Aging.
Types of support: Continuing support, research.
Limitations: Giving primarily in OR and WA. No grants to individuals.
Application information: Application form required.
Initial approach: Letter
Deadline(s): None
Trustees: C. Gordon Childs, U.S. National Bank of Oregon.
Number of staff: None.
EIN: 936176402

821
Fohs Foundation

P.O. Box 1001
Roseburg 97470 (541) 440-1587
Contact: Rose Mary Cooper, Secy.-Treas.

Trust established in 1937 in NY.
Donor(s): F. Julius Fohs,‡ Cora B. Fohs.‡
Financial data (yr. ended 12/31/94): Assets, $10,671,696 (M); expenditures, $609,395; qualifying distributions, $514,132, including $507,700 for 23 grants (high: $150,000; low: $1,000).
Purpose and activities: To promote science, art, education, health, healthful recreation and good citizenship of children and adults; research in general, charitable, humanitarian, sociological and educational problems; support for Ella Fohs children's and senior citizens' camps in CT; grants for Jewish-sponsored educational institutions, particularly in Israel.
Fields of interest: Arts/cultural programs; Higher education; Education; Recreation; Human services; Youth, services; Aging, centers & services; Jewish agencies & temples; Aging; Israel.
Types of support: Endowment funds, scholarship funds.
Application information: Application form not required.
Initial approach: Letter
Copies of proposal: 1
Deadline(s): None
Board meeting date(s): Apr. or May
Officers and Trustees:* Frances F. Sohn,* Chair.; Fred Sohn,* Vice-Chair.; Rose Mary Cooper, Secy.-Treas.; Edward Sohn, Howard Sohn, Ruth Sohn.
Number of staff: 1 part-time support.
EIN: 746003165

822
J & S Foundation

c/o James A. Thompsen
0333 S.W. Flower St.
Portland 97201 (503) 244-1333

Donor(s): Joan C. Wilcox, Stephen S. Wilcox.
Financial data (yr. ended 12/31/93): Assets, $607,867 (M); gifts received, $50,000; expenditures, $49,300; qualifying distributions, $48,267, including $48,227 for 12 grants (high: $15,227; low: $500).
Purpose and activities: Provides funds for heating bills for low-income elderly.
Fields of interest: Aging, centers & services; Aging; Economically disadvantaged.
Types of support: Emergency funds.
Limitations: Giving primarily in OR and WA.
Application information:
Initial approach: Letter
Deadline(s): None
Directors: Joan C. Wilcox, Stephen S. Wilcox.
EIN: 930775960

823
The Jackson Foundation

c/o U.S. National Bank of Oregon, Trust Group
P.O. Box 3168
Portland 97208 (503) 275-6564
Contact: Robert H. Depew, Asst. V.P., U.S. National Bank of Oregon

Trust established in 1960 in OR; Philip Ludwell Jackson Charitable and Residual Trusts were merged into The Jackson Foundation in 1981.
Donor(s): Maria C. Jackson.‡
Financial data (yr. ended 06/30/95): Assets, $12,440,172 (M); expenditures, $446,011; qualifying distributions, $384,990, including $337,601 for grants (average: $1,000-$25,000).
Purpose and activities: Support for adult care counseling and training, education, children and youth programs, arts and humanities, medical issues, civic affairs and the environment, domestic violence, and food, fuel and shelter.
Fields of interest: Performing arts; Humanities; Arts/cultural programs; Education; Environment; Health care; Substance abuse, services; Health organizations; Housing/shelter, development; Human services; Children & youth, services; Youth, services; Aging, centers & services; Women, centers & services; Minorities/immigrants, centers & services; Minorities; Disabled; Aging; Women.
Types of support: Continuing support, capital campaigns, endowment funds, research, program-related investments/loans, matching funds.
Limitations: Giving limited to OR. No support for churches or temples. No grants to individuals, or for matching gifts, scholarships, fellowships, or building or equipment funds for religious organizations; no loans to individuals.
Publications: Annual report.
Application information: Application form required.
Initial approach: Request for application form
Copies of proposal: 3
Deadline(s): Sept. 30, Dec. 31, Mar. 31, and June 30
Board meeting date(s): July, Oct., Jan., and Apr.
Final notification: 4 to 6 weeks
Trustees: Milo E. Ormseth, Julie Vigeland, U.S. National Bank of Oregon.
Number of staff: 3
EIN: 936020752

824
The Samuel S. Johnson Foundation

P.O. Box 356
Redmond 97756 (541) 548-8104
Contact: Elizabeth Hill Johnson, Pres.
FAX: (541) 548-2014

Incorporated in 1948 in CA.
Donor(s): Samuel S. Johnson,‡ Elizabeth Hill Johnson, Robert W. Hill.‡
Financial data (yr. ended 05/31/95): Assets, $4,983,491 (M); gifts received, $17,000; expenditures, $297,445; qualifying distributions, $284,955, including $258,397 for 141 grants (high: $10,000; low: $100).
Purpose and activities: Giving for education, including adult literacy, assistance to mature and returning students, medical education benefitting nonurban areas, preschool/daycare enrichment and school readiness, excellence in teaching, employment readiness, outreach programs, music and distance learning; medical, including projects benefitting rural areas, hospice and home health care, promotion of medical ethics and preventive care; domestic violence, including shelters and services to victims and families; youth development programs, including scouting, leadership and reading programs; voluntarism, and self-help; emergency food assistance; public safety/crime prevention, including drug and alcohol treatment and prevention programs emphasizing self-discipline; religious organizations, including outreach, but no giving to projects promoting sectarian views; humane societies, including programs for neutering, adoption and providing animal companions for elderly, blind and other handicapped; and historical and museum projects. Support primarily for field of interest grants, along with emergency, nonrecurring grants primarily to nonprofits located in or benefitting residents of OR.
Fields of interest: Museums; Humanities; Literature; Historic preservation/historical societies; Elementary/secondary education; Early childhood education; Vocational education; Higher education; Dental school/education; Medical school/education; Nursing school/education; Adult education—literacy & basic skills; Reading; Family planning; Nursing care; Substance abuse, services; Cancer; Heart/circulatory disease; Domestic violence prevention; Human services; Children & youth, services; Family services; Hospices; Aging, centers & services; Women, centers & services; Reproductive rights; Rural development; Community development; Voluntarism promotion; Science, public education; Public policy, research; Leadership development; Christian agencies & churches; Religion; Minorities; Native Americans; Disabled; Economically disadvantaged.
Types of support: General/operating support, continuing support, equipment, emergency funds, program development, conferences/seminars, publication, seed money, curriculum development, scholarship funds, matching funds, student loans—to individuals.
Limitations: Giving primarily in the Pacific Northwest and northern CA. No support for foreign organizations. No grants for annual campaigns, deficit financing, construction, sole underwriting of major proposals or projects, or endowments.
Publications: Application guidelines.
Application information: Application form not required.
Initial approach: Letter
Copies of proposal: 1
Deadline(s): June 1 for July meeting and Nov. 15 for Jan. meeting
Board meeting date(s): July and Jan.
Final notification: 2 to 3 weeks after board meeting
Officers and Directors:* Elizabeth Hill Johnson,* Pres.; Elizabeth K. Johnson-Helm,* V.P. and Secy.; Mary A. Krenowicz, Exec. Secy.-Treas.; Patricia C. Johnson,* C.F.O.; Karen K. Creason, John C. Helm.
Number of staff: 1 part-time professional.
EIN: 946062478

825
Sophia Byers McComas Foundation

c/o U.S. National Bank of Oregon, Trust Dept.
P.O. Box 3168
Portland 97208-3168 (503) 275-5718
Contact: Robert H. Depew, Trust Officer, U.S. National Bank of Oregon
For additional information contact: (503) 275-6564

Established in 1943 in OR.
Financial data (yr. ended 06/30/95): Assets, $1,726,639 (M); gifts received, $58,998; expenditures, $79,196; qualifying distributions, $69,713, including $63,975 for grants to individuals.
Purpose and activities: "Net income to be used for the care and maintenance of indigent aged people who are OR residents in suitable homes or institutions in the state". Individuals already receiving welfare assistance are not eligible for aid.
Fields of interest: Aging, centers & services; Aging.
Types of support: Continuing support.
Limitations: Giving limited to OR.
Application information: Applicants recommended by church groups, social service agencies, or similar groups.
Initial approach: Letter
Deadline(s): None
Trustee: U.S. National Bank of Oregon.
Number of staff: None.
EIN: 936019602

826
Meyer Memorial Trust

(Formerly Fred Meyer Charitable Trust)
1515 S.W. Fifth Ave., Suite 500
Portland 97201 (503) 228-5512
Contact: Charles S. Rooks, Exec. Dir.

Trust established by will in 1978; obtained IRS status in 1982 in OR.
Donor(s): Fred G. Meyer.‡
Financial data (yr. ended 03/31/96): Assets, $352,096,621 (M); expenditures, $18,774,525; qualifying distributions, $17,406,761, including $16,906,761 for grants (high: $1,000,000; low: $250; average: $100,000-$200,000) and $500,000 for program-related investments.
Purpose and activities: The trust provides general purpose grants, primarily in OR for education, the arts and humanities, health, and social welfare. Under general purpose, the trust operates the Small Grants Program, which provides awards of $500 to $8,000 for small projects in OR. The Support for Teacher Initiatives Program provides awards of up to $7,000 to teachers in OR.
Fields of interest: Museums; Performing arts; Humanities; Historic preservation/historical societies; Arts/cultural programs; Child development, education; Higher education; Education; Natural resource conservation & protection; Environment; Health care; Health organizations; Delinquency prevention/services; Housing/shelter, development; Human services; Children & youth, services; Youth, services; Child development, services; Family services; Aging, centers & services; Community development; Aging.
Types of support: General/operating support, capital campaigns, building/renovation, equipment, program development, seed money, research, technical assistance, program-related investments/loans, matching funds.
Limitations: Giving primarily in OR and that part of WA located in the greater metropolitan Portland area. No support for sectarian or religious organizations for religious purposes. No grants to individuals (except for Support for Teacher Initiatives Program), or for endowment funds, annual campaigns, deficit financing, scholarships, fellowships, or indirect or overhead costs, except as specifically and essentially related to the grant project; occasional program-related loans only.
Publications: Annual report, informational brochure (including application guidelines), program policy statement, application guidelines.
Application information: Special guidelines for Small Grants Program and Support for Teacher Initiatives. The Support for Children at Risk Program, a regional program covering 5 states, was terminated in 1996. Proposals related to children and youth may be submitted under the trust's General Purpose Program. Application form required.
Initial approach: Proposal
Copies of proposal: 1
Deadline(s): Jan. 15, Apr. 15, July 15, and Oct. 15 for Small Grants Program; Feb. 1 for Support for Teacher Initiatives; no set deadline for other grants
Board meeting date(s): Monthly
Final notification: 3 to 5 months for General Purpose proposals that pass first screening; 1 to 2 months for those that do not; 6 to 8 weeks for Small Grants; 8 to 10 weeks for Support for Teacher Initiatives
Officers and Trustees:* Gerry Pratt,* Chair.; Wayne G. Pierson, Treas.; Charles S. Rooks, Exec. Dir.; Debbie F. Craig, Travis Cross, Warne Nunn, Oran B. Robertson.
Staff: Alice McCartor, Prog. Officer; Charline McDonald, Prog. Officer; Victor Merced, Prog. Officer.
Number of staff: 5 full-time professional; 5 full-time support; 1 part-time support.
EIN: 930806316
Grants for Aging:

Ecumenical Ministries of Oregon, Portland, OR, $115,000. For new elevator to improve access for residents of Patton Home, residential care facility for elderly and disabled people. 96.
Enterprise for Progress in the Community, Yakima, WA, $144,300. For crisis nursery services and emergency respite care for low-income families in Wapato-Toppenish area of Yakima Valley. 96.
Family Friends, Grants Pass, OR, $26,000. For start-up of project designed to generate revenue for agency's treatment programs for abused children. 96.
Tillamook County General Hospital, Tillamook, OR, $134,000. For family support workers for Healthy Families project, which provides home visits to families with newborns. 96.
Vancouver Childrens Therapy Center, Clark Care and Development Center, Vancouver, WA, $10,000. For day care and respite program that serves infants and young children, including many with disabilities. 96.

827
The Oregon Community Foundation

621 S.W. Morrison, Suite 725
Portland 97205 (503) 227-6846
Contact: Gregory A. Chaille, Pres.

Established in 1973 in OR.
Foundation type: Community
Financial data (yr. ended 06/30/95): Assets, $125,597,029 (M); gifts received, $15,247,658; expenditures, $11,357,167, including $8,907,369 for 917 grants (high: $255,899; low: $1,000; average: $2,000-$25,000), $583,681 for 310 grants to individuals, $209,625 for 1 foundation-administered program and $411,800 for 1 program-related investment.
Purpose and activities: To meet educational, cultural, medical, social and civic needs in all areas and at all levels of society throughout the state of Oregon.
Fields of interest: Arts/cultural programs; Adult education—literacy & basic skills; Reading; Education; Health care; Health organizations; Youth development, services; Human services; Youth, services; Aging, centers & services; Community development; Voluntarism promotion; Government/public administration; Leadership development; Aging; Economically disadvantaged.
Types of support: General/operating support, building/renovation, equipment, land acquisition, program development, seed money, scholarship funds, technical assistance, matching funds.
Limitations: Giving limited to OR. No support for religious organizations for religious purposes. No grants to individuals (except for scholarships), or for emergency funding, endowments, annual campaigns, deficit financing, research, publications, films, or conferences, unless so designated by a donor; no loans.
Publications: Annual report, newsletter, program policy statement, application guidelines.
Application information: Application form required.
Initial approach: Letter or telephone to request grant guidelines; for scholarship guidelines contact Education Program Officer
Copies of proposal: 12
Deadline(s): Mar. 15 and Aug. 15 for Small Grants; inquiry letters for Targeted Grants accepted at any time
Board meeting date(s): Jan., June, Sept., and Nov.
Final notification: 3 months; several months for Targeted Grants
Officers and Directors:* Sally McCracken,* Chair.; Alex M. Byler,* Chair.; C. Morton Bishop, Jr., Vice-Chair.; Gregory A. Chaille, Pres.; Kathleen Cornett, V.P., Progs.; Ethel Simon-McWilliams, Secy.; John C. Hampton, Treas.; Clifford N. Carlsen, Jr., Sue Hollern, Mary K. Mark, Carolyn McMurchie, James A. Meyer, Matthew Prophet, David A. Rhoten, William Thorndike, Jr., Janet Webster, Donna P. Woolley.
Investment Managers: The Bank of California, N.A., First Interstate Bank of Oregon, N.A., Provident Investment Counsel, Scudder, Stevens, Clark, U.S. National Bank of Oregon.
Staff: Susan McLaughlin, Prog. Officer, Education/Special Funds; Don Neureuther, Dir., Neighborhood Partnership Fund; Laura Recko, Prog. Assoc., Neighborhood Partnership Fund; Laura Winter, Grants Administrator; Christine Tomlinson, Exec. Dir., Oregon Child Devel. Fund; Roberta Wood, Prog. Dir., Oregon Child Devel. Fund.
Number of staff: 7 full-time professional; 2 part-time professional; 3 full-time support.
EIN: 237315673
Grants for Aging:
Clackamas County Senior Citizens Council, Oregon City, OR, $10,000. 95.

828
Portland General Electric Co. Corporate Contributions

121 Southwest Salmon St.
Portland 97204 (503) 464-8535
Contact: Kathy Carlson, Mgr., Community Resources

Financial data (yr. ended 12/31/95): Total giving, $1,500,000, including .
Purpose and activities: Portland General's corporate contributions are focused on healthy families, children, education, cultural diversity, and environmental stewardship.
Fields of interest: Arts, cultural/ethnic awareness; Visual arts; Museums; Performing arts; Theater; Humanities; Arts/cultural programs; Early childhood education; Elementary school/education; Higher education; Adult education—literacy & basic skills; Libraries/library science; Reading; Education; Energy; Environment; Wildlife preservation & protection; Health care; Substance abuse, services; Legal services; Crime/law enforcement; Youth development, services; Youth development, citizenship; Human services; Children & youth, services; Children, services; Youth, services; Family services; Aging, centers & services; Women, centers & services; Minorities/immigrants, centers & services; Homeless, human services; Community development; Economics; Government/public administration; Public affairs, citizen participation; Leadership development; Public affairs; Minorities; Aging; Women; Economically disadvantaged; Homeless.
Types of support: General/operating support, capital campaigns, building/renovation, program development, scholarship funds, research, employee volunteer services, use of facilities, donated equipment, in-kind gifts, matching funds.
Limitations: Giving primarily in company areas. No grants to individuals.
Publications: Annual report, application guidelines.
Application information: Include 501(c)(3) status, description and goals of organization and project, project budget, list of directors and contributors. Application form not required.
Initial approach: Letter and proposal to headquarters
Copies of proposal: 1
Deadline(s): Sept.
Board meeting date(s): Quarterly
Final notification: 6 weeks
Administrators: Kathy Carlson, Mgr., Community Resources; Christine Crossland, Community Resources Specialist.
Number of staff: 2 full-time professional; 1 full-time support.

829
The Hubert & Ludmila Schlesinger Foundation

400 Yamhill Plaza
815 S.W. Second Ave.
Portland 97204
Contact: Andrew H. Josephson, Trustee

Established in 1986 in OR.
Financial data (yr. ended 12/31/94): Assets, $1,091,085 (M); expenditures, $72,756; qualifying distributions, $58,959, including $39,000 for 6 grants of $6,500 each.
Fields of interest: Orchestra (symphony); Higher education; Children, services; Aging, centers & services.
Limitations: Giving limited to OR. No grants to individuals.
Application information:
Initial approach: Letter
Deadline(s): None
Trustees: Christopher Bocci, Andrew H. Josephson, Susan K. Josephson.
EIN: 930900123

830
Swiss Aid Society

732 S.E. 166th Place
Portland 97233-4399

Foundation type: Operating
Financial data (yr. ended 12/31/94): Assets, $8,551 (M); gifts received, $1,495; expenditures, $2,869; qualifying distributions, $2,869, including $275 for 5 grants (high: $75; low: $25) and $1,821 for grants to individuals.
Purpose and activities: Aid to needy, sick and elderly of Swiss descent who reside in the Portland, OR, area; some support for organizations.
Fields of interest: Aging, centers & services; Aging; Economically disadvantaged.
Types of support: Grants to individuals.

Limitations: Applications not accepted. Giving limited to the Portland, OR, area.
Officers: Frank L. Truttman, Pres.; Al Odermott, V.P.; Mary Amstad, Secy.; Edna Truttman, Treas.
EIN: 936032292

831
The Tennant Foundation
(Formerly John J. Tennant Foundation)
P.O. Box 1658
Portland 97207

Established in 1967 in OR.
Donor(s): John J. Tennant.
Financial data (yr. ended 12/31/95): Assets, $308,018 (M); gifts received, $1,300; expenditures, $39,698; qualifying distributions, $38,075, including $38,075 for 33 grants (high: $11,000; low: $75).
Fields of interest: Arts/cultural programs; Secondary school/education; Higher education; Health care; Aging, centers & services; General charitable giving.
Limitations: Applications not accepted. Giving primarily in Portland, OR. No grants to individuals.
Application information: Contributes only to pre-selected organizations.
Trustees: John J. Tennant, Jr., Joseph P. Tennant.
EIN: 936042963

PENNSYLVANIA

832
Joseph & Lena Abramson Family Foundation
1105 Industrial Hwy.
Southampton 18966

Established in 1990 in PA.
Donor(s): Joseph Abramson, Stuart Licht.
Financial data (yr. ended 12/31/94): Assets, $19,921 (M); expenditures, $42; qualifying distributions, $42.
Fields of interest: Higher education; Aging, centers & services; Jewish agencies & temples; Aging.
Types of support: Research.
Limitations: Applications not accepted. Giving primarily in PA. No grants to individuals.
Application information: Contributes only to pre-selected organizations. No grants paid in 1994.
Officers: Joseph Abramson, Pres.; Barry Abramson, V.P.; Alan Harris, Secy.; Stuart Licht, Treas.
EIN: 232587965

833
Allegheny Ludlum Foundation
1000 Six PPG Place
Pittsburgh 15222-5479
Contact: Jon D. Walton, Esq., Trustee

Established in 1981 in PA.
Donor(s): Allegheny Ludlum Corp.
Foundation type: Company-sponsored
Financial data (yr. ended 12/31/95): Assets, $1,900,546 (M); gifts received, $1,000,000; expenditures, $1,044,663; qualifying distributions, $1,038,663, including $1,038,663 for 110 grants (high: $383,002; low: $500; average: $1,000-$10,000).
Purpose and activities: Giving primarily for community funds, youth agencies, and hospitals and medical research; some support for higher and other education, cultural programs, including the fine and performing arts, and social services benefiting the aged, the disabled, minorities, and women.
Fields of interest: Visual arts; Performing arts; Arts/cultural programs; Elementary/secondary education; Higher education; Libraries/library science; Hospitals (general); Medical care, rehabilitation; Substance abuse, services; Cancer; Medical research; Human services; Children & youth, services; Family services; Hospices; Aging, centers & services; Women, centers & services; Minorities/immigrants, centers & services; Community development; Federated giving programs.
Types of support: Continuing support, annual campaigns, capital campaigns, building/renovation, emergency funds, program development, publication, scholarship funds, employee-related scholarships.
Limitations: Giving primarily in PA, IN, CT, NY, and OK. No support for private foundations. No grants to individuals.
Application information: Application form not required.
Initial approach: Letter
Copies of proposal: 1
Deadline(s): None
Trustees: J.L. Murdy, R.P. Simmons, Jon D. Walton, PNC Bank, N.A.
Number of staff: None.
EIN: 256228755

834
The Arcadia Foundation
105 East Logan St.
Norristown 19401-3058 (610) 275-8460
Contact: Marilyn Lee Steinbright, Pres.

Incorporated in 1964 in PA.
Donor(s): Edith C. Steinbright,‡ Marilyn Lee Steinbright.
Financial data (yr. ended 09/30/95): Assets, $42,839,584 (M); gifts received, $4,389,124; expenditures, $3,797,427; qualifying distributions, $3,608,688, including $3,608,688 for 207 grants (high: $500,000; low: $400; average: $1,000-$20,000).
Purpose and activities: Emphasis on hospitals and hospital building funds, health agencies and services, nursing, hospices, early childhood, adult and higher education, libraries, child development and welfare agencies, youth organizations, and social service and general welfare agencies, including care of the handicapped, aged, and hungry; support also for family services, the environment and conservation, wildlife and animal welfare, religious organizations, historical preservation, and music organizations.
Fields of interest: Music; Historic preservation/historical societies; Early childhood education; Child development, education; Higher education; Adult/continuing education; Libraries/library science; Education; Natural resource conservation & protection; Environment; Animal welfare; Wildlife preservation & protection; Hospitals (general); Nursing care; Health care; Health organizations; Food services; Human services; Children & youth, services; Youth, services; Child development, services; Family services; Hospices; Aging, centers & services; Christian agencies & churches; Protestant agencies & churches; Religion; Disabled; Aging; Economically disadvantaged; General charitable giving.
Types of support: General/operating support, continuing support, annual campaigns, capital campaigns, building/renovation, equipment, endowment funds, program development, scholarship funds, research.
Limitations: Giving limited to eastern PA organizations whose addresses have zip codes of 18000 - 19000. Generally, low support for cultural programs. No grants to individuals, or for deficit financing, land acquisition, fellowships, demonstration projects, publications, or conferences; no loans.
Publications: Application guidelines.
Application information: Application form not required.
Initial approach: Letter or proposal (not exceeding 2 pages; otherwise entire proposal will be discarded)
Copies of proposal: 1
Deadline(s): Submit proposal only between June 1 and Aug. 15; deadline Aug. 15 for the following calendar year
Board meeting date(s): Dec.
Final notification: Up to 3 months after Aug. 15
Officers and Directors:* Marilyn Lee Steinbright,* Pres.; Tanya Hashorva,* V.P.; David P. Sandler,* Secy.; Harvey S.S. Miller,* Treas.; Edward L. Jones, Jr., Kathleen Shellington.
Number of staff: None.
EIN: 236399772
Grants for Aging:
Alzheimers Disease and Related Disorders Association of Greater Philadelphia, Philadelphia, PA, $15,000. For unrestricted support. 95.
Camilla Hall, Immaculata, PA, $10,000. For unrestricted support. 95.
Hayes Manor, Philadelphia, PA, $20,000. For unrestricted support. 95.
Holy Family Home, Philadelphia, PA, $10,000. For unrestricted support. 95.
Philadelphia Senior Center, Philadelphia, PA, $25,000. For unrestricted support. 95.

835
Claneil Foundation, Inc.
630 West Germantown Pike, Suite 400
Plymouth Meeting 19462-1059
Contact: Dr. Henry A. Jordan, Exec. Dir.

Incorporated in 1968 in DE.
Donor(s): Henry S. McNeil,‡ Langhorne B. Smith, Marjorie M. Findlay, Claniel Enterprises, Inc.
Financial data (yr. ended 12/31/94): Assets, $9,296,313 (M); gifts received, $719,884; expenditures, $452,314; qualifying distributions, $378,414, including $373,270 for 79 grants

(high: $25,000; low: $500; average: $500-$25,000).
Fields of interest: Visual arts; Historic preservation/historical societies; Arts/cultural programs; Early childhood education; Secondary school/education; Higher education; Medical school/education; Natural resource conservation & protection; Environment; Family planning; Health care; Domestic violence prevention; Child abuse prevention; Human services; Family services; Aging, centers & services; Reproductive rights; Community development; Women; Economically disadvantaged.
Types of support: Capital campaigns, building/renovation, equipment, research, exchange programs.
Limitations: Giving primarily in PA. No grants to individuals.
Publications: Informational brochure (including application guidelines).
Application information: Applications accepted between Jan. 1 and Mar. 31, and July 1 and Sept. 30; accepts Delaware Valley Grantmakers Common Grant Application. Application form not required.
Initial approach: Proposal
Copies of proposal: 1
Deadline(s): Sept. 30 and Mar. 31
Board meeting date(s): Oct. and Apr.
Final notification: Nov. and May
Officers and Directors:* Lois F. McNeil,* Pres.; Barbara M. Jordan,* V.P.; Henry A. Jordan,* Secy. and Exec. Dir.; Langhorne B. Smith,* Treas.; Marjorie M. Findlay, Robert D. McNeil.
Number of staff: None.
EIN: 236445450

836
The Anne L. and George H. Clapp Charitable and Educational Trust

(Formerly G. H. Clapp Dec'd Charitable and Educational Trust)
c/o Mellon Bank, N.A.
Three Mellon Bank Ctr., Rm. 4000
Pittsburgh 15259 (412) 234-1634
Contact: Annette Calgaro, Trust Officer, Mellon Bank, N.A.

Established around 1981.
Donor(s): George H. Clapp.‡
Financial data (yr. ended 09/30/95): Assets, $15,593,317 (M); expenditures, $815,372; qualifying distributions, $763,877, including $738,000 for 71 grants (high: $30,000; low: $1,500).
Purpose and activities: Primary areas of interest include child welfare, education, social services, and community funds; limited support for arts and conservation.
Fields of interest: Arts/cultural programs; Education; Environment; Human services; Aging; Economically disadvantaged.
Limitations: Giving limited to southwestern, PA. No grants to individuals.
Application information: Application form not required.
Initial approach: Proposal not exceeding 10 pages
Copies of proposal: 2
Deadline(s): May 31
Board meeting date(s): Late summer
Final notification: Sept.
Trustees: William E. Collin, William A. Galbraith, Jr., Mellon Bank, N.A.
EIN: 256018976

837
Andrew R. & Dorothy L. Cochrane Foundation

210 Field Club Rd.
Pittsburgh 15238 (412) 963-8218
Contact: Andrew R. Cochrane, Trustee, or Christine Cochrane Yukevich, Trustee

Established about 1968.
Donor(s): Andrew R. Cochrane, Wise Machine Co., Inc., Arch Engineering Co.
Financial data (yr. ended 12/31/95): Assets, $814,023 (M); gifts received, $26,821; expenditures, $46,938; qualifying distributions, $46,938, including $45,772 for grants (high: $5,100).
Fields of interest: Human services; Youth, services; Aging, centers & services; Christian agencies & churches; Aging; Economically disadvantaged.
Limitations: Giving primarily in Pittsburgh, PA. No grants to individuals.
Application information: Application form not required.
Deadline(s): None
Trustees: Andrew R. Cochrane, Christine Cochrane Yukevich.
Number of staff: None.
EIN: 256093648
Grants for Aging:
Vintage, Pittsburgh, PA, $3,000. 94.

838
Charles S. & Mary Coen Family Foundation

1100 West Chestnut St.
Washington 15301

Established in 1959 in PA.
Donor(s): C.S. Coen,‡ Mary Coen,‡ Charles R. Coen, C.S. Coen Land Co.
Financial data (yr. ended 02/28/95): Assets, $6,050,722 (M); gifts received, $36,000; expenditures, $326,255; qualifying distributions, $317,544, including $314,275 for 80 grants (high: $100,000; low: $100).
Fields of interest: Higher education; Hospitals (general); Health associations; Human services; Aging, centers & services; Aging.
Limitations: Applications not accepted. Giving primarily in PA. No grants to individuals.
Application information: Contributes only to pre-selected organizations.
Trustees: Mona Thompson, Lawrence A. Withum, Jr.
EIN: 256033877
Grants for Aging:
California Senior Center, California, PA, $5,000. 95.
Presbyterian Association on Aging, Oakmont, PA, $100,000. 95.

839
Columbia Gas of Pennsylvania Corporate Giving Program

650 Washington Rd.
Pittsburgh 15228 (412) 572-7104
Contact: Rosemary Martinelli, Mgr., Community Rels.

Financial data (yr. ended 12/31/94): Total giving, $150,000, including $130,000 for 200 grants (average: $900) and $20,000 for in-kind gifts.
Fields of interest: Arts education; Museums; Performing arts; Dance; Theater; Music; Historic preservation/historical societies; Secondary school/education; Education, special; Adult education—literacy & basic skills; Reading; Natural resource conservation & protection; Energy; Environmental education; Health care clinics & centers; Substance abuse, services; Mental health, treatment; Mental health/crisis services; Crime/law enforcement; Employment, services; Food services; Housing/shelter, development; Housing/shelter, homeless; Youth development, services; Family services; Aging, centers & services; Mentally disabled, centers & services; Race/intergroup relations; Business & industry; Philanthropy/voluntarism; Federated giving programs; Transportation; Consumer protection.
Types of support: General/operating support, continuing support, capital campaigns, building/renovation, endowment funds, conferences/seminars, publication, employee volunteer services, donated equipment, in-kind gifts.
Limitations: Giving primarily in Pittsburgh/Allegheny County and in the southwest, northwest, central, and eastern PA, areas. No support for fraternal, political, veterans, athletics, or non-501(c)(3) organizations.
Application information: Application form not required.
Initial approach: Letter
Deadline(s): None
Final notification: Varies
Number of staff: 1 full-time professional; 1 full-time support.

840
Connelly Foundation

One Tower Bridge, Suite 1450
West Conshohocken 19428 (610) 834-3222
Contact: Victoria K. Flaville, V.P.

Incorporated in 1955 in PA.
Donor(s): John F. Connelly,‡ Josephine C. Connelly.
Financial data (yr. ended 12/31/94): Assets, $362,232,772 (M); expenditures, $19,900,296; qualifying distributions, $19,324,498, including $18,780,865 for grants.
Purpose and activities: Giving to higher education; Christian religious institutions, including churches, schools and colleges, and welfare programs; hospitals; and social services.
Fields of interest: Arts/cultural programs; Elementary/secondary education; Early childhood education; Child development, education; Elementary school/education; Secondary school/education; Higher education;

Adult/continuing education; Education; Hospitals (general); Substance abuse, services; Cancer; AIDS; Alcoholism; Cancer research; AIDS research; Youth development, citizenship; Human services; Children & youth, services; Youth, services; Child development, services; Aging, centers & services; Women, centers & services; Homeless, human services; Community development; Federated giving programs; Roman Catholic federated giving programs; Religious federated giving programs; Government/public administration; Public affairs, citizen participation; Christian agencies & churches; Protestant agencies & churches; Roman Catholic agencies & churches; Religion; Minorities; Disabled; Aging; Women; Economically disadvantaged; Homeless.
Types of support: General/operating support, capital campaigns, building/renovation, endowment funds, emergency funds, program development, scholarship funds.
Limitations: Giving primarily in the Philadelphia, PA, and Delaware Valley areas. No grants to individuals, or for research; no loans.
Publications: 990-PF, application guidelines, annual report.
Application information: Accepts Delaware Valley Grantmakers Common Grant Application and Common Report Form. Application form not required.
Initial approach: Proposal
Copies of proposal: 1
Deadline(s): None
Board meeting date(s): Jan., Mar., Aug., Oct., and Dec.
Final notification: 3 to 6 months after receiving proposal
Officers and Trustees:* Josephine C. Connelly,* Chair.; Josephine C. Mandeville,* Pres. and C.E.O.; Emily L. Riley,* Exec. V.P., Progs.; Victoria K. Flaville, V.P. and Secy.; Chester C. Hilinski,* V.P. and General Counsel; Lewis W. Bluemle, Jr.,* V.P., Finance; Reda Amiry, Treas.; William J. Avery, Christine C. Connelly, Danielle Connelly, Thomas S. Connelly, Philippe Delouvrier, Thomas J. Farrell, Christopher C. Riley, Thomas A. Riley.
Number of staff: 5 full-time professional; 3 part-time professional; 3 part-time support.
EIN: 236296825

841
The Crels Foundation

5917 Main St.
East Petersburg 17520 (717) 581-8130
Contact: George C. Delp, Chair.

Trust established in 1953 in PA.
Donor(s): Edwin B. Nolt.‡
Financial data (yr. ended 12/31/94): Assets, $7,841,088 (M); gifts received, $930,565; expenditures, $425,793; qualifying distributions, $392,758, including $379,000 for 49 grants (high: $50,000; low: $1,000; average: $1,000-$45,000).
Purpose and activities: Support for hospitals, nursing homes, Mennonite-related religious associations, and parochial elementary education.
Fields of interest: Elementary/secondary education; Elementary school/education; Education; Hospitals (general); Aging, centers & services; Protestant agencies & churches; Religion; Aging.
Types of support: General/operating support, capital campaigns, building/renovation, equipment, debt reduction.
Limitations: Giving primarily in the Lancaster County, PA, area. No grants to individuals, or for endowment funds, research programs, scholarships, fellowships, continuing support, annual campaigns, seed money, emergency funds, land acquisition, renovation projects, publications, conferences, matching gifts, or special projects; no loans.
Application information: Applications not encouraged. Application form not required.
Initial approach: Letter
Copies of proposal: 1
Deadline(s): Sept. 15
Board meeting date(s): Oct. and as required
Officers and Trustees:* George C. Delp,* Chair.; Kenneth N. Burkholder,* Vice-Chair.; Clarence J. Nelson,* Secy.; Eugene N. Burkholder, Leon Ray Burkholder.
Number of staff: 1 part-time professional.
EIN: 236243577
Grants for Aging:
Fairmount Rest Home, Ephrata, PA, $15,000. 94.

842
Dolfinger-McMahon Foundation

c/o Duane, Morris & Heckscher
One Liberty Place
Philadelphia 19103-7396 (215) 979-1768
Contact: Marlene Valcich, Exec. Secy.

Trust established in 1957 in PA, and originally comprised of four separate trusts: T/W of Henry Dolfinger as modified by will of Mary McMahon; 1935 D/T of Henry Dolfinger as modified by will of Caroline D. McMahon; Residuary T/W of Caroline D. McMahon; Dolfinger-McMahon Trust for Greater Philadelphia. In 1986 the 1935 D/T of H. Dolfinger was merged with the residuary T/W of C. McMahon.
Donor(s): Caroline D. McMahon,‡ Mary M. McMahon.‡
Financial data (yr. ended 09/30/95): Assets, $14,470,335 (M); expenditures, $625,959; qualifying distributions, $479,200, including $478,100 for 113 grants (high: $12,000; low: $1,000).
Purpose and activities: Primary areas of interest include community development, the disadvantaged, education, the handicapped, and health. Emphasis on experimental, demonstration, or "seed money" projects in race relations, aid to the handicapped, higher and secondary education, social and urban programs, church programs, and health agencies. Emergency funding will be made rarely and, once made, will disqualify the agency from receiving any additional funding for the succeeding three years. Grants limited to $20,000 in any one year to a single project or program.
Fields of interest: Museums; Performing arts; Dance; Theater; Music; Humanities; Arts/cultural programs; Elementary/secondary education; Early childhood education; Child development, education; Elementary school/education; Secondary school/education; Vocational education; Higher education; Theological school/education; Adult/continuing education; Adult education—literacy & basic skills; Reading; Education; Natural resource conservation & protection; Energy; Environment; Animal welfare; Hospitals (general); Family planning; Nursing care; Health care; Substance abuse, services; Mental health/crisis services; AIDS; Alcoholism; Health organizations; AIDS research; Delinquency prevention/services; Legal services; Crime/law enforcement; Employment; Food services; Nutrition; Recreation; Youth development, services; Human services; Children & youth, services; Youth, services; Child development, services; Family services; Aging, centers & services; Women, centers & services; Minorities/immigrants, centers & services; Homeless, human services; Race/intergroup relations; Urban/community development; Community development; Voluntarism promotion; Religious federated giving programs; Government/public administration; Transportation; Leadership development; Public affairs; Religion; Minorities; Disabled; Aging; Women; Economically disadvantaged; Homeless.
Types of support: Debt reduction, emergency funds, program development, conferences/seminars, publication, seed money, matching funds.
Limitations: Giving limited to the greater Philadelphia, PA, area. No support for special interest advocacy through legislative lobbying or solicitation of government agencies. No grants to individuals, or for endowment funds, physical facilities, ordinary operating expenses, renovations or building repairs, building funds, scholarships, medical or scientific research, or fellowships.
Publications: Annual report (including application guidelines), application guidelines.
Application information: See guidelines for format required for requests. Application form not required.
Initial approach: Letter requesting guidelines, followed by proposal
Copies of proposal: 1
Deadline(s): Submit proposal preferably in Mar. or Sept.; must actually be received on or before Apr. 1 or Oct. 1 (or the preceding Friday if the 1st falls on a weekend)
Board meeting date(s): Late spring, late fall, and as required
Final notification: 2 to 4 weeks following semiannual meeting
Officer: Marlene Valcich, Exec. Secy.
Trustees: Martin A. Heckscher, Roland Morris.
Number of staff: None.
EIN: 236207346
Grants for Aging:
Chestnut Hill Hospital Healthcare, Philadelphia, PA, $7,080. To evaluate Senior Care Center implementation. 94.

843
Bright & Christella Erichson Charitable Trust

1735 Market St., Suite 3800
Philadelphia 19103-7598
Contact: Harvey N. Shapiro, Trustee

Established in 1980 in PA.
Financial data (yr. ended 10/31/95): Assets, $1,495,543 (M); expenditures, $71,703; qualifying distributions, $67,002, including $65,020 for 7 grants (high: $13,000; low: $1,000).
Purpose and activities: Support primarily to organizations which benefit the needy and the elderly.
Fields of interest: Nursing home/convalescent facility; Human services; Aging, centers & services; Aging.
Limitations: Applications not accepted. Giving limited to Philadelphia, PA. No grants to individuals.
Application information: Contributes only to pre-selected organizations.
Trustees: Rev. Gonzalo Correa Santa Cruz, Harvey N. Shapiro.
EIN: 236697739
Grants for Aging:
CARIE, Philadelphia, PA, $1,000. 95.
Golden Slipper Club Uptown Home for the Aged, Philadelphia, PA, $13,000. 95.
Holy Family Home, Philadelphia, PA, $12,000. 95.
Immaculate Mary Home, Philadelphia, PA, $12,000. 95.
Saint Ignatius Nursing Home, Philadelphia, PA, $12,000. 95.

844
Female Association of Philadelphia

c/o PNC Bank, N.A.
1632 Chestnut St.
Philadelphia 19103 (610) 525-6234

Established in 1810 in PA.
Financial data (yr. ended 09/30/94): Assets, $2,067,794 (M); gifts received, $3,523; expenditures, $106,635; qualifying distributions, $91,555, including $91,310 for 154 grants to individuals (high: $322; low: $200; average: $200-$800).
Purpose and activities: Modest, individual grants awarded only to women over 60 years of age, who reside in the Philadelphia area with a per annum income under $10,000 and not on Social Security Income.
Fields of interest: Aging; Women; Economically disadvantaged.
Types of support: Grants to individuals.
Limitations: Applications not accepted. Giving limited to the Philadelphia, PA, area.
Publications: 990-PF.
Application information:
Board meeting date(s): Apr. and Oct.
Trustee: PNC Bank, N.A.
Number of staff: None.
EIN: 236214961

845
Greensburg Foundation

P.O. Box 71
Greensburg 15601 (412) 834-8090
Contact: Judith R. Myers, Dir.

Established in 1947 in PA.
Foundation type: Community
Financial data (yr. ended 12/31/95): Assets, $3,000,000 (M); expenditures, $143,580, including $132,576 for grants (high: $6,000; low: $400).
Purpose and activities: Primary areas of interest include education, community development, family services, health associations, and youth.
Fields of interest: Visual arts; Museums; Performing arts; Arts/cultural programs; Elementary school/education; Secondary school/education; Higher education; Libraries/library science; Education; Health associations; Safety/disasters; Recreation; Youth, services; Family services; Aging, centers & services; Women, centers & services; Community development; Aging; Women; General charitable giving.
Types of support: General/operating support, capital campaigns, equipment, program development, scholarship funds.
Limitations: Giving limited to Greensburg, PA, and surrounding areas sharing Greensburg zip code (15601).
Application information: Application form not required.
Initial approach: Letter
Copies of proposal: 1
Deadline(s): Dec. 30 and June 30
Board meeting date(s): Feb. and Aug.
Officer and Directors:* Hugh Dempsey,* Chair.; Judith R. Myers.
Number of staff: 1 part-time support.
EIN: 256052355

846
The Hassel Foundation

1600 Market St., 34th Fl.
Philadelphia 19103 (215) 751-2526
Contact: Michael H. Krekstein, Esq., Trustee

Trust established in 1961 in PA.
Donor(s): Morris Hassel,‡ Calvin Hassel.‡
Financial data (yr. ended 12/31/95): Assets, $6,295,384 (M); expenditures, $220,369; qualifying distributions, $203,575, including $185,000 for 18 grants (high: $62,500; low: $1,000) and $8,500 for 5 grants to individuals (high: $2,000; low: $1,500).
Purpose and activities: Support primarily for higher and other education, the elderly and a museum; scholarships are awarded annually to graduating seniors of specific high schools.
Fields of interest: Museums; Higher education; Education; Aging.
Types of support: General/operating support, building/renovation, scholarships—to individuals.
Limitations: Giving primarily in PA. No grants to individuals (except for scholarships at specified high schools).
Application information: Scholarship applications are available from the high school principal's office; no application form for grants.
Initial approach: Letter
Deadline(s): None
Board meeting date(s): June and as required
Trustees: Barbara Cohen, Elizabeth Cohen, Sarle H. Cohen, Andrew Goldberg, Jay L. Goldberg, Maxine Goldberg, Marilyn Khoury, Michael H. Krekstein, Ephraim Royfe, Merle Wolfson.
EIN: 236251862
Grants for Aging:
Philadelphia Geriatric Center, Philadelphia, PA, $20,000. For caregiving project. 95.

847
Edward W. Helfrick Senior Citizens Trust

c/o First National Trust Bank
400 Market St.
Sunbury 17801-2336

Financial data (yr. ended 12/31/95): Assets, $20,359 (M); expenditures, $2,123; qualifying distributions, $2,123, including $1,500 for 3 grants to individuals of $500 each.
Purpose and activities: Financial aid to senior citizens as a result of fire damages or illness.
Fields of interest: Aging.
Types of support: Emergency funds, grants to individuals.
Limitations: Giving limited to residents of the 107th Legislative District in PA.
Application information: Application form required.
Deadline(s): None
Trustee: First National Trust Bank.
Committee Members: O.A. Rosini, Rev. C.R. Slough, L.E. Stibitz.
EIN: 232018916

848
The Hillman Foundation, Inc.

2000 Grant Bldg.
Pittsburgh 15219 (412) 338-3466
Contact: Ronald W. Wertz, Pres.

Incorporated in 1951 in DE.
Donor(s): John Hartwell Hillman, Jr.,‡ J.H. Hillman & Sons Co., Hillman Land Co., and family-owned corporations.
Financial data (yr. ended 12/31/95): Assets, $81,008,269 (M); expenditures, $4,381,175; qualifying distributions, $3,944,360, including $3,641,900 for 69 grants (high: $300,000; low: $2,500; average: $25,000-$100,000).
Purpose and activities: Program areas include cultural advancement and the arts, education, health and medicine, civic affairs, community development, conservation, religion, social welfare and youth.
Fields of interest: Arts/cultural programs; Higher education; Education; Health care; Health organizations; Domestic violence prevention; Human services; Youth, services; Community development; Government/public administration; Religion; Disabled; Aging; Women; People with AIDS (PWAs); Economically disadvantaged; Homeless.
Types of support: Continuing support, capital campaigns, building/renovation, equipment, land acquisition, endowment funds, program development, professorships, seed money, matching funds.

Limitations: Giving primarily in Pittsburgh and southwestern PA. No grants to individuals, or for operating budgets, annual campaigns, deficit financing, travel, or conferences; no loans.
Publications: Annual report (including application guidelines), 990-PF.
Application information: Application form not required.
Initial approach: Letter
Copies of proposal: 1
Deadline(s): None
Board meeting date(s): Apr., June, Oct., and Dec., and an annual meeting in May
Officers and Directors:* Henry L. Hillman,* Chair.; Ronald W. Wertz, Pres.; C.G. Grefenstette,* V.P.; H. Vaughan Blaxter III,* Secy.; Lawrence M. Wagner,* Treas.; Elsie H. Hillman.
Number of staff: 1 full-time professional; 1 full-time support.
EIN: 256011462
Grants for Aging:
Asbury Heights Foundation, Pittsburgh, PA, $30,000. Toward construction of Asbury Place, housing facility for persons with dementia. 95.

849
The William Talbott Hillman Foundation, Inc.
2000 Grant Bldg.
Pittsburgh 15219 (412) 338-3466
Contact: Ronald W. Wertz, Secy.

Established in 1986 in PA.
Donor(s): William Talbott Hillman, Henry Lea Hillman Charitable Lead Trust.
Financial data (yr. ended 12/31/95): Assets, $6,001,160 (M); gifts received, $39,920; expenditures, $236,732; qualifying distributions, $213,174, including $208,360 for 75 grants (high: $25,000; low: $150; average: $500-$5,000).
Fields of interest: Arts/cultural programs; Higher education; Education; Natural resource conservation & protection; Family planning; AIDS; Medical research; AIDS research; Abuse prevention; Disabled; Aging; People with AIDS (PWAs); Economically disadvantaged; Homeless.
Types of support: General/operating support, continuing support, annual campaigns, capital campaigns, building/renovation, program development, seed money.
Limitations: Giving primarily in Pittsburgh, PA. No grants to individuals.
Publications: Application guidelines, 990-PF.
Application information: Application form not required.
Initial approach: Proposal
Copies of proposal: 1
Deadline(s): None
Board meeting date(s): May and Dec.
Officers and Directors:* William Talbott Hillman,* Pres.; Mark Laskow,* V.P.; Ronald W. Wertz,* Secy.; Lawrence M. Wagner,* Treas.
Number of staff: 1 part-time professional.
EIN: 251536657

850
Arnold & Bette Hoffman Family Foundation
1464 Hunter Rd.
Rydal 19046

Established in 1985 in PA.
Donor(s): Arnold S. Hoffman, Bette Hoffman.
Financial data (yr. ended 07/31/95): Assets, $87,777 (M); gifts received, $25,625; expenditures, $49,293; qualifying distributions, $47,836, including $47,836 for 7 grants (high: $16,500; low: $500).
Fields of interest: Higher education; Geriatrics; Jewish agencies & temples; General charitable giving.
Limitations: Applications not accepted. Giving primarily in PA. No grants to individuals.
Application information: Contributes only to pre-selected organizations.
Trustees: Louis W. Fryman, Arnold S. Hoffman, Bette Hoffman.
EIN: 222702299

851
Esther Gowen Hood Trust
c/o Mellon Bank, N.A.
P.O. Box 7899
Philadelphia 19101-7899 (215) 553-3208
Contact: Patricia Kling, Mgr.

Financial data (yr. ended 09/30/94): Assets, $1,555,632 (M); expenditures, $74,227; qualifying distributions, $69,091, including $66,500 for 33 grants (high: $7,000; low: $1,000).
Fields of interest: Health associations; Human services; Children & youth, services; Aging, centers & services; Women, centers & services; Aging; Women.
Types of support: General/operating support.
Limitations: Giving limited to Philadelphia, PA. No grants to individuals.
Application information:
Initial approach: Proposal
Deadline(s): Apr. 15
Officer: Pat Kling, Mgr.
Trustee: Mellon Bank, N.A.
EIN: 236223619

852
Horsehead Community Development Fund, Inc.
P.O. Box 351
Palmerton 18071 (610) 826-3878
Contact: Charles H. Campton, Exec. Consultant

Established in 1989 in PA.
Donor(s): Horsehead Resources Development Corp.
Foundation type: Operating
Financial data (yr. ended 12/31/95): Assets, $131,533 (M); gifts received, $213,437; expenditures, $246,043; qualifying distributions, $246,043, including $237,375 for 53 grants (high: $25,000; low: $600).
Purpose and activities: Giving primarily to a hospital and a library association; support also for community development and sports activities for youth.
Fields of interest: Performing arts; Libraries/library science; Natural resource conservation & protection; Environment; Hospitals (general); Recreation; Youth, services; Community development; Federated giving programs; Disabled; Aging.
Types of support: Capital campaigns, building/renovation, equipment, emergency funds, program development.
Limitations: Giving limited to the Palmerton, PA, area. No grants for start-up funds.
Publications: Annual report (including application guidelines), informational brochure (including application guidelines), 990-PF, grants list, occasional report, program policy statement.
Application information: Grants must be used in same year awarded. Application form required.
Initial approach: Letter or telephone
Copies of proposal: 1
Deadline(s): Apr. 1, July 1, Sept. 1, and Dec. 1
Board meeting date(s): Quarterly
Final notification: After board meeting
Officers and Directors:* William Bechdolt,* Chair.; Fred L. Masenheimer, Vice-Chair; Richard Hager,* Secy.; Willard Doll, Treas.; Charles H. Campton, Exec. Consultant; Joseph Bechtel, Mary Elizabeth Cyr, Michael R. Harleman.
Number of staff: 1 part-time professional.
EIN: 232588172
Grants for Aging:
Palmerton Over 60 Administration Committee, Palmerton, PA, $1,000. 94.

853
The Stewart Huston Charitable Trust
76 South First Ave.
Coatesville 19320 (610) 384-2666
Contact: Louis J. Beccaria, Ph.D., Exec. Dir.

Established in 1989 in PA.
Donor(s): Stewart Huston.‡
Financial data (yr. ended 12/31/95): Assets, $18,400,000 (M); expenditures, $1,456,721; qualifying distributions, $1,343,471, including $1,138,425 for grants (average: $200-$60,000).
Fields of interest: Performing arts; Historic preservation/historical societies; Arts/cultural programs; Early childhood education; Vocational education; Adult education—literacy & basic skills; Reading; Education; Natural resource conservation & protection; Environment; Medical care, rehabilitation; Health care; Substance abuse, services; AIDS; Alcoholism; Health organizations; Employment; Food services; Housing/shelter, development; Recreation; Youth development, services; Human services; Children & youth, services; Family services; Hospices; Aging, centers & services; Homeless, human services; Peace; Community development; Voluntarism promotion; Public policy, research; Leadership development; Public affairs; Christian agencies & churches; Disabled; Aging; Economically disadvantaged; Homeless; General charitable giving.
Types of support: General/operating support, continuing support, capital campaigns, building/renovation, equipment, emergency

funds, program development, seed money, technical assistance, matching funds.
Limitations: Giving primarily in Coatesville and Chester County, PA, and the Savannah, GA, area.
Publications: Informational brochure (including application guidelines).
Application information: Accepts Delaware Valley Grantmakers Common Grant Application and Common Report Form. Application form required.
Initial approach: Telephone or office visit
Copies of proposal: 1
Deadline(s): Mar. 15 and Sept. 15
Board meeting date(s): June and Dec.
Final notification: June and Dec.
Trustees: Samuel A. Cann, Charles L. Huston III, Louis N. Seltzer.
Number of staff: 1 full-time professional; 1 full-time support.
EIN: 232612599

854
Agnes and Sophie Dallas Irwin Memorial Fund

c/o PNC Bank, N.A.
1632 Chestnut St.
Philadelphia 19103

Financial data (yr. ended 12/31/95): Assets, $1,013,030 (M); expenditures, $37,308; qualifying distributions, $32,443, including $8,935 for 1 grant and $23,400 for 6 grants to individuals (high: $10,000; low: $1,000).
Purpose and activities: To provide opportunities for travel, study, and research to retiring teachers in private schools for girls.
Fields of interest: Education; Pensions, teacher funds; Aging.
Types of support: Grants to individuals.
Application information:
Initial approach: Letter
Deadline(s): None
Directors: Richard Drayton, Saranne B. DuBois, Meta L. Neilson, Adele G. Sands, Maraban Sparkman.
Trustee: PNC Bank, N.A.
EIN: 236207350

855
Fred J. Jaindl Foundation

c/o PNC Bank, N.A.
P.O. Box 937
Scranton 18501
Contact: David Jaindl, Trustee
Application address: 3150 Coffetown Rd., Orefield, PA 18069; Tel.: (610) 395-3333

Established in 1988 in PA.
Financial data (yr. ended 12/31/95): Assets, $1,069,611 (M); expenditures, $68,042; qualifying distributions, $64,706, including $61,000 for 22 grants (high: $30,000; low: $250).
Fields of interest: Education; Housing/shelter, development; Aging, centers & services; Disabled; Aging.
Limitations: Giving primarily in Lehigh Valley, PA.
Application information: Application form not required.
Initial approach: Letter
Deadline(s): 90 days prior to date when funds are needed
Trustees: David Jaindl, PNC Bank, N.A.
Number of staff: None.
EIN: 232495124
Grants for Aging:
Holy Family Manor, Bethlehem, PA, $30,000. 95.
Phoebe-Devitt Home, Allentown, PA, $500. 95.

856
The Jewish Healthcare Foundation of Pittsburgh

Centre City Tower, Suite 2550
650 Smithfield St.
Pittsburgh 15222 (412) 261-1400
Contact: Karen Wolk Feinstein, Ph.D., Pres.

Established in 1990 in PA.
Donor(s): Presbyterian University Health Systems, Inc.
Financial data (yr. ended 12/31/95): Assets, $100,517,275 (M); gifts received, $1,471,607; expenditures, $6,267,588; qualifying distributions, $4,189,154, including $3,489,097 for 78 grants (high: $687,500; low: $2,000; average: $5,000-$750,000).
Purpose and activities: To support and foster the provision of health care services, health care education, and to respond to the health-related needs of the elderly, underprivileged, indigent, and underserved populations in western PA. The foundation will assist in the treatment and care of those who are elderly, sick, infirm, or in any way afflicted with physical or mental disease, in both the Jewish and general community. Current foundation priorities include: 1) the health of children at risk; 2) special needs of the elderly and chronically ill; and 3) women's health.
Fields of interest: Hospitals (general); Health care; Mental health/crisis services; AIDS; Health organizations; AIDS research; Nutrition; Human services; Family services, single parents; Aging, centers & services; Women, centers & services; Jewish federated giving programs; Aging; Women.
Types of support: Emergency funds, program development, conferences/seminars, seed money, technical assistance, program-related investments/loans, matching funds.
Limitations: Giving limited to western PA. No grants to individuals (including scholarships or fellowships), or for research or travel, general operations, endowment programs, capital needs, operating deficits, or retirement of debt.
Publications: Annual report, application guidelines, newsletter, occasional report, program policy statement.
Application information: Application form not required.
Initial approach: Preliminary letter of intent (no more than 6 pages)
Copies of proposal: 4
Deadline(s): None
Officers and Trustees:* David Shapira,* Chair.; Stephen Halpern,* Vice-Chair.; Leon Netzer,* Vice-Chair.; Karen Wolk Feinstein, Ph.D.,* Pres.; Judith Palkovitz,* Secy.; Robert A. Paul,* Treas.; and 51 additional trustees.
Staff: Kenneth Segel, Prog. Officer; Nancy Zionts, Prog. Officer.
Number of staff: 5 full-time professional; 1 part-time professional; 3 full-time support.
EIN: 251624347
Grants for Aging:
Alliance for Aging Research, DC, $30,000. For caregiver training initiatives including manual for elderly and their caregivers, curriculum for students in health care professions and use of geriatric assessments as part of Moderating the Effects of Aging initiative. 94.
California Area Senior Center, California, PA, $18,000. For pilot program, A New Model of Activities for Impaired Older Adults. 94.
Eastern Area Adult Services, Pittsburgh, PA, $18,000. For Hospital Liaison Project. 94.
Housing Authority of the City of Pittsburgh, Pittsburgh, PA, $30,000. For Adopt-A-High-Rise program, demonstration project between area businesses and senior high rises to provide health and social services for residents. 94.
Interfaith Volunteer Caregivers, Pittsburgh, PA, $60,000. For A Move to Independence. 94.
Jewish Association on Aging (JAA), Pittsburgh, PA, $200,000. For Renaissance Campaign. 94.
Jewish Association on Aging (JAA), Pittsburgh, PA, $80,000. For challenge grant to establish Elderlink program. 94.
Jewish Association on Aging (JAA), Pittsburgh, PA, $75,000. For Renaissance Campaign. 94.
Jewish Association on Aging (JAA), Pittsburgh, PA, $10,000. For continuum of services for Jewish elderly. 94.
National Council of Jewish Women, Pittsburgh, PA, $25,000. For Council Care Adult Day Care. 94.
OMG Center for Institutional Learning, Philadelphia, PA, $30,000. For nutrition programs for frail elderly. 94.
Pittsburgh Mercy Foundation, Pittsburgh, PA, $40,000. For Fallsfree, falls prevention program for elderly. 94.
Riverview Towers, Pittsburgh, PA, $16,700. For home-based services for frail elders including fall prevention training. 94.
Riverview Towers, Pittsburgh, PA, $13,750. For home-based services for frail elders including fall prevention training. 94.
Southwestern Pennsylvania Partnership for Aging, Warrendale, PA, $15,000. To build regional approach to services for elderly. 94.
United Jewish Federation of Greater Pittsburgh, Pittsburgh, PA, $37,855. For Phase II of Continuum of Care for Jewish Seniors. 94.
University of Pittsburgh Medical Center, Pittsburgh, PA, $15,000. For Ladies Hospital Aid Society Follow-Me-Home Project. 94.

857
Donald P. Jones Foundation

P.O. Box 58910
Philadelphia 19102-8910
Contact: Arthur W. Jones, Trustee

Established in 1953 in PA.
Donor(s): Donald P. Jones.
Financial data (yr. ended 12/31/95): Assets, $1,591,243 (M); expenditures, $87,697; qualifying distributions, $77,290, including $75,725 for 89 grants (high: $3,000; low: $150).
Fields of interest: Education; Children & youth, services; Aging, centers & services.

Types of support: General/operating support, continuing support.
Limitations: Giving primarily in Delaware County, PA. No grants to individuals.
Application information: Application form not required.
Initial approach: Letter
Deadline(s): None
Trustees: Elizabeth J. Gilson, Arthur W. Jones, Lawrence T. Jones.
Number of staff: None.
EIN: 236259820
Grants for Aging:
Retired Senior Volunteer Program (RSVP) of Delaware County, Lansdowne, PA, $850. 94.

858
Kohn Foundation
1101 Market St., Suite 2400
Philadelphia 19107-2924 (215) 238-1700
Contact: Harold E. Kohn, Treas.

Established in 1965 in PA.
Donor(s): Harold E. Kohn.
Financial data (yr. ended 12/31/95): Assets, $612,688 (M); expenditures, $141,940; qualifying distributions, $139,763, including $137,374 for 40 grants (high: $50,000; low: $100).
Fields of interest: Theater; Higher education; Law school/education; Education; Hospitals (general); Aging, centers & services; Jewish agencies & temples; Aging; Israel.
Types of support: Annual campaigns, endowment funds, seed money, scholarship funds.
Limitations: Giving primarily in Philadelphia, PA, and Israel.
Application information: Application form not required.
Initial approach: Letter
Copies of proposal: 1
Deadline(s): None
Officers and Directors:* Edith Kohn,* Pres.; Joseph C. Kohn,* V.P. and Secy.; Harold E. Kohn,* Treas.; Ellen E. Goddard, Amy K. Goldberg.
Number of staff: None.
EIN: 236398546
Grants for Aging:
Philadelphia Geriatric Center, Philadelphia, PA, $10,000. 95.

859
John R. McCune Charitable Trust
1104 Commonwealth Bldg.
316 Fourth Ave.
Pittsburgh 15222 (412) 644-7796
Contact: James M. Edwards, Exec. Dir.

Established in 1972 in PA.
Donor(s): John R. McCune IV.‡
Financial data (yr. ended 11/30/94): Assets, $66,035,745 (M); expenditures, $3,683,498; qualifying distributions, $3,522,403, including $3,318,400 for 99 grants (high: $300,000; low: $5,000; average: $10,000-$50,000).
Purpose and activities: Emphasis on secondary and higher education, health services, church-related institutions, and social services.
Fields of interest: Secondary school/education; Higher education; Health care; Human services; Protestant agencies & churches; Aging.
Types of support: General/operating support, continuing support, capital campaigns, building/renovation, endowment funds, seed money.
Limitations: Giving primarily in southwestern PA.
Publications: Application guidelines.
Application information: Unsolicited proposals usually not accepted. Application form not required.
Initial approach: 2-page letter of inquiry
Copies of proposal: 1
Deadline(s): Feb. 1
Board meeting date(s): Annually
Final notification: Nov.
Dispensing Committee: David L. Edwards, Chair.; Janet McCune Edwards Anti, Molly McCune Cathey, James M. Edwards, John H. Edwards, Michael M. Edwards, Carrie McCune Katigan, Laurie M. Lewis, Sarah McCune Losinger, John R. McCune VI.
Trustee: Integra Trust Co., N.A.
Number of staff: 1 part-time professional; 1 part-time support.
EIN: 256160722

860
McCune Foundation
1104 Commonwealth Bldg.
316 Fourth Ave.
Pittsburgh 15222 (412) 644-8779
Contact: Henry S. Beukema, Exec. Dir.
FAX: (412) 644-8059

Established in 1979 in PA.
Donor(s): Charles L. McCune.‡
Financial data (yr. ended 09/30/95): Assets, $343,895,982 (M); expenditures, $15,443,260; qualifying distributions, $14,712,470, including $13,825,050 for 99 grants (high: $1,000,000; low: $2,500; average: $50,000-$500,000).
Purpose and activities: Following the donor's granting interests, the foundation emphasizes two major program areas: independent higher education and human services. The foundation also recognizes the importance of civic, cultural, and community-based organizations that are working to remedy the effects of economic dislocation, while addressing future issues. The foundation is particularly interested in collaborative approaches among groups involved in similar activities with similar purposes.
Fields of interest: Museums; Performing arts; Historic preservation/historical societies; Arts/cultural programs; Higher education; Adult education—literacy & basic skills; Libraries/library science; Health care; Medical research; Employment; Housing/shelter, development; Youth development, services; Human services; Youth, services; Aging, centers & services; Urban/community development; Community development; Leadership development; Public affairs; Aging.
Types of support: Capital campaigns, building/renovation, equipment, endowment funds, program development.
Limitations: Giving primarily in southwestern PA, with emphasis on the Pittsburgh area. No grants to individuals, or for general operating purposes; no loans.
Publications: Annual report (including application guidelines), application guidelines.
Application information: Applicants are encouraged to wait at least 3 years after receiving a grant before reapplying. Application form not required.
Initial approach: Letter of inquiry
Copies of proposal: 1
Deadline(s): None
Board meeting date(s): Apr., June, Sept., and Dec.
Final notification: 90 days
Officers: Henry S. Beukema, Exec. Dir.; Martha J. Perry, Assoc. Exec. Dir.
Distribution Committee: Richard D. Edwards, Chair.; James M. Edwards, John R. McCune, Jr.
Trustee: Integra Trust Co., N.A.
Staff: Elizabeth R. Lynn, Prog. Officer; Graham N. McGinnis, Grants Administrator.
Number of staff: 4 full-time professional; 2 full-time support.
EIN: 256210269
Grants for Aging:
Overbrook Community Council and Senior Citizen Center, Philadelphia, PA, $10,000. 94.
Southwestern Pennsylvania Partnership for Aging, Warrendale, PA, $150,000. 94.
Vintage, Pittsburgh, PA, $100,000. 94.

861
William V. and Catherine A. McKinney Charitable Foundation
c/o Integra Trust Co., N.A.
300 Fourth Ave.
Pittsburgh 15278-2241 (412) 644-8332
Contact: William M. Schmidt, V.P., Integra Trust Co., N.A.

Established in 1990 in PA.
Donor(s): Catherine A. McKinney.‡
Financial data (yr. ended 03/31/95): Assets, $2,898,395 (M); gifts received, $500,000; expenditures, $274,095; qualifying distributions, $261,163, including $251,600 for 22 grants (high: $50,000; low: $1,000).
Purpose and activities: Giving limited to organizations in western PA whose activities aid the elderly, disadvantaged youth and/or the disabled and support the arts.
Fields of interest: Performing arts; Children & youth, services; Aging, centers & services; Disabled; Aging.
Types of support: General/operating support, capital campaigns, endowment funds, program development, matching funds.
Limitations: Giving limited to western PA. No grants to individuals.
Application information: Application form not required.
Initial approach: Letter
Copies of proposal: 1
Deadline(s): None
Board meeting date(s): Varies
Trustee: Integra Trust Co., N.A.
Number of staff: None.
EIN: 251641619
Grants for Aging:
Saint Clair Hospital Foundation, Pittsburgh, PA, $10,000. For geriatric services endowment fund. 94.

862
Millard Foundation
P.O. Box 572
Wayne 19087
Contact: Marion Thompson, Secy.

Established around 1987.
Financial data (yr. ended 12/31/95): Assets, $273,396 (M); expenditures, $21,253; qualifying distributions, $19,742, including $4,881 for 4 grants (high: $3,000; low: $45) and $14,861 for 14 grants to individuals (high: $3,000; low: $383).
Fields of interest: Human services, special populations; Disabled; Aging.
Types of support: Grants to individuals.
Limitations: Giving primarily in PA.
Application information:
Initial approach: Letter
Deadline(s): None
Officers: John N. Irwin, Pres.; Marsha Solmssen, Secy.; Marion Thompson, Secy.; Philip Cohen, Treas.
EIN: 232452507

863
Charles M. Morris Charitable Trust
c/o Integra Trust Co., N.A., I.D.C. No. 1-021
300 Fourth Ave.
Pittsburgh 15278-2241
Contact: Joanna M. Mayo, V.P., Integra Trust Co., N.A.

Established in 1988 in PA.
Donor(s): Charles M. Morris.‡
Financial data (yr. ended 12/31/94): Assets, $21,183,323 (M); gifts received, $82,232; expenditures, $1,161,370; qualifying distributions, $1,089,963, including $1,045,900 for 29 grants (high: $600,000; low: $400; average: $400-$600,000).
Purpose and activities: Giving primarily to a Jewish home and hospital for the elderly.
Fields of interest: Family services; Aging, centers & services; Homeless, human services; Federated giving programs; Jewish agencies & temples; Religion; Aging; Homeless; General charitable giving.
Types of support: General/operating support, continuing support, capital campaigns, building/renovation, equipment.
Limitations: Giving primarily in Pittsburgh, PA. No grants to individuals.
Publications: 990-PF.
Application information: Application form required.
Initial approach: Letter
Copies of proposal: 4
Board meeting date(s): Varies
Final notification: Following board meetings
Trustee: Integra Trust Co., N.A.
Number of staff: None.
EIN: 256312920

864
The 1957 Charity Trust
P.O. Box 540
Plymouth Meeting 19462 (610) 828-8145
Contact: Judith L. Bardes, Mgr.

Trust established in 1957 in PA.
Donor(s): Elizabeth R. Moran.
Financial data (yr. ended 06/30/95): Assets, $16,234,346 (M); expenditures, $733,342; qualifying distributions, $771,510, including $688,051 for 170 grants (average: $1,000-$10,000).
Purpose and activities: Primary areas of interest include projects benefiting human service and social welfare organizations, youth, and early childhood education; giving also for environmental concerns, health care for the indigent, education, conservation, and culture.
Fields of interest: Early childhood education; Child development, education; Elementary school/education; Adult education—literacy & basic skills; Reading; Education; Natural resource conservation & protection; Environment; Medical care, rehabilitation; Health care; Substance abuse, services; Health associations; Housing/shelter, development; Youth development, services; Human services; Children & youth, services; Child development, services; Aging, centers & services; Homeless, human services; Community development; Leadership development; Minorities; Disabled; Aging; Economically disadvantaged; Homeless.
Types of support: General/operating support, continuing support, annual campaigns, capital campaigns, building/renovation, equipment, endowment funds, program development, seed money.
Limitations: Giving primarily in the five-county region in southeastern PA. No grants to individuals; no loans.
Publications: Application guidelines, program policy statement.
Application information: Accepts Delaware Valley Grantmakers Common Grant Application and Common Report Form.
Initial approach: Proposal
Copies of proposal: 1
Deadline(s): Jan. 15, May 15, and Sept. 15
Board meeting date(s): Feb., June, and Oct.
Final notification: Within 3 weeks
Committee Members and Trustees:* Elizabeth R. Moran,* Member; James M. Moran, Jr.,* Member; Frances M. Abbott, Caroline M. Lawrence, Elizabeth M. Legnini, Ranney Robert Moran, Roderic Zengeri, Mellon PSFS.
Number of staff: 1 part-time professional.
EIN: 236227603

865
Novak Family Foundation
2400 South Weccacoe Ave.
Philadelphia 19148
Contact: Everett Novak, Trustee

Established in 1986 in PA.
Financial data (yr. ended 11/30/95): Assets, $69,080 (M); expenditures, $2,113; qualifying distributions, $1,799, including $1,375 for grants.
Fields of interest: Jewish agencies & temples; Aging.
Limitations: Giving primarily in the Philadelphia, PA, area. No grants to individuals.
Application information: Generally contributes to pre-selected organizations, but unsolicited applications are reviewed by the trustees. Application form not required.
Deadline(s): None
Trustees: Ann Marie Novak, Everett Novak.
EIN: 222774823

866
PECO Energy Company Giving Program
(Formerly Philadelphia Electric Company Giving Program)
2301 Market St., 513-1
Philadelphia 19103 (215) 841-5555
Contact: Gwendolyn S. King, Sr. V.P.

Financial data (yr. ended 12/31/92): Total giving, $2,500,000, including $2,500,000 for grants.
Fields of interest: Arts/cultural programs; Higher education; Education; Health care; Health organizations; Human services; Aging, centers & services; Government/public administration; Disabled; Aging.
Types of support: General/operating support, capital campaigns, scholarship funds.
Limitations: Giving primarily in headquarters city and major operating locations. No grants to individuals.
Application information: Application form not required.
Initial approach: Letter
Board meeting date(s): Monthly
Final notification: 6 to 8 weeks

867
The Pew Charitable Trusts
One Commerce Sq.
2005 Market St., Suite 1700
Philadelphia 19103-7017 (215) 575-9050
Contact: Rebecca W. Rimel, Pres.
FAX: (215) 575-4939;
URL: http://www.pewtrusts.com

Pew Memorial Trust, J.N. Pew, Jr. Charitable Trust, J. Howard Pew Freedom Trust, Mabel Pew Myrin Trust, Medical Trust, Knollbrook Trust, and Mary Anderson Trust established in 1948, 1956, 1957, 1957, 1979, 1965, and 1957 respectively.
Donor(s): Mary Ethel Pew,‡ Mabel Pew Myrin,‡ J. Howard Pew,‡ Joseph N. Pew, Jr.‡
Financial data (yr. ended 12/31/95): Assets, $3,778,481,571 (M); expenditures, $208,930,383; qualifying distributions, $205,452,522, including $194,049,238 for grants (high: $5,000,000; low: $5,000; average: $200,000-$500,000), $16,178 for 148 employee matching gifts, $834,000 for 2 program-related investments and $79,636 for 65 in-kind gifts.
Purpose and activities: The Pew Charitable Trusts support the work of nonprofit organizations in the fields of culture, education, the environment, health and human services, public policy and religion. Through their grantmaking, the trusts seek to encourage individual development and personal achievement, cross-disciplinary problem solving, and innovative, practical approaches to meeting the changing needs of a global community. The trusts are based in Philadelphia and maintain a special commitment to the city and its neighboring region.

Fields of interest: Visual arts; Museums; Performing arts; Dance; Theater; Music; Humanities; Language & linguistics; Literature; Historic preservation/historical societies; Arts/cultural programs; Education, association; Education, research; Elementary/secondary education; Child development, education; Secondary school/education; Higher education; Theological school/education; Adult education—literacy & basic skills; Reading; Education; Natural resource conservation & protection; Energy; Environment; Wildlife preservation & protection; Family planning; Health care; Health associations; Biomedicine; Health organizations; Employment; Nutrition; Housing/shelter, development; Youth development, services; Youth development, citizenship; Human services; Youth, services; Child development, services; Family services; Aging, centers & services; Minorities/immigrants, centers & services; Homeless, human services; Human rights (international); International affairs; Civil rights; Urban/community development; Rural development; Community development; Voluntarism promotion; Engineering & technology; Biological sciences; Science; Social sciences; Population studies; International studies; Public policy, research; Government/public administration; Public affairs, citizen participation; Leadership development; Public affairs; Religion, research; Christian agencies & churches; Protestant agencies & churches; Religion; Minorities; African Americans; Latinos; Native Americans; Disabled; Aging; Women; Immigrants/refugees; Economically disadvantaged; Homeless; Caribbean; Eastern Europe; Africa; Latin America.
Types of support: General/operating support, continuing support, capital campaigns, building/renovation, program development, conferences/seminars, publication, seed money, fellowships, internships, research, technical assistance, consulting services, program-related investments/loans, exchange programs, matching funds.
Limitations: Giving primarily in Philadelphia, PA, and its neighboring region; giving also on a national and international basis. No grants to individuals, or for endowment funds, deficit financing, scholarships, or fellowships (except those identified or initiated by the trusts).
Publications: Annual report, grants list, occasional report, application guidelines.
Application information: Contact foundation for brochure on specific guidelines and limitations in each program area. Application form required.
Initial approach: Letter of inquiry (2 to 3 pages)
Copies of proposal: 1
Board meeting date(s): Mar., June, Sept., and Dec.
Final notification: Approximately 4 to 6 weeks after board meetings
Officers and Board Members:* Rebecca W. Rimel,* Pres. and C.E.O.; Nadya K. Shmavonian, Exec. V.P.; Susan W. Catherwood, Thomas W. Langfitt, M.D., Robert E. McDonald, Graham McKelvy Walker, J. Howard Pew II, J.N. Pew III, Joseph N. Pew IV, M.D., R. Anderson Pew, Sandy Pew.
Trustee: The Glenmede Trust Co.
Staff: Carolyn H. Asbury, Dir., Health and Human Services; Joel A. Carpenter, Dir., Religion; Marian A. Godfrey, Dir., Culture; Paul Light, Dir., Public Policy; Keith McKeown, Dir., Communications; Timothy F. Murray, Dir., Finance and Administration; Joshua S. Reichert, Dir., Environment; Robert B. Schwartz, Dir., Education; Peter Szanton, Interim Dir., Research and Eval.
Number of staff: 72 full-time professional; 3 part-time professional; 38 full-time support; 2 part-time support.
Grants for Aging:
Adult Care of Chester County, West Chester, PA, $50,000. For continued general operating support for adult day care services. 95.
Aid for Friends, Philadelphia, PA, $80,000. For continued general operating support to provide home-delivered meals and friendly visiting to homebound elderly people. 95.
Alzheimers Disease and Related Disorders Association of Greater Philadelphia, Philadelphia, PA, $100,000. For continued support of education and support services for families of Alzheimer's disease patients in African American communities in Philadelphia and Delaware counties. 95.
American Cancer Society, Philadelphia Division, Philadelphia, PA, $90,000. For continued support of homemaker and home health aide services for elderly, low-income cancer patients in Philadelphia and Montgomery Counties. 95.
Bucks County Opportunity Council, Doylestown, PA, $80,000. For continued support of health- and safety-related repairs to homes of elderly residents of Bucks County. 95.
California Association for Health Services at Home Foundation, Sacramento, CA, $385,000. To develop patient database on home health care costs and utilization that could serve as basis for developing managed care agreements. 95.
Center in the Park, Philadelphia, PA, $125,000. For continued general operating support to deliver in-home care, counseling and health promotion services to elderly people in city's northwest region. 95.
Central Montgomery Mental Health/Mental Retardation Center, Norristown, PA, $129,000. For mental health services for elderly people. 95.
Coalition of Advocates for the Rights of the Infirm Elderly (CARIE), Philadelphia, PA, $147,000. For continued support of CARIE LINE, telephone problem-solving service for vulnerable elderly people and their caregivers. 95.
Community Health Affiliates, Ardmore, PA, $190,000. For Continuum of Independent Living program, which provides array of long-term care services to elderly people living in subsidized housing. 95.
Community Legal Services, Philadelphia, PA, $50,000. For continued support of Hispanic Outreach Project for Elderly. 95.
Contact Bucks County, Richboro, PA, $30,000. For continued support of Reassurance CONTACT program to provide telephone reassurance and companionship to frail elderly people in Bucks County. 95.
Downingtown Senior Center, Downingtown, PA, $10,000. For continued general operating support. 95.
Energy Coordinating Agency of Philadelphia, Philadelphia, PA, $97,000. For Home Energy Fitness Program for elderly. 95.
Episcopal Community Services of the Diocese of Pennsylvania, Philadelphia, PA, $195,000. For continued support of in-home health, mental health and social services to low-income frail elderly people in Philadelphia. 95.
Family and Community Service of Delaware County, Media, PA, $84,000. For continued support of Older Adults Counseling Service project, to provide mental health counseling to isolated elderly persons. 95.
Family Service of Montgomery County, Norristown, PA, $80,000. For continued support of Project Hearth, to provide in-home services to fragile elderly persons in Pottstown. 95.
Horizons Unlimited Geriatric Education Corporation, Media, PA, $40,000. For continued support to provide cognitive stimulation to frail and isolated elderly people in Philadelphia nursing homes, senior centers and adult day care facilities. 95.
Jewish Community Centers of Greater Philadelphia, Philadelphia, PA, $110,000. For continued support of home-delivered meals, meals coordinator, and on-site nurse and social worker. 95.
Jewish Family and Childrens Service of Greater Philadelphia, Philadelphia, PA, $170,000. For continued support of Enhanced Home Services Project for frail elderly people. 95.
Korean Community Development Services Center, Philadelphia, PA, $80,000. To continue providing support services to low-income elderly Asian people. 95.
Lincoln Center for Family and Youth, Bridgeport, PA, $115,000. For continued support of Project Aspect to provide counseling support for elderly people and their caregivers during periods of life transition and crisis. 95.
Little Brothers Friends of the Elderly, Philadelphia, PA, $50,000. For Mental Health Outreach project for isolated elderly Philadelphians. 95.
Lower Merion-Narberth Coalition on Aging and Adult Services, Bryn Mawr, PA, $30,000. For continued general operating support to provide range of support services to needy elderly people. 95.
Lutheran Home at Germantown, HomeLink, Philadelphia, PA, $100,000. To expand home-delivered meals program in Philadelphia. 95.
Mid-County Senior Services, Newtown Square, PA, $80,000. For continued support of Community Resource Development Program to provide home support services to low-income, fragile elderly people. 95.
Montgomery County Association for the Blind, Norristown, PA, $60,000. For continued support of case management, and orientation and mobility training for blind and visually impaired elderly people. 95.
National Academy of Sciences, Institute of Medicine, DC, $25,000. To identify issues and develop recommendations to help ensure that managed care organizations provide quality care to Medicare beneficiaries, and that

elderly consumers can make well-informed decisions about participating in such plans. 95.
Neighborhood Health Agencies, West Chester, PA, $40,000. For continued support of Healthlink, program to monitor health status of elderly people discharged from skilled home care and to prevent avoidable rehospitalization. 95.
Oxford Area Neighborhood Services Center, Oxford, PA, $12,000. For continued support of Adopt-a-Friend, program to link homebound elderly people with volunteers and community-based services. 95.
Pennsylvania Association for the Blind, Delaware County Branch, Chester, PA, $65,000. For continued support of Homebound Rehabilitation program that teaches communication skills, home management and leisure time activities to visually impaired and blind elderly people in Delaware County. 95.
Pennsylvania Care Management Institute, Norristown, PA, $54,000. For continued operating support to provide training to care managers and other professionals who provide community-based care to needy elderly persons. 95.
Philadelphia Geriatric Center, Philadelphia, PA, $182,000. For continued support of Counseling for Caregivers Program. 95.
Philadelphia Senior Center, Philadelphia, PA, $132,000. For continued support of Financial Management Service Program. 95.
Retired Senior Volunteer Program (RSVP) of Montgomery County, Plymouth Meeting, PA, $70,000. For continued support of Eldercare Corps, which provides in-home services to elderly people. 95.
Retired Senior Volunteer Program (RSVP) of Montgomery County, Plymouth Meeting, PA, $12,000. For Volunteer Executive Consultants program to provide technical assistance to small nonprofit organizations in Montgomery County. 95.
Roxborough Memorial Hospital, Philadelphia, PA, $75,000. For Home Safety Assessment and Intervention Program for elderly. 95.
Salvation Army of Philadelphia, Divisional Headquarters, Philadelphia, PA, $90,000. To support Elderly Home Repair and Equipment Program. 95.
Senior Adult Activities Center of Montgomery County, Norristown, PA, $30,000. For continued support of adult day care services for frail elderly people. 95.
Senior Citizen Judicare Project of Philadelphia, Philadelphia, PA, $70,000. For continued support of Homeowner's Assistance Program. 95.
Senior Community Services, Folsom, PA, $100,000. To support Center without Walls Program. 95.
Senior Victim Services of Delaware County, Folsom, PA, $20,000. For continued general operating support to serve elderly victims of crime. 95.
Supportive Older Womens Network, Philadelphia, PA, $50,000. For continued operating support to establish support groups that serve elderly women. 95.
Temple University, Center for Intergenerational Learning, Philadelphia, PA, $120,000. For continued support of Time Out program to train and place college students as providers of respite care and home support services for infirm elderly and their caregivers. 95.
Tenants Action Group of Philadelphia, Philadelphia, PA, $85,000. For continued support of housing and financial counseling for elderly people. 95.
Thomas Jefferson University, Department of Family Medicine, Philadelphia, PA, $161,000. For continued support of Geriatric Assessment and Treatment Program. 95.
Trinity Memorial Church, Philadelphia, PA, $16,000. For continued support of Communicare, which provides friendly visiting to elderly people. 95.
United Polish American Social Services, Philadelphia, PA, $70,000. For continued general operating support to provide information, referral and benefits counseling services to frail elderly people, with focus on Eastern Europeans with language and cultural barriers. 95.
United Seniors Health Cooperative, DC, $375,000. For partially matching grant for Cooperative Caring Network demonstration project to expand volunteer services to elderly in greater Washington, DC area. 95.
University of Pennsylvania, School of Nursing, Philadelphia, PA, $97,000. For continued support of Collaborative Assessment and Rehabilitation for Elderly program. 95.
University of Pennsylvania, University of Pennsylvania Health System, Philadelphia, PA, $185,000. To provide in-home primary care and support services for elderly people who live in West and Southwest Philadelphia. 95.
Visiting Nurse Association of Greater Philadelphia, Philadelphia, PA, $95,000. For continued support of in-home nursing care management and mental health nursing services for frail elderly people. 95.
VNA Community Services, Abington, PA, $90,000. For continued support of in-home personal care and home support services to low-income elderly people in Montgomery and portions of Bucks and Philadelphia Counties. 95.

868
The Potamkin Foundation

130 Spruce St., Suite 30B
Philadelphia 19106

Established in 1985 in PA.
Donor(s): Members of the Potamkin family.
Financial data (yr. ended 05/31/95): Assets, $8,914 (M); expenditures, $45,747; qualifying distributions, $44,495, including $44,495 for grants.
Fields of interest: Law school/education; Hospitals (general); Health associations; Aging, centers & services.
Limitations: Applications not accepted. Giving primarily in Philadelphia, PA. No grants to individuals.
Application information: Contributes only to pre-selected organizations.
Directors: Alan Potamkin, Robert Potamkin, Victor Potamkin.
EIN: 236800690

869
PQ Corporation

P.O. Box 840
Valley Forge 19482 (610) 651-4205
Contact: Cora D. Barrow, Contribs. Administrator

Established in 1831.
Financial data (yr. ended 12/31/94): Total giving, $439,800, including $129,600 for 36 grants (high: $10,000; low: $500; average: $500-$1,000) and $271,520 for 752 employee matching gifts.
Purpose and activities: To assist the corporation in fulfilling its responsibility to institutions and community programs in areas in which it operates and abetting like efforts by individual employees, retirees, and shareholders.
Fields of interest: Arts/cultural programs; Employment; Food services; Youth development; Human services; Homeless, human services; Disabled; Aging; Economically disadvantaged; Homeless.
Types of support: General/operating support, capital campaigns, program development, employee matching gifts.
Limitations: Giving primarily in areas of company operations. No support for religious, political, or foreign organizations. No grants to individuals.
Publications: Informational brochure.
Application information: Executive Dept. handles giving. Application form not required.
Initial approach: Letter stating financial need to nearest company facility
Copies of proposal: 1
Deadline(s): None
Board meeting date(s): Four times a year
Number of staff: 1 part-time support.

870
Harry A. Robinson Foundation

Ponllyn Pike
P.O. Box 1233
Blue Bell 19422

Financial data (yr. ended 09/30/94): Assets, $134,653 (M); expenditures, $7,239; qualifying distributions, $6,500, including $6,500 for grants.
Fields of interest: Aging, centers & services; Aging.
Limitations: Applications not accepted.
Application information: Contributes only to pre-selected organizations.
Trustees: Fred Robinson, Herman Robinson.
EIN: 236243440

871
Lawrence Saunders Fund

c/o First Fidelity Bank, N.A., PA
Broad & Walnut Sts.
Philadelphia 19109
Contact: Maureen Evans, Trust Officer, First Fidelity Bank, N.A., PA

Established in 1970 in PA.
Financial data (yr. ended 12/31/95): Assets, $1,795,861 (M); expenditures, $82,295; qualifying distributions, $62,393, including $62,387 for 37 grants (high: $3,000; low: $500).

Fields of interest: Music; Historic preservation/historical societies; Arts/cultural programs; Elementary/secondary education; Child development, education; Family planning; Human services; Child development, services; Family services; Aging, centers & services; Protestant federated giving programs; Protestant agencies & churches; Aging.
Types of support: General/operating support, program development, seed money.
Limitations: Giving primarily in Philadelphia and Chester and Montgomery counties, PA. No grants to individuals.
Application information: Application form required.
Initial approach: Letter
Copies of proposal: 1
Deadline(s): None
Board meeting date(s): As needed
Trustees: Isaac H. Clothier IV, Esq., Kenneth W. Gemmill, Esq., Anne B. Kellett, First Fidelity Bank, N.A., PA.
Number of staff: 1 part-time professional.
EIN: 236488524
Grants for Aging:
Dolphins of Delaware County, Gladwyne, PA, $3,000. 94.
Dolphins of Delaware County, Gladwyne, PA, $2,000. 95.
Philadelphia Senior Center, Philadelphia, PA, $1,500. 94.
Saint Marys Family Respite Center, Philadelphia, PA, $2,000. 95.

872
Shaffer Family Charitable Trust
3548 Bingen Rd.
Bethlehem 18015

Established in 1987 in PA.
Donor(s): David Shaffer, Susan Shaffer, Jack M. Shaffer,‡ Cecile Shaffer, Rose Shaffer.
Financial data (yr. ended 12/31/95): Assets, $8,205,197 (M); gifts received, $425,000; expenditures, $303,974; qualifying distributions, $277,835, including $277,049 for 21 grants (high: $70,000; low: $750).
Purpose and activities: Support for capital and special projects not funded through normal income sources to social service agencies in the Lehigh Valley, PA, area.
Fields of interest: Human services; Children & youth, services; Aging, centers & services.
Types of support: Capital campaigns, building/renovation, program development, seed money.
Limitations: Giving primarily in Lehigh Valley, PA. No grants to individuals, or for ongoing operations.
Application information: Application form not required.
Initial approach: Proposal
Copies of proposal: 1
Deadline(s): None
Board meeting date(s): Quarterly
Trustees: Cecile Shaffer, David Shaffer, Rose Shaffer, Susan Shaffer.
Number of staff: None.
EIN: 232502319
Grants for Aging:
Bethlehem Senior Citizens Center, Bethlehem, PA, $10,000. 95.

873
Shenango Valley Foundation
272 East Connelly Blvd.
Sharon 16146 (412) 981-0900
Contact: Robert C. Jazwinski, Exec. V.P.
FAX: (412) 981-2154

Established in Oct. 1981.
Donor(s): Paul O'Brien, Tina O'Brien.
Foundation type: Community
Financial data (yr. ended 12/31/95): Assets, $9,990,916 (M); gifts received, $383,671; expenditures, $470,786, including $170,701 for 37 grants (high: $60,000; low: $200), $69,770 for 29 grants to individuals (high: $5,000; low: $50) and $671,350 for 137 loans to individuals.
Fields of interest: Early childhood education; Higher education; Education; Medical care, rehabilitation; Food services; Recreation; Homeless, human services; Community development; Disabled; Aging; Economically disadvantaged; General charitable giving.
Types of support: General/operating support, building/renovation, emergency funds, program development, scholarship funds, employee-related scholarships, grants to individuals, scholarships—to individuals, matching funds, student loans—to individuals.
Limitations: Giving limited to the Shenango Valley and Mercer County, PA, area, and Trumbull County, OH.
Publications: Informational brochure.
Application information: Application form required.
Initial approach: Letter
Copies of proposal: 1
Deadline(s): 2 weeks prior to Board meeting
Board meeting date(s): Quarterly
Final notification: 3 to 4 days after Board meeting
Officers and Trustees:* James E. Winner,* Pres.; Robert C. Jazwinski,* Exec. V.P.; James A. O'Brien,* V.P.; Karen Winner Hale,* Secy.; Ronald R. Anderson, Henry G. Evans, James E. Feeney, Mel Grata, Paul E. O'Brien, Albert R. Puntureri, William J. Strimbu, James T. Weller, Sr.
Number of staff: 1 part-time support.
EIN: 251407396

874
Shusterman Foundation
c/o Fox Rothschild Obrien & Frankel
2000 Market St., 10th Fl.
Philadelphia 19103-3231 (215) 299-2026
Contact: Murray H. Shusterman, Mgr.
Additional application address: c/o Robert J. Shusterman, Esq., 1608 Walnut St., 18th Fl., Philadelphia, PA 19103; Tel.: (215) 772-0200

Established in 1981.
Donor(s): Murray H. Shusterman.
Financial data (yr. ended 06/30/95): Assets, $1,207,737 (M); gifts received, $22,700; expenditures, $78,732; qualifying distributions, $76,311, including $76,311 for 44 grants (high: $40,100; low: $25).
Purpose and activities: Giving primarily for education, community funds, and general charitable giving.
Fields of interest: Historic preservation/historical societies; Arts/cultural programs; Higher education; Law school/education; Adult/continuing education; Education; Aging, centers & services; Civil rights; Federated giving programs; Jewish agencies & temples; Aging; General charitable giving.
Types of support: Continuing support, annual campaigns, capital campaigns, building/renovation, curriculum development, scholarship funds, research.
Limitations: Giving primarily in the Philadelphia, PA, and New York, NY, areas through local and national organizations.
Application information: Application form not required.
Initial approach: Letter
Copies of proposal: 1
Deadline(s): None
Officer and Directors:* Murray H. Shusterman,* Mgr.; Robert J. Shusterman.
Number of staff: 1
EIN: 232187215
Grants for Aging:
Philadelphia Geriatric Center, Philadelphia, PA, $400. 95.

875
The Juliet L. Hillman Simonds Foundation, Inc.
2000 Grant Bldg.
Pittsburgh 15219 (412) 338-3466
Contact: Ronald W. Wertz, Secy.

Established in 1986 in PA.
Donor(s): Juliet Lea Hillman Simonds, Henry Lea Hillman Charitable Lead Trust.
Financial data (yr. ended 12/31/95): Assets, $5,889,023 (M); gifts received, $539,920; expenditures, $280,330; qualifying distributions, $255,819, including $251,000 for 36 grants (high: $70,000; low: $500; average: $250-$15,000).
Fields of interest: Museums; Arts/cultural programs; Secondary school/education; Higher education; Domestic violence prevention; Disabled; Aging; Women; People with AIDS (PWAs); Economically disadvantaged; Homeless.
Types of support: General/operating support, capital campaigns, building/renovation, equipment, endowment funds, program development.
Limitations: Giving primarily in Pittsburgh, PA. No grants to individuals.
Publications: 990-PF, application guidelines.
Application information: Application form not required.
Initial approach: Proposal
Copies of proposal: 1
Deadline(s): None
Board meeting date(s): May and Dec.
Officers and Directors:* Juliet Lea Hillman Simonds,* Pres.; Mark Laskow,* V.P.; Ronald W. Wertz,* Secy.; Lawrence M. Wagner,* Treas.
Number of staff: 1 part-time professional.
EIN: 251536654

876
W. W. Smith Charitable Trust
10 South Bryn Mawr Ave.
Bryn Mawr 19010 (610) 525-9667

Contact: Frances R. Pemberton, Trust Administrator

Trust established in 1976 in PA.
Donor(s): William Wikoff Smith.‡
Financial data (yr. ended 06/30/95): Assets, $109,039,578 (M); expenditures, $4,937,392; qualifying distributions, $4,586,641, including $4,586,641 for 105 grants (high: $158,000; low: $5,000; average: $5,000-$100,000).
Purpose and activities: Support for college financial aid programs for qualified needy undergraduate students at accredited universities and colleges, and for basic scientific medical research programs dealing with cancer, AIDS, and heart disease, and programs of organizations providing shelter, food, and clothing for children and the aged.
Fields of interest: Higher education; Education; Hospitals (general); Health care; Cancer; Heart/circulatory disease; AIDS; Biomedicine; Health organizations; Medical research; Cancer research; Heart/circulatory research; AIDS research; Food services; Housing/shelter, development; Human services; Children & youth, services; Youth, services; Aging, centers & services; Women, centers & services; Minorities/immigrants, centers & services; Homeless, human services; Minorities; Aging; Women; Economically disadvantaged; Homeless.
Types of support: General/operating support, continuing support, building/renovation, equipment, emergency funds, program development, seed money, scholarship funds, research, matching funds.
Limitations: Giving primarily in the Delaware Valley, including Philadelphia, PA, and its six neighboring counties; grants to colleges by invitation only. No grants to individuals, or for deficit financing, existing endowment funds, or retroactive funding for non-emergencies; no grants over three consecutive years; no funding of events such as dinners, golf tournaments, and program ads.
Publications: Biennial report (including application guidelines).
Application information: College financial aid programs by invitation only; applications for medical research grants must be submitted in quadruplicate; application forms required for medical research only; accepts Delaware Valley Grantmakers Common Grant Application and Common Report Form.
Initial approach: Proposal, letter, or telephone requesting guidelines
Copies of proposal: 1
Deadline(s): No deadline for social service programs; for college scholarships, May 1; for cancer and AIDS research, June 15; and for heart research, Sept. 15
Board meeting date(s): For medical care, Mar.; social services, Mar. and Sept.; scholarships, June; cancer and AIDS research, Sept.; heart research, Dec.
Final notification: 1 month after trustees meet
Trustees: Mary L. Smith, CoreStates Bank, N.A.
Staff: Frances R. Pemberton, Trust Administrator; Louise A. Havens, Grant Administrator; Gloria J. Massucci, Account Administrator.
Number of staff: None.
EIN: 236648841

877
Hoxie Harrison Smith Foundation

(Formerly Smith Foundation)
210 Fairlamb Ave.
Havertown 19083 (610) 446-4651
Contact: Joseph H. Barber, Secy.-Treas.

Incorporated in 1920 in PA.
Donor(s): W. Hinckle Smith,‡ H. Harrison Smith.‡
Financial data (yr. ended 12/31/95): Assets, $7,863,193 (M); expenditures, $424,410; qualifying distributions, $391,554, including $366,050 for 52 grants (high: $37,000; low: $200).
Purpose and activities: To aid the sick, aged, and poor, as well as to aid in the education of needy boys and girls through local organizations engaged in such work; grants for hospitals, child welfare, the aged, and the handicapped.
Fields of interest: Education; Hospitals (general); Children & youth, services; Aging, centers & services; Disabled; Aging.
Types of support: Building/renovation, equipment, program development.
Limitations: Giving limited to southeastern PA, including Bucks, Chester, Delaware, Montgomery, and Philadelphia counties. No grants to individuals, or for endowment funds.
Publications: Annual report.
Application information: Application form not required.
Initial approach: Letter
Copies of proposal: 1
Deadline(s): Before Sept. 1
Board meeting date(s): Semiannually
Officers and Directors:* Roger P. Hollingsworth,* Pres.; Robert L. Strayer,* V.P.; Joseph H. Barber,* Secy.-Treas.; Charles P. Barber, Bruce M. Brown, Philip C. Burnham, Howard W. Busch, William Buchanan Gold, Jr., William Powell, Francis R. Veale.
Trustee Bank: Philadelphia National Bank.
EIN: 236238148

878
Snee-Reinhardt Charitable Foundation

2101 One Mellon Bank Ctr.
500 Grant St.
Pittsburgh 15219 (412) 471-2944
Contact: Joan E. Szymanski, Admin. Assoc.

Established in 1987 in PA.
Donor(s): Katherine E. Snee.
Financial data (yr. ended 12/31/95): Assets, $6,402,836 (M); gifts received, $233,928; expenditures, $305,638; qualifying distributions, $282,166, including $255,490 for 36 grants (high: $20,000; low: $500).
Fields of interest: Arts/cultural programs; Libraries/library science; Education; Environment; Health care; Substance abuse, services; Health associations; Cancer; Cancer research; Children & youth, services; Aging, centers & services; Community development; Aging.
Types of support: Building/renovation, program development, seed money.
Limitations: Giving primarily in PA (especially the southwestern region), northeast WV, and northern MD. No support for sectarian or religious organizations or organizations that promote abortion or euthanasia. No grants to individuals, or for capital improvement, endowment funds, or general operating expenses.
Publications: 990-PF, application guidelines, informational brochure (including application guidelines), grants list.
Application information: Application form required.
Initial approach: Telephone for guidelines
Copies of proposal: 1
Deadline(s): Varies
Board meeting date(s): May, Sept., and Nov.
Final notification: 2 weeks after board meeting
Officer and Directors:* Paul A. Heasley,* Chair.; Virginia M. Davis, Karen L. Heasley, Timothy Heasley, James W. Ummer, Richard T. Vail.
Trustee: Mellon Bank, N.A.
Number of staff: 2 full-time support.
EIN: 256292908

879
St. Benedict's Charitable Society

1663 Bristol Pike
Bensalem 19020 (215) 244-9900
Contact: Margaret Kuehmstedt, Treas.

Financial data (yr. ended 12/31/95): Assets, $226,477 (M); gifts received, $3,000; expenditures, $12,966; qualifying distributions, $12,966, including $10,700 for 42 grants (high: $1,300; low: $100) and $1,970 for 2 grants to individuals (high: $1,200; low: $770).
Purpose and activities: Relief assistance to aged, infirm, needy people for basic living, medical and funeral expenses; support also for Catholic churches, organizations and scholarship funds.
Fields of interest: Higher education; Aging, centers & services; Roman Catholic agencies & churches; Aging; Economically disadvantaged.
Types of support: Scholarship funds, grants to individuals.
Limitations: Applications not accepted. Giving on a national basis.
Application information: No new applications are being considered.
Officers: Sister Monica Loughlin, Pres.; Roger A. Johnsen, V.P.; Sister Beatrice Jeffries, Secy.; Margaret Kuehmstedt, Treas.
EIN: 236256990

880
James Sutton Home for Aged & Infirm Men Trust

c/o Robert W. Hall, CPA
39 Public Sq., Suite 300
Wilkes-Barre 18701
Contact: Secy. to the Trustees

Established in 1917 in PA.
Financial data (yr. ended 06/30/94): Assets, $1,839,976 (M); expenditures, $108,615; qualifying distributions, $102,803, including $26,000 for 4 grants of $6,500 each and $76,803 for 6 foundation-administered programs.
Purpose and activities: Support primarily for hospitals, churches, and social services; also operates a program that provides partial support

to aged and infirm men residing in Luzerne County, PA.
Fields of interest: Hospitals (general); Human services; Aging, centers & services; Protestant agencies & churches; Aging.
Limitations: Giving primarily in Wilkes-Barre, PA.
Application information: Application form required.
Deadline(s): None
Trustees: James I. Alexander, Richard Hogaboom, George Johnson.
EIN: 240795490

881
Teleflex Foundation
155 South Limerick Rd.
Limerick 19468-1699 (610) 948-5100
Contact: Robert Bertschy, Treas.

Established in 1980 in PA.
Donor(s): Teleflex, Inc.
Foundation type: Company-sponsored
Financial data (yr. ended 12/31/95): Assets, $993,413 (M); gifts received, $200,000; expenditures, $259,375; qualifying distributions, $259,267, including $259,267 for 245 grants (high: $30,250; low: $25; average: $1,000-$5,000).
Purpose and activities: Support for higher, elementary, and vocational education, literacy programs; hospitals and health, medical research, cancer care, rehabilitation programs for alcohol and drug abuse, science and technology; community funds and social services, including women and child welfare, family planning, and the handicapped; public affairs and policies; culture, especially fine and performing arts; environmental issues; and urban and civic affairs.
Fields of interest: Visual arts; Museums; Performing arts; Dance; Theater; Music; Historic preservation/historical societies; Arts/cultural programs; Elementary school/education; Vocational education; Higher education; Business school/education; Engineering school/education; Adult education—literacy & basic skills; Libraries/library science; Reading; Education; Natural resource conservation & protection; Environment; Wildlife preservation & protection; Hospitals (general); Family planning; Medical care, rehabilitation; Health care; Substance abuse, services; Mental health/crisis services; Health associations; Cancer; Alcoholism; Medical research; Cancer research; Crime/law enforcement; Food services; Human services; Children & youth, services; Family services; Hospices; Aging, centers & services; Women, centers & services; Minorities/immigrants, centers & services; Human rights (international); Urban/community development; Community development; Federated giving programs; Engineering & technology; Engineering; Science; Public policy, research; Government/public administration; Public affairs; Minorities; Disabled; Aging; Women; Economically disadvantaged.
Types of support: General/operating support, endowment funds, program development, seed money, curriculum development, employee matching gifts, matching funds.
Limitations: Applications not accepted. Giving primarily in areas of plant locations in CA, ME, MI, OH, PA, TX, CT, VA, MD, FL, AL, and UT.
Publications: Application guidelines.
Application information:
Board meeting date(s): Fall and spring
Officers: Lennox K. Black, Pres.; Bonnie Groff, Secy.; Robert Bertschy, Treas.
Directors: Chris Black, Thomas Byrne, M.C. Chisholm, Thelma Fretz, Diane Fukuda, William Haussmann, Anita Piacentino, Palmer Retzlaff.
Number of staff: 1 part-time professional; 1 part-time support.
EIN: 232104782

882
Harry C. Trexler Trust
33 South Seventh St., Suite 205
Allentown 18101 (610) 434-9645
Contact: Thomas H. Christman, Secy. to the Trustees
FAX: (610) 437-5721

Trust established in 1934 in PA.
Donor(s): Harry C. Trexler,‡ Mary M. Trexler.‡
Financial data (yr. ended 03/31/95): Assets, $72,914,705 (M); expenditures, $3,516,075; qualifying distributions, $3,081,493, including $2,897,477 for 120 grants (high: $932,812; low: $835; average: $2,000-$75,000).
Purpose and activities: The will provides that one-fourth of the income shall be added to the corpus, one-fourth paid to the City of Allentown for park purposes, and the remainder distributed to such charitable organizations and objects as shall be "of the most benefit to humanity," but limited to Allentown and Lehigh County, particularly for hospitals, churches, institutions for the care of the crippled and orphans, youth agencies, social services, cultural programs, and support of ministerial students at two named PA institutions.
Fields of interest: Arts/cultural programs; Higher education; Education; Hospitals (general); Recreation; Human services; Youth, services; Aging, centers & services; Disabled; Aging; Economically disadvantaged.
Types of support: General/operating support, continuing support, capital campaigns, building/renovation, equipment, land acquisition, matching funds.
Limitations: Giving limited to Lehigh County, PA. No grants to individuals, or for endowment funds, research, scholarships, or fellowships; no loans.
Publications: Occasional report, application guidelines.
Application information: Application form not required.
Initial approach: Letter
Copies of proposal: 1
Deadline(s): Dec. 31 for consideration at annual fund distribution
Board meeting date(s): Monthly; however, grant distribution takes place annually after Mar. 31
Final notification: June 1
Trustees: Dexter F. Baker, Philip I. Berman, Carl J.W. Hessinger, Kathryn Stephanoff, Richard K. White, M.D.
Staff: Thomas H. Christman, Secy. to the Trustees.
Number of staff: 2 full-time professional.
EIN: 231162215

883
Rae S. Uber Trust
c/o Mellon Bank, N.A.
P.O. Box 7236
Philadelphia 19101-7236 (215) 553-3208
Contact: Patricia Kling, Trust Officer, Mellon Bank, N.A.

Financial data (yr. ended 06/30/95): Assets, $771,861 (M); expenditures, $36,828; qualifying distributions, $34,591, including $33,250 for grants.
Purpose and activities: Awards grants for relief of the following groups: blind persons, crippled children, aged persons, and mentally disturbed, and also for cancer research.
Fields of interest: Mental health/crisis services; Cancer; Cancer research; Aging, centers & services; Disabled; Aging.
Limitations: Giving primarily in Philadelphia, PA. No grants to individuals.
Application information:
Initial approach: Proposal
Deadline(s): Nov. 15
Trustee: Mellon Bank, N.A.
EIN: 236578512

884
Visiting Nurse Association Foundation of Lebanon County
P.O. Box 1203
Lebanon 17042
Contact: Bonnie Yocum, Pres.

Foundation type: Operating
Financial data (yr. ended 06/30/95): Assets, $616,175 (M); expenditures, $32,895; qualifying distributions, $28,070, including $28,070 for grants.
Fields of interest: Nursing home/convalescent facility; Sexual abuse prevention; Mentally disabled, centers & services.
Types of support: General/operating support, equipment.
Limitations: Giving limited to Lebanon County, PA.
Application information:
Initial approach: Letter
Deadline(s): None
Officers: Bonnie Yocum, Pres.; Marion Cook, V.P.; Kathy Wolfson, Secy.; Brenda Denisar, Treas.
EIN: 231365981

885
A. H. and Helen L. Weiss Foundation
c/o PSFS Bldg.
12 South 12th St., 24th Fl.
Philadelphia 19107 (215) 351-2050
Contact: Edward N. Polisher, Trustee

Established about 1956.
Financial data (yr. ended 09/30/95): Assets, $301,731 (M); expenditures, $294,588; qualifying distributions, $283,889, including $283,889 for 46 grants (high: $159,035; low: $25).

Fields of interest: Language & linguistics; Literature; Elementary/secondary education; Higher education; Law school/education; Medical school/education; Theological school/education; Hospitals (general); Human services; Aging, centers & services; Women, centers & services; Jewish agencies & temples; Religion; Aging; Women.
Types of support: General/operating support, continuing support, internships.
Limitations: Giving primarily in Philadelphia, PA. No grants to individuals.
Application information: Application form not required.
Deadline(s): None
Trustees: Charles Lazrow, Edward N. Polisher, Helen L. Weiss.
EIN: 236298302
Grants for Aging:
Philadelphia Geriatric Center, Philadelphia, PA, $159,035. 95.

886
Henrietta Tower Wurts Memorial

c/o First Fidelity Bank, N.A., PA
Broad and Walnut Sts.
Philadelphia 19109 (215) 985-8712
Contact: Cecelia Lumsden, Asst. V.P., First Fidelity Bank, N.A., PA

Incorporated in 1934 in PA.
Donor(s): Henrietta Tower Wurts.‡
Financial data (yr. ended 12/31/95): Assets, $4,295,485 (M); expenditures, $144,935; qualifying distributions, $112,566, including $112,250 for grants (average: $2,000).
Purpose and activities: To contribute to nonsectarian corporate institutions which are engaged in helping or caring for people in need, or alleviating the conditions under which they live; grants primarily for the elderly, women, family and child welfare services, community development, and health services.
Fields of interest: Early childhood education; Education; Health care; Human services; Children & youth, services; Family services; Aging, centers & services; Women, centers & services; Homeless, human services; Community development; Minorities; Aging; Women; Economically disadvantaged; Homeless.
Types of support: General/operating support, continuing support, annual campaigns, equipment, emergency funds, seed money.
Limitations: Giving limited to Philadelphia, PA. No grants to individuals, or for endowment funds, scholarships, fellowships, or matching gifts; no loans.
Publications: Application guidelines, annual report (including application guidelines).
Application information: Application form required.
Initial approach: Letter
Copies of proposal: 9
Deadline(s): Submit proposal preferably before Jan. 1, May 1, or Sept. 30
Board meeting date(s): Feb., June, and Oct.
Final notification: 2 weeks after meeting
Officers and Directors:* S. Stoney Simons,* Pres.; Mrs. Henry T. Reath,* V.P.; Fay C. Potter, Treas.; Allison Anderson, Pamela G. Model, Nan Beth Rosso, Richard Ferree Smith.
Number of staff: 1 full-time professional; 1 full-time support.
EIN: 236297977
Grants for Aging:
Coalition of Advocates for the Rights of the Infirm Elderly (CARIE), Philadelphia, PA, $1,000. 94.

PUERTO RICO

887
Puerto Rico Community Foundation

Royal Bank Ctr. Bldg., Suite 1417
Hato Rey 00917 (809) 751-3822
Contact: Eliuth M. Alvarez, Administrator
Additional tel.: (809) 751-3885;
FAX: (809) 751-3297

Incorporated in 1984 in PR; began operations in 1985.
Foundation type: Community
Financial data (yr. ended 12/31/95): Assets, $15,041,030 (M); gifts received, $1,085,810; expenditures, $1,926,221, including $422,523 for grants and $947,893 for foundation-administered programs.
Purpose and activities: The foundation "seeks to contribute to the achievement of a healthier economy and enhance quality of life in Puerto Rico"; giving in areas such as economic development, educational associations, the elderly, community development, science and technological innovation, health, including AIDS programs, drug and alcohol abuse programs, arts and cultural activities, including dance and fine arts, criminal justice, agriculture, animal welfare, and civic affairs.
Fields of interest: Visual arts; Architecture; Performing arts; Dance; Arts/cultural programs; Education, association; Early childhood education; Child development, education; Adult/continuing education; Education; Natural resource conservation & protection; Animal welfare; Health care; Substance abuse, services; Health associations; AIDS; Alcoholism; AIDS research; Delinquency prevention/services; Crime/law enforcement; Agriculture; Human services; Child development, services; Aging, centers & services; Civil rights; Community development; Engineering & technology; Computer science; Science; Anthropology & sociology; Economics; Government/public administration; Minorities; Aging; Economically disadvantaged.
Types of support: General/operating support, continuing support, emergency funds, conferences/seminars, professorships, publication, research, technical assistance, consulting services, program-related investments/loans, matching funds.
Limitations: Giving limited to Puerto Rico. No support for religious organizations or commonly accepted community services. No grants to individuals, or for annual campaigns, seed money, endowments, deficit financing, or scholarships; generally no grants for building funds.
Publications: Annual report, newsletter, informational brochure (including application guidelines), 990-PF, financial statement.
Application information: Application form required.
Initial approach: Letter
Deadline(s): None
Board meeting date(s): June, Sept., Dec., and Mar.
Final notification: Within 2 weeks after board meetings
Officers and Directors:* Jaime R. Escalona,* Chair.; Nestor M. Mendez Gomez,* Vice-Chair.; Ethel Rios de Betancourt, Pres.; Mabel Burckhart,* Secy.; Ana Irma Villa,* Treas.; and 14 additional directors.
Staff: Eliuth Alvarez, Administrator; Nelson I. Colon, Prog. Dir.; Matilde Urrutia de Torres, Development Officer; Luis Vizoso, Prog. Dir.
Number of staff: 4 full-time professional; 5 full-time support.
EIN: 660413230

RHODE ISLAND

888
Edward Austin Trust

c/o Fleet Bank of Massachusetts, N.A.
Fleet Investment Svcs., P.O. Box 14777
East Providence 02914
Contact: Sarah Whitaker, V.P., Fleet Bank of Massachusetts, N.A.
Application address: c/o Fleet Bank of Massachusetts, N.A., 75 State St., Boston, MA 02109; Tel.: (617) 346-2484

Donor(s): Edward Austin.‡
Financial data (yr. ended 12/31/95): Assets, $378,821 (M); expenditures, $14,430; qualifying distributions, $12,809, including $10,000 for 2 grants of $5,000 each.
Fields of interest: Aging, centers & services; Aging; Economically disadvantaged.
Limitations: Giving primarily in the Boston, MA, area.
Application information: 2 copies of Grant Coversheet must be submitted.
Initial approach: Proposal
Copies of proposal: 1
Deadline(s): Sept. 15
Trustee: Fleet Bank of Massachusetts, N.A.
EIN: 046024257

889
Bristol Home for Aged Women

c/o Hospital Trust National Bank
P.O. Box 1597, T-05-01
Providence 02901-1597 (401) 278-8752
Contact: Deirdre W.S. Martin, V.P., Hospital Trust National Bank

Established in 1873 in RI.
Financial data (yr. ended 06/30/95): Assets, $1,266,946 (M); expenditures, $83,208; qualifying distributions, $72,024, including $70,838 for 10 grants (high: $15,000; low: $800).
Purpose and activities: Support primarily for needy, elderly women who are residents of Bristol County, RI, through service organizations.

Fields of interest: Food services; Human services; Aging, centers & services; Women, centers & services; Aging; Women.
Types of support: General/operating support.
Limitations: Giving limited to Bristol County, RI.
Application information: Application form required.
Initial approach: Letter
Copies of proposal: 1
Deadline(s): May 1
Board meeting date(s): June
Final notification: June
Officers: Mrs. Ralph Peters, Pres.; Mrs. Walter J. St. Germain, V.P.; Mrs. John B. McGregor, Secy.; Mrs. Alfred E. Newton, Treas.
Trustee: Hospital Trust National Bank.
EIN: 050262707
Grants for Aging:
East Bay Geriatric Center, Riverside, RI, $2,000. 95.
Meals on Wheels, $15,000. 94.
Meals on Wheels of Rhode Island, Providence, RI, $15,000. 95.
Senior Companion Program of Rhode Island, Providence, RI, $12,505. 94.
Senior Companion Program of Rhode Island, Providence, RI, $12,000. 95.
Senior Companion Program of Rhode Island, Providence, RI, $6,000. 94.
United Methodist Retirement and Health Care Centers, Providence, RI, $6,038. 95.

890
Hattie L. Carr Trust
c/o Fleet Bank of Massachusetts, N.A.
Fleet Investment Svcs., P.O. Box 14777
East Providence 02914

Financial data (yr. ended 12/31/95): Assets, $71,566 (M); expenditures, $4,728; qualifying distributions, $3,981, including $2,500 for grants.
Fields of interest: Human services; Aging, centers & services; Disabled; Aging.
Limitations: Giving limited to Brookline, MA.
Application information:
Initial approach: Letter
Deadline(s): Monthly
Trustee: Fleet Bank of Massachusetts, N.A.
EIN: 046051688

891
The Champlin Foundations
410 South Main St.
Providence 02903 (401) 421-3719
Contact: David A. King, Exec. Dir.

Trusts established in 1932, 1947, and 1975 in DE.
Donor(s): George S. Champlin,‡ Florence C. Hamilton,‡ Hope C. Neaves.‡
Financial data (yr. ended 12/31/95): Assets, $345,070,672 (M); gifts received, $13,223,643; expenditures, $14,025,138; qualifying distributions, $12,800,436, including $12,271,981 for 203 grants (high: $1,000,000; low: $600; average: $15,000-$70,000).
Purpose and activities: Giving primarily for conservation; higher, secondary, and other education, including libraries; health and hospitals; cultural activities, including historic preservation; scientific activities; and social and family services, including programs for youth and the elderly.
Fields of interest: Historic preservation/historical societies; Arts/cultural programs; Secondary school/education; Higher education; Libraries/library science; Education; Natural resource conservation & protection; Environment; Animal welfare; Hospitals (general); Family planning; Health care; Health organizations; Human services; Youth, services; Aging, centers & services; Engineering & technology; Science; Aging.
Types of support: Capital campaigns, building/renovation, equipment, land acquisition.
Limitations: Giving primarily in RI. No support for religious schools, books, films, videos, plays. No grants to individuals, or for general support, program or operating budgets, matching gifts, special projects, research, publications, conferences, or continuing support; no loans.
Publications: Program policy statement, application guidelines, annual report, grants list.
Application information: Application form not required.
Initial approach: 1-page letter
Copies of proposal: 1
Deadline(s): Submit proposal preferably between Apr. 1 and Aug. 31; deadline Aug. 31
Board meeting date(s): Nov.
Final notification: After Nov. meeting
Distribution Committee: David A. King, Exec. Dir.; Francis C. Carter, John Gorham, Louis R. Hampton, Earl W. Harrington, Jr., Robert W. Kenyon, Norma B. LaFreniere, John W. Linnell.
Trustee: PNC Bank, N.A.
Number of staff: 1 full-time professional; 2 part-time professional; 2 part-time support.
Grants for Aging:
Bethany Home of Rhode Island, Providence, RI, $52,000. 95.
Elizabeth Higginson Weeden Home for Indigent and Infirm Females, Pawtucket, RI, $20,000. 95.
Hattie Ide Chaffee Nursing Home, East Providence, RI, $80,000. 95.
Saint Elizabeth Home, Westminster Place, Providence, RI, $41,754. 95.
Steere House-Home for the Aged, Providence, RI, $100,000. 95.

892
Robert B. Cranston/Theophilus T. Pitman Fund
55 Memorial Blvd.
Newport 02840 (401) 847-0217
Contact: Vernon A. Harvey, Trustee
Application address: 18 Market Sq., Newport, RI 02840; Tel.: (401) 847-4260

Financial data (yr. ended 12/31/94): Assets, $1,451,550 (M); expenditures, $60,178; qualifying distributions, $48,532, including $46,532 for 206 grants to individuals.
Purpose and activities: Support for the aged, the temporarily indigent, indigent individuals, and organizations which assist them.
Fields of interest: Aging; Economically disadvantaged.
Types of support: General/operating support, grants to individuals.
Limitations: Giving limited to Newport County, RI.
Application information: Application form not required.
Initial approach: Personal appearance or reference from local welfare agencies
Deadline(s): None
Trustees: Allen S. Harlow, Vernon A. Harvey, Wilbur Nelson.
EIN: 056008897

893
George W. Davenport Charitable Trust
c/o Fleet National Bank of Massachusetts
P.O. Box 14777
East Providence 02914
Application address: Christa Keefe, Fleet National Bank of Massachusetts, Springfield, MA 01101; Tel.: (413) 772-4917

Financial data (yr. ended 12/31/95): Assets, $425,480 (M); expenditures, $28,106; qualifying distributions, $24,623, including $18,032 for 17 grants to individuals (high: $6,184; low: $64).
Purpose and activities: Grants for needy elderly women or couples living in Bernardston, Leyden, or Greenfield, MA.
Fields of interest: Aging, centers & services; Aging; Economically disadvantaged.
Types of support: Grants to individuals.
Limitations: Giving limited to residents of Bernardston, Leydon, and Greenfield, MA. No grants for direct charitable activities or program-related investments.
Application information: Application form required.
Deadline(s): None
Trustees: Stanley L. Cummings, Margaret P. Haigis, Irmarie Jones, Fleet National Bank of Massachusetts.
EIN: 046312563

894
Marvin and Roberta Holland Family Foundation
Four Woodland Terr.
Providence 02906-5808

Established in 1986 in RI.
Donor(s): Betsy Holland, Bruce Holland, Marvin S. Holland, Roberta Holland, American Chemical Works.
Financial data (yr. ended 12/31/94): Assets, $83,360 (M); gifts received, $22,000; expenditures, $37,734; qualifying distributions, $37,421, including $37,045 for grants.
Fields of interest: Higher education; Health care; Health organizations; Human services; Aging, centers & services; Jewish federated giving programs; Jewish agencies & temples; Aging.
Types of support: Scholarship funds.
Limitations: Applications not accepted. Giving primarily in Providence, RI. No grants to individuals.
Application information: Contributes only to pre-selected organizations.

Trustees: Bruce S. Holland, Marvin S. Holland, Roberta Holland.
EIN: 056080166

895
Horace A. Kimball and S. Ella Kimball Foundation

c/o The Washington Trust Co.
23 Broad St.
Westerly 02891 (401) 364-3565
Contact: Thomas F. Black III, Pres.
Application address: 130 Woodville Rd., Hope Valley, RI 02832

Incorporated in 1956 in DE.
Donor(s): H. Earle Kimball.‡
Financial data (yr. ended 09/30/95): Assets, $5,504,207 (M); expenditures, $197,573; qualifying distributions, $159,744, including $148,771 for 22 grants (high: $30,000; low: $500).
Fields of interest: Arts/cultural programs; Secondary school/education; Education; Natural resource conservation & protection; Environment; Animal welfare; Health care; Health associations; Human services; Youth, services; Aging, centers & services; Homeless, human services; Disabled; Aging; Economically disadvantaged; Homeless; General charitable giving.
Types of support: General/operating support, emergency funds, seed money, matching funds.
Limitations: Giving limited to RI, with emphasis on South County. No grants to individuals.
Publications: 990-PF.
Application information: Application form required.
Copies of proposal: 3
Deadline(s): None
Board meeting date(s): Varies
Officers and Trustees:* Thomas F. Black III,* Pres.; Norman D. Baker, Jr.,* Secy.-Treas.; F. Thomas Lenihan.
Number of staff: 1 part-time support.
EIN: 056006130
Grants for Aging:
Meals on Wheels of Rhode Island, Providence, RI, $10,000. For equipment. 95.

896
Margaret W. Leighton Trust

c/o Fleet Bank of Massachusetts, N.A.
Fleet Investment Svcs., P.O. Box 14777
East Providence 02914
Application address: c/o Fleet Bank of Massachusetts, N.A., 75 State St., Boston, MA 02109

Financial data (yr. ended 12/31/95): Assets, $170,200 (M); expenditures, $11,127; qualifying distributions, $10,249, including $8,710 for 67 grants to individuals of $130 each.
Purpose and activities: Grants only for residents of nursing homes in Newburyport, MA.
Fields of interest: Aging, centers & services; Aging.
Types of support: Grants to individuals.
Limitations: Giving limited to residents of Newburyport, MA.
Application information:
Initial approach: Letter
Deadline(s): Nov. 15
Trustee: Fleet Bank of Massachusetts, N.A.
EIN: 046025524

897
The Rhode Island Foundation

70 Elm St.
Providence 02903 (401) 274-4564
Contact: Ronald Thorpe, V.P., Progs.

Incorporated in 1916 in RI (includes The Rhode Island Community Foundation in 1984).
Foundation type: Community
Financial data (yr. ended 12/31/95): Assets, $231,543,675 (M); gifts received, $3,860,000; expenditures, $11,626,099, including $9,691,037 for 795 grants (high: $250,000; low: $56).
Purpose and activities: To promote educational and charitable activities which will tend to improve the living conditions and well-being of the inhabitants of RI; grants for capital and operating purposes principally to agencies working in the fields of education, health care, the arts and cultural affairs, youth, the aged, social services, urban affairs, historic preservation, and the environment. Some restricted grants for scholarships and medical research.
Fields of interest: Performing arts; Historic preservation/historical societies; Arts/cultural programs; Libraries/library science; Education; Natural resource conservation & protection; Environment; Animal welfare; Hospitals (general); Health care; Health associations; AIDS; Alcoholism; AIDS research; Legal services; Food services; Human services; Children & youth, services; Family services; Aging, centers & services; Minorities/immigrants, centers & services; Homeless, human services; Community development; Voluntarism promotion; Government/public administration; Public affairs; Minorities; Aging; Immigrants/refugees; Economically disadvantaged; Homeless.
Types of support: General/operating support, capital campaigns, building/renovation, equipment, land acquisition, emergency funds, program development, conferences/seminars, publication, seed money, fellowships, scholarship funds, research, technical assistance, consulting services, matching funds.
Limitations: Giving limited to RI. No support for religious organizations for sectarian purposes (except as specified by donors). No grants to individuals (except designated funds), or for endowment funds, annual campaigns, or deficit financing; no loans.
Publications: Annual report (including application guidelines), program policy statement, application guidelines, newsletter, informational brochure.
Application information: Priority given to first 25 applications received prior to each board meeting. Application form not required.
Initial approach: Letter (3- to 4-pages)
Copies of proposal: 5
Deadline(s): Approximately 2 months prior to board meetings
Board meeting date(s): Mar., July, and Nov.
Final notification: One week after board meeting
Officers: Ronald V. Gallo, Pres.; Carol Golden, V.P., Development; Robert D. Rosendale, V.P., Finance and Administration; Ronald D. Thorpe, Jr., V.P., Progs.
Distribution Committee and Board of Directors: Melvin G. Alperin, Chair.; Ann F. Conner, Vice-Chair.; Paul J. Choquette, Jr., B. Jae Clanton, William H. Heisler III, Edward L. Maggiacomo, Norman Estes McCulloch, Jr., Pablo Rodriguez, John W. Wall.
Trustees: Citizens Bank, Fleet Bank, N.A., Hospital Trust National Bank, Van Liew Trust Co., The Washington Trust Co.
Staff: Melvin J. Bell, Jr., Prog. Officer; Nellie M. Gorbea, Prog. Officer; Ruth Hersh, Prog. Officer; Karen Voci, Prog. Officer; Catherine B. Walsh, Prog. Officer; Gregory Duyck, Donor Services Officer; Rick Schwartz, Dir., Communications; Carol Scott, Special Funds Officer.
Number of staff: 6 full-time professional; 3 part-time professional; 4 full-time support; 1 part-time support.
EIN: 050208270
Grants for Aging:
Central Adult Day Care Services, Warwick, RI, $10,000. For general support. 94.
East Bay Geriatric Center, Riverside, RI, $10,000. For asbestos removal. 94.
New England Gerontology Academy, Warwick, RI, $15,000. For general support. 94.
Saint Francis Home, Woonsocket, RI, $10,720. For general support. 94.
Tockwotton Home, Providence, RI, $11,900. For general support. 94.
Tockwotton Home, Providence, RI, $11,860. For general support. 94.

898
Charles Nelson Robinson Fund

c/o Fleet Investment Svcs.
P.O. Box 14777
East Providence 02914 (860) 244-6871
Contact: Diane O. Stables, Investment Svcs. Officer

Trust established in 1928 in CT.
Donor(s): Charles Nelson Robinson.‡
Financial data (yr. ended 06/30/95): Assets, $2,943,850 (M); expenditures, $102,950; qualifying distributions, $94,912, including $77,780 for 26 grants (high: $5,000; low: $500).
Purpose and activities: To aid "organized charities having a principal office in the City of Hartford"; support for social service agencies, including aid for the aged and youth, secondary education, and cultural programs.
Fields of interest: Arts/cultural programs; Secondary school/education; Human services; Children & youth, services; Aging, centers & services; Aging.
Types of support: Program development.
Limitations: Giving primarily in Hartford, CT. No grants to individuals, or for endowment funds.
Publications: Application guidelines.
Application information: Application form required.
Initial approach: Letter
Copies of proposal: 6

Deadline(s): Feb. 15 and Aug. 15
Board meeting date(s): Apr. and Oct.
Trustee: Fleet Bank, N.A.
EIN: 066029468
Grants for Aging:
Big Brothers/Big Sisters, Nutmeg/Foster Grandparents, Hartford, CT, $5,000. 94.

899
Townsend Aid for the Aged
c/o Helen Tennant
Eight Eadie St.
Newport 02840
Application address: 12 Madeline Dr., Newport, RI 02840

Established in 1882 in RI.
Financial data (yr. ended 04/30/95): Assets, $1,822,474 (M); expenditures, $100,530; qualifying distributions, $94,462, including $83,350 for grants to individuals.
Purpose and activities: Provides aid to the needy elderly.
Fields of interest: Aging, centers & services; Aging; Economically disadvantaged.
Types of support: Grants to individuals.
Limitations: Applications not accepted. Giving limited to residents of the City of Newport, RI.
Application information: Foundation initiates application process.
Officers: Helen S. Tennant, Pres.; Carolyn Kaull, V.P.; Janice M. Barrows, Treas.
EIN: 056009549

900
The Wikstrom Foundation
c/o Fleet Trust Co., Fleet Investment Svcs.
P.O. Box 14777
East Providence 02914
Additional address: c/o Fleet Trust Co., One Clinton Sq., Syracuse, NY 13221

Established in 1960 in NY.
Donor(s): A.S. Wikstrom,‡ Wikstrom Liquidating Trust.
Financial data (yr. ended 12/31/95): Assets, $1,476,062 (M); gifts received, $150,087; expenditures, $115,133; qualifying distributions, $111,860, including $108,500 for 19 grants (high: $15,000; low: $500).
Fields of interest: Arts/cultural programs; Higher education; Aging, centers & services; Aging; Christian agencies & churches.
Types of support: General/operating support, continuing support, annual campaigns, capital campaigns.
Limitations: Giving limited to NY, with emphasis on Onondaga and Monroe counties. No grants to individuals; no loans.
Application information:
Deadline(s): None
Trustee: Fleet Trust Co.
Number of staff: None.
EIN: 146014286

SOUTH CAROLINA

901
The Abney Foundation
1214 North Main St., Suite D
Anderson 29621 (864) 964-9201
Contact: Carl T. Edwards, Exec. Dir.

Trust established in 1957 in SC.
Donor(s): John S. Abney,‡ Susie M. Abney.‡
Financial data (yr. ended 12/31/95): Assets, $32,090,649 (M); expenditures, $1,418,347; qualifying distributions, $1,297,152, including $1,246,000 for grants (high: $250,000; low: $2,900; average: $5,000-$100,000).
Purpose and activities: Support primarily for higher education; some grants for social service and youth organizations.
Fields of interest: Higher education; Human services; Youth, services; Aging.
Types of support: General/operating support, continuing support, annual campaigns, building/renovation, equipment, land acquisition, endowment funds, emergency funds, professorships, seed money, fellowships, internships, scholarship funds, research.
Limitations: Giving primarily in SC, with emphasis on the Anderson area. No grants to individuals, or for matching gifts; no loans.
Publications: Application guidelines.
Application information: Application form not required.
Initial approach: Letter to request application guidelines
Copies of proposal: 1
Deadline(s): Submit proposal preferably during the 1st half of the year; no set deadline
Board meeting date(s): June and Dec.
Officers and Trustees:* J.R. Fulp, Jr.,* Chair.; Carl T. Edwards,* Vice-Chair. and Exec. Dir.; William N. Bobo,* Secy.; D. Wellsman Johnson,* Treas.; Lebrena F. Campbell, John R. Fulp III, Carlette F. Holmes, Sally A. Rose.
Number of staff: 1 full-time professional; 1 part-time support.
EIN: 576019445

902
The Bailey Foundation
P.O. Box 494
Clinton 29325 (803) 833-1910
Contact: H. William Carter, Jr., Administrator

Trust established in 1951 in SC.
Donor(s): M.S. Bailey & Son, Bankers, Clinton Investment Co.
Financial data (yr. ended 08/31/95): Assets, $4,795,748 (M); gifts received, $73,125; expenditures, $257,961; qualifying distributions, $235,280, including $185,100 for grants (high: $35,000; low: $100), $24,000 for 9 grants to individuals (high: $4,000; low: $1,500; average: $3,000) and $26,180 for 16 employee matching gifts.
Purpose and activities: Support primarily for higher education, including a scholarship program for graduating seniors at local high schools accepted in a degree-granting four-year college or university; support also for churches, community services, libraries, museums, and social services including child welfare and development and the elderly.
Fields of interest: Higher education; Libraries/library science; Education; Human services; Children & youth, services; Child development, services; Aging, centers & services; Community development; Religion; Aging.
Types of support: Capital campaigns, building/renovation, endowment funds, scholarship funds, employee matching gifts, matching funds.
Limitations: Giving primarily in Laurens County, SC. No grants to individuals (except scholarships for students attending local high schools), or for operating expenses.
Publications: Annual report, informational brochure (including application guidelines), 990-PF.
Application information: Applications for students available from guidance counselors at Clinton High School and Laurens High School. Application form not required.
Initial approach: For grants, write administrator
Copies of proposal: 1
Deadline(s): For scholarships, Apr. 15 of applicant's senior year in high school
Board meeting date(s): Periodically
Final notification: May 15
Trustee: M.S. Bailey & Son, Bankers.
Advisory Committee: Emily F. Bailey, George H. Cornelson, C. Bailey Dixon, Toccoa W. Switzer, Robert M. Vance, James Von Hollen.
Grants Advisory Committee: Joseph O. Nixon, Chair.; Linwood Floyd, W.E. Little, Virginia McMurray, Susan Polson, Donny Ross, Donny Wilder.
Number of staff: None.
EIN: 576018387
Grants for Aging:
Laurens Memorial Home for the Aged, Laurens, SC, $500. 94.

903
Central Carolina Community Foundation
P.O. Box 11222
Columbia 29211-1222 (803) 254-5601
Contact: Mary Choate

Incorporated in 1984 in SC.
Foundation type: Community
Financial data (yr. ended 06/30/95): Assets, $15,946,679 (M); gifts received, $1,223,966; expenditures, $924,804, including $570,442 for 115 grants (high: $22,500; low: $25; average: $3,000-$5,000).
Purpose and activities: Giving primarily for the arts, education, health services, the disadvantaged, and youth; support also for community development, literacy programs, delinquency and child welfare, child development and family services, family planning, and recreation.
Fields of interest: Music; Arts/cultural programs; Early childhood education; Child development, education; Elementary school/education; Adult education—literacy & basic skills; Reading; Education; Family planning; Health care; Substance abuse, services; Health associations; AIDS; Delinquency prevention/services; Crime/law enforcement; Nutrition;

Housing/shelter, development; Recreation; Human services; Children & youth, services; Child development, services; Family services; Aging, centers & services; Homeless, human services; Community development; Government/public administration; Aging; Economically disadvantaged; Homeless.
Types of support: Equipment, program development, seed money, matching funds.
Limitations: Giving limited to Calhoun, Clarendon, Fairfield, Kershaw, Lee, Lexington, Newberry, Orangeburg, Richland, Saluda, and Sumter counties, SC. No grants to individuals (except for designated awards or prizes), or for endowments, debt reduction, fundraising projects, medical research, publications, annual appeals, or routine operating expenses.
Publications: Annual report (including application guidelines), application guidelines, newsletter, grants list.
Application information: Application form required.
Initial approach: Letter or telephone
Copies of proposal: 1
Deadline(s): None
Board meeting date(s): Quarterly
Final notification: May, Oct., and Dec.
Officers and Directors:* Francis P. Mood,* Pres.; John W. Folsom,* V.P.; Robert E. Staton,* V.P.; E. Perry Palmer,* Secy.-Treas.; J. Mac Bennett, Exec. Dir.; and 30 additional directors.
Staff: Mary Wyatt Choate, Assoc. Dir.; Cindy S. Conrads, Financial Officer; Ann Lyons, Admin. Asst.
Number of staff: 2 full-time professional; 1 part-time professional; 1 full-time support.
EIN: 570793960
Grants for Aging:
Council on Aging of the Midlands, Columbia, SC, $5,000. For Neighborcare project. 94.

904
Colonial Life and Accident Insurance Company Contributions Program

1200 Colonial Life Blvd. West
Columbia 29210 (803) 798-7000
Contact: Robert E. Staton, Sr. V.P.
Application address: P.O. Box 1365, Columbia, SC 29202

Established in 1939 in SC.
Financial data (yr. ended 12/31/92): Total giving, $475,000, including $475,000 for grants.
Purpose and activities: Primary support for education, especially K-12; giving also for a variety of other programs.
Fields of interest: Visual arts; Performing arts; Humanities; Historic preservation/historical societies; Arts/cultural programs; Education, association; Education, research; Education, fund raising; Early childhood education; Elementary school/education; Business school/education; Adult/continuing education; Libraries/library science; Natural resource conservation & protection; Environment; Animal welfare; Hospitals (general); Family planning; Nursing care; Health care; Substance abuse, services; Mental health/crisis services; Cancer; Heart/circulatory disease; AIDS; Alcoholism; Health organizations; Cancer research; Heart/circulatory research; AIDS research; Crime/law enforcement; Food services; Housing/shelter, development; Youth development, citizenship; Human services; Children & youth, services; Family services; Aging, centers & services; Human rights (international); Civil rights; Government/public administration; Public affairs, citizen participation; Minorities; Disabled; Aging; Economically disadvantaged.
Types of support: General/operating support, continuing support, annual campaigns, capital campaigns, building/renovation, land acquisition, endowment funds, emergency funds, conferences/seminars, fellowships, internships, scholarship funds, employee volunteer services, loaned talent, use of facilities, employee matching gifts.
Limitations: Giving limited to cities and counties in SC, with emphasis on headquarters area.
Application information: Contributions handled by office of Vice-Chair.
Initial approach: Send requests to headquarters
Number of staff: 1 full-time professional; 1 full-time support.

905
Edgefield County Foundation

108 1/2 Courthouse Sq.
P.O. Box 388
Edgefield 29824

Established in 1991 in SC.
Donor(s): Bettis C. Rainsford.
Financial data (yr. ended 12/31/93): Assets, $579,094 (M); gifts received, $44,500; expenditures, $181,556; qualifying distributions, $177,986, including $106,333 for 4 grants (high: $77,639; low: $1,000).
Fields of interest: Historic preservation/historical societies; Arts/cultural programs; Education; Aging, centers & services.
Limitations: Applications not accepted. Giving limited to Edgefield, SC.
Application information: Contributes only to pre-selected organizations.
Officers and Trustees:* Bettis C. Rainsford,* Chair.; Nancy Thurmond, Pres.; Joseph F. Anderson, Butler C. Derrick, Jr., Albert E. Rainsford, Jr., J. Strom Thurmond, Jr.
EIN: 570945737

906
Francis Nathaniel and Katheryn Padgett Kennedy Foundation

933 Sunset Dr.
Greenwood 29646
Contact: Dr. Don Johnson, Admin. Asst.

Established in 1973 in SC.
Donor(s): Katheryn Padgett Kennedy,‡ Francis Nathaniel Kennedy.‡
Financial data (yr. ended 06/30/95): Assets, $1,320,400 (M); expenditures, $73,403; qualifying distributions, $63,100, including $40,800 for 10 grants (high: $14,000; low: $300; average: $300-$14,000) and $22,300 for 46 grants to individuals (high: $1,000; low: $300; average: $300-$1,000).
Purpose and activities: Grants largely for higher education and missionary programs; scholarships to young men and women primarily in the Piedmont section of SC studying at an accredited college for the ministry in the Southern Baptist Church and for foreign mission work or Christian education in their local church; support also for youth agencies and a church.
Fields of interest: Higher education; Theological school/education; Education; Human services; Children & youth, services; Youth, services; Hospices; Aging, centers & services; International economic development; Protestant federated giving programs; Christian agencies & churches; Protestant agencies & churches; Religion; Aging.
Types of support: Continuing support, annual campaigns, scholarship funds, scholarships—to individuals.
Limitations: Giving primarily in Laurens County and the upper Piedmont sections of SC. No grants for capital needs; no loans.
Publications: Informational brochure (including application guidelines), application guidelines.
Application information: Application form required for scholarships for ministry students, available upon written request. Application form required.
Initial approach: Letter
Copies of proposal: 1
Deadline(s): Mar. 15 for scholarships
Board meeting date(s): Oct., June, and as required
Final notification: Prior to July 10
Officer and Trustees:* John P. Faris,* Chair.; James E. Bryan, Jr., L. Leon Patterson, John C. Sharp, Sam M. Smith.
Number of staff: 1 part-time professional.
EIN: 237347655
Grants for Aging:
Martha Franks Retirement Home, Laurens, SC, $2,760. 94.

907
The Self Foundation

P.O. Drawer 1017
Greenwood 29648 (803) 941-4036
Contact: Frank J. Wideman III, Pres.

Incorporated in 1942 in SC.
Donor(s): James C. Self.‡
Financial data (yr. ended 12/31/95): Assets, $34,010,327 (M); gifts received, $100; expenditures, $1,706,419; qualifying distributions, $1,451,824, including $1,278,902 for 18 grants (high: $342,000; low: $750; average: $20,000).
Purpose and activities: Primary interest in health care and higher education. Support also for civic and community service, activities for youth and the elderly, and cultural and historical activities; grants mainly for capital or special purposes.
Fields of interest: Arts/cultural programs; Education; Health care; Youth, services; Aging, centers & services; Community development, neighborhood development; Aging.
Types of support: Equipment, emergency funds, program development, seed money, technical assistance, matching funds.
Limitations: Giving limited to SC, with primary emphasis on Greenwood. No grants to individuals, or for endowment funds, land

acquisition, operating budgets, continuing support, annual campaigns, deficit financing, publications, conferences, scholarships, fellowships, or research-related programs; no loans.
Publications: Annual report (including application guidelines).
Application information: Application form not required.
Initial approach: Proposal
Copies of proposal: 1
Deadline(s): Submit proposal preferably in the 2 months prior to board meetings; deadlines, 1st day of month in which board meets
Board meeting date(s): 3rd week in Mar., June, Sept., and Dec.
Final notification: 10 days after board meeting
Officers and Trustees:* Virginia S. Brennan,* Chair.; W.M. Self,* Vice-Chair.; Frank J. Wideman III, Pres.; Sally S. Harley, M.D.,* Secy.; William B. Allin, Treas.; G.W. Ballentine, David L. Bell, J.C. Self III, Paul E. Welder.
Number of staff: 1 full-time professional.
EIN: 570400594
Grants for Aging:
Greenwood Methodist Home, Greenwood, SC, $125,000. For Health Center rehabilitation. 94.

908
The Stringer Foundation
Nine Burbridge Court
Greenville 29605
Contact: John S. Rainey, Chair.

Established in 1947.
Financial data (yr. ended 12/31/94): Assets, $733,812 (M); expenditures, $43,411; qualifying distributions, $33,994, including $31,452 for grants.
Fields of interest: Higher education; Human services; Protestant agencies & churches; Aging.
Limitations: Giving primarily in SC.
Application information:
Initial approach: Letter
Deadline(s): Sept. 10
Officer and Trustees:* John S. Rainey,* Chair. and Pres.; Mary R. Belser, Nancy Crowley, Robert M. Rainey, Leila Stringer, W.K. Stringer III.
EIN: 576022719

SOUTH DAKOTA

909
Alzheimers and Other Charities Fund
(Formerly Larry Pressler Charitable Foundation)
513 South Main Ave.
Sioux Falls 57102-0992 (605) 336-2880
Contact: Dave Knutson

Established in 1988 in SD.
Donor(s): Larry Pressler.
Financial data (yr. ended 12/31/94): Assets, $11,648 (M); gifts received, $5,500; expenditures, $2,772; qualifying distributions, $2,520, including $2,520 for 17 grants (high: $300; low: $25).
Fields of interest: Arts/cultural programs; Alzheimer's disease; Disasters, preparedness & services; Human services; Religion; Disabled; Aging.
Limitations: Giving primarily in SD. No grants to individuals.
Application information:
Initial approach: Letter or proposal
Deadline(s): None
Officers: Larry Pressler, Pres.; Harriet Pressler, V.P.; Richard Cutler, Secy.-Treas.
EIN: 363627215

910
Sheldon F. Reese Foundation
P.O. Box 89704
Sioux Falls 57105-9057

Established about 1980 in SD.
Donor(s): Sheldon F. Reese.‡
Financial data (yr. ended 12/31/94): Assets, $2,983,116 (M); expenditures, $155,694; qualifying distributions, $128,130, including $126,000 for grants.
Fields of interest: Human services; Children & youth, services; Aging, centers & services; Community development; Aging.
Types of support: General/operating support.
Limitations: Giving primarily in SD, with some emphasis on Sioux Falls.
Application information: Application form required.
Deadline(s): Apr. 30
Final notification: May 31
Officers: John Quello, Pres. and Treas.; Oscar M. Austad, V.P.; Virginia Pavelka Luke, Secy.
Directors: Ernest G. Carlsen, Vance Goldammer.
EIN: 460358682

TENNESSEE

911
Aladdin Industries Foundation, Inc.
703 Murfreesboro Rd.
Nashville 37210-4521 (615) 748-3360
Contact: L.B. Jenkins, Secy.-Treas.

Incorporated in 1964 in TN.
Donor(s): Aladdin Industries.
Foundation type: Company-sponsored
Financial data (yr. ended 12/31/92): Assets, $2,198,296 (M); gifts received, $100,000; expenditures, $139,557; qualifying distributions, $132,479, including $132,395 for 58 grants (high: $33,750; low: $100).
Fields of interest: Music; Education; Substance abuse, services; Youth, services; Aging, centers & services; Business & industry; Aging.
Types of support: General/operating support, seed money, employee-related scholarships.
Limitations: Giving primarily in TN. No grants to individuals.
Application information:
Initial approach: Letter
Deadline(s): Current calendar year
Board meeting date(s): Quarterly
Officer and Directors:* Lillian B. Jenkins,* Secy.-Treas.; V.S. Johnson III, Frederick R. Meyer.
EIN: 620701769

912
Dantzler Bond Ansley Foundation
c/o SunTrust Bank, Nashville, N.A.
P.O. Box 305110, Mail Code NA-6410
Nashville 37230-5110 (615) 748-4234
Contact: Kim Williams, Trust Officer, SunTrust Bank, Nashville, N.A.

Incorporated in 1980 in TN.
Donor(s): Mildred B. Ansley.‡
Financial data (yr. ended 04/30/94): Assets, $7,307,800 (M); expenditures, $316,165; qualifying distributions, $294,388, including $272,500 for 44 grants (high: $50,000; low: $100).
Fields of interest: Arts/cultural programs; Secondary school/education; Higher education; Health care; Alcoholism; Health organizations; Medical research; Human services; Aging; Homeless.
Types of support: General/operating support, scholarship funds.
Limitations: Giving primarily in central TN, including Nashville.
Application information: Application form not required.
Copies of proposal: 3
Deadline(s): May 31
Trustees: Frank Drowota, Thomas F. Frist, Fred Russell, SunTrust Bank, Nashville, N.A.
EIN: 592111990

913
The Jeniam Clarkson Foundation
270 Bremington Place
Memphis 38111
Contact: Charlotte Giannini, Exec. Dir.
Application address: 3030 Poplar Ave., Memphis, TN 38111; Tel.: (901) 485-7175

Established in 1992 in TN.
Donor(s): Andrew M. Clarkson, Carole G. Clarkson.
Financial data (yr. ended 12/31/94): Assets, $5,598,616 (M); gifts received, $120,000; expenditures, $228,474; qualifying distributions, $228,474, including $225,054 for 21 grants (high: $40,000; low: $250).
Fields of interest: Arts, multipurpose centers/programs; Museums (children's); Education; Natural resource conservation & protection; Nursing home/convalescent facility; Camps; Youth development, services; Aging.
Types of support: Capital campaigns, building/renovation, equipment, seed money, research.
Limitations: Giving on a national basis for conservation, in TN for art, and in CT for education and the aging. No grants to individuals, or for ongoing operating support.
Publications: Informational brochure (including application guidelines), 990-PF.
Application information: Contact Exec. Dir. for application guidelines.
Initial approach: 1- to 2-page letter
Deadline(s): None
Board meeting date(s): Varies
Officer: Charlotte Giannini, Exec. Dir.
Trustee: Andrew M. Clarkson.
Advisory Board: Carole G. Clarkson, Jennifer M. Clarkson.
Number of staff: 1 part-time professional.

EIN: 621516244

914
The Community Foundation of Greater Chattanooga, Inc.

736 Market St., Suite 1701
Chattanooga 37402 (423) 265-0586
Contact: Peter T. Cooper, Exec. Dir.

Incorporated in 1963 in TN.
Foundation type: Community
Financial data (yr. ended 12/31/95): Assets, $24,155,934 (M); gifts received, $4,284,561; expenditures, $1,966,787, including $1,339,396 for 277 grants (high: $100,000; low: $21; average: $1,500-$100,000) and $229,621 for 129 grants to individuals (high: $28,014; low: $150; average: $500-$5,000).
Purpose and activities: "To promote and enhance the well-being of the inhabitants of the greater Chattanooga area." Primary areas of interest include education, community development, youth and child development, and the arts.
Fields of interest: Performing arts; Dance; Arts/cultural programs; Early childhood education; Child development, education; Elementary school/education; Higher education; Education; Natural resource conservation & protection; Environment; Medical care, rehabilitation; Health care; Substance abuse, services; Mental health/crisis services; Health associations; Children & youth, services; Child development, services; Family services; Aging, centers & services; Urban/community development; Community development; Minorities; Disabled; Aging; General charitable giving; Japan.
Types of support: Capital campaigns, building/renovation, equipment, program development, seed money, scholarships—to individuals, exchange programs.
Limitations: Giving limited to the greater Chattanooga, TN, area. No support for private schools or religious causes. No loans.
Publications: Annual report, application guidelines, newsletter.
Application information: The foundation has a new application form available; do not use previous form. Application form required.
Initial approach: Brief letter, visit, or application form
Copies of proposal: 18
Deadline(s): Jan. 25, Apr. 25, July 25, and Oct. 25
Board meeting date(s): Quarterly; grants committee meets in Feb., May, Aug., and Nov.
Final notification: 4 to 5 weeks after meeting
Officers and Directors:* Jane W. Harbaugh,* Pres.; Svan Davenport, V.P.; Ruth Holmberg, V.P.; Phillip B. Whitaker, V.P.; Liston Bishop, Secy.; Robert J. Sudderth,* Treas.; J. Guy Beatty, L.H. Caldwell III, Emmy Casey, Al Chapman, Kay K. Chitty, Claudie Clark, Jr., Alan Edgar, R. Allan Edgar, Zan Guerry, Elaine Hill, Richard Houck, James D. Kennedy, Jr., Grant Law, Charles Love, Lyda McKuldin, Sharon Mills, Yuji Noma, David P. Phillips, Helen S. Pregulman, Hilda Roddy, Frances Smith, Yvonne Smith, Robert J. Sudderth, Jr., Lynn Woodworth.
Number of staff: 3 full-time professional; 1 full-time support.
EIN: 626045999

915
H. W. Durham Foundation

5050 Poplar Ave., Suite 1522
Memphis 38157 (901) 683-3583
Contact: Jenks McCrory, Prog. Dir.

Incorporated in 1955 in TN.
Donor(s): H.W. Durham.‡
Financial data (yr. ended 12/31/94): Assets, $10,040,639 (M); expenditures, $733,292; qualifying distributions, $598,713, including $450,921 for grants (average: $1,500-$6,410).
Purpose and activities: Giving primarily for the elderly and issues relating to the aging process.
Fields of interest: Arts/cultural programs; Aging.
Types of support: Program development, conferences/seminars, publication, seed money, fellowships, scholarship funds, research, technical assistance, program-related investments/loans.
Limitations: Giving primarily in Memphis, TN, and the Mid-South region of the U.S.
Publications: Application guidelines, informational brochure (including application guidelines).
Application information: Application form required.
Initial approach: Letter
Copies of proposal: 5
Deadline(s): Jan. 1, Apr. 1, and Aug. 1
Board meeting date(s): Feb., May, and Sept.
Final notification: Immediately after board meeting
Officers and Directors:* Thomas H. Durham, Jr.,* Pres.; Ralph Lawrence,* V.P.; Jo Scott,* Secy.; Jenks McCrory,* Treas. and Prog. Dir.; Kaye Brooksbank, Robert Burns, Evertt Huffard, Al J. Kelly, Hugh McHenry, Linda Nichols.
Number of staff: 2 full-time professional; 1 part-time support.
EIN: 620583854

916
Federal Express Corporate Giving Program

2005 Corporate Ave.
Memphis 38132-1854 (901) 395-3478
Contact: Thomas L. Hollands, Mgr., Investor Rels.
Mailing Address: P.O. Box 727, Memphis, TN 38194

Financial data (yr. ended 05/31/92): Total giving, $1,704,810, including $1,704,810 for grants (high: $142,857; low: $100).
Fields of interest: Arts/cultural programs; Higher education; Education; Natural resource conservation & protection; Health care; Health organizations; Crime/law enforcement; Youth, services; Aging, centers & services; Civil rights; Community development; Government/public administration; Disabled; Aging.
Types of support: General/operating support, continuing support, annual campaigns, capital campaigns, building/renovation, endowment funds, emergency funds, scholarship funds, research, technical assistance, consulting services, employee volunteer services, loaned talent, donated equipment, donated products, in-kind gifts.
Limitations: Giving primarily in major operating areas. No support for political organizations, unionized organizations or religious groups, except for interdenominational activities. No grants to individuals, or for sponsorships or advertising.
Publications: Corporate giving report (including application guidelines) (including program policy statement).
Application information: Send requests to headquarters. Application form not required.
Initial approach: Proposal
Deadline(s): Applications accepted throughout year
Board meeting date(s). Monthly
Number of staff: 2 full-time professional.

917
Magdovitz Family Foundation

P.O. Box 650
Memphis 38101

Established in 1975 in TN.
Donor(s): Joseph A. Magdovitz, Earl J. Magdovitz.
Financial data (yr. ended 06/30/94): Assets, $1,405,348 (M); gifts received, $7,500; expenditures, $70,293; qualifying distributions, $68,146, including $62,078 for grants (high: $21,588).
Purpose and activities: Support primarily for Jewish welfare organizations; support also for the fine arts, including museums and other arts groups, religion, conservation, wildlife and animal welfare, family and social service agencies, health associations, including cancer programs and AIDS research, community development and civic affairs, and early childhood and elementary education.
Fields of interest: Visual arts; Museums; Performing arts; Theater; Music; Arts/cultural programs; Elementary/secondary education; Early childhood education; Elementary school/education; Education; Natural resource conservation & protection; Animal welfare; Wildlife preservation & protection; Health care; Substance abuse, services; Health associations; Cancer; Heart/circulatory disease; AIDS; Biomedicine; Health organizations; Medical research; Cancer research; Heart/circulatory research; AIDS research; Crime/law enforcement; Recreation; Human services; Youth, services; Family services; Aging, centers & services; Community development; Federated giving programs; Jewish federated giving programs; Government/public administration; Public affairs; Jewish agencies & temples; Religion; Aging; Economically disadvantaged; General charitable giving; Israel.
Limitations: Applications not accepted. Giving limited to the Memphis, TN, area. No grants to individuals.
Officers and Trustees:* Joseph A. Magdovitz,* Pres. and Treas.; Earl J. Magdovitz,* V.P. and Secy.
Number of staff: None.
EIN: 510164695

918
Nashville Community Foundation, Inc.

210 23rd Ave. North
Nashville 37203-1502 (615) 321-4939
Contact: Ellen Lehman, Exec. Dir.
FAX: (615) 327-2746

Established in 1991 in TN.
Foundation type: Community
Financial data (yr. ended 12/31/95): Assets, $23,443,554 (M); gifts received, $5,328,486; expenditures, $1,113,231, including $906,390 for 293 grants (high: $191,000; low: $25; average: $256-$191,000) and $32,527 for in-kind gifts.
Fields of interest: Humanities; Historic preservation/historical societies; Arts/cultural programs; Education; Natural resource conservation & protection; Environment; Health care; Health organizations; Employment; Housing/shelter, development; Human services; Aging, centers & services; Community development, neighborhood development; Community development; Aging.
Types of support: Program development, seed money, in-kind gifts.
Limitations: Giving limited to Nashville and central TN. No support for private foundations, religious or sectarian purposes, private schools, or biomedical or clinic studies. No grants for fundraising events, debt retirement, annual and capital campaigns, general operations, advertising, trips, or conferences.
Publications: Annual report, newsletter, informational brochure, application guidelines.
Application information: Application form not required.
Initial approach: Proposal
Copies of proposal: 3
Deadline(s): May 1
Board meeting date(s): Feb., Apr., June, Sept., Nov., and Dec.
Final notification: Sept. 15
Officers and Directors:* Betty M. Brown,* Chair.; Robert K. Zelle,* Vice-Chair; Jamye C. Williams,* Secy.; William W. McInnes,* Treas.; Ellen E. Lehman,* Exec. Dir.; and 18 additional directors.
Number of staff: 3 full-time professional.
EIN: 621471789

919
Washington Foundation

(Formerly Church of Christ Foundation, Inc.)
P.O. Box 159057
Nashville 37215
Contact: Paul A. Hargis, Pres.

Incorporated in 1946 in TN.
Donor(s): G.L. Comer.
Financial data (yr. ended 12/31/92): Assets, $13,784,450 (M); expenditures, $644,844; qualifying distributions, $584,115, including $564,100 for 133 grants (high: $60,000; low: $200).
Purpose and activities: Support mainly for Church of Christ-related organizations, including churches, schools, and colleges; grants also for health and welfare.
Fields of interest: Elementary/secondary education; Higher education; Health care; Human services; Aging, centers & services; Federated giving programs; Christian agencies & churches; Religion; Aging.
Types of support: General/operating support.
Limitations: Giving limited to U.S. for Church of Christ-related organizations; support primarily in the Nashville, TN, area for health and welfare. No grants to individuals.
Application information:
Initial approach: Letter
Deadline(s): Dec. 1
Board meeting date(s): Quarterly
Officers and Trustees:* Paul A. Hargis,* Pres.; E.M. Shepherd,* V.P.; R. Hix Clark,* Secy.; Paschal H. Young,* Treas.; Howard R. Amacher, Andrew Benedict, William W. Berry, James N. Denton III, F. Miles Ezell, Jr., Harold Hazelip, Neal L. Jennings, Robert C. Taylor.
Number of staff: 1
EIN: 620649477

TEXAS

920
Abell-Hanger Foundation

P.O. Box 430
Midland 79702 (915) 684-6655
Contact: David L. Smith, Exec. Dir.

Incorporated in 1954 in TX.
Donor(s): George T. Abell,‡ Gladys H. Abell.‡
Financial data (yr. ended 06/30/95): Assets, $113,388,381 (M); expenditures, $5,944,549; qualifying distributions, $5,365,328, including $4,833,856 for 136 grants (high: $400,000; low: $250; average: $10,000-$50,000).
Purpose and activities: Support primarily for higher education, youth activities, cultural programs, health services, the handicapped, and social welfare agencies.
Fields of interest: Arts/cultural programs; Higher education; Business school/education; Nursing school/education; Nursing care; Health care; Substance abuse, services; Human services; Youth, services; Family services; Aging, centers & services; Community development; Voluntarism promotion; Government/public administration; Disabled; Aging; Economically disadvantaged.
Types of support: General/operating support, continuing support, annual campaigns, capital campaigns, building/renovation, equipment, endowment funds, program development, seed money, scholarship funds, research, matching funds.
Limitations: Giving limited to TX, preferably within the Permian Basin. No grants to individuals, or for individual scholarships or fellowships; no loans.
Publications: Annual report (including application guidelines).
Application information: Application form required.
Initial approach: Letter
Copies of proposal: 1
Deadline(s): May 30, Feb. 28, Nov. 15, and Aug. 30
Board meeting date(s): June 30, Mar. 30, Dec. 30, and Sept. 30
Final notification: 1 month
Officers and Trustees:* Arlen L. Edgar,* Pres.; James I. Trott,* V.P.; Lester Van Pelt, Jr.,* Secy.-Treas.; David L. Smith, Exec. Dir.; Jerome M. Fullinwider, Robert L. Leibrock, Charles M. Younger.
Number of staff: 1 full-time professional; 2 part-time professional; 2 full-time support.
EIN: 756020781
Grants for Aging:
Christmas in April, Midland, TX, $40,000. For housing materials. 95.
Community and Senior Services of Midland, Midland, TX, $45,000. For unrestricted operating support. 95.
Community and Senior Services of Midland, Midland, TX, $15,000. For close-captioned television decoders. 95.
Meals on Wheels of Odessa, Odessa, TX, $10,000. For expansion of services to additional clients. 95.

921
Aged & Indigent Old Folks of El Paso County Foundation

c/o Texas Commerce Bank, N.A.
P.O. Drawer 140
El Paso 79980 (915) 546-2454
Contact: Pat Sandford, V.P., Texas Commerce Bank, N.A.

Financial data (yr. ended 06/30/95): Assets, $689,878 (M); expenditures, $37,856; qualifying distributions, $30,444, including $26,600 for grants.
Fields of interest: Salvation Army; Aging, centers & services; Aging.
Types of support: Capital campaigns.
Limitations: Giving limited to El Paso County, TX.
Application information:
Initial approach: Letter
Deadline(s): None
Trustee: Texas Commerce Bank, N.A.
EIN: 746033945

922
Amarillo Area Foundation, Inc.

700 First National Place I
801 South Fillmore
Amarillo 79101 (806) 376-4521
Contact: Jim Allison, Pres. and Exec. Dir.
FAX: (806) 373-3656

Established as a trust in 1957 in TX.
Foundation type: Community
Financial data (yr. ended 12/31/95): Assets, $36,651,664 (M); gifts received, $8,410,958; expenditures, $13,554,461, including $13,193,188 for 71 grants (high: $6,912,361; low: $100; average: $500-$35,000).
Purpose and activities: Giving primarily for education, arts and cultural programs, and health and human services.
Fields of interest: Arts/cultural programs; Education; Health care; Human services; Youth, services; Aging, centers & services; Economically disadvantaged.
Types of support: Building/renovation, equipment, land acquisition, program

development, seed money, scholarship funds, matching funds.
Limitations: Giving limited to the 26 most northern counties of the TX Panhandle. No support for private or parochial schools. No grants to individuals (except for limited scholarships from designated funds), or for operating budgets, annual campaigns, deficit financing, endowment funds, publications, or conferences; no loans.
Publications: Annual report, application guidelines, newsletter, 990-PF.
Application information: Specific application format required. Application form required.
Initial approach: Proposal (no more than 8 pages)
Copies of proposal: 1
Deadline(s): Quarterly - Jan., Mar., July, and Sept.
Board meeting date(s): Board meets bimonthly - Feb., Apr., June, Aug., Oct., and Dec; executive committee meets bimonthly - Mar., May, July, Sept., and Nov.
Final notification: Mar., June, Aug., and Dec.
Officers and Directors:* John Marmaduke,* Chair.; Danny Conklin,* 1st Vice-Chair.; Don Powell,* 2nd Vice-Chair.; Jim Allison, Pres. and Exec. Dir.; Beth Duke,* Secy.; Ron McVean,* Treas.; and 19 additional directors.
Number of staff: None.
EIN: 750978220
Grants for Aging:
Donley County Senior Citizens, Clarendon, TX, $13,484. 94.

923
M. D. Anderson Foundation
P.O. Box 2558
Houston 77252-8037 (713) 658-2316
Contact: Elizabeth A. Calvert, Secy.-Treas.

Trust established in 1936 in TX.
Donor(s): M.D. Anderson.‡
Financial data (yr. ended 12/31/94): Assets, $92,383,135 (M); expenditures, $3,497,382; qualifying distributions, $3,026,151, including $2,958,428 for 92 grants (high: $200,000; low: $1,000; average: $10,000-$50,000).
Purpose and activities: Support for the establishment, support and maintenance of hospitals, homes, and institutions for the care of the sick, the young, the aged, the incompetent and the helpless; the promotion of health science, and education; and the improvement of living conditions among workers and people generally or in particular sections or local. Support for a large local medical center and for educational and related projects.
Fields of interest: Education; Health care; Health organizations; Human services; Youth, services; Aging, centers & services; Public policy, research; Government/public administration; Aging.
Types of support: Building/renovation, equipment, seed money, research, matching funds.
Limitations: Giving limited to TX, primarily the Houston area. No grants to individuals, or for endowment funds or operating budgets.
Publications: Multi-year report, application guidelines.
Application information: Application form not required.
Initial approach: Letter
Copies of proposal: 5
Deadline(s): None
Board meeting date(s): Third Tuesday of each month
Final notification: 1 month
Officers: Gibson Gayle, Jr., Pres.; Uriel E. Dutton, V.P.; Charles W. Hall, V.P.; Jack Trotter, V.P.; Elizabeth A. Calvert, Secy.-Treas.
Number of staff: None.
EIN: 746035669
Grants for Aging:
Holly Hall, Houston, TX, $25,000. To renovate retirement facility. 94.
Saint James House of Baytown, Baytown, TX, $10,000. For nursing equipment. 94.

924
Barber Foundation
133 Wall St.
Abilene 79603-6430 (915) 698-0186
Contact: Harwell Barber, Mgr.

Established in 1966 in TX.
Donor(s): Harwell Barber, Rita Barber.‡
Financial data (yr. ended 12/31/94): Assets, $971,147 (M); expenditures, $58,161; qualifying distributions, $54,749, including $54,749 for 86 grants (high: $6,285; low: $100).
Purpose and activities: Giving to Catholic organizations; support excludes individual scholarship grants; limited scholarships available only to mortuary schools, which decide recipients based on financial need.
Fields of interest: Human services; Aging, centers & services; Community development; Religion; Aging; Economically disadvantaged; General charitable giving.
Types of support: General/operating support, capital campaigns.
Limitations: Giving primarily in Abilene, TX. No grants to individuals.
Application information:
Initial approach: Letter
Deadline(s): None
Officer: Harwell Barber, Mgr.
Trustees: Carolyn Barber, Rita C. Barber Hampton.
Number of staff: None.
EIN: 756067600

925
Mary E. Bivins Foundation
6214 Elmhurst
Amarillo 79106
Contact: Mr. Lindy Ward, Dir.

Incorporated in 1949 in TX.
Donor(s): Mary E. Bivins Trust, and others.
Foundation type: Operating
Financial data (yr. ended 08/31/95): Assets, $63,153,711 (M); gifts received, $7,939,795; expenditures, $7,774,988; qualifying distributions, $7,946,015, including $424,372 for 15 grants (high: $150,000; low: $1,000), $12,902 for grants to individuals and $7,508,741 for 2 foundation-administered programs.
Purpose and activities: A private operating foundation; operates nursing homes for the aged; also giving for social service agencies and Christian colleges, including scholarships.
Fields of interest: Higher education; Human services; Aging, centers & services; Christian agencies & churches; Aging.
Types of support: General/operating support, scholarships—to individuals.
Limitations: Giving primarily in TX.
Application information:
Initial approach: Letter
Deadline(s): Oct. 31
Officers and Directors:* Clyde Israel,* Pres.; Miles Childers,* V.P.; Tom Bivins,* Secy.; Patrick Dunne, Patrick Oles, Larry Pickens, Lindy L. Ward.
Number of staff: 3 full-time professional.
EIN: 750842370
Grants for Aging:
Amarillo Multiservice Center for the Aging, Amarillo, TX, $150,000. For construction. 95.
Amarillo Senior Citizens Association, Amarillo, TX, $50,000. 95.

926
Carrie Morton Brown Foundation
c/o Texas Commerce Bank, N.A.
P.O. Box 140
El Paso 79980 (915) 546-2454
Contact: Pat Sandford, Administrator, Texas Commerce Bank, N.A.

Financial data (yr. ended 06/30/95): Assets, $565,546 (M); expenditures, $34,701; qualifying distributions, $27,639, including $24,000 for grants.
Purpose and activities: Support for programs in El Paso County, TX which benefit the elderly.
Fields of interest: Health associations; Aging, centers & services; Aging.
Limitations: Giving limited to El Paso County, TX. No grants to individuals.
Application information:
Initial approach: Letter
Deadline(s): None
Trustee: Texas Commerce Bank, N.A.
EIN: 742111392

927
Burlington Resources Foundation
5051 Westheimer St., Suite 1400
Houston 77056 (713) 624-9898
Contact: Gavin H. Smith, Pres.

Established in 1989.
Donor(s): Burlington Resources, Inc., and its subsidiaries.
Foundation type: Company-sponsored
Financial data (yr. ended 12/31/94): Assets, $645,835 (M); gifts received, $1,698,000; expenditures, $2,665,444; qualifying distributions, $2,658,947, including $2,407,443 for 174 grants (high: $250,000; low: $500; average: $5,000-$100,000) and $251,504 for 82 employee matching gifts.
Purpose and activities: Giving in the following areas: 1) community funds and other federated organizations; 2) educational institutions, both public and private, primarily at the college level, preferably directed toward the improvement of

the quality of education; 3) youth organizations; 4) hospitals and medical facilities, including hospital building funds and equipment; 5) cultural programs, including performing and visual arts, historical centers, and public and educational broadcasting; and 6) human service agencies, including chemical dependency treatment and prevention, senior citizens, runaway youth, spouse and child abuse, offender programs, and women's programs.
Fields of interest: Arts/cultural programs; Higher education; Education; Hospitals (general); Substance abuse, services; Human services; Youth, services; Aging, centers & services; Women, centers & services; Federated giving programs; Aging; Women.
Types of support: Building/renovation, equipment, employee matching gifts.
Limitations: Giving primarily in areas of company operations. No support for religious groups for religious purposes, veterans' or fraternal service organizations, or national health organizations. No grants to individuals, or for endowment funds, fundraising events, or computers or computer-related projects.
Application information: Application form required.
Officers and Directors:* Thomas H. O'Leary,* Chair.; Gavin H. Smith,* Pres.; John E. Hagale,* V.P., Finance; Hays R. Warden, V.P. and Cont.; Wendi S. Zerwas, Secy.; Everett D. Dubois,* Treas.
EIN: 943096534

928
The Effie and Wofford Cain Foundation

4131 Spicewood Springs Rd., Suite A-1
Austin 78759 (512) 346-7490
Contact: Harvey L. Walker, Exec. Dir.
FAX: (512) 346-7490

Incorporated in 1952 in TX.
Donor(s): Effie Marie Cain, R. Wofford Cain.‡
Financial data (yr. ended 10/31/95): Assets, $70,295,586 (M); gifts received, $400,000; expenditures, $3,560,134; qualifying distributions, $3,057,005, including $2,827,648 for 75 grants (high: $500,000; low: $598; average: $1,000-$50,000).
Purpose and activities: Giving primarily for higher and secondary education, medical research, and public service organizations; grants also for religious organizations and aid to the handicapped.
Fields of interest: Elementary/secondary education; Early childhood education; Child development, education; Secondary school/education; Higher education; Law school/education; Medical school/education; Nursing school/education; Education; Hospitals (general); Health care; Biomedicine; Health organizations; Medical research; Crime/law enforcement; Youth development, services; Human services; Child development, services; Community development; Religious federated giving programs; Biological sciences; Government/public administration; Leadership development; Religion; African Americans; Latinos; Disabled; Aging; Economically disadvantaged; Homeless.
Types of support: General/operating support, continuing support, annual campaigns, capital campaigns, building/renovation, equipment, endowment funds, program development, professorships, seed money, curriculum development, fellowships, internships, scholarship funds, research, matching funds.
Limitations: Giving primarily in TX. No grants to individuals.
Publications: Application guidelines.
Application information:
Initial approach: Telephone call or 1-page letter of inquiry prepared in accordance with instructions provided upon contact
Copies of proposal: 1
Deadline(s): None; budget usually fully committed by July 31
Board meeting date(s): Oct. (annual meeting); 6 to 8 interim meetings (dates vary)
Final notification: Varies
Officers and Directors:* Franklin W. Denius,* Exec. V.P.; James B. Cain,* V.P.; Harvey L. Walker, Secy.-Treas. and Exec. Dir.; John C. Cain, F. Wofford Denius, Charmaine D. McGill.
Number of staff: 2 full-time professional; 1 full-time support.
EIN: 756030774
Grants for Aging:
University of Texas Southwestern Medical Center, Dallas, TX, $300,000. Toward endowed Alzheimer's Disease Research Chair and Center. 94.

929
Harry S. and Isabel C. Cameron Foundation

c/o NationsBank of Texas, N.A.
P.O. Box 2518
Houston 77252-2518 (713) 247-7435
Contact: Carl W. Schumacher, Jr.

Established in 1966 in TX.
Donor(s): Isabel C. Cameron.‡
Financial data (yr. ended 06/30/94): Assets, $18,187,424 (M); gifts received, $2,500,025; expenditures, $2,091,560; qualifying distributions, $1,930,506, including $1,901,750 for 201 grants (high: $245,500; low: $500; average: $1,000-$15,000).
Purpose and activities: Giving primarily for elementary, secondary, and higher education, religious organizations, and human services.
Fields of interest: Elementary school/education; Secondary school/education; Higher education; Natural resource conservation & protection; Environment; Nursing care; Health care; Substance abuse, services; Mental health/crisis services; AIDS; Health organizations; AIDS research; Food services; Human services; Youth, services; Hospices; Aging, centers & services; Homeless, human services; Roman Catholic federated giving programs; Roman Catholic agencies & churches; Aging; Homeless.
Types of support: General/operating support, building/renovation, equipment, research.
Limitations: Giving primarily in TX, especially Houston. No grants to individuals, or for operating support, endowment funds, or matching gifts; no loans.
Application information: Application form not required.
Initial approach: Letter
Copies of proposal: 6
Deadline(s): Prior to board meetings
Board meeting date(s): Apr., Aug., and Dec.
Final notification: 2 weeks after board meetings, when action is favorable
Directors: Priscilla Bormet, David W. Cameron, Sylvia J. Cameron, Estelle Cameron Maloney, Frances Cameron Miller.
Trustee: NationsBank of Texas, N.A.
Number of staff: None.
EIN: 746073312

930
Carlile Foundation, Inc.

(Formerly Carlile & Howell Foundation, Inc.)
P.O. Box 2069
Marshall 75671

Classified as a private operating foundation in 1987.
Donor(s): Quinton B. Carlile, Kenneth Q. Carlile, Steve B. Carlile.
Foundation type: Operating
Financial data (yr. ended 10/31/95): Assets, $3,663 (M); gifts received, $19,631; expenditures, $32,257; qualifying distributions, $32,257, including $28,070 for 7 grants (high: $15,235; low: $25).
Fields of interest: Higher education; Aging; Economically disadvantaged.
Types of support: Scholarship funds, grants to individuals.
Limitations: Applications not accepted. Giving primarily in Marshall, TX.
Officers and Trustees:* Quinton B. Carlile,* Pres.; Kenneth Q. Carlile,* V.P.; Steve B. Carlile,* Secy.-Treas.; Penny F. Carlile, Mgr.
EIN: 751729109

931
Amon G. Carter Foundation

500 West Seventh St., Suite 1212
P.O. Box 1036
Fort Worth 76101 (817) 332-2783
Contact: John H. Robinson, Exec. V.P., Grant Administration

Incorporated in 1945 in TX.
Donor(s): Amon G. Carter,‡ N.B. Carter,‡ Star-Telegram Employees Fund, Carter Foundation Production Co.
Financial data (yr. ended 12/31/94): Assets, $174,294,629 (M); expenditures, $11,097,209; qualifying distributions, $9,585,360, including $9,341,402 for 182 grants (high: $4,572,891; low: $500; average: $1,000-$100,000).
Purpose and activities: Grants primarily for the visual and performing arts, education, health care, social service and youth agencies, programs for the aged, and civic and community endeavors that enhance the quality of life. The foundation sponsors and largely supports an art museum.
Fields of interest: Museums; Performing arts; Arts/cultural programs; Higher education; Education; Hospitals (general); Health care; Human services; Youth, services; Aging, centers & services; Government/public administration; Aging.
Types of support: General/operating support, continuing support, annual campaigns, capital

campaigns, building/renovation, equipment, land acquisition, endowment funds, emergency funds, program development, professorships, seed money, research, matching funds.
Limitations: Giving largely restricted to Fort Worth and Tarrant County, TX. No grants to individuals, or for ongoing operating budgets, deficit financing, publications, or conferences; no loans.
Publications: Program policy statement, annual report.
Application information: Grants outside local geographic area usually initiated by board. Application form not required.
Initial approach: Letter
Copies of proposal: 1
Deadline(s): None
Board meeting date(s): Apr., Sept., and Dec.
Final notification: Within 10 days of board meeting
Officers and Directors:* Ruth Carter Stevenson,* Pres.; W. Patrick Harris, Exec. V.P., Investments; John H. Robinson, Exec. V.P., Grant Administration; Robert W. Brown, M.D.,* V.P.; J. Lee Johnson IV, Secy.; Mark L. Johnson, Treas.
Number of staff: 3 full-time professional; 3 full-time support.
EIN: 756000331
Grants for Aging:
Alzheimers Disease and Related Disorders Association, Fort Worth, TX, $25,000. For special program. 94.
Meals on Wheels of Fort Worth, Fort Worth, TX, $35,000. For general support. 94.

932
The CH Foundation
P.O. Box 16458
Lubbock 79490 (806) 799-3250
Contact: Nelda Thompson, Secy.

Established in 1976 in TX.
Donor(s): Christine DeVitt.‡
Financial data (yr. ended 12/31/95): Assets, $33,203,690 (M); expenditures, $1,647,719; qualifying distributions, $1,365,110, including $1,289,441 for 45 grants (high: $150,000; low: $1,000).
Purpose and activities: Giving primarily for education, arts and cultural organizations, medicine, and human services.
Fields of interest: Museums; Elementary/secondary education; Higher education; Medical school/education; Nursing school/education; Hospitals (general); Domestic violence prevention; human services; Disabled; Aging; Women; Economically disadvantaged.
Types of support: General/operating support, annual campaigns, capital campaigns, building/renovation, equipment, publication, curriculum development, scholarship funds, research, matching funds.
Limitations: Giving primarily in the South Plains, TX, area.
Application information: Application form not required.
Initial approach: Proposal
Copies of proposal: 1
Deadline(s): June 1
Board meeting date(s): As necessary
Officers and Trustees:* L. Edwin Smith,* Pres.; Nelda Thompson,* Secy.; Louise Willson Arnold,* Treas.; Don Graf, Kay Sanford.
Number of staff: 1 full-time professional.
EIN: 751534816

933
The Cockrell Foundation
1600 Smith, Suite 4600
Houston 77002-7348 (713) 209-7500
Contact: Nancy Williams, Exec. V.P.

Trust established in 1957 in TX; incorporated in 1966.
Donor(s): Dula Cockrell,‡ Ernest Cockrell, Jr.,‡ Virginia H. Cockrell.‡
Financial data (yr. ended 12/31/94): Assets, $73,654,466 (M); expenditures, $4,114,076; qualifying distributions, $3,726,170, including $3,665,876 for 45 grants (high: $2,010,000; low: $250; average: $1,000-$50,000).
Purpose and activities: Giving for higher education; support also for cultural programs, social services, youth, religion, and hospitals.
Fields of interest: Museums; Arts/cultural programs; Higher education; Hospitals (general); Domestic violence prevention; Human services; Children & youth, services; Christian agencies & churches; Disabled; Aging; Women.
Types of support: Annual campaigns, capital campaigns, building/renovation, land acquisition, endowment funds, program development, professorships, fellowships, scholarship funds, research, matching funds.
Limitations: Giving primarily in Houston, TX. No grants to individuals.
Publications: Annual report, 990-PF.
Application information: Application form not required.
Initial approach: Proposal
Copies of proposal: 1
Deadline(s): None
Board meeting date(s): Mar. and Oct.
Final notification: 6 weeks
Officers and Directors:* Ernest H. Cockrell,* Pres.; Nancy Williams, Exec. V.P.; Milton T. Graves, V.P. and Assoc. Dir.; W.F. Wright, Jr., Secy.-Treas. and Assoc. Dir.; Janet S. Cockrell, Carol Cockrell Curran, Richard B. Curran, Charles W. Hubbard, J. Webb Jennings III, Laura Jennings Turner.
Number of staff: None.
EIN: 746076993
Grants for Aging:
Holly Hall, Houston, TX, $10,000. For general support. 94.

934
The Community Foundation of Metropolitan Tarrant County
Fort Worth Club Bldg.
306 West Seventh St., Suite 702
Fort Worth 76102 (817) 877-0702
Contact: Homer M. Dowd, Pres.
FAX: (817) 877-1215

Established in 1981 in TX as a program of the United Way; status changed to independent community foundation in 1989.
Foundation type: Community
Financial data (yr. ended 12/31/95): Assets, $34,652,361 (L); gifts received, $2,536,214; expenditures, $2,141,359, including $1,573,218 for 312 grants (high: $80,000; average: $500-$100,000) and $150,297 for 2 foundation-administered programs.
Purpose and activities: Support for community development, social services, education, youth, health, and arts and cultural programs; emphasis on one-time grants to new and innovative programs.
Fields of interest: Arts/cultural programs; Education; Health care; AIDS; Health organizations; AIDS research; Human services; Youth, services; Community development; Disabled; Aging; Women; People with AIDS (PWAs); Gays/lesbians; Economically disadvantaged; Homeless.
Types of support: General/operating support, building/renovation, program development, seed money, internships, scholarship funds, technical assistance.
Limitations: Giving primarily in the Fort Worth Metroplex, TX. No support for secular, religious, or fraternal organizations. No grants to individuals, or for annual or capital campaigns, deficit financing, endowments or emergency funds, matching grants, publications, research, continuing support, or conferences and seminars.
Publications: Application guidelines, annual report, informational brochure, 990-PF.
Application information: Application form not required.
Initial approach: Letter requesting guidelines
Copies of proposal: 1
Deadline(s): Apr. 15 and Oct. 15; letter of intent due Sept. 1 and Mar. 1
Board meeting date(s): Mar., June, Sept., and Dec.
Final notification: June 30 and Dec. 31
Officers and Directors:* Edgar H. Keltner, Jr.,* Chair.; Garland M. Lasater, Jr.,* Vice-Chair.; Homer M. Dowd,* Pres. and Exec. Dir.; Alann Bedford Sampson,* Secy.; Clifton H. Morris, Jr.,* Treas.; Carol Alexander, Ronald Clinkscale, Tom Cravens, Robert W. Decker, Leland Hodges, R.B. Kelley III, William Landreth, Jr., Joe B. Macchia, Joseph A. Monteleone, Joe K. Pace, Douglas A. Stroud, George S. Walls, Lloyd J. Weaver.
Number of staff: 1 full-time professional; 2 full-time support; 2 part-time support.
EIN: 752267767
Grants for Aging:
James L. West Presbyterian Special Care Center, Fort Worth, TX, $10,500. 94.

935
J. Paul Craig Foundation
c/o Amarillo National Bank, Trust Dept.
P.O. Box 1
Amarillo 79105 (806) 378-8334
Contact: Trust Officer, Amarillo National Bank

Donor(s): Gertrude Craig,‡ J. Paul Craig,‡ Norah Craig.‡
Financial data (yr. ended 09/30/95): Assets, $2,519,836 (M); expenditures, $130,193; qualifying distributions, $106,414, including $106,268 for 12 grants (high: $20,268; low: $1,000).

Fields of interest: Human services; Children & youth, services; Youth, services; Aging, centers & services; Aging.
Types of support: General/operating support.
Limitations: Giving limited to the Texas Panhandle area. No grants to individuals.
Application information: Application form not required.
Deadline(s): Sept. 1
Distribution Committee: J. Walter Browers, William L. Dickey, L.R. Hammer, Jr., William K. Irwin, Warren Jordan.
Trustee: Amarillo National Bank.
EIN: 756196164
Grants for Aging:
Amarillo Senior Citizens Association, Amarillo, TX, $15,000. 94.
Amarillo Senior Citizens Association, Amarillo, TX, $15,000. 95.
Board of Pensions, Northwest Texas Conference, Amarillo, TX, $3,000. For endowment fund. 95.
Jan Werner Adult Day Care Center, Amarillo, TX, $10,000. 94.
Jan Werner Adult Day Care Center, Amarillo, TX, $10,000. 95.
Meals on Wheels of Amarillo, Amarillo, TX, $10,000. 94.
Meals on Wheels of Amarillo, Amarillo, TX, $10,000. 95.
Sears Methodist Retirement System, Abilene, TX, $20,268. 95.

936
Dalkowitz Charitable Trust
c/o NationsBank of Texas, N.A.
P.O. Box 121
San Antonio 78291-0121 (210) 270-5314
Contact: Jay Higginson, V.P., NationsBank of Texas, N.A.

Established in 1993 in TX.
Donor(s): Nathalie Dalkowitz.
Financial data (yr. ended 07/31/95): Assets, $295,089 (M); gifts received, $114,503; expenditures, $72,172; qualifying distributions, $69,120, including $68,474 for 6 grants (high: $17,224; low: $1,000).
Fields of interest: Museums (art); Arts/cultural programs; Aging, centers & services; Jewish federated giving programs.
Limitations: Giving limited to Bexar County, TX.
Application information: Application form required.
Initial approach: Letter
Copies of proposal: 10
Deadline(s): June 1
Board meeting date(s): 3rd Thursday in July
Trustee: NationsBank of Texas, N.A.
Number of staff: None.
EIN: 746410360
Grants for Aging:
Golden Manor Jewish Home for the Aged, San Antonio, TX, $17,224. For hydrosound therapy bathing units installation. 95.

937
The Dallas Foundation
400 South Record St., Suite 600
Dallas 75202-4818 (214) 977-6676
Contact: Mary M. Jalonick, Exec. Dir.
FAX: (214) 977-7781

Established in 1929 in TX.
Foundation type: Community
Financial data (yr. ended 12/31/94): Assets, $28,515,092 (M); gifts received, $3,120,298; expenditures, $2,611,605, including $2,098,746 for 130 grants (high: $100,000; low: $100; average: $5,000-$100,000).
Purpose and activities: Giving to promote charitable, educational, cultural, civic, and health programs, including those for the disadvantaged, through grants to community organizations and agencies, principally for capital purposes.
Fields of interest: Arts/cultural programs; Nursing school/education; Education; Health care; Health organizations; Human services; Government/public administration; African Americans; Disabled; Aging; Economically disadvantaged.
Types of support: Capital campaigns, building/renovation, equipment, program development, matching funds.
Limitations: Giving limited to the City and County of Dallas, TX. No grants to individuals, or for endowment or emergency funds, operating budgets, annual campaigns, seed money, land acquisition, conferences and seminars, continuing support, publications, deficit financing, consulting services, technical assistance, research, scholarships, or fellowships; no loans.
Publications: Annual report, program policy statement, application guidelines, informational brochure, grants list.
Application information: Application form not required.
Initial approach: 1-page proposal
Copies of proposal: 1
Deadline(s): Apr. 15 and Oct. 1
Board meeting date(s): Mar., May, Aug., and Nov.
Final notification: Following Nov. board meeting
Officer: Mary M. Jalonick, Exec. Dir.
Governors: Caren H. Prothro, Chair.; Ruben E. Esquivel, Rev. Zan W. Holmes, Jr., Ward L. Huey, Jr., Erle Nye, Peggy S. Oglesby, Sidney Stahl, J. McDonald Williams, Linus Wright.
Trustee Banks: Bank One, Texas, N.A., Bankers Trust Co. of the Southwest, NationsBank of Texas, N.A.
Number of staff: 2 full-time professional; 1 full-time support.
EIN: 756038529

938
Alice Gist Dunaway Foundation
P.O. Box 9938
Amarillo 79105-5938
Contact: Geraldine Anderson, Pres.
Application address: 101 Clover, Ruidoso, NM 88345

Established in 1981 in TX.
Foundation type: Operating
Financial data (yr. ended 12/31/95): Assets, $215,257 (M); expenditures, $63,470; qualifying distributions, $47,000, including $47,000 for 4 grants (high: $30,000; low: $5,000).
Fields of interest: Aging, centers & services; Christian agencies & churches.
Types of support: Continuing support, capital campaigns, program development.
Limitations: Giving primarily in TX.
Publications: 990-PF.
Application information: Application form required.
Copies of proposal: 2
Deadline(s): None
Board meeting date(s): Nov.
Officers: Geraldine Anderson, Pres.; Susan A. Frawley, V.P.; Evelyn Marshall, Secy.-Treas.
Directors: Robert W. Anderson, Judy Dotson.
Number of staff: None.
EIN: 751676023

939
Early Foundation, Inc.
6319 Mimosa Ln.
Dallas 75230 (214) 373-7114
Contact: Mrs. Jeannette B. Early, Pres.

Established in 1963 in TX.
Donor(s): Jeannette B. Early.
Financial data (yr. ended 05/31/95): Assets, $2,758,882 (M); expenditures, $210,231; qualifying distributions, $210,231, including $185,250 for 42 grants (high: $16,000; low: $500).
Purpose and activities: "To achieve growth in areas such as social services where governmental support is insufficient to accomplish worthwhile goals." Support also for Presbyterian and other Christian schools and organizations.
Fields of interest: Arts/cultural programs; Early childhood education; Higher education; Nursing home/convalescent facility; Youth development, centers & clubs; Human services; Protestant agencies & churches; Aging.
Types of support: General/operating support, capital campaigns, building/renovation, land acquisition, endowment funds, emergency funds, conferences/seminars, fellowships, internships, scholarship funds, exchange programs.
Limitations: Giving primarily in Dallas, TX. No grants to individuals.
Application information: Application form required.
Initial approach: Letter
Copies of proposal: 1
Deadline(s): None
Board meeting date(s): June 10
Officers: Jeannette B. Early, Pres.; Patti Rose Early Toifet, V.P. and Secy.
EIN: 756011853
Grants for Aging:
Grace Presbyterian Village Ministries, Dallas, TX, $10,000. 95.

940
El Paso Natural Gas Foundation
P.O. Box 1492
El Paso 79978
Contact: Lesley J. Gosling, Pres.

Established in 1992 in TX.
Donor(s): El Paso Natural Gas Co.
Foundation type: Company-sponsored

Financial data (yr. ended 12/31/94): Assets, $3,801,116 (M); gifts received, $2,069,057; expenditures, $1,598,879; qualifying distributions, $1,598,879, including $1,598,859 for 172 grants (high: $148,042; low: $50).
Fields of interest: Media/communications; Performing arts; Arts/cultural programs; Higher education; Business school/education; Hospitals (general); Substance abuse, services; Human services; Youth, services; Aging, centers & services; Community development; Federated giving programs; Government/public administration; Aging.
Types of support: Building/renovation, scholarship funds.
Limitations: Giving limited to AZ, NM, OK, TX, and UT. No support for religious organizations for religious purposes, or for political, veterans' and fraternal organizations, or national health organizations, including local chapters. No grants to individuals; or for endowment funds, fundraising events, or for computers or computer-related projects.
Publications: Informational brochure (including application guidelines).
Application information: Application form required.
Deadline(s): None
Officers and Directors:* William A. Wise,* Chair.; Lesley J. Gosling, Pres.; Luino Dell'Osso, Jr.,* Sr. V.P.; H. Brent Austin,* V.P. and Treas.; Joel Richards III, V.P.; Britton White, Jr., V.P.; Stacy J. James, Secy.
EIN: 742638185

941
Estill Foundation
700 Everhart Terr., J-1
Corpus Christi 78411-1906 (512) 851-2813
Contact: Jeannette Holloway, Pres.

Donor(s): Gentry Estill,‡ Jeannette Holloway.
Financial data (yr. ended 09/30/95): Assets, $257,127 (M); gifts received, $35,000; expenditures, $34,081; qualifying distributions, $34,021, including $26,800 for 2 grants (high: $25,000; low: $1,800) and $1,800 for 1 grant to an individual.
Fields of interest: Human services; Aging, centers & services; Aging; Economically disadvantaged.
Types of support: Grants to individuals.
Limitations: Giving primarily in TX.
Application information:
Initial approach: Letter
Deadline(s): None
Officers and Directors:* Jeannette Holloway,* Pres.; Ann Lockhart,* V.P.; Vicki Cochran,* Secy.-Treas.
EIN: 741892894

942
Thelma Emil and Edmund Fahrenkamp Memorial Trust
c/o Bank One, Texas, N.A.
P.O. Box 2050
Fort Worth 76113-2050 (817) 884-4248
Contact: Jay Bartley, Trust Officer, Bank One, Texas, N.A.

Established in 1994 in TX.
Financial data (yr. ended 05/31/95): Assets, $52,496 (M); gifts received, $51,083; expenditures, $130; qualifying distributions, $7.
Fields of interest: Alzheimer's disease.
Limitations: Giving limited to Fort Worth, TX.
Application information: First year of operation, 1994-95; no grants paid.
Initial approach: Proposal
Deadline(s): Feb.
Trustee: Bank One, Texas, N.A.
EIN: 756466013

943
Jerry and Nanette Finger Foundation
2600 Citadel Plaza Dr., Suite 600
Houston 77008

Established in 1986 in TX.
Donor(s): Jerry E. Finger, Nanette B. Finger, and other members of the Finger family.
Financial data (yr. ended 11/30/95): Assets, $192,097 (M); gifts received, $91,000; expenditures, $43,906; qualifying distributions, $43,860, including $43,800 for 16 grants (high: $12,500; low: $500).
Fields of interest: Museums; Arts/cultural programs; Higher education; Education; Aging, centers & services; Jewish federated giving programs; Jewish agencies & temples; Aging.
Types of support: General/operating support, annual campaigns, building/renovation, endowment funds, scholarship funds.
Limitations: Applications not accepted. Giving primarily in Aspen, CO, and Houston, TX. No grants to individuals.
Publications: 990-PF.
Application information: Contributes only to pre-selected organizations.
Officers and Directors:* Jerry E. Finger,* Pres.; Nanette B. Finger,* V.P.; Walter G. Finger,* Secy.-Treas.; Sherrie Gibson, Mgr.
Number of staff: None.
EIN: 760209018

944
Foresight Foundation
2605 Pecan Dr.
Temple 76502
Contact: Alan C. Jones, M.D., Pres.

Established in 1986 in TX.
Donor(s): Alan C. Jones, M.D., Lillian McKibbin.
Financial data (yr. ended 11/30/94): Assets, $975,049 (M); gifts received, $1,100; expenditures, $62,215; qualifying distributions, $54,000, including $54,000 for 11 grants (high: $20,000; low: $1,000; average: $1,000-$50,000).
Purpose and activities: Awards and grants are limited to institutions where primary activities are to support senior centers in central TX; provide sight saving programs in developing counties; and for local schools and colleges, local United Ways and Rotary Foundations; also some support in developing countries.
Fields of interest: Higher education; Eye disease; Health organizations; Eye research; Human services; Aging, centers & services; Federated giving programs; Religious federated giving programs; Government/public administration; Latinos; Aging; Africa; Latin America; Mexico; Honduras.
Types of support: Capital campaigns, building/renovation, equipment, endowment funds, program development, seed money, matching funds.
Limitations: Giving limited to central TX. Generally, no support for program operations.
Publications: Informational brochure.
Application information: Application form not required.
Initial approach: Proposal
Deadline(s): Oct. 1
Board meeting date(s): Nov.
Final notification: Nov.
Officer and Trustees:* Alan C. Jones, M.D.,* Pres. and Secy.; John M. Burrough, David Fischer, Charles Harrel, Ginger Jones, Scott MacEwan.
Number of staff: None.
EIN: 742444567
Grants for Aging:
Senior Center, $6,000. For endowment fund. 94.
Senior Center, $2,000. 94.

945
C. J. & Syble Fowlston Charitable Trust
c/o First Bank of Southwest
2201 Civic Circle, Suite 715
Amarillo 79109 (806) 358-4513
Contact: U.C. Sterquell, Trustee

Donor(s): Syble Fowlston, C.J. Fowlston.‡
Financial data (yr. ended 12/31/94): Assets, $2,061,433 (M); gifts received, $30,125; expenditures, $145,921; qualifying distributions, $109,757, including $92,656 for 7 grants (high: $50,000; low: $2,000).
Fields of interest: Health associations; Human services; Aging, centers & services; Human services.
Limitations: Giving limited to the top twenty counties of the TX Panhandle. No grants to individuals.
Application information:
Initial approach: Letter
Deadline(s): None
Final notification: Within two months
Trustees: Joyce Perkins, U.C. Sterquell.
EIN: 756281596
Grants for Aging:
Alzheimers Disease and Related Disorders Association, Amarillo, TX, $5,000. 94.
Amarillo Senior Citizens Association, Amarillo, TX, $12,156. For capital improvements. 94.
Meals on Wheels of Amarillo, Amarillo, TX, $10,000. 94.

946
Kenneth P. Gifford Foundation
c/o Texas Commerce Trust Co.
P.O. Drawer 140
El Paso 79980
Contact: Pat Sandford

Established in 1977.
Financial data (yr. ended 09/30/95): Assets, $1,592,966 (M); expenditures, $108,397; qualifying distributions, $90,350, including

$88,500 for 3 grants (high: $62,500; low: $4,000).
Purpose and activities: Emphasis on organizations concerned with care for the aged and youth; supports a scholarship program sponsored by El Paso Community Foundation for students of local high schools for undergraduate study at the University of Texas-El Paso.
Fields of interest: Higher education; Youth, services; Aging, centers & services; Federated giving programs; Aging.
Types of support: General/operating support, scholarship funds.
Limitations: Giving primarily in El Paso County, TX. No grants to individuals.
Application information: Application form not required.
Initial approach: Letter
Copies of proposal: 1
Deadline(s): Mar. 1
Board meeting date(s): Mar.
Trustee: Texas Commerce Trust Co.
EIN: 741977400

947
Meyer and Ida Gordon Foundation
2401 Fountain View, Suite 350
Houston 77057

Incorporated in 1950 in TX.
Donor(s): Members of the Gordon family, Gordon's Jewelry Co.
Financial data (yr. ended 12/31/95): Assets, $7,246,729 (M); expenditures, $139,259; qualifying distributions, $136,883, including $136,883 for 16 grants (high: $100,000; low: $50).
Purpose and activities: Giving primarily to a children's hospital, a Jewish welfare fund, and a geriatric center.
Fields of interest: Hospitals (general); Nursing home/convalescent facility; Human services; Jewish federated giving programs; Jewish agencies & temples.
Limitations: Applications not accepted. Giving primarily in Houston, TX. No grants to individuals.
Application information: Contributes only to pre-selected organizations.
Officers: Harry B. Gordon, Pres.; James C. Gordon, V.P. and Secy.; Aron S. Gordon, V.P. and Treas.
EIN: 746046795
Grants for Aging:
Seven Acres Jewish Geriatric Center, Houston, TX, $100,000. 94.

948
Leon and Beatrice Obenhaus Grodhaus Foundation
420 Walnut
P.O. Box 867
Columbus 78934
Contact: James H. Whitcomb, Secy.-Treas.

Established in 1984 in TX.
Financial data (yr. ended 12/31/94): Assets, $1,332,425 (M); expenditures, $72,078; qualifying distributions, $65,600, including $65,600 for 10 grants (high: $25,000; low: $1,000).
Purpose and activities: Giving primarily for welfare programs for needy families, the elderly, and health organizations; support also for education.
Fields of interest: Education; Hospitals (general); Health associations; Human services; Family services; Aging, centers & services; Aging.
Types of support: Endowment funds, scholarship funds.
Limitations: Giving limited to the Weimar, Colorado County, TX, area.
Application information: Application form not required.
Initial approach: Letter
Deadline(s): None
Officer and Trustees:* James H. Whitcomb,* Secy.-Treas.; F.T. Barfield, Alfred Flournoy, Gus H. Miller, Jr., Harvey Vornsand.
EIN: 746328959

949
Paul and Mary Haas Foundation
P.O. Box 2928
Corpus Christi 78403 (512) 887-6955
Contact: Karen L. Wesson, Exec. Dir.

Trust established in 1954 in TX.
Donor(s): Paul R. Haas, Mary F. Haas.
Financial data (yr. ended 12/31/95): Assets, $1,275,087 (M); gifts received, $200,000; expenditures, $376,834, qualifying distributions, $332,052, including $332,052 for 102 grants (high: $24,600; low: $100; average: $5,000).
Purpose and activities: Primary areas of interest include social services, the disadvantaged and the homeless, higher and other education, and civic affairs. Grants also for youth agencies, housing, child development, alcohol abuse programs, early childhood, and adult education, the fine arts and other cultural programs, and community funds; scholarships only to Corpus Christi High School graduates entering freshman year; limited medical support, including cancer and other medical research.
Fields of interest: Visual arts; Performing arts; Dance; Music; Arts/cultural programs; Education, association; Early childhood education; Child development, education; Elementary school/education; Secondary school/education; Higher education; Adult/continuing education; Adult education—literacy & basic skills; Reading; Education; Animal welfare; Hospitals (general); Family planning; Medical care, rehabilitation; Health care; Substance abuse, services; Cancer; AIDS; Alcoholism; Health organizations; Cancer research; AIDS research; Delinquency prevention/services; Food services; Housing/shelter, development; Youth development, services; Human services; Children & youth, services; Child development, services; Family services; Aging, centers & services; Women, centers & services; Homeless, human services; Civil rights; Community development; Federated giving programs; Government/public administration; Leadership development; Disabled; Aging; Women; Economically disadvantaged; Homeless; General charitable giving.
Types of support: General/operating support, continuing support, annual campaigns, equipment, emergency funds, program development, conferences/seminars, seed money, scholarship funds, scholarships—to individuals, matching funds.
Limitations: Giving primarily in the Corpus Christi, TX, area. No grants to individuals (except for student aid); no support for graduate students.
Publications: Annual report (including application guidelines), application guidelines, 990-PF, grants list, financial statement.
Application information: Application form required for scholarship applicants only. Application form not required.
Initial approach: Proposal
Copies of proposal: 1
Deadline(s): For scholarships, Nov. of senior high school year; none for other grants
Board meeting date(s): 1st quarter of the year
Final notification: Within a few weeks of receipt of proposal
Officers and Trustees:* Paul R. Haas,* Pres.; Rheta Haas Page,* Secy.; Mary F. Haas, Raymond P. Haas, Rene Haas.
Number of staff: 1 part-time professional.
EIN: 746031614

950
The Curtis & Doris K. Hankamer Foundation
9039 Katy Freeway, Suite 530
Houston 77024-1623
Contact: Gregory A. Herbst

Established in 1981 in TX.
Donor(s): Doris K. Hankamer, Earl Curtis Hankamer, Jr.‡
Financial data (yr. ended 12/31/94): Assets, $7,007,655 (M); expenditures, $589,013; qualifying distributions, $475,602, including $470,000 for 11 grants (high: $300,000; low: $2,500).
Purpose and activities: Giving primarily to a medical school for geriatrics fellowships and cancer research; some support also for ministry programs.
Fields of interest: Cancer; Medical research; Cancer research; Aging, centers & services; Christian agencies & churches; Aging.
Types of support: General/operating support, fellowships.
Limitations: Applications not accepted. Giving primarily in Houston, TX. No grants to individuals.
Application information: Contributes only to pre-selected organizations.
Trustees: S. Terry Bracken, Doris K. Hankamer, Scott Hunsaker.
Number of staff: None.
EIN: 760022687
Grants for Aging:
Meals on Wheels of Houston, Houston, TX, $15,000. 94.
Saint Joseph Hospital Foundation, Houston, TX, $50,000. For senior services. 94.

951
Hardin Foundation for Wichita County
P.O. Drawer 97511
Wichita Falls 76307-7511
Contact: Joseph N. Sherrill, Jr., Chair.
Scholarship application address: Judy Simmons, Financial Aid Office, Midwestern State Univ., 3400 Taft Blvd., Wichita Falls, TX 76308

Established in 1934 in TX.
Financial data (yr. ended 12/31/95): Assets, $625,818 (M); expenditures, $33,935; qualifying distributions, $27,161, including $25,006 for grants.
Purpose and activities: Professorship and scholarship restricted to faculties and students of Midwestern University, TX; some support for youth, civic affairs and the elderly.
Fields of interest: Education; Aging, centers & services; Government/public administration; Aging.
Types of support: Professorships, scholarship funds, scholarships—to individuals.
Limitations: Giving primarily in Wichita County, TX.
Publications: 990-PF.
Application information: Application form for scholarship required.
Initial approach: Letter
Copies of proposal: 1
Deadline(s): Apr. 1, July 1, and Nov. 1 for scholarship
Board meeting date(s): Dec. 1
Final notification: Dec. 15
Trustees: Joseph N. Sherrill, Jr., Chair.; R. Caven Crosnoe.
Number of staff: 1 part-time professional; 1 part-time support.
EIN: 751106480

952
The Don and Sybil Harrington Foundation
700 First National Place I
801 South Fillmore
Amarillo 79101 (806) 373-8353
Contact: Jim Allison, Pres. and Exec. Dir.

Trust established in 1951 in TX; incorporated in 1971; supporting organization of Amarillo Area Foundation, Inc.
Donor(s): Donald D. Harrington,‡ Sybil B. Harrington.
Financial data (yr. ended 12/31/95): Assets, $78,990,251 (M); expenditures, $4,978,456; qualifying distributions, $4,842,566, including $4,471,080 for 36 grants (high: $1,342,157; low: $1,000; average: $10,000-$250,000) and $71,486 for 1 foundation-administered program.
Purpose and activities: Interests include hospitals and health agencies, the arts and cultural programs, higher and other education, including scholarship funds, youth agencies, social services, and civic affairs.
Fields of interest: Arts/cultural programs; Early childhood education; Education; Health care; Human services; Youth, services; Child development, services; Aging, centers & services; Human services.
Types of support: Building/renovation, equipment, program development, scholarship funds, technical assistance, matching funds.
Limitations: Giving limited to the 26 northernmost counties of the Texas Panhandle. No grants to individuals, or for operating support, annual campaigns, deficit financing, endowment funds, publications, or conferences; no loans.
Publications: Application guidelines.
Application information: Application form required.
Initial approach: Letter or telephone
Copies of proposal: 1
Deadline(s): Quartery; Jan., Mar., July, and Sept.
Board meeting date(s): Board meets quarterly Mar., May, Aug., and Dec.
Final notification: 2 months following submission deadline
Officers and Directors:* Richard Ware II,* Chair.; Don Powell,* Vice-Chair.; Jim Allison, Pres. and Exec. Dir.; Jack Shelton, Secy.-Treas.; and 4 additional directors.
Number of staff: None.
EIN: 751336604
Grants for Aging:
ACT for the Elderly, Amarillo, TX, $76,605. 94.
Amarillo Multiservice Center for the Aging, Amarillo, TX, $350,000. 94.

953
John Herman Hasenbeck Trust
500 Elizabeth Rd.
San Antonio 78209 (210) 225-5964
Contact: George A. Olson, Trustee

Financial data (yr. ended 12/31/95): Assets, $689,660 (M); expenditures, $44,581; qualifying distributions, $44,581, including $17,000 for 8 grants (high: $4,000; low: $1,000).
Fields of interest: Health associations; Christian agencies & churches; Aging.
Limitations: Giving primarily in San Antonio, TX.
Application information:
Initial approach: Letter
Deadline(s): Oct. 1
Trustee: George A. Olson.
EIN: 746327096

954
Ed and Mary Heath Foundation
P.O. Box 338
Tyler 75710 (903) 597-7436
Contact: Charlotte Schaefers, Asst. to Chair.

Established in 1954 in TX.
Donor(s): J.E. Heath,‡ Mary M. Heath.‡
Financial data (yr. ended 12/31/94): Assets, $2,348,076 (M); expenditures, $278,190; qualifying distributions, $117,531, including $77,856 for 122 grants (high: $6,000; low: $25).
Purpose and activities: Giving primarily for human services, including programs to train youth in leadership and work skills, and small rural churches in Smith County, TX.
Fields of interest: Arts/cultural programs; Education; Housing/shelter, development; Youth development, services; Human services; Youth, services; Aging, centers & services; Christian agencies & churches; Aging; Economically disadvantaged.
Types of support: General/operating support, annual campaigns, building/renovation, equipment, emergency funds, program development, conferences/seminars, seed money, curriculum development, scholarship funds, matching funds.
Limitations: Giving limited to Smith County, TX. No support for private schools. No grants to individuals, or for endowment funds.
Publications: Newsletter, occasional report.
Application information: Application form not required.
Initial approach: Brief letter
Copies of proposal: 1
Deadline(s): None
Board meeting date(s): Mar., June, Sept., and Dec.
Final notification: Dec.
Officers and Directors:* W.R. Smith, Chair.; Jack Jackson,* Secy.-Treas.; Charlotte Smith Shaefers,* Prog. Officer; Russell Cooper, L.H. Reese, Margaret Smith, Charles White.
Staff: Gregg Bonham, C.P.A., Accountant.
Number of staff: 3 full-time professional; 1 part-time professional.
EIN: 756021506

955
Wilton & Effie Mae Hebert Foundation
P.O. Box 908
Port Neches 77651
Contact: Pauline Womack, Dir.
Application address: 802 West Dr., Port Neches, TX 77651

Established in 1992 in TX.
Donor(s): Wilton P. Hebert,‡ Effie Mae Hebert.‡
Financial data (yr. ended 12/31/95): Assets, $3,316,979 (M); expenditures, $764,519; qualifying distributions, $656,175, including $632,070 for 23 grants (high: $125,000; low: $4,000).
Fields of interest: Literature; Libraries/library science; Education; Aging, centers & services; Science; Religion; Aging.
Types of support: General/operating support, building/renovation.
Limitations: Giving primarily in Port Neches, TX. No grants to individuals.
Application information: Application form required.
Copies of proposal: 6
Deadline(s): None
Board meeting date(s): Mar., June, Sept., and Dec.
Directors: Earl Black, James Black, Joe Hebert, Ed Hughes, Joe Vernon, Pauline Womack.
Number of staff: 1 full-time professional; 1 part-time professional.
EIN: 760065521
Grants for Aging:
Groves Senior Citizens Foundation, Groves, TX, $15,000. 95.
Mid-County Senior Citizens Foundation, Port Neches, TX, $15,000. 95.

956
Hillcrest Foundation
c/o NationsBank of Texas, N.A., Trust Div.
P.O. Box 830241
Dallas 75283-0241 (214) 508-1965
Contact: Daniel Kelly, V.P., NationsBank of Texas, N.A.

Trust established in 1959 in TX.
Donor(s): Mrs. W.W. Caruth, Sr.‡
Financial data (yr. ended 05/31/95): Assets, $135,621,469 (M); expenditures, $8,767,596; qualifying distributions, $7,831,207, including $7,746,079 for 232 grants (high: $500,000; low: $1,000; average: $10,000-$50,000).
Purpose and activities: To relieve poverty, advance education, and promote health; support for higher and other education, health and hospitals, social services, including programs for youth and child welfare, drug abuse, rehabilitation and housing.
Fields of interest: Education, fund raising; Secondary school/education; Vocational education; Higher education; Business school/education; Adult/continuing education; Education; Hospitals (general); Dental care; Medical care, rehabilitation; Health care; Substance abuse, services; Cancer; Health organizations; Medical research; Cancer research; Food services; Housing/shelter, development; Human services; Children & youth, services; Aging, centers & services; Disabled; Aging.
Types of support: General/operating support, continuing support, capital campaigns, building/renovation, equipment, land acquisition, program development, research, matching funds.
Limitations: Giving limited to TX, with emphasis on Dallas. No grants to individuals, or for endowment funds, scholarships, or fellowships; no loans.
Publications: Application guidelines, informational brochure (including application guidelines).
Application information: Application form required.
Initial approach: Letter
Copies of proposal: 2
Deadline(s): End of Mar., Aug., and Nov.
Board meeting date(s): As required, usually 3 times annually; May, Oct., and Jan.
Final notification: Within 30 days after meeting
Trustees: D. Harold Byrd, Jr., Mabel P. Caruth, Harry A. Shuford, Chas P. Storey, NationsBank of Texas, N.A.
Number of staff: 1 part-time professional; 2 part-time support.
EIN: 756007565
Grants for Aging:
Assistance League of Dallas, Dallas, TX, $16,000. For improvements and maintenance of senior citizens facility. 94.
Grace Presbyterian Village Ministries, Dallas, TX, $60,000. For Alzheimer's personal care unit conversion to provide safe and active environment for residents. 94.
Hearts and Hammers, Dallas, TX, $10,000. To repair and improve housing for elderly and low income families. 94.
Juliette Fowler Homes, Dallas, TX, $25,000. For community based youth program to provide counseling and education to emotionally, mentally, behaviorally disturbed youth, children and their families. 94.
Salvation Army of Dallas, Dallas, TX, $23,000. For van for Cedar Crest Corps Community Center for youth and senior citizen programs. 94.

957
Hoblitzelle Foundation
5956 Sherry Ln., Suite 901
Dallas 75225-6522 (214) 373-0462
Contact: Paul W. Harris, Exec. V.P.

Trust established in 1942 in TX; incorporated in 1953.
Donor(s): Karl St. John Hoblitzelle,‡ Esther T. Hoblitzelle.‡
Financial data (yr. ended 04/30/95): Assets, $81,841,822 (M); gifts received, $18,892; expenditures, $4,687,667; qualifying distributions, $4,440,427, including $4,006,436 for 76 grants (high: $250,000; low: $250; average: $25,000-$50,000).
Purpose and activities: Grants for higher, secondary, vocational, and medical education, hospitals and health services, youth agencies, cultural programs, social services, and community development.
Fields of interest: Visual arts; Performing arts; Historic preservation/historical societies; Arts/cultural programs; Secondary school/education; Vocational education; Higher education; Medical school/education; Adult/continuing education; Adult education—literacy & basic skills; Reading; Education; Hospitals (general); Medical care, rehabilitation; Health care; AIDS; Alcoholism; AIDS research; Housing/shelter, development; Human services; Children & youth, services; Aging, centers & services; Community development; Minorities; Aging; Economically disadvantaged.
Types of support: General/operating support, capital campaigns, building/renovation, equipment, land acquisition, program development, seed money, matching funds.
Limitations: Giving limited to TX, primarily Dallas. No support for religious organizations for sectarian purposes. No grants to individuals; only occasional board-initiated support for operating budgets, debt reduction, research, scholarships, or endowments; no loans.
Publications: Annual report (including application guidelines), program policy statement, newsletter.
Application information: Application form not required.
Initial approach: Letter
Copies of proposal: 1
Deadline(s): May 15, Sep. 15, and Jan. 15
Board meeting date(s): Later part of May, Sept., and Jan.
Final notification: After next board meeting
Officers and Directors:* James W. Keay,* Chair.; Gerald W. Fronterhouse, Pres.; Paul W. Harris, Exec. V.P.; Mary L. Stacy, Secy.; George A. Shafer, Treas.; Lillian M. Bradshaw, Dorothy R. Cullum, Charles C. Sprague, M.D.
Number of staff: 1 full-time professional; 1 full-time support.
EIN: 756003984
Grants for Aging:
Grace Presbyterian Village Ministries, Dallas, TX, $59,750. To renovate clinic, medical evaluation and professional training areas. 95.

958
M. G. and Lillie A. Johnson Foundation, Inc.
P.O. Box 2269
Victoria 77902 (512) 575-7970
Contact: Robert Halepeska, Exec. V.P.

Incorporated in 1958 in TX.
Donor(s): M.G. Johnson,‡ Lillie A. Johnson.‡
Financial data (yr. ended 11/30/95): Assets, $35,573,948 (M); expenditures, $1,948,277; qualifying distributions, $1,679,098, including $1,672,105 for 40 grants (high: $175,000; low: $2,229; average: $20,000-$100,000).
Purpose and activities: Primary emphasis on medical and allied health purposes and institutions of higher education.
Fields of interest: Higher education; Nursing school/education; Education; Hospitals (general); Nursing care; Health care; Health organizations; Human services; Aging, centers & services; Community development.
Types of support: Capital campaigns, building/renovation, equipment, land acquisition, scholarship funds, matching funds.
Limitations: Giving limited primarily to TX. Recently giving exclusively to the Gulf Coast area located between San Patricio and Wharton counties. No grants to individuals, or for general support, operating budgets, endowment funds, fellowships, research, special projects, publications, or conferences; no loans.
Publications: Application guidelines.
Application information: Application form not required.
Initial approach: Proposal
Copies of proposal: 1
Deadline(s): Submit proposal 1 month before meetings; no set deadline
Board meeting date(s): Mar., July, and Oct.
Final notification: Varies
Officers and Trustees:* Irving Moore, Jr.,* Pres.; Robert Halepeska, Exec. V.P.; Jack R. Morrison,* V.P.; Rev. M.H. Lehnhardt,* Secy.; M.H. Brock, Dick Koop, Lloyd Rust, Munson Smith.
Number of staff: 1 full-time professional; 1 part-time support.
EIN: 746076961
Grants for Aging:
Lavaca, County of, Hallettsville, TX, $40,000. Toward building Nutrition Center in Moulton for Lavaca County Senior Citizens Center. 94.

959
Robert W. Knox, Sr. and Pearl Wallis Knox Charitable Foundation
c/o NationsBank of Texas, N.A.
P.O. Box 298502
Houston 77298-0502 (713) 787-4553
Contact: Carl Schumacher, Sr. V.P., NationsBank of Texas, N.A.

Established in 1964 in TX.
Donor(s): Robert W. Knox, Jr.‡
Financial data (yr. ended 08/31/94): Assets, $3,968,831 (M); expenditures, $236,289;

qualifying distributions, $200,558, including $190,600 for 74 grants (high: $15,000; low: $100; average: $500-$5,000).
Fields of interest: Performing arts; Historic preservation/historical societies; Adult education—literacy & basic skills; Reading; Substance abuse, services; Mental health/crisis services; AIDS; AIDS research; Food services; Human services; Children & youth, services; Youth, services; Family services; Aging, centers & services; Voluntarism promotion; Disabled; Aging; Economically disadvantaged.
Limitations: Giving primarily in Houston, TX. No grants to individuals.
Application information: Application form not required.
Initial approach: Letter
Copies of proposal: 1
Deadline(s): None
Board meeting date(s): Monthly
Trustee Bank: NationsBank of Texas, N.A.
EIN: 746064974
Grants for Aging:
Jewish Community Center of Houston, Houston Day Center for Older Adults, Houston, TX, $1,000. 94.

960
Arnold J. and Irene B. Kocurek Family Foundation, 1986

562 PR 2635
Rio Medina 78066 (210) 751-2881
Contact: Arnold J. Kocurek

Established in 1986 in TX.
Donor(s): Arnold J. Kocurek, Irene B. Kocurek.
Financial data (yr. ended 02/28/95): Assets, $127,692 (M); gifts received, $111,888; expenditures, $62,204; qualifying distributions, $62,204, including $60,000 for 27 grants (high: $5,000; low: $1,000).
Fields of interest: Education, research; Elementary/secondary education; Higher education; Theological school/education; Education; Hospitals (general); Health care; Substance abuse, services; Health associations; Cancer; Alcoholism; Cancer research; Human services; Children & youth, services; Hospices; Aging, centers & services; Homeless, human services; Community development; Federated giving programs; Roman Catholic federated giving programs; Religious federated giving programs; Christian agencies & churches; Roman Catholic agencies & churches; Disabled; Aging; Economically disadvantaged; Homeless; General charitable giving.
Types of support: Professorships, fellowships, research, matching funds.
Limitations: Giving limited to TX, with emphasis on San Antonio.
Application information: Application form not required.
Initial approach: Letter
Copies of proposal: 1
Deadline(s): None
Trustee: Frost National Bank.
Number of staff: 1 part-time support.
EIN: 746345100
Grants for Aging:
Respite Care of San Antonio, San Antonio, TX, $2,000. 95.

961
Marcia & Otto Koehler Foundation

c/o NationsBank of Texas, N.A.
P.O. Box 121
San Antonio 78291-0121 (210) 270-5313
Contact: J.A. Higginson, Jr., V.P., NationsBank of Texas, N.A.

Established in 1980 in TX.
Donor(s): Marcia Koehler.‡
Financial data (yr. ended 07/31/95): Assets, $7,637,180 (M); expenditures, $563,653; qualifying distributions, $492,647, including $492,647 for 49 grants (high: $50,000; low: $500).
Fields of interest: Arts/cultural programs; Higher education; Nursing school/education; Human services; Youth, services; Disabled; Aging; Economically disadvantaged.
Types of support: General/operating support, building/renovation, research.
Limitations: Giving limited to Bexar County, TX. No grants to individuals.
Application information: Application form required.
Initial approach: Letter
Copies of proposal: 10
Deadline(s): June 1
Board meeting date(s): July 31
Final notification: Aug.
Trustee: NationsBank of Texas, N.A.
Number of staff: None.
EIN: 742131195

962
Lula Hasam McAfee Trust

c/o Texas Commerce Bank, N.A.
P.O. Drawer 140
El Paso 79980 (915) 546-2454
Contact: Pat Sandford, V.P., Texas Commerce Bank, N.A.

Financial data (yr. ended 07/31/95): Assets, $768,297 (M); expenditures, $43,953; qualifying distributions, $33,864, including $29,400 for grants.
Purpose and activities: Supports programs for the elderly.
Fields of interest: Aging, centers & services; Protestant agencies & churches; Aging.
Limitations: Giving limited to El Paso County, TX.
Application information:
Initial approach: Letter
Deadline(s): None
Trustee: Texas Commerce Bank, N.A.
EIN: 746109154

963
Meadows Foundation, Inc.

Wilson Historic Block
3003 Swiss Ave.
Dallas 75204-6090 (214) 826-9431
Contact: Bruce Esterline, V.P., Grants

Incorporated in 1948 in TX.
Donor(s): Algur Hurtle Meadows,‡ Virginia Meadows.‡
Financial data (yr. ended 12/31/94): Assets, $559,077,594 (M); expenditures, $37,747,367; qualifying distributions, $31,238,347, including $25,198,912 for grants (average: $10,000-$1,000,000), $2,971,590 for 2 foundation-administered programs and $700 for 1 program-related investment.
Purpose and activities: Support for the arts, social services, community and rural development, health, education, and civic and cultural programs. Operates a historic preservation investment-related program using a cluster of Victorian homes as offices for nonprofit agencies.
Fields of interest: Media/communications; Film/video; Architecture; Museums; Humanities; History & archaeology; Historic preservation/historical societies; Arts/cultural programs; Early childhood education; Child development, education; Medical school/education; Adult/continuing education; Adult education—literacy & basic skills; Libraries/library science; Reading; Education; Natural resource conservation & protection; Environment; Wildlife preservation & protection; Dental care; Medical care, rehabilitation; Nursing care; Health care; Substance abuse, services; Mental health/crisis services; AIDS; Alcoholism; AIDS research; Crime/law enforcement; Employment; Agriculture; Nutrition; Housing/shelter, development; Safety/disasters; Recreation; Youth development, services; Human services; Children & youth, services; Child development, services; Family services; Hospices; Aging, centers & services; Homeless, human services; International affairs, goodwill promotion; Race/intergroup relations; Urban/community development; Rural development; Community development; Voluntarism promotion; Government/public administration; Transportation; Leadership development; Public affairs; Christian agencies & churches; Aging; Economically disadvantaged; Homeless.
Types of support: General/operating support, continuing support, capital campaigns, building/renovation, equipment, land acquisition, endowment funds, debt reduction, emergency funds, program development, conferences/seminars, professorships, publication, seed money, curriculum development, fellowships, internships, research, technical assistance, consulting services, program-related investments/loans, matching funds.
Limitations: Giving limited to TX. No grants to individuals; generally, no grants for annual fundraising appeals, biomedical research projects, professional conferences and symposia, or travel expenses for groups to perform or compete outside of TX.
Publications: Annual report (including application guidelines), program policy statement, application guidelines.
Application information: Application form not required.
Initial approach: Proposal
Copies of proposal: 1
Deadline(s): None
Board meeting date(s): Grants review committee meets monthly; full board meets 2 or 3 times a year to act on major grants
Final notification: 3 to 4 months
Officers and Directors:* Robert A. Meadows,* Chair. and V.P.; Linda P. Evans,* Pres.; G. Tomas

Rhodus, V.P. and Secy.; Robert E. Wise, V.P., Finance, C.F.O., and Treas.; Bruce Esterline, V.P., Grants; Evy Kay Ritzen,* V.P., Opers.; Judy B. Culbertson, V.P.; Eloise Meadows Rouse,* V.P.; Robert E. Weiss, V.P.; John W. Broadfoot, J.W. Bullion, Daniel Chapman, John A. Hammack, Sally R. Lancaster, P. Mike McCullough, Mark Meadows, Sally C. Miller, Dorothy C. Wilson.
Staff: Michael K. McCoy, Sr. Prog. Officer; D. Matteson Pascal, Sr. Prog. Officer; Esmer Garza Wear, Prog. Officer.
Number of staff: 18 full-time professional; 3 part-time professional; 24 full-time support; 2 part-time support.
EIN: 756015322
Grants for Aging:
Christopher House, Austin, TX, $45,000. Toward start-up support for home health services for persons with AIDS. 95.
Friendly Door, Iowa Park, TX, $14,284. For heating and air conditioning system for new senior citizens activities center. 95.
Gathering Place, Houston, TX, $40,000. Toward continuation of support services for mentally ill adults. 95.
Gem of the Hills Senior Citizens Community Center, Blanco, TX, $25,310. For kitchen equipment and supplies for new center. 95.
Hill Country Senior Citizens Center, Dripping Springs, TX, $26,458. Toward construction of new facility to relocate thrift store. 95.
Senior Citizens Center of Dawson County, Lamesa, TX, $44,546. To retire debt incurred in facility updating. 95.
University of Texas Health Science Center, San Antonio, TX, $90,000. For annual biomedical research awards to junior investigators and post-doctoral research fellows working in research on aging. 95.
YMCA of Beaumont, Beaumont, TX, $235,000. Toward renovation of historic building for housing for low-income elderly persons. 95.

964
The Moody Foundation
2302 Postoffice St., Suite 704
Galveston 77550 (409) 763-5333
Contact: Peter M. Moore, Grants Officer

Trust established in 1942 in TX.
Donor(s): William Lewis Moody, Jr.,‡ Libbie Shearn Moody.‡
Financial data (yr. ended 12/31/95): Assets, $330,735,000 (M); gifts received, $13,292,000; expenditures, $18,099,000; qualifying distributions, $15,042,023, including $15,364,000 for 37 grants (high: $5,845,636; low: $5,000) and $350,000 for grants to individuals.
Purpose and activities: Funds to be used for historic restoration projects, performing arts organizations, and cultural programs; promotion of health, science, and education; community and social services; and the field of religion.
Fields of interest: Performing arts; Arts/cultural programs; Medical school/education; Education; Health care; AIDS; Medical research; AIDS research; Human services; Community development; Engineering & technology; Science; Religion; Disabled; Aging; Economically disadvantaged.
Types of support: Capital campaigns, building/renovation, equipment, land acquisition, program development, conferences/seminars, publication, seed money, scholarship funds, research, technical assistance, matching funds.
Limitations: Giving limited to TX. No grants to individuals (except for students covered by one scholarship program in Galveston County), or for operating budgets (except for start-up purposes), continuing support, annual campaigns, or deficit financing; no loans.
Publications: Annual report, application guidelines, 990-PF, financial statement.
Application information: Foundation will send application guidelines if project is of interest. For scholarship application form and submission deadlines contact Nelda Davis. Application form not required.
Initial approach: Letter or telephone
Copies of proposal: 1
Deadline(s): 6 weeks prior to board meetings
Board meeting date(s): Quarterly
Final notification: 3 weeks after board meetings
Officers and Trustees:* Frances Moody Newman,* Chair.; Robert L. Moody,* Vice-Chair.; Robert E. Baker, Secy. and Exec. Administrator; Ross R. Moody,* Treas.; Harold C. MacDonald, Compt.
Staff: Peter M. Moore, Grant Officer; Allan Matthews, Prog. Officer; Gerald J. Smith, Prog. Officer.
Number of staff: 7 full-time professional; 7 full-time support.
EIN: 741403105
Grants for Aging:
Harbourview Care Center, League City, TX, $441,624. To continue operating support of Harbourview Sleep Laboratory as both competitive research facility studying sleep abnormalities in elderly and respiratory function during sleep and as clinical sleep laboratory providing therapeutic interventions. 95.
University of Texas Medical Branch, Galveston, TX, $163,075. For Director of Sleep Laboratory and Director of Behavioral Research for their continued investigation of sleep disorders in elderly and other special populations as collaborative effort with Harbourview Care Center Sleep Laboratory. 95.

965
Louise L. Morrison Trust
c/o Frost National Bank, Trust Dept.
P.O. Box 2950
San Antonio 78299-2950 (210) 220-4449
Contact: William T. Clyborne, Jr., V.P., Frost National Bank

Donor(s): Louise L. Morrison.‡
Financial data (yr. ended 09/30/95): Assets, $1,893,808 (M); expenditures, $85,205; qualifying distributions, $74,219, including $66,280 for 6 grants (high: $28,408; low: $4,734).
Fields of interest: Higher education; Human services; Aging, centers & services; Aging.
Limitations: Giving limited to San Antonio, TX.
Application information:
Initial approach: Proposal
Deadline(s): Sept. 30
Trustee: Frost National Bank.
Number of staff: 2 part-time professional.
EIN: 741386236
Grants for Aging:
Sarah Roberts French Home, San Antonio, TX, $7,218. 94.
Sarah Roberts French Home, San Antonio, TX, $4,734. 95.

966
Oshman Foundation
P.O. Box 230234
Houston 77223-8234

Established in 1958.
Donor(s): Oshman Sporting Goods, Jeanette Oshman Efron.
Foundation type: Company-sponsored
Financial data (yr. ended 11/30/95): Assets, $3,385,565 (M); gifts received, $40,000; expenditures, $143,590; qualifying distributions, $139,404, including $138,542 for 58 grants (high: $37,000; low: $250).
Purpose and activities: Support primarily for Jewish giving; support also for the aged, cultural programs, and a college of medicine.
Fields of interest: Elementary/secondary education; Medical school/education; Recreation, community facilities; Children & youth, services; Aging, centers & services; Jewish agencies & temples; Aging.
Limitations: Applications not accepted. Giving primarily in Houston, TX. No grants to individuals.
Application information: Contributes only to pre-selected organizations.
Officers and Directors:* Jeanette Oshman Efron,* Pres.; Marilyn O. Lubetkin,* V.P.; Judy O. Margolis,* V.P.; Marvin Aronowitz, Alvin N. Lubetkin.
EIN: 746039864
Grants for Aging:
Seven Acres Jewish Geriatric Center, Houston, TX, $36,000. 94.
Seven Acres Jewish Geriatric Center, Houston, TX, $15,000. 95.

967
David D. & Nona S. Payne Foundation, Inc.
Hughes Bldg., Suite 436
Pampa 79065 (806) 665-7281
Contact: Vanessa G. Buzzard, Pres.
Application address: c/o Adelaide S. Colwell, Secy., 2000 Charles, Pampa, TX 79065; Tel.: (806) 665-3488

Established in 1980 in TX.
Donor(s): Nona S. Payne.‡
Financial data (yr. ended 06/30/95): Assets, $2,040,685 (M); gifts received, $47,327; expenditures, $120,329; qualifying distributions, $110,180, including $110,180 for 23 grants (high: $26,000; low: $500; average: $1,000-$10,000).
Purpose and activities: Primary areas of interest include the fine arts, education, social services, the elderly, and youth.

Fields of interest: Visual arts; Museums; Performing arts; Adult education—literacy & basic skills; Libraries/library science; Reading; Education; Mental health/crisis services; Human services; Youth, services; Hospices; Aging, centers & services; Government/public administration; Christian agencies & churches; Aging.
Types of support: General/operating support, building/renovation, equipment, emergency funds, matching funds.
Limitations: Giving primarily in the TX Panhandle area. No grants to individuals.
Application information: Application form required.
Initial approach: Letter or telephone
Copies of proposal: 3
Deadline(s): Sept. 23 and Mar. 23; grant awards are made semiannually in Apr. and Oct.
Board meeting date(s): 1st Tuesday of each calendar quarter
Final notification: 2 weeks
Officers and Trustees:* Vanessa G. Buzzard,* Pres.; Rebecca L. Holmes,* V.P. and Treas.; Adelaide S. Colwell,* Secy.
EIN: 751736339

968
Pearle Vision Foundation, Inc.
2534 Royal Ln.
Dallas 75229 (972) 277-5993
Contact: Trina Parasiliti, Administrator
Application address: P.O. Box 227175, Dallas, TX 75222

Established in 1986 in CA.
Donor(s): Pearle, Inc.
Foundation type: Operating
Financial data (yr. ended 09/30/95): Assets, $526,203 (M); gifts received, $388,627; expenditures, $394,432; qualifying distributions, $394,432, including $334,386 for 46 grants (high: $35,000; low: $400) and $29,986 for 18 grants to individuals (high: $2,500; low: $424).
Purpose and activities: Support for vision-oriented giving, including surgery for needy individuals, eye exams and eyeglass assistance programs and equipment for testing and improving vision.
Fields of interest: Eye disease; Eye research; Human services; Aging; Economically disadvantaged; Homeless.
Types of support: Equipment, program development, research, grants to individuals.
Limitations: Giving limited to the U.S.
Publications: Program policy statement, application guidelines, informational brochure.
Application information: Applications not accepted from individuals for routine eye exams or eyeglasses. Application form required.
Initial approach: Write or telephone for application form
Copies of proposal: 1
Deadline(s): Mar. 21, June 20, Sept. 19, and Dec. 21 for individual grants; Dec. 15, June 15 for block grants
Board meeting date(s): Jan., Apr., July, and Oct.
Final notification: Mid-Apr., mid-July, mid-Oct., and mid-Jan.
Officers and Directors:* Barbara McAninch,* Chair.; Trina Parasiliti, Secy.; Daniel Crowley, Treas.; Jeff Smith, O.D., Exec. Dir.; James Benning, O.D., Alan D. Davis, M.D., Stanley C. Pearle, O.D.
Number of staff: 1 part-time professional.
EIN: 752173714
Grants for Aging:
Associated Catholic Charities, Memphis, TN, $10,000. For low-income aged eyeglass and exam program. 95.
Vision Foundation, Watertown, MA, $4,000. For Visually Impaired Elders project. 95.

969
Leo Potishman Foundation
c/o Bank One, Texas, N.A.
P.O. Box 2050
Fort Worth 76113-2050 (817) 884-4153
Contact: Lesley Atkinson

Established in 1983 in TX.
Financial data (yr. ended 06/30/95): Assets, $4,187,668 (M); gifts received, $1,000; expenditures, $123,096; qualifying distributions, $93,563, including $92,000 for 7 grants (high: $50,000; low: $2,000; average: $2,500-$50,000).
Fields of interest: Higher education; Health associations; Youth, services; Aging; Economically disadvantaged; Homeless; General charitable giving.
Types of support: Continuing support, annual campaigns, capital campaigns, equipment.
Limitations: Giving primarily in TX. No grants to individuals.
Application information: Application form not required.
Initial approach: Letter
Copies of proposal: 1
Deadline(s): Sept.
Board meeting date(s): As needed
Trustee: Bank One, Texas, N.A.
EIN: 756314202

970
Potterhouse Foundation
5001 South Hulen, Suite 106
Fort Worth 76132 (817) 346-4416
Contact: A.E. Dumois, Dir.

Donor(s): A.E. Dumois.
Financial data (yr. ended 05/31/95): Assets, $91,104 (M); gifts received, $20,000; expenditures, $8,408; qualifying distributions, $8,424, including $7,950 for 8 grants (high: $5,000; low: $100).
Fields of interest: Aging, centers & services; Christian agencies & churches; Aging; Economically disadvantaged.
Types of support: Grants to individuals.
Limitations: Giving primarily in Fort Worth, TX.
Application information: Application form required for rental assistance.
Deadline(s): Feb 1.
Directors: A.E. Dumois, Sherry Lynn Dumois, Stephen E. Geis.
EIN: 751824677

971
The Powell Foundation
2121 San Felipe, Suite 110
Houston 77019-5600 (713) 523-7557
Contact: Ms. Nancy Powell Moore, Managing Trustee

Established in 1967 in TX.
Donor(s): Ben H. Powell, Jr.,‡ Kitty King Powell.
Financial data (yr. ended 12/31/95): Assets, $8,860,152 (M); expenditures, $344,839; qualifying distributions, $344,839, including $315,607 for 71 grants (high: $25,000; low: $200; average: $2,000-$5,000).
Fields of interest: Arts/cultural programs; Education, association; Education, research; Early childhood education; Higher education; Law school/education; Education; Environment; Health care; Medical research; Human services; Human services; Aging, centers & services; Minorities; Aging; Economically disadvantaged; General charitable giving.
Types of support: General/operating support.
Limitations: Giving primarily in Harris, Walker, and Travis counties, TX. No support for private foundations, or religious organizations for religious purposes. No grants to individuals, or for testimonial dinners, fundraising events, advertising, or debt retirement.
Publications: Informational brochure (including application guidelines).
Application information: Application form not required.
Initial approach: Letter
Copies of proposal: 1
Deadline(s): Varies
Board meeting date(s): Varies
Final notification: Positive replies only
Officers and Trustees:* Kitty King Powell,* Chair.; Nancy Powell Moore,* Secy. and Mgr.; Antonia Scott Day, Ben H. Powell V.
Number of staff: 1 part-time professional.
EIN: 746104592

972
Lulu Bryan Rambaud Charitable Trust
c/o Houston Trust Co.
1001 Fannin, Suite 1500
Houston 77002-6714

Financial data (yr. ended 12/31/95): Assets, $1,045,292 (M); expenditures, $39,110; qualifying distributions, $20,720, including $20,000 for 3 grants (high: $10,000; low: $5,000) and $720 for 1 grant to an individual.
Purpose and activities: Giving only for the benefit of elderly, indigent women.
Fields of interest: Aging, centers & services; Women, centers & services; Aging; Women; Economically disadvantaged.
Types of support: General/operating support, grants to individuals.
Limitations: Giving limited to Houston and Harris County, TX.
Application information: Individuals are referred by Sheltering Arms, Houston, TX. Application form not required.
Initial approach: Proposal
Copies of proposal: 1
Deadline(s): None
Trustees: James A. Elkins, Jr., Stuart A. Hellman, A.J. Hurt, Jr., NationsBank of Texas, N.A.

Number of staff: None.
EIN: 746033114

973
N. D. & Mary Redmon Foundation, Inc.

P.O. Box 88
Tulia 79088-0088 (806) 995-3528
Contact: George Jennings, Jr., Dir.

Financial data (yr. ended 12/31/94): Assets, $975,426 (M); expenditures, $54,386; qualifying distributions, $49,090, including $47,900 for 14 grants (high: $7,000; low: $500).
Fields of interest: Museums; Historic preservation/historical societies; Medical care, rehabilitation; Youth, services; Aging, centers & services; Community development; Aging.
Types of support: General/operating support, capital campaigns.
Limitations: Giving primarily in the Swisher County, TX, area. No grants to individuals.
Application information: Application form required.
Deadline(s): None
Board meeting date(s): Fall
Directors: Earl Bell Cosby, Kenneth B. Godwin, George J. Jennings, Jr.
EIN: 751333002

974
Redwine Foundation

P.O. Box 391
San Angelo 76902

Established in 1992.
Donor(s): Bruce A. Redwine.
Financial data (yr. ended 06/30/95): Assets, $63,545 (M); gifts received, $25,000; expenditures, $43,535; qualifying distributions, $43,535, including $36,876 for 7 grants (high: $18,500; low: $150).
Fields of interest: Higher education; Health care, emergency transport services; Housing/shelter, development; Human services; Aging, centers & services.
Types of support: Scholarship funds.
Limitations: Giving primarily in TX.
Application information:
Initial approach: Letter
Deadline(s): None
Trustees: G.E. Cannon, Thomas E. Covington, Bruce A. Redwine, Sharon Redwine, M.D. Schall, B.R. Williams.
EIN: 752441030

975
RGK Foundation

1301 West 25th St., Suite 300
Austin 78705-4236 (512) 474-9298
Contact: Gregory A. Kozmetsky, Pres.

Incorporated in 1966 in TX.
Donor(s): George Kozmetsky, Ronya Kozmetsky.
Financial data (yr. ended 12/31/94): Assets, $52,895,545 (M); gifts received, $9,637,300; expenditures, $2,544,589; qualifying distributions, $2,495,645, including $2,063,303 for 101 grants (high: $300,000; low: $25; average: $1,000-$10,000) and $19,008 for in-kind gifts.
Purpose and activities: Grants to higher educational institutions, with emphasis on medical and educational research; support also for business and economic issues.
Fields of interest: Education, research; Higher education; Medical research; Business & industry; Economics; Aging; Women.
Types of support: Program development, conferences/seminars, publication, research, matching funds.
Limitations: No grants to individuals, or for deficit financing, building or endowment funds, indirect costs, or equipment; no loans.
Publications: Informational brochure (including application guidelines).
Application information: Proposals for medical research must follow NIH guidelines. Application form required.
Initial approach: Letter or telephone
Copies of proposal: 1
Deadline(s): Submit proposal before Dec.; no set deadline
Board meeting date(s): Annually
Final notification: 2 to 3 months
Officers and Trustees:* Gregory A. Kozmetsky,* Chair. and Pres.; Cynthia Kozmetsky,* V.P. and Secy.-Treas.; Nadya Kozmetsky Scott,* V.P.; Charles Hurwitz, George Kozmetsky, Ronya Kozmetsky.
Number of staff: 2 full-time support.
EIN: 746077587
Grants for Aging:
American Occupational Therapy Foundation, Rockville, MD, $15,000. For continued support to supplement federal, university and private sector funding to undertake study at University of Southern California to investigate effectiveness of community-based occupational therapy treatment program in helping elderly people maintain independence and remain in their homes. 94.
Johns Hopkins University, Dana Center for Preventive Ophthalmology, Baltimore, MD, $18,394. To study effect of B-complex vitamin (D-pantethine) on cataract formation in Emory mouse, animal model for human age-related cataracts. 94.

976
Rockwell Fund, Inc.

1360 Post Oak Blvd., Suite 780
Houston 77056 (713) 629-9022
Contact: R. Terry Bell
FAX: (713) 629-7702

Trust established in 1931; incorporated in 1949 in TX; merged with Rockwell Brothers Endowment, Inc. in 1981.
Donor(s): Members of the James M. Rockwell family, Rockwell Bros. & Co., Rockwell Lumber Co.
Financial data (yr. ended 12/31/95): Assets, $81,675,993 (M); expenditures, $3,462,891; qualifying distributions, $3,242,674, including $3,062,575 for 203 grants (high: $50,000; low: $75; average: $2,000-$25,000).
Purpose and activities: Giving primarily for charitable, religious, educational, medical, arts and humanities, and civic purposes.
Fields of interest: Visual arts; Museums; Performing arts; Theater; Music; Humanities; Historic preservation/historical societies; Arts/cultural programs; Early childhood education; Child development, education; Elementary school/education; Secondary school/education; Higher education; Adult/continuing education; Adult education—literacy & basic skills; Libraries/library science; Reading; Education; Natural resource conservation & protection; Environment; Animal welfare; Hospitals (general); Family planning; Medical care, rehabilitation; Nursing care; Health care; Health associations; Cancer; AIDS; Biomedicine; Health organizations; Delinquency prevention/services; Crime/law enforcement; Food services; Human services; Children & youth, services; Youth, services; Child development, services; Homeless, human services; Protestant federated giving programs; Government/public administration; Christian agencies & churches; Protestant agencies & churches; Minorities; Disabled; Aging; Homeless; General charitable giving.
Types of support: General/operating support, continuing support, annual campaigns, building/renovation, equipment, land acquisition, program development, professorships, publication, seed money, curriculum development, scholarship funds, matching funds.
Limitations: Giving primarily in TX, with emphasis on Houston. No grants to individuals; no loans; grants awarded on a year-to-year basis only; no future commitments; no multi-year grants.
Publications: Application guidelines.
Application information: Applicants should not submit more than 1 proposal per year. Application form required.
Initial approach: Letter
Copies of proposal: 1
Deadline(s): None
Board meeting date(s): Quarterly
Final notification: After each quarterly meeting
Officers and Trustees:* R. Terry Bell,* Pres.; Helen N. Sterling,* V.P.; Mary Jo Loyd,* Secy.; Bennie Green,* Treas.
Number of staff: 1 full-time professional; 2 part-time professional; 1 full-time support.
EIN: 746040258
Grants for Aging:
Alzheimers Disease and Related Disorders Association, Houston, TX, $10,000. For patient and family service programs. 94.
Gathering Place, Houston, TX, $15,000. For training programs. 94.
Holly Hall, Houston, TX, $15,000. For building renovation. 94.
Methodist Retirement Services, The Woodlands, TX, $15,000. For capital campaign. 94.
Northwest Assistance Ministries, Houston, TX, $15,000. For pediatric health care program. 94.
Saint James House of Baytown, Baytown, TX, $15,000. For financial assistance program. 94.
Sheltering Arms, Houston, TX, $25,000. For programs for elderly. 94.

977
The Arch and Stella Rowan Foundation, Inc.

307 West Seventh St., No. 1900
Fort Worth 76102-5118 (817) 336-2679
Contact: Alice B. Myatt, Secy.

Established in 1963 in TX.
Donor(s): Stella S. Rowan,‡ Arch H. Rowan.‡
Financial data (yr. ended 08/31/95): Assets, $1,746,871 (M); expenditures, $66,664; qualifying distributions, $65,931, including $65,199 for 41 grants (high: $12,000; low: $250; average: $250-$12,000).
Purpose and activities: Grants for arts and cultural programs, higher education, hospitals, medical research, child development, the aged, and civic affairs.
Fields of interest: Museums; Music; Arts/cultural programs; Child development, education; Higher education; Business school/education; Nursing school/education; Education; Hospitals (general); Nursing care; Cancer; AIDS; Alcoholism; Medical research; Cancer research; AIDS research; Child development, services; Aging, centers & services; Biological sciences; Aging; Homeless.
Types of support: General/operating support, annual campaigns, scholarship funds.
Limitations: Giving limited to TX. No grants to individuals.
Application information: Application form not required.
Initial approach: Letter
Copies of proposal: 1
Deadline(s): None
Board meeting date(s): Varies
Officers: Alice B. Myatt, Secy.
Number of staff: None.
EIN: 756030348
Grants for Aging:
Meals on Wheels of Fort Worth, Fort Worth, TX, $2,000. 94.
Senior Citizens Services of Greater Tarrant County, Fort Worth, TX, $1,000. 94.
Senior Citizens Services of Greater Tarrant County, Fort Worth, TX, $500. 95.

978
San Antonio Area Foundation

530 McCullough, Suite 650
San Antonio 78215 (210) 225-2243
Contact: Lori McNealy, Fiscal and Admin. Officer
Mailing address: P.O. Box 120366, San Antonio, TX 78212-9566; FAX: (210) 227-0310

Established in 1964 in TX.
Foundation type: Community
Financial data (yr. ended 09/30/94): Assets, $26,785,153 (M); gifts received, $4,086,078; expenditures, $2,199,746, including $1,760,662 for 721 grants (high: $106,400; low: $25; average: $1,000-$10,000).
Purpose and activities: To improve the lives of the people in the San Antonio community by increasing the permanent, unrestricted endowment in order to respond to emerging, changing community needs in the fields of arts, culture, community and social services, education, environment, health, and biomedical research.
Fields of interest: Media/communications; Visual arts; Museums; Performing arts; Dance; Theater; Historic preservation/historical societies; Arts/cultural programs; Education, research; Education, fund raising; Early childhood education; Child development, education; Higher education; Medical school/education; Nursing school/education; Adult/continuing education; Adult education—literacy & basic skills; Reading; Education; Natural resource conservation & protection; Environment; Animal welfare; Wildlife preservation & protection; Family planning; Medical care, rehabilitation; Health care; Substance abuse, services; Cancer; Heart/circulatory disease; AIDS; Alcoholism; Health organizations; Medical research; Cancer research; Heart/circulatory research; AIDS research; Domestic violence prevention; Human services; Children & youth, services; Youth, services; Child development, services; Family services; Hospices; Aging, centers & services; Homeless, human services; Community development; Federated giving programs; Computer science; Biological sciences; Government/public administration; Roman Catholic agencies & churches; Religion; Minorities; African Americans; Latinos; Disabled; Aging; Women; Economically disadvantaged; Homeless.
Types of support: General/operating support, continuing support, annual campaigns, building/renovation, equipment, land acquisition, emergency funds, program development, professorships, publication, seed money, curriculum development, scholarship funds, research, scholarships—to individuals, matching funds.
Limitations: Giving limited to the San Antonio, TX area, except when otherwise specified by donor. No support for individual churches, congregations, or parishes (unless projects benefit community at large). No grants to individuals (except for designated scholarship funds), or for deficit financing, endowment funds, seminars or conferences, or salaries (except as part of a project); no loans.
Publications: Annual report, 990-PF, newsletter, application guidelines, financial statement, grants list.
Application information: Application form required.
Initial approach: Letter or telephone
Copies of proposal: 8
Deadline(s): Letter of intent, Jan. 15; full proposal, Apr. 1
Board meeting date(s): Monthly
Final notification: Late May or early June
Officers and Board of Directors:* Mary Beth Williamson,* Chair.; Edward M. Polansky,* Vice-Chair.; Candes P. Chumney, Secy. and Exec. Dir.; Pete R. Martinez,* Treas.; Margaret F. Anderson, Arthur H. Bayern, AudreyJane Castro, Marilyn Cockburn, Kenneth L. Farrimond, M.D., Sylvia P. Fernandez, Ph.D., Larry D. Franklin, Leonard E. Lawrence, M.D., Aaronetta Pierce, Robert S. Rosow.
Trustee Banks: Bank One, Texas, N.A., Broadway National Bank, Citizens State Bank, Frost National Bank, Groos Bank, Jefferson Bank, Kelly Field National Bank, NationsBank of Texas, N.A., Texas Commerce Bank-El Paso, N.A.
Staff: Carolina Flores, Administrator; William M. Kromer, Grants and Scholarships Mgr.
Number of staff: 2 full-time professional; 1 full-time support; 1 part-time support.
EIN: 746065414
Grants for Aging:
Visiting Nurse Association of San Antonio, San Antonio, TX, $20,000. For Homemaker Health Aides training classes. 94.

979
Lura Sira Sanders Trust

c/o NationsBank of Texas, N.A.
P.O. Box 831041
Dallas 75283-1041
Application address: c/o NationsBank of Texas, N.A., Specialized Portfollo Svcs., P.O. Box 830259, Dallas, TX 75283-0259; Tel.: (214) 508-5000

Financial data (yr. ended 05/31/95): Assets, $215,556 (M); expenditures, $24,559; qualifying distributions, $21,833, including $20,657 for grants.
Purpose and activities: "Support for the care, maintenance, and health of elderly people who are otherwise unable to recieve such care and maintenance."
Fields of interest: Aging, centers & services; Aging.
Limitations: Giving limited to Dallas, TX. No grants to individuals.
Application information: Generally contributes only to pre-selected organizations.
Initial approach: Letter
Deadline(s): None
Trustees: M. Robert Blakeney, NationsBank of Texas, N.A.
EIN: 756045901

980
Walter Benona Sharp Memorial Foundation

c/o NationsBank of Texas, N.A.
P.O. Box 2518
Houston 77252-2518

Established in 1953 in TX.
Donor(s): Sharp Family Trust, Honey Sharp Lippmann.
Financial data (yr. ended 12/31/94): Assets, $39,021 (M); gifts received, $40,000; expenditures, $57,261; qualifying distributions, $53,795, including $53,795 for 18 grants (high: $10,000; low: $100).
Fields of interest: Alzheimer's disease; Medical research; Neighborhood centers; Community development.
Types of support: Annual campaigns.
Limitations: Giving primarily in Houston, TX. No grants to individuals.
Application information: Application form not required.
Deadline(s): None
Trustees: Tina C. Sharp, NationsBank of Texas, N.A.
EIN: 746033150

981
Southwestern Public Service Company Giving Program

c/o Jim Michel
P.O. Box 1261
Amarillo 79170 (806) 378-2121

Financial data (yr. ended 12/31/95): Total giving, $248,142, including $248,142 for grants.
Purpose and activities: Supports civic activities, economic development, and environmental issues.
Fields of interest: Environment; Health associations; Human services; Youth, services; Aging, centers & services; Economics; Government/public administration; Aging; Economically disadvantaged.
Types of support: General/operating support, curriculum development, employee volunteer services.
Limitations: Giving primarily in areas of company operations.
Application information:
Initial approach: Contact nearest local branch manager

982
Sparks Charitable Trust

(Formerly Helen Gertrude Sparks Charitable Trust)
c/o NationsBank of Texas, N.A.
P.O. Box 831041
Dallas 75283-1041
Contact: Pamela Bradley, V.P., NationsBank of Texas, N.A.
Application address: c/o NationsBank of Texas, N.A., P.O. Box 1317, Fort Worth, TX 76101

Financial data (yr. ended 05/31/95): Assets, $546,857 (M); expenditures, $27,125; qualifying distributions, $17,026, including $15,850 for grants.
Fields of interest: Arts/cultural programs; Education; Youth, services; Aging, centers & services; Disabled; Aging.
Limitations: Giving limited to the Fort Worth, TX, area.
Application information:
Initial approach: Proposal
Deadline(s): May 31
Trustee: NationsBank of Texas, N.A.
EIN: 756167997

983
B. A. and Elinor Steinhagen Benevolent Trust

c/o Texas Commerce Bank-Beaumont, N.A.
P.O. Box 3928
Beaumont 77704 (409) 880-1415
Contact: Jean Moncla, V.P. and Trust Officer, Texas Commerce Bank-Beaumont, N.A.

Trust established in 1939 in TX.
Donor(s): B.A. Steinhagen,‡ Elinor Steinhagen.‡
Financial data (yr. ended 08/31/95): Assets, $4,604,795 (M); expenditures, $297,138; qualifying distributions, $263,059, including $263,059 for 18 grants (high: $62,500; low: $3,059; average: $10,000-$20,000).
Purpose and activities: Giving for the housing and general assistance of the elderly and the helpless and afflicted of any age.
Fields of interest: Arts/cultural programs; Education; Health care; Housing/shelter, development; Human services; Aging, centers & services; Disabled; Aging; Economically disadvantaged.
Types of support: Building/renovation, equipment, program development, publication, seed money, research, matching funds.
Limitations: Giving limited to Jefferson County, TX. No grants to individuals, or for operating budgets, continuing support, annual campaigns, emergency funds, deficit financing, conferences, scholarships, or fellowships; no loans.
Publications: Application guidelines.
Application information: Application form required.
Initial approach: Letter
Copies of proposal: 1
Deadline(s): May 31
Board meeting date(s): Annually
Final notification: Aug.
Trustee: Texas Commerce Bank-Beaumont, N.A.
Number of staff: None.
EIN: 746039544

984
Hesta Stuart Christian Charitable Trust

c/o Bank One, Texas, N.A.
P.O. Box 2050
Fort Worth 76113 (817) 884-4151
Contact: Robert Lansford

Established in 1973 in TX.
Financial data (yr. ended 06/30/95): Assets, $3,689,960 (M); expenditures, $427,817; qualifying distributions, $382,689, including $381,000 for 16 grants (high: $75,000; low: $10,000; average: $1,000-$50,000).
Purpose and activities: Grants to Methodist organizations, including orphanages, hospitals, educational institutions, churches, homes for unwed mothers, and homes for the elderly; grants also for Methodist Church support.
Fields of interest: Higher education; Human services; Christian agencies & churches; Protestant agencies & churches; African Americans; Native Americans; Disabled; Aging; Homeless.
Types of support: General/operating support, matching funds.
Limitations: Giving primarily in TX. No grants to individuals.
Application information: Application form not required.
Initial approach: 2- to 3-page letter or proposal
Copies of proposal: 1
Deadline(s): Sept. 30
Board meeting date(s): Nov.
Final notification: Prior to Dec. 31
Trustee: Bank One, Texas, N.A.
Number of staff: None.
EIN: 756177306

985
Swalm Foundation

8707 Katy Freeway, Suite 300
Houston 77024 (713) 464-1321
Contact: Miriam Minkoff, Grants Administrator

Established in 1980 in TX.
Donor(s): Dave C. Swalm, Texas Olefins Co.
Financial data (yr. ended 11/30/94): Assets, $55,705,308 (M); gifts received, $6,760,000; expenditures, $2,675,812; qualifying distributions, $2,373,594, including $2,306,022 for 78 grants (high: $300,000; low: $850; average: $500-$200,000).
Purpose and activities: Giving primarily for human service organizations, education, and health.
Fields of interest: Education, research; Education, fund raising; Early childhood education; Child development, education; Elementary school/education; Higher education; Engineering school/education; Adult/continuing education; Adult education—literacy & basic skills; Libraries/library science; Reading; Education; Medical care, rehabilitation; Health care; Substance abuse, services; Mental health/crisis services; Skin disorders; AIDS; Alcoholism; Skin research; AIDS research; Food services; Nutrition; Housing/shelter, development; Human services; Children & youth, services; Youth, services; Child development, services; Family services; Hospices; Aging, centers & services; Women, centers & services; Homeless, human services; Engineering; Christian agencies & churches; Minorities; Disabled; Aging; Women; Economically disadvantaged; Homeless; General charitable giving.
Types of support: General/operating support, building/renovation, endowment funds, emergency funds, scholarship funds, matching funds.
Limitations: Giving primarily in TX.
Publications: Informational brochure (including application guidelines), 990-PF.
Application information: Application form required.
Initial approach: Call or write for application form
Copies of proposal: 1
Deadline(s): 90 days prior to board meetings for consideration in current quarter
Board meeting date(s): Mar., June, Sept., and Jan.
Officers and Trustees:* JoBeth Camp Swalm,* Pres.; Dave C. Swalm,* V.P.; Mark C. Mendelovitz,* Secy.
Number of staff: 1 part-time professional; 1 part-time support.
EIN: 742203536

986
Tenneco Corporate Contributions Program

P.O. Box 2511
Houston 77252-2511 (713) 757-3930
Contact: Jo Ann Swinney, Dir., Community Affairs

Established in 1952 in TX.
Financial data (yr. ended 12/31/94): Total giving, $5,726,361, including $4,631,550 for grants (high: $100,000; low: $1,000; average: $1,000-$10,000), $794,811 for 2,048 employee matching gifts and $300,000 for in-kind gifts.
Purpose and activities: Emphasis on elementary and secondary education, including a Tenneco

Presidential Scholarship Program for students at Jefferson Davis High School in Houston's inner city. The scholarship carries a maximum award of $4,000 for those ninth graders who are able to maintain a 2.5 grade point average and meet other academic requirements. To be eligible, students must also attend two summer enrichment sessions, which Tenneco helped develop under the sponsorship of a local philanthropic foundation and a local university.
Fields of interest: Museums; Theater; Humanities; Historic preservation/historical societies; Arts/cultural programs; Education, association; Education, research; Early childhood education; Elementary school/education; Secondary school/education; Higher education; Engineering school/education; Adult education—literacy & basic skills; Libraries/library science; Reading; Education; Natural resource conservation & protection; Environment; Hospitals (general); Health care; Alcoholism; Health organizations; Medical research; Crime/law enforcement; Food services; Housing/shelter, development; Youth development, services; Human services; Youth, services; Hospices; Aging, centers & services; Women, centers & services; Homeless, human services; Urban/community development; Community development; Engineering; Public policy, research; Government/public administration; Leadership development; Minorities; Aging; Women; Economically disadvantaged; Homeless; United Kingdom.
Types of support: Capital campaigns, building/renovation, professorships, fellowships, internships, scholarship funds, research, employee volunteer services, use of facilities, employee matching gifts, donated equipment, donated products, in-kind gifts, matching funds.
Limitations: Giving primarily in areas of company operations in TX, WI, IL, VA, and TN; also in Canada and England. No grants to individuals, or for political, religious, fraternal or veterans' organizations.
Publications: Corporate report, informational brochure (including application guidelines).
Application information: Company has a staff that only handles contributions. Application form not required.
Initial approach: Initial contact by letter on letterhead stationery; write to nearest company facility
Copies of proposal: 1
Deadline(s): Prior to Aug. 15 for consideration in next calendar year's budget
Board meeting date(s): 2nd Tuesday in Jan. each year
Final notification: 4 weeks after submission of application
Administrators: JoAnn Hogg, Sr. Contribs. Asst.; Ethel Samuels, Sr. Contribs. Coord.
Number of staff: 1 full-time professional; 1 full-time support.

987
Texas Commerce Bank Foundation, Inc.

(Formerly Texas Commerce Bank Foundation of Texas Commerce Bank-Houston, Inc.)
c/o Texas Commerce Bank-Houston, N.A.
P.O. Box 2558
Houston 77252
Contact: Jana Gunter

Incorporated in 1952 in TX.
Donor(s): Texas Commerce Bank-Houston, N.A.
Foundation type: Company-sponsored
Financial data (yr. ended 12/31/95): Assets, $281,018 (M); gifts received, $1,042,781; expenditures, $1,283,881; qualifying distributions, $1,283,881, including $1,283,881 for 230 grants (high: $505,000; low: $25) and $42,151 for 60 employee matching gifts.
Purpose and activities: Primary areas of interest include the arts, community development, housing, and civic affairs. Giving for a community fund, higher education, and health and medical research organizations; support also for social service agencies, including programs for minorities, child welfare, the homeless, and drug abuse.
Fields of interest: Museums; Performing arts; Arts/cultural programs; Early childhood education; Elementary school/education; Secondary school/education; Higher education; Adult education—literacy & basic skills; Libraries/library science; Reading; Education; Hospitals (general); Health care; Substance abuse, services; Mental health/crisis services; Health associations; Cancer; Alcoholism; Biomedicine; Medical research; Cancer research; Food services; Housing/shelter, development; Recreation; Human services; Family services; Hospices; Aging, centers & services; Minorities/immigrants, centers & services; Homeless, human services; Race/intergroup relations; Community development; Voluntarism promotion; Government/public administration; Public affairs; Minorities; Disabled; Aging; Homeless.
Types of support: General/operating support, continuing support, annual campaigns, capital campaigns, building/renovation, equipment, endowment funds, program development, conferences/seminars, research, employee matching gifts, in-kind gifts.
Limitations: Giving limited to Houston, TX. No grants to individuals.
Publications: Application guidelines.
Application information: Application form not required.
Initial approach: Formal letter of request
Copies of proposal: 1
Board meeting date(s): 3 times annually
Officers and Trustees:* Shelaghmichael Lents,* Chair. and Pres.; Melanie McKittrick, Secy.; Beverly McCaskill,* Treas.; Belinda Griffin, Sarah Peterson.
Number of staff: None.
EIN: 746036696

988
Ella B. Thompson Trust

c/o NationsBank of Texas, N.A.
P.O. Box 2518, TX4-213-31-09
Houston 77252-2518

Financial data (yr. ended 12/31/94): Assets, $496,027 (M); expenditures, $28,026; qualifying distributions, $22,047, including $20,375 for 9 grants to individuals (high: $4,075; low: $500).
Fields of interest: Aging.
Types of support: Grants to individuals, scholarships—to individuals.
Limitations: Applications not accepted. Giving limited to Galveston County, TX.
Trustee: NationsBank of Texas, N.A.
EIN: 746082981

989
Turner Charitable Foundation

811 Rusk, Suite 205
Houston 77002-2811 (713) 237-1117
Contact: Eyvonne Moser, Asst. Secy.

Incorporated in 1956 in TX.
Donor(s): Isla Carroll Turner,‡ P.E. Turner.‡
Financial data (yr. ended 12/31/94): Assets, $21,131,975 (M); expenditures, $900,232; qualifying distributions, $842,630, including $812,267 for 67 grants (high: $166,667; low: $750; average: $1,000-$5,000).
Purpose and activities: Giving for higher and secondary education, social services, youth, the elderly, fine and performing arts groups and other cultural programs, Catholic, Jewish, and Protestant church support and religious programs, hospitals, health services, AIDS research, hospices, programs for women and children, minorities, the homeless, the handicapped, urban and community development, civic and urban affairs, libraries, and conservation programs.
Fields of interest: Visual arts; Museums; Performing arts; Theater; Historic preservation/historical societies; Arts/cultural programs; Education, association; Education, research; Education, fund raising; Elementary/secondary education; Child development, education; Secondary school/education; Higher education; Adult education—literacy & basic skills; Libraries/library science; Reading; Natural resource conservation & protection; Animal welfare; Hospitals (general); Medical care, rehabilitation; Health care; Substance abuse, services; Mental health/crisis services; Cancer; Heart/circulatory disease; AIDS; Cancer research; Heart/circulatory research; AIDS research; Domestic violence prevention; Food services; Recreation; Children & youth, services; Youth, services; Child development, services; Family services; Hospices; Minorities/immigrants, centers & services; Homeless, human services; Civil rights, minorities; Civil rights, disabled; Civil rights, women; Civil rights, aging; Civil rights, gays/lesbians; Community development, business promotion; Community development; Federated giving programs; Government/public administration; Protestant agencies & churches; Roman Catholic agencies & churches; Jewish

agencies & temples; Religion; Minorities; African Americans; Latinos; Aging; Women; People with AIDS (PWAs); Homeless.
Types of support: General/operating support, continuing support, annual campaigns, capital campaigns, building/renovation, equipment, land acquisition, endowment funds, emergency funds, program development, conferences/seminars, professorships, seed money, curriculum development, fellowships, scholarship funds, research, matching funds.
Limitations: Giving limited to TX. No grants to individuals.
Application information: Application form not required.
Initial approach: Written request
Copies of proposal: 1
Deadline(s): Mar. 15
Board meeting date(s): Apr.
Final notification: Positive responses only
Officers and Trustees:* T.R. Reckling III,* Pres.; Bert F. Winston, Jr.,* V.P.; Clyde J. Verheyden,* Secy.; Isla C. Reckling,* Treas.; Thomas E. Berry, Carroll R. Goodman, Chaille W. Hawkins, Christiana R. McConn, James S. Reckling, Stephen M. Reckling, T.R. "Cliffe" Reckling IV, Blake W. Winston.
Number of staff: 1 full-time professional.
EIN: 741460482

990
The Vale-Asche Foundation
1010 River Oaks Bank Bldg.
2001 Kirby Dr.
Houston 77019-6033 (713) 520-7334
Contact: Mrs. Vale Asche Russell, Pres.

Incorporated in 1956 in DE.
Donor(s): Ruby Vale,‡ Fred B. Asche.‡
Financial data (yr. ended 11/30/95): Assets, $7,865,931 (M); expenditures, $341,901; qualifying distributions, $322,839, including $320,480 for 20 grants (high: $40,000; low: $2,500).
Purpose and activities: Grants for medical research, health care, child welfare, and aid to the aged and the handicapped; support also for secondary education and cultural programs, and projects that benefit the homeless.
Fields of interest: Arts/cultural programs; Secondary school/education; Education; Medical care, rehabilitation; Health care; Substance abuse, services; Mental health/crisis services; Eye disease; AIDS; Medical research; Eye research; AIDS research; Food services; Human services; Children & youth, services; Aging, centers & services; Homeless, human services; Community development; Minorities; Disabled; Aging; People with AIDS (PWAs); Economically disadvantaged; Homeless.
Types of support: Equipment, program development, research.
Limitations: Giving primarily in Houston, TX. No grants to individuals, or for operating funds.
Application information: Request reviewed mid-Aug. through Oct. Application form not required.
Initial approach: Letter
Deadline(s): Aug. 15
Board meeting date(s): Early Sept. and early Oct.
Officers and Trustees:* Mrs. Vale Asche Russell,* Pres.; Bettyann Asche Murray,* V.P.; William E. Blummer,* Secy.-Treas.; Asche Ackerman.
EIN: 516015320
Grants for Aging:
Sheltering Arms, Houston, TX, $25,000. For training and volunteer recruitment video production. 95.

991
The Gil and Dody Weaver Foundation
500 West Seventh St., Suite 1714
Fort Worth 76102 (817) 877-1712
Contact: Mrs. Debbie L. Cain, Mgr.

Established in 1980 in TX.
Donor(s): Galbraith McF. Weaver.
Financial data (yr. ended 09/30/95): Assets, $4,074,683 (M); expenditures, $286,634; qualifying distributions, $237,066, including $235,000 for 53 grants (high: $18,000; low: $20).
Purpose and activities: Primary areas of interest include women, children and youth, the elderly, and the handicapped.
Fields of interest: Human services; Children & youth, services; Child development, services; Aging, centers & services; Women, centers & services; Disabled; Aging; Women; Economically disadvantaged; General charitable giving.
Types of support: General/operating support, equipment.
Limitations: Giving limited to TX, NM, OK, LA, KS, PA, and WV; emphasis on the Fort Worth/Tarrant County, TX, area. No support for the arts. No grants to individuals, or for seed money, emergency funds, deficit financing, land acquisition, renovation projects, endowment funds, matching gifts, scholarships, fellowships, publications, or conferences; no loans.
Application information: Application form not required.
Initial approach: Letter or proposal
Copies of proposal: 1
Deadline(s): July 31
Board meeting date(s): Sept.
Final notification: Sept. 30
Trustees: Galbraith McF. Weaver, William R. Weaver, M.D.
Number of staff: 1
EIN: 751729449
Grants for Aging:
Meals on Wheels of Fort Worth, Fort Worth, TX, $15,000. 94.
Meals on Wheels of Fort Worth, Tarrant County, Fort Worth, TX, $16,000. 95.
Senior Citizen Services of Greater Tarrant County, Fort Worth, TX, $3,000. For low-income senior citizen meal program. 95.
W.H.Grove Home for the Aged, Fort Worth, TX, $4,500. For equipment and supplies. 94.
W.H.Grove Home for the Aged, Fort Worth, TX, $4,000. For equipment and supplies. 95.

992
Jasper L. & Jack Denton Wilson Charitable Foundation
P.O. Box 2558
Houston 77252-2558

Established in 1989 in TX.
Donor(s): Mrs. Jack D. Wilson.
Financial data (yr. ended 12/31/94): Assets, $0 (M); gifts received, $50,000; expenditures, $50,417; qualifying distributions, $50,000, including $50,000 for 1 grant.
Fields of interest: Medical school/education; Health care; Alzheimer's disease research.
Limitations: Applications not accepted. Giving primarily in TX. No grants to individuals.
Application information: Contributes only to pre-selected organizations.
Trustees: Joseph A. Denton, J. Denton DeWitt, Timothy R. Vaughan, Mrs. Jack D. Wilson, Texas Commerce Bank, N.A.
EIN: 760285403

993
Ann Berger Wolens Foundation
P.O. Box 2235
Corsicana 75151-2235 (903) 874-2961
Contact: Dean Milkes, Trustee

Established in 1991.
Donor(s): Anne Berger Wolens.‡
Financial data (yr. ended 12/31/94): Assets, $2,742,742 (M); gifts received, $162,804; expenditures, $114,093; qualifying distributions, $96,100, including $96,100 for 8 grants (high: $51,100; low: $500).
Fields of interest: Human services; Jewish federated giving programs; Jewish agencies & temples; Aging.
Limitations: Giving primarily in TX. No grants to individuals.
Application information:
Initial approach: Letter
Deadline(s): None
Trustees: Matt Dawson, Dean Milkes.
EIN: 752328477
Grants for Aging:
Dallas Home for Jewish Aged, Dallas, TX, $51,100. For endowment fund. 94.

994
Lola Wright Foundation, Inc.
P.O. Box 1138
Georgetown 78627-1138 (512) 869-2574
Contact: Patrick H. O'Donnell, Pres.
Austin tel.: (512) 255-5353

Incorporated in 1954 in TX.
Donor(s): Johnie E. Wright.‡
Financial data (yr. ended 12/31/95): Assets, $11,339,399 (M); expenditures, $767,016; qualifying distributions, $603,339, including $574,812 for 55 grants (high: $25,000; low: $999; average: $1,500-$25,000).
Purpose and activities: Emphasis on social services, including drug and alcohol abuse programs, family services and planning, organizations providing assistance to minorities, the aged and youth; legal services; community funds; and health services and hospitals, including rehabilitation programs, AIDS research, diseases of the heart, and organizations serving the handicapped. Support also for the arts and culture, including fine and performing arts; early childhood, adult, higher and other education; media and communications; and the environment.

Fields of interest: Media/communications; Visual arts; Museums; Performing arts; Arts/cultural programs; Education, association; Early childhood education; Child development, education; Higher education; Adult/continuing education; Adult education—literacy & basic skills; Reading; Education; Environment; Animal welfare; Hospitals (general); Family planning; Medical care, rehabilitation; Health care; Substance abuse, services; Health associations; Heart/circulatory disease; AIDS; Alcoholism; Heart/circulatory research; AIDS research; Legal services; Human services; Children & youth, services; Child development, services; Family services; Hospices; Aging, centers & services; Minorities/immigrants, centers & services; Homeless, human services; Federated giving programs; Minorities; Disabled; Aging; Homeless.
Types of support: Continuing support, building/renovation, equipment, program development, research, matching funds.
Limitations: Giving limited to within a 50-mile radius of Austin, TX. No grants to individuals; generally no support for operating budgets.
Publications: Annual report, application guidelines.
Application information: Application form not required.
Initial approach: Letter
Copies of proposal: 9
Deadline(s): Feb. 28 and Aug. 31
Board meeting date(s): May and Nov.
Final notification: May 15 and Nov. 15
Officers and Directors:* Patrick H. O'Donnell,* Pres.; William Hilgers,* V.P.; Vivian E. Todd,* Secy.-Treas.; Wilford Flowers, Juan J. Gonzalez, James Meyers, Ron Oliveira, Carole Rylander.
Number of staff: None.
EIN: 746054717
Grants for Aging:
Alzheimers Disease and Related Disorders Association, Austin, TX, $5,000. For furniture. 95.

995
George & Fay Young Foundation, Inc.
5520 LBJ Freeway, Suite 545
Dallas 75240 (972) 386-8581
Contact: Carol Young Marvin, Pres.

Established in 1993 in TX as successor to George & Fay Young Charitable Foundation.
Donor(s): George Young,‡ Fay Cameron Young.
Financial data (yr. ended 11/30/95): Assets, $5,072,026 (M); gifts received, $180,001; expenditures, $416,650; qualifying distributions, $308,000, including $308,000 for 26 grants (high: $100,000; low: $500).
Fields of interest: Education; Health care; Human services; Children & youth, services; Aging, centers & services; Protestant agencies & churches.
Types of support: General/operating support, continuing support, annual campaigns, capital campaigns, building/renovation, land acquisition, endowment funds, debt reduction, curriculum development, matching funds.
Limitations: Giving primarily in TX. No grants to individuals.
Publications: Annual report.
Application information: Application form not required.
Initial approach: Proposal
Board meeting date(s): Nov.
Officers and Directors:* Carol Young Marvin,* Pres.; Walton Grayson III,* V.P.; Sandra Lindsey, Secy.; L. Edward Marvin.
Number of staff: None.
EIN: 752478225
Grants for Aging:
C. C. Young Memorial Home, Dallas, TX, $5,000. 94.

UTAH

996
R. Harold Burton Private Foundation
c/o First Security Bank of Utah, N.A.
P.O. Box 30007
Salt Lake City 84130-0007
Contact: David L. Buchman, Administrator

Established in 1985 in UT.
Donor(s): Robert H. Burton.‡
Financial data (yr. ended 12/31/95): Assets, $24,330,592 (M); gifts received, $5,996; expenditures, $960,029; qualifying distributions, $899,754, including $890,697 for 18 grants (high: $150,000; low: $3,000; average: $3,000-$150,000).
Fields of interest: Media/communications; Arts/cultural programs; Secondary school/education; Higher education; Natural resource conservation & protection; Hospitals (general); Aging.
Types of support: Continuing support, building/renovation, equipment, emergency funds, program development, conferences/seminars, scholarship funds, scholarships—to individuals, matching funds.
Limitations: Giving primarily in Salt Lake County, UT.
Publications: Application guidelines.
Application information: Application form required.
Copies of proposal: 4
Deadline(s): Apr. 15 and Sept. 1
Board meeting date(s): Varies
Members: Richard Robert Burton, Chair.; Frederick A. Moreton, Jr., Judith Burton Moyle.
Trustee: First Security Bank of Utah, N.A.
Number of staff: None.
EIN: 742425567

997
Harold & Ruth Dance Charitable Foundation
1044 North 1600 East
Logan 84321
Contact: Harold W. Dance, Trustee
Application address: 360 North Main, Logan, UT 84321; Tel.: (801) 752-8484

Donor(s): Harold W. Dance.
Financial data (yr. ended 12/31/94): Assets, $245,350 (M); expenditures, $12,941; qualifying distributions, $12,600, including $12,600 for grants.
Fields of interest: Higher education; Education; Aging.
Limitations: Applications not accepted. Giving limited to Logan, UT. No grants to individuals.
Application information: Contributes only to pre-selected organizations.
Trustees: Harold W. Dance, Ruth B. Dance.
EIN: 870440689

998
Marriner S. Eccles Foundation
701 Deseret Bldg.
79 South Main St.
Salt Lake City 84111 (801) 322-0116
Contact: Erma E. Hogan, Mgr.

Established in 1973 in Utah.
Donor(s): Marriner S. Eccles.‡
Financial data (yr. ended 03/31/95): Assets, $21,944,169 (M); gifts received, $78,944; expenditures, $1,204,943; qualifying distributions, $1,128,557, including $1,077,130 for 82 grants (high: $164,800; low: $1,000; average: $2,000-$20,000).
Purpose and activities: Giving primarily for higher education; health, hospitals, and medical research; arts and culture, including the performing arts, fine arts, and museums; and family and social services, including programs for rehabilitation, the aged, drug and alcohol abuse, welfare, youth, women, and the homeless.
Fields of interest: Visual arts; Museums; Performing arts; Dance; Theater; Humanities; Arts/cultural programs; Education, research; Higher education; Medical school/education; Education; Hospitals (general); Family planning; Medical care, rehabilitation; Nursing care; Health care; Substance abuse, services; Mental health/crisis services; Health associations; Cancer; AIDS; Alcoholism; Biomedicine; Medical research; Cancer research; AIDS research; Crime/law enforcement; Food services; Housing/shelter, development; Human services; Children & youth, services; Family services; Aging, centers & services; Women, centers & services; Homeless, human services; Voluntarism promotion; Federated giving programs; Roman Catholic federated giving programs; Engineering & technology; Science; Aging; Women; Economically disadvantaged; Homeless.
Types of support: General/operating support, equipment, scholarship funds, research, matching funds.
Limitations: Giving limited to UT. No grants to individuals, or for capital expenditures for construction of buildings.
Application information: Application form not required.
Initial approach: Proposal
Copies of proposal: 7
Deadline(s): None
Board meeting date(s): 3 to 4 meetings annually, usually beginning in July
Final notification: Within a week after meeting
Officers and Committee Members:* Sara M. Eccles,* Chair.; Alonzo W. Watson, Jr.,* Secy.; John D. Eccles, Spencer F. Eccles, Harold J. Steele, Elmer D. Tucker.
Trustee: First Security Bank of Utah, N.A.
Number of staff: 1 full-time professional.

EIN: 237185855
Grants for Aging:
Saint Joseph Villa, Salt Lake City, UT, $30,000. 94.

999
Eldred Sunset Manor Foundation, Inc.

P.O. Box 1387
Provo 84603
Contact: Sidney Gilbert, Pres.
Application address: 190 West 800 North, Provo, UT 84601

Financial data (yr. ended 12/31/95): Assets, $1,168,090 (M); gifts received, $100; expenditures, $33,106; qualifying distributions, $32,120, including $32,120 for 16 grants (high: $4,500; low: $420).
Fields of interest: Human services; Aging, centers & services; Aging.
Limitations: Giving primarily in UT.
Application information: Application form required.
Deadline(s): None
Officer: Sidney S. Gilbert, Pres.
EIN: 870232411

1000
Ben B. and Iris M. Margolis Charitable Foundation for Medical Research

c/o First Security Bank of Utah, N.A.
P.O. Box 30007
Salt Lake City 84130
Contact: Julie Webster

Established in 1979 in UT.
Donor(s): Iris M. Margolis,‡ Ben B. Margolis.‡
Financial data (yr. ended 03/31/95): Assets, $1,838,212 (M); gifts received, $54,524; expenditures, $81,971; qualifying distributions, $70,226, including $70,000 for 2 grants (high: $50,000; low: $20,000).
Purpose and activities: Gifts are generally made to specific areas of medical research in the state of UT designated by trustee.
Fields of interest: Medical research; Cystic fibrosis research; Arthritis research; Epilepsy research; AIDS research; Alzheimer's disease research; Diabetes research; Geriatrics research; Pediatrics research.
Types of support: Research.
Limitations: Giving primarily in UT. No grants to individuals, or for scholarships, fellowships, or endowments; no loans.
Application information: Grants currently made upon trustee's request. Application form not required.
Initial approach: Proposal
Copies of proposal: 1
Deadline(s): None
Board meeting date(s): Semiannually
Trustee: First Security Bank of Utah, N.A.
Number of staff: None.
EIN: 876180864
Grants for Aging:
University of Utah, Salt Lake City, UT, $10,000. For geriatric research. 94.
University of Utah, Salt Lake City, UT, $8,000. For Alzheimer's disease research. 94.
University of Utah, School of Medicine, Salt Lake City, UT, $50,000. For pulmonary and Alzheimer's research. 95.

1001
The Margaret E. Oser Foundation

7070 Pinebrook Rd.
Park City 84098
Contact: Carl Mitchell, Pres.

Established in 1986 in CA.
Donor(s): Margaret E. Oser.‡
Financial data (yr. ended 12/31/95): Assets, $7,846,938 (M); gifts received, $8,198; expenditures, $463,680; qualifying distributions, $463,680, including $374,350 for 26 grants (high: $33,000; low: $1,000).
Fields of interest: Performing arts; Education; Hospitals (general); Health care; Biomedicine; Medical research; Domestic violence prevention; Children & youth, services; Biological sciences; Aging; Women; Homeless.
Types of support: Equipment, emergency funds, program development, seed money, scholarship funds.
Limitations: Giving primarily in Southern CA. No grants to individuals.
Publications: Annual report (including application guidelines).
Application information: Application form not required.
Initial approach: Letter
Copies of proposal: 1
Deadline(s): Dec. 1
Board meeting date(s): Dec.
Final notification: Dec. 31
Officers: Carl Mitchell, Pres.; Edith M. Doyle, Secy.-Treas.
Number of staff: None.
EIN: 330210168
Grants for Aging:
Alzheimers Disease and Related Disorders Association of Orange County, Costa Mesa, CA, $3,000. 94.
Senior Gleaners, North Highlands, CA, $5,000. 95.

1002
Questar Corporate Giving Program

180 East First South St.
P.O. Box 45433
Salt Lake City 84145-0433 (801) 534-5435
Contact: Janice Bates, Dir., Community Affairs

Financial data (yr. ended 12/31/94): Total giving, $650,000, including $650,000 for grants.
Fields of interest: Museums; Performing arts; Humanities; Arts/cultural programs; Higher education; Business school/education; Engineering school/education; Education; Animal welfare; Hospitals (general); Health care; Health organizations; Food services; Human services; Children & youth, services; Family services; Aging, centers & services; Homeless, human services; Community development; Voluntarism promotion; Engineering; Disabled; Aging; Economically disadvantaged; Homeless; General charitable giving.
Types of support: Continuing support, annual campaigns, building/renovation, emergency funds, program development, scholarship funds, employee volunteer services, loaned talent, in-kind gifts.
Limitations: Giving primarily in service and operating locations in CO, OK, UT and WY. No support for religious or fraternal organizations. No grants for group trips, exhibitions, or operating expenses.
Application information: Community Rels. Dept. handles giving. Application form not required.
Initial approach: Letter; send to nearest company facility
Copies of proposal: 1
Board meeting date(s): Every 6 to 8 weeks
Number of staff: 1 part-time professional; 1 part-time support.

VERMONT

1003
Copley Fund

P.O. Box 696
Morrisville 05661
Contact: Richard C. Sargent, Trustee

Financial data (yr. ended 12/31/93): Assets, $1,821,189 (M); expenditures, $98,289; qualifying distributions, $92,840, including $25,000 for 2 grants (high: $15,000; low: $10,000) and $67,482 for 134 grants to individuals.
Purpose and activities: Support for housing assistance for the elderly of Lamoille County, VT.
Fields of interest: Housing/shelter, development; Aging, centers & services; Aging; Economically disadvantaged.
Types of support: General/operating support, grants to individuals.
Limitations: Giving limited to Lamoille County, VT.
Application information:
Initial approach: Letter
Deadline(s): Dec. 31
Trustees: Robert Parker, Richard C. Sargent.
EIN: 036006013

1004
Corry Memorial Fund

c/o Chittenden Bank
P.O. Box 820
Burlington 05402-0820

Established in 1993 in VT.
Donor(s): Vera Corry.‡
Financial data (yr. ended 12/31/94): Assets, $1,575,722 (M); expenditures, $154,728; qualifying distributions, $100,000, including $100,000 for 2 grants of $50,000 each.
Fields of interest: Secondary school/education; Aging, centers & services.
Limitations: Applications not accepted. Giving primarily in Montpelier, VT. No grants to individuals.
Application information: Contributes only to pre-selected organizations.
Trustee: Chittenden Bank.
EIN: 036057859
Grants for Aging:

Montpelier Senior Center, Montpelier, VT, $50,000. For maintenance fund. 94.

1005
Green Mountain Fund, Inc.

R.R. 1, Box 295
Machia Hill Rd.
Westford 05494 (802) 879-0288
Contact: Will Miller, Secy.-Treas.

Established in 1988 in VT.
Donor(s): Charles MacMartin.
Financial data (yr. ended 12/31/95): Assets, $202,728 (M); gifts received, $10,000; expenditures, $65,835; qualifying distributions, $65,835, including $49,000 for 14 grants (high: $7,500; low: $500).
Purpose and activities: Giving to "community organizing and education to bring about fundamental social change toward a genuinely democratic, socialist feminist society."
Fields of interest: Environment; Animal welfare; Health care; AIDS; AIDS research; Labor unions/organizations; Agriculture, farm cooperatives; Food services; Housing/shelter, development; Children & youth, services; Aging, centers & services; Women, centers & services; Homeless, human services; Peace; Civil rights, advocacy; Civil rights, gays/lesbians; Reproductive rights; Community development, neighborhood development; African Americans; Native Americans; Disabled; Aging; Women; People with AIDS (PWAs); Gays/lesbians; Homeless; Ireland; Southern Africa; Global programs; Developing countries; Central America.
Types of support: General/operating support, publication.
Limitations: Giving limited to VT and the Champlain Valley Watershed, NY. No grants to individuals.
Publications: Informational brochure (including application guidelines).
Application information: Does not contribute to organizations with budgets over $100,000. Application form required.
Initial approach: Letter or telephone
Copies of proposal: 8
Deadline(s): Feb. 15, June 15, and Oct. 15
Board meeting date(s): After Feb. 15, June 15, and Oct. 15
Officers and Directors:* Ann Lipsitt,* Pres.; Will Miller,* Secy.-Treas.; Michael Cassidy, Beth Mintz, Eric Sakai.
Number of staff: None.
EIN: 030316083

1006
The Kelsey Trust

c/o Vermont Community Foundation
P.O. Box 30
Middlebury 05753 (802) 462-3355

Established in 1988 in MA.
Donor(s): Sally P. Johnson.
Financial data (yr. ended 06/30/95): Assets, $3,033,145 (M); expenditures, $145,860; qualifying distributions, $138,220, including $130,720 for 16 grants (high: $44,220; low: $1,000; average: $1,000-$10,000).
Purpose and activities: Primary areas of interest include education, health, the environment, and children and families.
Fields of interest: Child development, education; Vocational education; Adult education—literacy & basic skills; Reading; Education; Natural resource conservation & protection; Environment; Family planning; Health care; Health organizations; Nutrition; Children & youth, services; Family services; Aging.
Types of support: General/operating support, land acquisition, emergency funds, program development, seed money, scholarship funds, matching funds.
Limitations: Giving limited to the Lake Champlain Valley drainage basin: eastern Adirondacks, in NY, and western VT, north of Rutland.
Publications: Program policy statement, application guidelines.
Application information: Application form required.
Initial approach: Letter requesting application material
Copies of proposal: 1
Deadline(s): Oct. and Apr.
Board meeting date(s): Nov. and May
Trustees: Paula D. Johnson, Sally P. Johnson, Stephen P. Johnson, Jonathan K. Woods.
Number of staff: None.
EIN: 046609917

1007
The Vermont Community Foundation

P.O. Box 30
Middlebury 05753 (802) 462-3355
Contact: Charlotte M. Stetson, Asst. Dir.

Established in 1986 in VT.
Foundation type: Community
Financial data (yr. ended 12/31/93): Assets, $10,921,401 (L); gifts received, $3,093,001; expenditures, $1,461,466, including $967,982 for 334 grants (high: $30,000; low: $40; average: $40-$30,000).
Purpose and activities: Support for the arts and humanities, education, the environment, health, historic preservation, public affairs and community development, and social services. The foundation is interested in projects which increase citizens' commitment to community needs, increase efficiency of nonprofit agencies, eliminate duplication of services, develop self-reliance, and emphasize prevention as well as treatment.
Fields of interest: Historic preservation/historical societies; Arts/cultural programs; Early childhood education; Child development, education; Elementary school/education; Secondary school/education; Higher education; Adult/continuing education; Libraries/library science; Natural resource conservation & protection; Environment; Animal welfare; Family planning; Substance abuse, services; Mental health/crisis services; AIDS; Alcoholism; Health organizations; Human services; Children & youth, services; Youth, services; Child development, services; Family services; Minorities/immigrants, centers & services; Homeless, human services; Civil rights; Community development; Public affairs; Disabled; Aging; Economically disadvantaged.
Types of support: Program development, seed money, scholarship funds, technical assistance, consulting services, program-related investments/loans.
Limitations: Giving limited to VT. No support for religious purposes. No grants to individuals, or for annual campaigns, building funds, continuing support, debt reduction, equipment and materials, general endowments, or operating budgets.
Publications: Annual report, multi-year report, application guidelines, 990-PF, financial statement, grants list, informational brochure (including application guidelines), program policy statement, occasional report.
Application information: Application form not required.
Initial approach: Letter
Copies of proposal: 3
Deadline(s): Apr. 1 and Oct. 1
Board meeting date(s): 8 times annually
Final notification: 2 months
Officers and Directors:* Richard M. Chapman,* Chair.; Karen N. Meyer,* Vice-Chair.; Jonathan N. Brownell, Paul Bruhn, Frederick W. Lapham III, John H. Marshall, Linda Morse, Stephen Terry, Alec Webb, Peggy R. Williams, Polly P. Wright.
Number of staff: 2 full-time professional; 1 part-time professional; 3 part-time support.
EIN: 222712160

1008
Ellen M. Willard Trust

153 Main St.
P.O. Box 517
Brattleboro 05302 (802) 254-4588
Contact: Robert T. Gannett, Trustee

Financial data (yr. ended 12/31/95): Assets, $322,843 (M); expenditures, $13,696; qualifying distributions, $13,196, including $11,000 for 9 grants (high: $2,500; low: $500).
Fields of interest: Youth, services; Aging, centers & services; Women, centers & services; Homeless, human services; Aging; Women; Homeless.
Limitations: Giving primarily in the southeastern Windham County, VT, area. No grants to individuals.
Application information:
Initial approach: Letter
Deadline(s): None
Trustees: Shirley H. Crockett, Robert T. Gannett, John A. Wallace.
EIN: 036005923

VIRGINIA

1009
American Society of Consultant Pharmacists Research & Education Foundation

1321 Duke St.
Alexandria 22314-3563 (703) 739-1300

Contact: Janice L. Feinberg, Dir.
FAX: (703) 739-1321

Incorporated in 1969 in MA.
Financial data (yr. ended 12/31/94): Assets, $4,101,000; gifts received, $3,071,000; expenditures, $5,930,000.
Purpose and activities: The foundation is the research and education affiliate of the American Society of Consultant Pharmacists. Its mission is to fund, coordinate, and conduct educational programs and research. The unique focus of the foundation is the integration and application of knowledge regarding drug use in the elderly and the practice of long-term care and consultant pharmacy to optimize health care outcomes. The foundation's areas of interest include geriatrics, the elderly, medications, drug therapy, long-term care, and pharmacy.
Fields of interest: Geriatrics; Aging, centers & services; Aging.
Types of support: Conferences/seminars, fellowships, research.
Publications: Annual report, informational brochure.
Application information: Unsolicited requests for funding not considered. Application form required.
Initial approach: Response to RFP only
Deadline(s): Varies
Officers and Directors:* Timothy Bien,* Chair.; Lynne Williams,* Pres.; Thomas Chamberlain,* V.P.; Robert Gale,* Secy.-Treas.
Number of staff: 1 full-time professional; 2 full-time support.

1010
Arlington Community Foundation, Inc.

2009 North 14th St., Suite 103
Arlington 22201 (703) 243-4785
Contact: Elizabeth Gawron, Exec. Dir.

Established in 1991 in VA.
Foundation type: Community
Financial data (yr. ended 12/31/93): Assets, $523,706 (M); gifts received, $293,372; expenditures, $137,754, including $20,450 for 10 grants (high: $3,000; low: $250) and $11,848 for in-kind gifts.
Fields of interest: Performing arts; Arts/cultural programs; Adult education—literacy & basic skills; Reading; Education; Health care; Human services; Children & youth, services; Youth, services; Aging, centers & services; Minorities/immigrants, centers & services; Community development; Government/public administration; Minorities; Aging; Economically disadvantaged.
Types of support: General/operating support, program development, seed money, scholarship funds, technical assistance, grants to individuals, matching funds.
Limitations: Giving limited to the Arlington, VA, area.
Publications: Financial statement, informational brochure, application guidelines, 990-PF.
Application information: Application form not required.
Initial approach: Letter or telephone
Copies of proposal: 1
Deadline(s): Jan. 1 and July 1
Board meeting date(s): Apr. and Sept.
Final notification: Within 90 days
Officers and Trustees:* Leslie Ariail,* Pres.; Ernst Volgenau,* V.P.; Audrey Wyatt,* Secy.; Frank Sands,* Treas.; Elizabeth Gawron, Exec. Dir.; Peter A. Arnston, Fred A. Burroughs III, Stephen P. Caruthers, Susan Jones Cooper, Charles B. DeLashmutt, David M. Guernsey, Hon. Claude M. Hilton, Charles T. Lindsay, Jr., Donald O. Manning, William F. Marman, Joseph Mirabella, Hon. William T. Newman, Jr., Charles McDonnell Radigan, Lola C. Reinsch, Sidney G. Simmonds, Evelyn Reid Syphax, Pamela Galloway Tabb, Raul Torres.
Number of staff: 1 full-time professional; 1 part-time support.
EIN: 541602838

1011
Beazley Foundation, Inc.

3720 Brighton St.
Portsmouth 23707-1788 (804) 393-1605
Contact: Lawrence W. I'Anson, Jr., Pres.
FAX: (804) 393-4708;
E-mail: beazley@norfolk.infi.net

Incorporated in 1948 in VA.
Donor(s): Fred W. Beazley,‡ Marie C. Beazley,‡ Fred W. Beazley, Jr.‡
Financial data (yr. ended 12/31/95): Assets, $55,531,250 (M); expenditures, $3,036,633; qualifying distributions, $2,327,616, including $2,002,811 for 74 grants (high: $217,574; low: $75; average: $10,000-$50,000) and $231,046 for 2 foundation-administered programs.
Purpose and activities: "To further the causes of charity, education, and religion." Grants for operation of community and senior citizens' centers and a dental clinic for the indigent. Support also for higher, secondary and medical education, youth agencies, community development, the aged, and other general charities, including health organizations and hospitals, the homeless, religion, recreation, and drug abuse prevention.
Fields of interest: Secondary school/education; Higher education; Medical school/education; Education; Hospitals (general); Health care; Substance abuse, services; Health organizations; Recreation; Youth, services; Aging, centers & services; Homeless, human services; Community development; Religion; Aging; Homeless; General charitable giving.
Types of support: General/operating support, continuing support, capital campaigns, building/renovation, program development, scholarship funds.
Limitations: Giving primarily in the South Hampton Roads area of VA. No grants to individuals.
Publications: Annual report, application guidelines, program policy statement.
Application information: Application form not required.
Initial approach: Request guidelines in writing before submitting proposal
Copies of proposal: 1
Deadline(s): 15th of the month preceeding board meetings
Board meeting date(s): Apr., July, Oct., and Jan.
Officers and Trustees:* Lawrence W. I'Anson, Jr.,* Pres.; John T. Kavanaugh,* V.P.; W. Ashton Lewis,* Secy.; Jeannette C. Bridgeman, Treas.; Richard S. Bray, Leroy T. Canoles, Jr., Mills E. Godwin, Jr., Mrs. Arnold B. McKinnon, P. Ward Robinett, Jr.
Number of staff: 1 full-time professional; 8 full-time support; 1 part-time support.
EIN: 540550100
Grants for Aging:
Eastern Virginia Medical School, Norfolk, VA, $85,000. For Geriatric Evaluation Clinic. 94.
Virginia Home, Richmond, VA, $25,000. For multi-purpose facility. 94.

1012
Camp Foundation

P.O. Box 813
Franklin 23851 (804) 562-3439
Contact: Bobby B. Worrell, Exec. Dir.

Incorporated in 1942 in VA.
Donor(s): James L. Camp,‡ P.D. Camp,‡ and their families.
Financial data (yr. ended 12/31/95): Assets, $14,647,883 (M); expenditures, $885,095; qualifying distributions, $865,132, including $723,350 for 63 grants (high: $127,900; low: $1,000; average: $1,000-$20,000) and $74,000 for 28 grants to individuals (high: $4,000; low: $2,500; average: $2,000-$4,000).
Purpose and activities: "To provide or aid in providing in or near the town of Franklin, VA,...parks, playgrounds, recreational facilities, libraries, hospitals, clinics, homes for the aged or needy, refuge for delinquent, dependent or neglected children, training schools, or other like institutions or activities." Grants also to select organizations statewide, with emphasis on youth agencies, safety programs, hospitals, mental illness, and nursing programs, higher and secondary education, including scholarships filed through high school principals, recreation, the environment, historic preservation, and cultural programs.
Fields of interest: Historic preservation/historical societies; Arts/cultural programs; Secondary school/education; Higher education; Libraries/library science; Education; Environment; Hospitals (general); Nursing care; Health care; Mental health/crisis services; Safety/disasters; Recreation; Children & youth, services; Aging, centers & services; Government/public administration; Aging.
Types of support: Annual campaigns, building/renovation, equipment, land acquisition, emergency funds, seed money, scholarship funds, research, scholarships—to individuals, matching funds.
Limitations: Giving primarily in Franklin, Southampton County, Isle of Wight County, and Tidewater, VA, and northeastern NC.
Publications: Informational brochure.
Application information: 4-year scholarships awarded to graduating high school seniors who are residents of the City of Franklin or the counties of Southampton and Isle of Wight. Application form not required.
Initial approach: Proposal
Copies of proposal: 7
Deadline(s): Submit proposal between June and Aug.; deadline Sept. 1; scholarship application deadlines Feb. 26 for filing with

high school principals; Mar. 15 for principals to file with foundation
Board meeting date(s): May and Nov.
Final notification: 3 months
Officers and Directors:* Robert C. Ray,* Chair.; Sol W. Rawls, Jr.,* Pres.; Westbrook Parker,* V.P.; John M. Camp, Jr.,* Treas.; Bobby B. Worrell,* Exec. Dir.; Christopher P. Camp, John M. Camp III, W.M. Camp, Jr., Clifford A. Cutchins III, William W. Cutchins, Mills E. Godwin, Jr., John R. Marks, Paul Camp Marks, J. Edward Moyler, Jr., John D. Munford, S. Waite Rawls, Jr., J.E. Ray III, Richard E. Ray, Toy D. Savage, Jr.
Number of staff: 1 full-time professional; 1 full-time support; 1 part-time support.
EIN: 546052488

1013
Ward K. Ensminger Charitable Trust

1603 Kenwood Ln.
Charlottesville 22901-3021
Contact: Virginia G. Shepherd, Trustee

Established in 1990 in VA.
Donor(s): Ward K. Ensminger.‡
Financial data (yr. ended 02/28/96): Assets, $2,689,926 (M); expenditures, $118,690; qualifying distributions, $114,500, including $110,000 for 16 grants (high: $30,000; low: $1,000).
Fields of interest: Adult education—literacy & basic skills; Reading; Education; Health care; Aging, centers & services; Engineering & technology; Science; Religion; Aging.
Types of support: General/operating support, continuing support, building/renovation.
Limitations: Giving limited to Charlottesville, VA. No grants to individuals or private foundations.
Application information: Application form not required.
Initial approach: Letter
Copies of proposal: 2
Deadline(s): None
Trustee: Virginia G. Shepherd.
EIN: 546287893
Grants for Aging:
Jefferson Area Board for the Aging, Charlottesville, VA, $30,000. 96.
Meals on Wheels, Community, Charlottesville, VA, $5,000. 96.
Ministry with the Aging, Charlottesville, VA, $5,000. 96.
Senior Center, Charlottesville, VA, $25,000. 96.

1014
Gannett Foundation, Inc.

(Formerly Gannett Communities Fund/Gannett Company, Inc.)
1100 Wilson Blvd., 30th Fl.
Arlington 22234
Contact: Irma Simpson, Mgr.

Established in 1991.
Donor(s): Gannett Co., Inc.
Foundation type: Company-sponsored
Financial data (yr. ended 12/31/94): Assets, $15,861,654 (M); gifts received, $20,463,593; expenditures, $5,308,950; qualifying distributions, $5,020,300, including $4,441,090 for 1,170 grants (high: $150,000; low: $236; average: $1,000-$10,000) and $579,210 for employee matching gifts.
Purpose and activities: The fund values projects that take a creative approach to such fundamental issues as education and neighborhood improvement, economic development, youth development, community problem-solving, assistance to people who are disadvantaged, environmental conservation, and cultural enrichment. The fund has an employee matching gift program for all levels of educational institutions in the U.S., its territories, and Canada.
Fields of interest: Arts/cultural programs; Vocational education; Adult education—literacy & basic skills; Reading; Education; Natural resource conservation & protection; Environment; Health care; Housing/shelter, development; Human services; Youth, services; Civil rights, aging; Community development; Voluntarism promotion; Asians/Pacific Islanders; African Americans; Latinos; Native Americans; Disabled; Aging; Women; People with AIDS (PWAs); Gays/lesbians; Immigrants/refugees; Economically disadvantaged; Homeless; Canada; Guam.
Types of support: General/operating support, capital campaigns, building/renovation, equipment, program development, seed money, technical assistance, employee matching gifts, matching funds.
Limitations: Giving limited to organizations in Gannett-served communities, including the U.S., Canada, and U.S. territories, including Guam and the Virgin Islands; no support for national or regional programs. No support for religious purposes, elementary or secondary schools (except special initiatives not provided by regular school budgets), medical or other research, fraternal or veterans' organizations, or athletic teams, bands, volunteer firefighters or similiar groups. No grants to individuals, or for endowments or multiple-year pledge campaigns.
Publications: Corporate report, informational brochure (including application guidelines).
Application information: Application form required.
Initial approach: Contact nearest Gannett newspaper, broadcast station, or outdoor advertising operation
Copies of proposal: 1
Deadline(s): Check with local executives for local deadlines
Board meeting date(s): Proposals reviewed four times a year, Feb.-Nov.
Final notification: Approximately 60 to 90 days after submission
Officers: John J. Curley,* Chair.; Douglas H. McCorkindale,* Pres.; Millicent A. Feller, V.P.; Thomas L. Chapple, Secy.; Jimmy L. Thomas, Treas.
Number of staff: 1 full-time professional; 1 full-time support.
EIN: 541568843
Grants for Aging:
Housing Options for Seniors Today, Ithaca, NY, $1,000. To help provide housing options for seniors through development of an elder cottage lease program. 94.
Perinatal Association of Delaware, Newark, DE, $16,000. Toward Resource Mother's project, providing home visitors to aid at-risk, pregnant women and their babies. 94.
Saint Vincent Senior Citizen Nutrition Program, Los Angeles, CA, $10,000. Toward installation of emergency generator and exhaust system so Meals on Wheels program can continue during disaster. 94.

1015
Ivakota Association, Inc.

c/o CMC, Inc.
901 North Pitt St.
Alexandria 22314 (703) 836-3344
Contact: Louis B. Rodenberg, Jr., Secy.-Treas.

Established in 1919 in VA.
Donor(s): Kate Waller Barrett.‡
Financial data (yr. ended 12/31/95): Assets, $3,824,374 (M); expenditures, $136,268; qualifying distributions, $109,567, including $101,500 for 39 grants (high: $5,000; low: $500; average: $1,500-$4,000).
Purpose and activities: Primary interest is support of needy women and children; grants also for higher and other education, including early childhood; housing; AIDS programs and hospices.
Fields of interest: Early childhood education; Child development, education; Higher education; Education; Delinquency prevention/services; Housing/shelter, development; Human services; Children & youth, services; Child development, services; Aging, centers & services; Women, centers & services; Minorities; Aging; Women; Economically disadvantaged.
Types of support: Continuing support, emergency funds, scholarship funds.
Limitations: Giving limited to Alexandria, VA. No grants to individuals.
Publications: Grants list, program policy statement, application guidelines.
Application information: Application form not required.
Initial approach: Proposal
Copies of proposal: 1
Deadline(s): Feb. 15
Board meeting date(s): 1st week in Mar.
Final notification: Apr. 15
Officers and Directors:* John T. Martyn, Jr.,* Pres.; David M. Burke,* V.P.; Louis B. Rodenberg, Jr.,* Secy.-Treas.; A. Hugo Blankingship, Douglas G. Lindsay, Viola G. Pope.
Number of staff: None.
EIN: 540505919
Grants for Aging:
Senior Citizens Employment and Services of Alexandria, Alexandria, VA, $5,000. 94.

1016
Kindt Christian Charitable Trust

5537 Wipledale Ave., N.W.
Roanoke 24019
Contact: June Ann Gibson, Trustee

Established in 1990.
Donor(s): Warren Kindt, Lois Kindt.
Financial data (yr. ended 12/31/94): Assets, $34,143 (M); expenditures, $128; qualifying distributions, $128.
Fields of interest: Housing/shelter, development; Aging, centers & services; Aging.

Application information: No grants paid in 1994. Application form not required.
Deadline(s): None
Trustees: June Ann Gibson, John W. Kindt.
EIN: 546296044

1017
Greater Lynchburg Community Trust
Central Fidelity Bank Bldg., 14th Fl.
P.O. Box 700
Lynchburg 24505 (804) 847-9417
Contact: William F. Quillian, Jr., Exec. Dir.
FAX: (804) 847-9491

Established as a community trust in 1972 in VA.
Foundation type: Community
Financial data (yr. ended 09/30/95): Assets, $3,164,406 (M); expenditures, $136,845, including $100,002 for 40 grants (high: $5,300; low: $500; average: $500-$5,300), $6,240 for 9 grants to individuals (high: $1,000; low: $50; average: $50-$1,000) and $50 for 1 employee matching gift.
Fields of interest: Arts/cultural programs; Libraries/library science; Education; Food services; Human services; Children & youth, services; Family services; Aging, centers & services; Women, centers & services; Homeless, human services; Community development; Social sciences; Disabled; Aging; Women; Economically disadvantaged; Homeless; General charitable giving.
Types of support: General/operating support, building/renovation, equipment, emergency funds, seed money, scholarship funds, technical assistance, grants to individuals, scholarships—to individuals, matching funds.
Limitations: Giving limited to Lynchburg, and Bedford City, and Amherst, Bedford, and Campbell counties, VA. No support for religious organizations for sectarian or religious purposes. No grants for continuing support, annual campaigns, deficit financing, employee matching gifts, or non-grant support; no loans or multiple year grants. Grants not ordinarily awarded to individuals.
Publications: Application guidelines, program policy statement, annual report, informational brochure.
Application information: Application form not required.
Initial approach: Letter (no more than 2 pages) or telephone
Copies of proposal: 1
Deadline(s): May 1 and Nov. 1
Board meeting date(s): June, Sept., Dec., Feb., and Apr.
Officers and Directors:* George T. Stewart,* Chair.; Carl W. Calandra,* Chair., Distribs. Comm.; Yuille Holt III,* Vice-Chair.; William F. Quillian, Jr., Exec. Dir.; James K. Candler, Mary Spencer Craddock, Carroll Freeman, Allethia J. Ingram, Patricia W. Leggett, William N. Mays, Adrian Mood, William E. Painter, Larry H. Redmond.
Trustee Banks: Central Fidelity Bank, Crestar Bank, N.A., First Community Bank, NationsBank of Virginia, N.A.
Number of staff: 1 full-time professional; 1 part-time professional.
EIN: 546112680

1018
The Claude Moore Charitable Foundation
11350 Random Hills Rd., No. 500
Fairfax 22030
Contact: Jesse B. Wilson III, Trustee
Application address: P.O. Box 208, Oakton, VA 22124

Established in 1987.
Financial data (yr. ended 12/31/95): Assets, $2,664,183 (M); gifts received, $173,000; expenditures, $208,079; qualifying distributions, $140,129, including $100,400 for 2 grants (high: $100,000; low: $400) and $39,729 for 1 program-related investment.
Fields of interest: Medical school/education; Aging.
Limitations: Applications not accepted. Giving primarily in VA.
Application information:
Board meeting date(s): Monthly
Trustees: Peter A. Arnston, Leigh B. Middleditch, Jr., Verlin W. Smith, Jesse B. Wilson III.
Number of staff: None.
EIN: 521558571
Grants for Aging:
University of Virginia, School of Medicine, Charlottesville, VA, $100,000. For Geriatrics chair. 95.

1019
The Norfolk Foundation
1410 NationsBank Ctr.
Norfolk 23510 (804) 622-7951
Contact: Lee C. Kitchin, Exec. Dir.

Established in 1950 in VA by resolution and declaration of trust.
Foundation type: Community
Financial data (yr. ended 12/31/95): Assets, $53,004,897 (M); gifts received, $1,348,592; expenditures, $2,226,049, including $1,470,148 for 52 grants (high: $200,000; low: $700; average: $5,000-$100,000) and $337,207 for 175 grants to individuals (high: $6,000; low: $300; average: $1,000-$3,500).
Purpose and activities: Support for local hospitals, higher, medical, and other educational institutions, family and child welfare agencies, a community fund, programs for drug abuse, the aged, the homeless, and the handicapped, and cultural and civic programs; certain donor-designated scholarships restricted by residence in nearby localities and/or area colleges, and payable directly to the school.
Fields of interest: Museums; Historic preservation/historical societies; Arts/cultural programs; Child development, education; Higher education; Medical school/education; Adult/continuing education; Adult education—literacy & basic skills; Libraries/library science; Reading; Education; Natural resource conservation & protection; Environment; Animal welfare; Hospitals (general); Family planning; Medical care, rehabilitation; Health care; Substance abuse, services; Mental health/crisis services; AIDS; Health organizations; Medical research; AIDS research; Youth development, services; Human services; Children & youth, services; Youth, services; Child development, services; Family services; Aging, centers & services; Homeless, human services; Community development; Voluntarism promotion; Government/public administration; Leadership development; Disabled; Aging; Economically disadvantaged; Homeless.
Types of support: Capital campaigns, building/renovation, equipment, land acquisition, seed money, scholarships—to individuals.
Limitations: Giving limited to Norfolk, VA, and a 50-mile area from its boundaries. No support for national or international organizations, or religious organizations for religious purposes. No grants to individuals (except for donor-designated scholarships), or for operating budgets, endowment funds, or deficit financing; no loans.
Publications: Annual report (including application guidelines), application guidelines, informational brochure, newsletter, financial statement, grants list.
Application information: Application form not required.
Initial approach: Letter or telephone
Copies of proposal: 1
Deadline(s): For scholarships only, Dec. 1 to Mar. 1
Board meeting date(s): 4 times a year
Final notification: 3 to 4 months
Officer: Lee C. Kitchin, Exec. Dir.
Distribution Committee: Toy D. Savage, Jr., Chair.; Joshua P. Darden, Jr., Vice-Chair.; Jean C. Bruce, Charles F. Burroughs, Jr., John H. Foster, H.P. McNeal, Kurt M. Rosenbach.
Number of staff: 1 full-time professional; 2 part-time professional; 1 part-time support.
EIN: 540722169

1020
The Frank H. Nott Foundation
P.O. Box 27225
Richmond 23261

Established in 1988 in VA.
Foundation type: Operating
Financial data (yr. ended 12/31/93): Assets, $332,550 (M); gifts received, $9,800; expenditures, $14,696; qualifying distributions, $39,676.
Fields of interest: Human services; Aging, centers & services; Homeless, human services; Roman Catholic agencies & churches; Religion; Aging; Homeless.
Limitations: Applications not accepted. Giving primarily in VA.
Application information: Contributes only to pre-selected organizations.
Officers and Directors:* P. Bradley Nott,* Pres.; W.J. Nott,* Treas.; W. Earle Murphy III, Frank J. Stumpf.
EIN: 541490235

1021
Perry Foundation, Inc.
P.O. Box 558
Charlottesville 22902 (804) 973-9441
Contact: Nancy Williams

Incorporated in 1946 in VA.

Donor(s): Hunter Perry,‡ Lillian Perry Edwards.‡
Financial data (yr. ended 12/31/95): Assets, $20,465,056 (M); expenditures, $644,877; qualifying distributions, $607,473, including $595,472 for 28 grants (high: $150,000; low: $1,000).
Purpose and activities: Support for higher and secondary education; grants also for a community fund and aid to the handicapped.
Fields of interest: Education, fund raising; Secondary school/education; Higher education; Education; Aging, centers & services; Federated giving programs; Disabled; Aging.
Types of support: Annual campaigns, building/renovation, equipment, matching funds.
Limitations: Giving limited to VA, with emphasis on Charlottesville and Albemarle. No grants to individuals, or for operating budgets.
Application information: Application form not required.
Initial approach: Proposal
Copies of proposal: 6
Deadline(s): 1st day of Mar., June, Sept., and Nov.
Board meeting date(s): Quarterly
Officers and Trustees:* George C. Palmer II,* Pres.; Francis H. Fife,* V.P.; Gary C. McGee,* Secy.; Edward D. Tayloe II,* Treas.; Roberta F. Brownfield, Susan M. Cabell.
Number of staff: 1 part-time support.
EIN: 546036446

1022
Kathryn & W. Harry Schwarzschild Fund

219 East Broad St.
Richmond 23219
Contact: W. Harry Schwarzchild, Jr., Secy.-Treas.
Application address: P.O. Box 27602, Richmond, VA 23261

Donor(s): W. Harry Schwarzschild, Jr.
Financial data (yr. ended 12/31/94): Assets, $1,015,383 (M); expenditures, $35,664; qualifying distributions, $35,664, including $31,744 for 66 grants (high: $7,200; low: $5).
Fields of interest: Arts/cultural programs; Health care; Human services; American Red Cross; Children & youth, services; Aging, centers & services; Jewish federated giving programs; Jewish agencies & temples.
Limitations: Giving primarily in Richmond, VA. No grants to individuals.
Application information: Application form not required.
Deadline(s): None
Officers: Kathryn E. Schwarzschild, Pres.; Kathrin S. Brown, V.P.; W. Harry Schwarzschild III, V.P.; W. Harry Schwarzschild, Jr., Secy.-Treas.
EIN: 546035733

1023
The Sophron Foundation

7404 Colshire Dr.
McLean 22102-7404
Contact: T.F. Rogers, Chair.

Established in 1980; classified as a private operating foundation in 1981.
Donor(s): Estelle E. Rogers, Thomas F. Rogers.
Foundation type: Operating
Financial data (yr. ended 11/30/95): Assets, $1,190,696 (M); expenditures, $45,680; qualifying distributions, $35,191, including $18,150 for 9 grants (high: $5,000; low: $100) and $5,600 for 4 grants to individuals (high: $1,200; low: $600).
Purpose and activities: Giving interests include ameliorating the problems of the very young and the very old, and space programs; some grants also for dental care.
Fields of interest: Dental care; Children & youth, services; Aging.
Limitations: Applications not accepted. Giving primarily in VA. No grants to individuals.
Publications: Annual report.
Application information: Contributes only to pre-selected organizations.
Board meeting date(s): Oct. and Nov.
Officers and Directors:* Thomas F. Rogers,* Chair. and Pres.; Estelle E. Rogers,* Vice-Chair. and V.P.; Robert E. Grove, Secy.-Treas.; Hope E. Grove, Judith L. Reynolds, Stephen A. Reynolds.
Number of staff: 1 part-time professional.
EIN: 521199140

1024
The Titmus Foundation, Inc.

P.O. Box 10
Sutherland 23885-0010 (804) 265-5834
Contact: Edward B. Titmus, Pres.

Incorporated in 1945 in VA.
Donor(s): Edward Hutson Titmus, Sr.‡
Financial data (yr. ended 01/31/96): Assets, $15,898,046 (M); expenditures, $704,753; qualifying distributions, $655,499, including $609,341 for 126 grants (high: $207,500; low: $100; average: $100-$162,941).
Purpose and activities: Emphasis on Baptist church support and religious organizations, higher education, health, cancer research, and child welfare.
Fields of interest: Museums; Performing arts; Historic preservation/historical societies; Education, fund raising; Elementary/secondary education; Child development, education; Elementary school/education; Higher education; Medical school/education; Nursing school/education; Education; Hospitals (general); Health care; Health associations; Cancer; Medical research; Cancer research; Domestic violence prevention; Human services; Children & youth, services; Youth, services; Engineering & technology; Science; Christian agencies & churches; Protestant agencies & churches; Religion; Disabled; Aging; People with AIDS (PWAs); Economically disadvantaged; Homeless; General charitable giving.
Types of support: Continuing support, capital campaigns, building/renovation, equipment, land acquisition, emergency funds, professorships, scholarship funds, research, matching funds.
Limitations: Giving primarily in VA. No grants to individuals.
Application information: Application form not required.
Initial approach: Proposal
Copies of proposal: 1
Deadline(s): None
Board meeting date(s): July
Officers: Edward B. Titmus, Pres. and Secy.; George M. Modlin, V.P.; John J. Muldowney, Treas.
Directors: William Dudley Allen III, Kimberly C. Titmus.
Number of staff: 1 full-time professional; 1 full-time support.
EIN: 546051332
Grants for Aging:
Baptist Retirement Homes of North Carolina, Winston-Salem, NC, $3,500. 96.

1025
The Virginia Beach Foundation

P.O. Box 4629
Virginia Beach 23454 (804) 422-5249
Contact: Ted Clarkson, Exec. Dir.
Application address: 1604 West Hilltop Executive Ctr., Suite 308, Virginia Beach, VA 23451

Incorporated in 1987 in VA.
Foundation type: Community
Financial data (yr. ended 09/30/95): Assets, $1,196,015 (M); gifts received, $353,944; expenditures, $259,054, including $161,501 for 61 grants (high: $12,000; low: $50).
Fields of interest: Arts/cultural programs; Education; Environment; Health care; Domestic violence prevention; Human services; Youth, services; Reproductive rights; Asians/Pacific Islanders; African Americans; Disabled; Aging; Women; People with AIDS (PWAs); Economically disadvantaged; Homeless.
Types of support: Emergency funds, program development, technical assistance, in-kind gifts, matching funds.
Limitations: Giving primarily within a 60-mile radius of Virginia Beach, VA. No grants to individuals, or for general operating support or seed money.
Publications: Newsletter, application guidelines, financial statement, informational brochure, 990-PF, grants list, annual report.
Application information: Application form required.
Initial approach: Letter
Copies of proposal: 2
Deadline(s): Mar.
Board meeting date(s): Semiannually
Final notification: June
Officers and Trustees:* Thomas R. Frantz,* Chair.; Macon F. Brock,* 1st Vice-Chair.; John Baillio,* 2nd Vice-Chair.; Margaret G. Campbell,* Secy.; Patrick M. Barberich,* Treas.; Lynne Farrell, Andrew S. Fine, Robert Goodman, Robert C. Goodman, Jr., Thomas J. Lyons, Jr., Robert C. Miller, Frederick J. Napolitano, Robin D. Ray, Craig Slingluff, Robert L. Stein.
Number of staff: 1 full-time professional; 1 full-time support; 1 part-time support.
EIN: 541553631
Grants for Aging:
M. E. Cox Center for the Elder Day Care, Virginia Beach, VA, $2,000. For Saturday health care service. 94.

1026
Lillian Wardman Trust
c/o Crestar Bank, N.A.
P.O. Box 27385
Richmond 23261-7385
Application address: Cheryl Williams, c/o Crestar Bank N.A., 15th and New York Ave., N.W., Washington, DC 20005

Established as a private foundation in 1989 in DC.
Financial data (yr. ended 12/31/95): Assets, $1,161,899 (M); expenditures, $69,472; qualifying distributions, $51,422, including $51,400 for 8 grants (high: $10,000; low: $2,500).
Fields of interest: Hospitals (general); Aging, centers & services; Aging.
Types of support: General/operating support, building/renovation.
Limitations: Giving primarily in Washington, DC. No grants to individuals.
Application information: Application form not required.
Initial approach: Letter
Copies of proposal: 1
Deadline(s): None
Trustee: Crestar Bank, N.A.
EIN: 526121876
Grants for Aging:
Aged Womens Home of Georgetown, DC, $7,500. For structural repairs. 95.
Christian Communities Group Homes, DC, $10,000. 95.
Iona Senior Services, DC, $2,500. 95.

WASHINGTON

1027
Norman Archibald Charitable Foundation
c/o First Interstate Bank of Washington, N.A.
P.O. Box 21927
Seattle 98111 (206) 292-3543
Contact: Stuart H. Prestrud, Secy., Board of Mgrs.

Established in 1976 in WA.
Donor(s): Norman Archibald.‡
Financial data (yr. ended 09/30/95): Assets, $8,257,840 (M); expenditures, $365,442; qualifying distributions, $306,753, including $268,750 for 100 grants (high: $15,000; low: $750).
Purpose and activities: Support primarily for youth and child development programs; support also for AIDS and other medical research, higher education and libraries, museums and the performing arts, social services for the aged and the handicapped, housing programs, and animal welfare and conservation.
Fields of interest: Museums; Performing arts; Theater; Music; History & archaeology; Arts/cultural programs; Child development, education; Higher education; Libraries/library science; Education; Natural resource conservation & protection; Environment; Animal welfare; Hospitals (general); Health care; Health associations; AIDS; Medical research; AIDS research; Housing/shelter, development; Youth development, services; Human services; Children & youth, services; Child development, services; Hospices; Aging, centers & services; Federated giving programs; Engineering & technology; Science; Leadership development; Christian agencies & churches; Native Americans; Disabled; Aging.
Types of support: General/operating support, building/renovation, equipment, land acquisition, program development, conferences/seminars, publication, seed money, research, program-related investments/loans.
Limitations: Giving primarily in the Puget Sound region of WA. No support for government entities or private foundations. No grants to individuals, or for deficit financing, endowment funds, scholarships, or fellowships; no loans.
Publications: Annual report, application guidelines.
Application information: Application form not required.
Initial approach: Letter or telephone
Copies of proposal: 3
Deadline(s): None
Board meeting date(s): Bimonthly from Sept. to May
Officers and Board of Mgrs.:* J. Shan Mullin,* Chair.; Stuart H. Prestrud,* Secy.; Durwood Alkire.
Trustee: First Interstate Bank of Washington, N.A.
Number of staff: None.
EIN: 911098014
Grants for Aging:
Buckley Senior Citizens, Buckley, WA, $1,000. 95.
East County Senior Center, Monroe, WA, $2,500. 95.

1028
Blue Mountain Area Foundation
11 South Second
P.O. Box 603
Walla Walla 99362 (509) 529-4371
Contact: Eleanor S. Kane, Administrator

Incorporated in 1984 in WA.
Foundation type: Community
Financial data (yr. ended 06/30/95): Assets, $5,649,588 (M); gifts received, $948,530; expenditures, $252,851, including $194,216 for grants and $39,254 for 60 grants to individuals.
Purpose and activities: Giving primarily for community projects, programs for organizations promoting welfare and education, social services, historical preservation, the arts, health, and animal welfare; support also for higher education through scholarship funds.
Fields of interest: Visual arts; Performing arts; Humanities; Historic preservation/historical societies; Higher education; Adult education—literacy & basic skills; Animal welfare; Family planning; Health care; Human services; Children & youth, services; Child development, services; Family services; Hospices; Aging, centers & services; Homeless, human services.
Types of support: Program development, seed money, scholarships—to individuals.
Limitations: Giving limited to Walla Walla, Columbia, Garfield, Benton and Franklin counties, WA, and Umatilla County, OR; discretionary funds for scholarships and grants limited to Walla Walla County, WA.
Publications: Annual report, application guidelines, newsletter, informational brochure.
Application information: Application form not required.
Initial approach: Letter
Copies of proposal: 1
Deadline(s): July 1
Final notification: Oct.
Officers and Trustees:* Mark C. Graves,* Pres.; Thomas K. Baffney,* V.P.; Vernon D. Kegley,* Secy.-Treas.; Louis B. Perry,* Exec. Dir.; Tom Baker, Sharon Colley, Arthur H. Griff, Vernon Marll, Judy Mulkerin, W.W. Peery, Wilbur Pribilsky, John M. Reese, Robert Zagelow.
Number of staff: 1 part-time professional.
EIN: 911250104

1029
The Boeing Company Corporate Giving Program
P.O. Box 3707, No. MS 11-83
Seattle 98124-2207 (206) 655-0803
Contact: Christine G. Jones, Mgr., Company Contribs.
FAX: (206) 655-2000

Financial data (yr. ended 12/31/94): Total giving, $35,461,136, including $26,142,266 for grants (high: $2,000,000; low: $500), $2,018,870 for 16,637 employee matching gifts and $7,300,000 for in-kind gifts.
Purpose and activities: "The Boeing commitment to corporate citizenship is a basic part of our approach to doing business. We believe that the true quality of any company is measured not only by the quality of its products and services, but by the strength of its partnership with the larger community. Boeing and its employees take great pride in supporting a wide range of educational, human service, civic, and cultural programs. In 1994, Boeing and its employees contributed over $60 million to community projects. Corporate gifts totaled $33.4 million, of which $26.1 million was donated in cash, and $7.3 million was given as in-kind donations, such as loaned executives, printing and computing services, and gifts of equipment and supplies. Boeing employees and retirees donated over $27 million in 1994 through the Boeing Employees Good Neighbor Fund and the company's gift-matching program. Employees also volunteered more than 1,000,000 hours of their own time to participate in hundreds of worthwhile projects."
Fields of interest: Theater; Humanities; Arts/cultural programs; Education, association; Early childhood education; Child development, education; Vocational education; Higher education; Adult/continuing education; Adult education—literacy & basic skills; Libraries/library science; Reading; Education; Natural resource conservation & protection; Health care; Substance abuse, services; AIDS; Alcoholism; Health organizations; AIDS research; Delinquency prevention/services; Food services; Housing/shelter, development; Youth development, services; Youth development, citizenship; Human services; Children & youth, services; Youth, services; Child development, services; Family services; Aging, centers & services; Women, centers & services; Minorities/immigrants, centers &

services; Homeless, human services; Urban/community development; Business & industry; Community development; Voluntarism promotion; Federated giving programs; Engineering & technology; Science; Government/public administration; Public affairs, citizen participation; Leadership development; Public affairs; Minorities; Disabled; Aging; Women; Homeless; General charitable giving; Canada.
Types of support: Continuing support, capital campaigns, building/renovation, equipment, emergency funds, conferences/seminars, professorships, seed money, fellowships, scholarship funds, research, technical assistance, consulting services, employee volunteer services, loaned talent, use of facilities, sponsorships, employee matching gifts, donated equipment, in-kind gifts, matching funds.
Limitations: Giving primarily in Huntsville, AL; Wichita, KS; Philadelphia, PA; Houston,TX; and Seattle, WA, and other operating locations including Winnipeg and Arnprior, Canada. No support for programs whose beneficiaries are not in the area where Boeing employees live or work, personal requests, grants for political candidates, committees or organizations, travel expenses for individuals or groups, religious organizations, hospital or medical research organizations, athletic organizations or events, agency-sponsored walk, runs, or gulf tournaments. No grants to individuals.
Publications: Corporate giving report (including application guidelines).
Application information: Company has a staff that only handles contributions. Application form required.
Initial approach: One- to two-page proposal letter to headquarters or nearest company facility
Copies of proposal: 1
Deadline(s): None
Board meeting date(s): No regular schedule
Final notification: 4 to 6 weeks for disposition
Number of staff: 6 full-time professional; 1 part-time professional; 3 full-time support.

1030
Ben B. Cheney Foundation
1201 Pacific Ave., Suite 1600
Tacoma 98402 (206) 572-2442
Contact: William O. Rieke, M.D., Exec. Dir.

Incorporated in 1955 in WA.
Donor(s): Ben B. Cheney,‡ Marian Cheney Olrogg.‡
Financial data (yr. ended 12/31/95): Assets, $69,149,833 (M); expenditures, $3,437,714; qualifying distributions, $2,976,427, including $2,588,650 for 175 grants (high: $100,000; low: $1,000; average: $5,000-$50,000).
Purpose and activities: Giving for education, health, social services, the elderly, the disabled, youth, recreation and cultural programs.
Fields of interest: Museums; Arts/cultural programs; Higher education; Education; Hospitals (general); Health care; Health organizations; Human services; Youth, services; Aging, centers & services; Disabled; Aging.
Types of support: General/operating support, building/renovation, equipment, emergency funds, program development, seed money, scholarship funds.
Limitations: Giving limited to WA, OR, and the seven northern-most CA counties. No support for religious organizations for sectarian purposes. No grants to individuals, or for operating budgets, basic research, endowment funds, conferences or seminars, or book, film, or video production; no loans.
Publications: Informational brochure (including application guidelines).
Application information: Application form required.
Initial approach: Letter
Copies of proposal: 5
Deadline(s): 5 weeks prior to board meetings
Board meeting date(s): Apr., June, Sept., and Dec.
Final notification: Within 3 months
Officers and Directors:* R. Gene Grant,* Pres.; Elgin E. Olrogg,* V.P.; John F. Hansler,* Secy.; Bradbury F. Cheney, Treas.; William O. Rieke, M.D., Exec. Dir.; Piper Cheney.
Staff: Kenneth I. Ristine, Prog. Officer.
Number of staff: 2 full-time professional; 1 full-time support.
EIN: 916053760
Grants for Aging:
Good Samaritan Outreach Services, Puyallup, WA, $30,000. For rural health care project for disabled seniors. 94.
Illinois Valley Senior Center, Cave Junction, OR, $15,000. To complete new senior center. 94.
Lutheran Social Services, Tacoma, WA, $10,000. For equipment to publish Senior Scene. 94.
Rogue Valley Manor Community Services, Medford, OR, $15,000. To establish foster grandparent program. 94.
Senior Services of South Sound, Olympia, WA, $17,500. To expand STARS program. 94.

1031
Comstock Foundation
819 Washington Trust Financial Ctr.
717 West Sprague Ave.
Spokane 99204 (509) 747-1527
Contact: Horton Herman, Trustee

Established in 1950 in WA.
Donor(s): Josie Comstock Shadle.‡
Financial data (yr. ended 12/31/94): Assets, $12,374,207 (M); expenditures, $887,566; qualifying distributions, $797,269, including $781,269 for 60 grants (high: $75,000; low: $537; average: $300-$35,000).
Purpose and activities: Emphasis on capital grants to recreational facilities and other community development projects, social service agencies, aid to the disadvantaged and handicapped, child welfare, and youth agencies. Giving also for health organizations and hospitals, the arts, including music and the performing arts, civic affairs, vocational and higher education, transportation, drug abuse programs, crime and law enforcement, hunger programs, Native Americans, and religious organizations.
Fields of interest: Arts/cultural programs; Vocational education; Higher education; Education; Hospitals (general); Health care; Substance abuse, services; Health associations; Cancer; Alcoholism; Cancer research; Food services; Recreation; Human services; Children & youth, services; Family services; Community development; Government/public administration; Religion; Disabled; Aging; Economically disadvantaged; General charitable giving.
Types of support: General/operating support, building/renovation, equipment, land acquisition, scholarship funds, research, matching funds.
Limitations: Giving limited to WA, with emphasis on the Spokane and Inland Empire areas. No grants to individuals, or for endowment funds or operating budgets; no loans. In general, no grants payable for reserve purposes, deficit financing, publications, films, emergency funds, conferences, or travel.
Publications: Informational brochure, program policy statement, application guidelines.
Application information: Application form required.
Initial approach: Proposal
Copies of proposal: 1
Deadline(s): None
Board meeting date(s): Weekly
Final notification: 10 days
Trustees: Harold W. Coffin, Horton Herman, Charles M. Leslie, Luke G. Williams.
Number of staff: 1 part-time support.
EIN: 911534637

1032
Daystar Northwest Trust, Inc.
P.O. Box 10538
Bainbridge Island 98110

Donor(s): Hilda Anderson.
Financial data (yr. ended 12/31/94): Assets, $337,333 (M); gifts received, $55,176; expenditures, $18,215; qualifying distributions, $18,115, including $24 for 1 grant and $14,954 for 2 grants to individuals (high: $9,000; low: $5,954).
Fields of interest: Aging.
Types of support: Grants to individuals.
Limitations: Applications not accepted. Giving primarily in Seattle, WA.
Officers and Directors:* Ethel Moore,* Pres.; Jerome Smith,* V.P.; Mary Dundon,* Secy.; Rachael Forney,* Treas.; Bryce Boers, Roy Kannitzer, Don Swanson.
EIN: 910782369

1033
Foundation Northwest
(Formerly Spokane Inland Northwest Community Foundation)
421 West Riverside Ave., No. 400
Spokane 99201-0403 (509) 624-2606
Contact: Peter A. Jackson, Pres.

Incorporated in 1974 in WA.
Foundation type: Community
Financial data (yr. ended 06/30/94): Assets, $7,353,497 (M); gifts received, $581,603; expenditures, $883,831, including $508,478 for 147 grants (average: $2,500-$7,500).
Purpose and activities: Primary areas of interest include the arts, education, community development, and social services.

Fields of interest: Historic preservation/historical societies; Arts/cultural programs; Education; Medical care, rehabilitation; Health care; Human services; Youth, services; Aging, centers & services; Community development; Government/public administration; Aging.
Types of support: General/operating support, program development, seed money, scholarship funds, technical assistance.
Limitations: Giving limited to the Inland Northwest (eastern WA and northern ID). No support for sectarian religious purposes. No grants to individuals, or for deficit financing, building funds, emergency funds, research, or matching grants; no loans.
Publications: Biennial report, informational brochure (including application guidelines), newsletter, application guidelines.
Application information: Scholarship awards paid to educational institutions. Application form required.
Initial approach: Letter or telephone requesting guidelines
Copies of proposal: 3
Deadline(s): Oct. 1 and Apr. 1 for grants; Mar. 1 for scholarships
Board meeting date(s): Sept. through June
Final notification: 3 months
Officers: Peter A. Jackson, Pres. and C.E.O.; Heidi B. Stanley, Secy.; Christine S. Schnug, Treas.
Directors: Craig R. Soehren, Chair.; Robert D. Fukai, Vice-Chair.; and 12 additional directors.
Staff: Candy Hanford, Prog. Dir.
Number of staff: 2 full-time professional; 1 full-time support.
EIN: 910941053
Grants for Aging:
Retired Senior Volunteer Program (RSVP), Spokane, WA, $2,000. 94.

1034
Glaser Foundation, Inc.

P.O. Box 6548
Bellevue 98008-0548
Contact: Joanne Van Sickle

Incorporated in 1952 in WA.
Donor(s): Paul F. Glaser.‡
Financial data (yr. ended 11/30/95): Assets, $9,068,731 (M); expenditures, $467,086; qualifying distributions, $384,942, including $364,568 for 71 grants (high: $25,000; low: $500; average: $3,000-$5,000).
Purpose and activities: Major focus on direct-line service agencies serving children, youth, the handicapped, the aged, and the indigent; support also for some arts organizations, substance abuse, and health services.
Fields of interest: Performing arts; Arts/cultural programs; Vocational education; Medical care, rehabilitation; Health care; Substance abuse, services; Mental health/crisis services; Health associations; Alcoholism; Biomedicine; Medical research; Delinquency prevention/services; Employment; Human services; Children & youth, services; Family services; Hospices; Aging, centers & services; Homeless, human services; Minorities; Disabled; Aging; Economically disadvantaged; Homeless.
Types of support: Program development, seed money, matching funds.
Limitations: Giving primarily in King County, WA, and immediately adjoining areas. No grants to individuals, or for general purposes, operating funds, building or endowment funds, scholarships, fellowships, publications, or conferences; no loans.
Publications: Application guidelines.
Application information: Application form required.
Initial approach: Letter
Copies of proposal: 2
Deadline(s): None
Board meeting date(s): Jan., Mar., May, July, Sept., and Nov.
Final notification: Last day in month of board meeting
Officers and Directors:* R.N. Brandenburg,* Pres.; Janet L. Politeo,* V.P.; R. William Carlstrom, Secy.; Walter Smith,* Treas.; R. Thomas Olson.
Number of staff: 1 part-time professional.
EIN: 916028694
Grants for Aging:
Counterpoint Community Mental Health Services, Everett, MA, $5,000. For Senior to Senior Peer Support. 95.
YMCA, Skagit Valley Family, Mount Vernon, WA, $5,700. For equipment for Active Older Adults program. 95.

1035
Kawabe Memorial Fund

(also known as Harry S. Kawabe Trust)
c/o Seafirst Bank
P.O. Box 24565
Seattle 98124-8824 (206) 358-0806
Contact: Mollie C. Determan, V.P., Seafirst Bank

Trust established in 1972 in WA.
Donor(s): Tomo Kawabe,‡ Harry Kawabe.‡
Financial data (yr. ended 12/31/94): Assets, $2,602,338 (M); expenditures, $138,790; qualifying distributions, $112,272, including $85,000 for 20 grants (high: $10,000; low: $500; average: $2,000-$5,000) and $6,000 for 2 grants to individuals of $3,000 each.
Purpose and activities: Giving for Buddhist and Protestant church support, including training teachers and clergy and improving facilities; support also for colleges and universities for research, and for institutions devoted to the care of the indigent, children, and the aged. Preference given to AK citizens and institutions for research; scholarships limited to graduating students in Seward, AK.
Fields of interest: Higher education; Theological school/education; Human services; Children & youth, services; Aging, centers & services; Protestant agencies & churches; Buddhism; Religion; Aging; Economically disadvantaged.
Types of support: General/operating support, continuing support, building/renovation, equipment, land acquisition, emergency funds, publication, seed money, research.
Limitations: Giving primarily in AK and the Seattle, WA, area; scholarships limited to graduating students in Seward, AK.
Publications: Application guidelines.
Application information: Application form not required.
Initial approach: Proposal
Copies of proposal: 1
Deadline(s): None
Board meeting date(s): Approximately 4 times a year with no set schedule
Allocation Committee: Yasue Brevig, Tsuyoshi Horike, Ruth S. Iwata, Jeanette Y. Otsuka, Rev. Sadmori Ouchi, Toru Sakahara, Terrance M. Toda, Chiyoko Yasutake, W.T. Yasutake.
Trustee: Seafirst Bank.
Number of staff: None.
EIN: 916116549

1036
Marilyn Moyer Charitable Trust

703 Broadway, Suite 605
Vancouver 98660 (360) 693-2886
Contact: Thomas Paul Moyer, Trustee

Established in 1991 in WA.
Donor(s): Thomas Paul Moyer.
Financial data (yr. ended 07/31/95): Assets, $841,479 (M); expenditures, $50,178; qualifying distributions, $37,872, including $5,000 for 1 grant and $26,980 for 8 grants to individuals (high: $5,000; low: $1,500).
Purpose and activities: Scholarships only to high school graduates of Ashland, OR, attending an OR State funded college or university. Grants to residents of WA, OR, CA, and ID, who are in need of basic care, not covered by insurance, social, or governmental agencies.
Fields of interest: Mental health, counseling/support groups; Youth, services; Aging.
Types of support: Grants to individuals.
Limitations: Giving limited to CA, ID, OR, and WA. Scholarships limited to OR.
Application information: Application form required.
Deadline(s): None
Officer and Trustees:* Kimberly Moyer Kassab,* Exec. Secy.; Thomas Paul Moyer, Thomas Peter Moyer, Timothy P. Moyer, Colleen Moyer Thrift.
EIN: 936238025

1037
The Norcliffe Foundation

(Formerly The Norcliffe Fund)
First Interstate Ctr.
999 Third Ave., Suite 1006
Seattle 98104
Contact: Ann P. Wyckoff, Pres.

Incorporated in 1952 in WA.
Donor(s): Theiline M. McCone.‡
Financial data (yr. ended 11/30/95): Assets, $35,622,724 (M); gifts received, $502,933; expenditures, $8,975,581; qualifying distributions, $8,944,679, including $8,862,981 for 151 grants (high: $5,250,700; low: $50; average: $1,000-$25,000).
Purpose and activities: Emphasis on arts and cultural activities, Roman Catholic church support and religious associations, hospitals, early childhood, higher and secondary education, and historic preservation; support also for medical research and health associations, hospices, the environment and conservation, and social services, including programs for the disabled, the homeless, child

welfare, and the aged, youth agencies, and wildlife organizations.
Fields of interest: Visual arts; Architecture; Performing arts; Theater; Music; Historic preservation/historical societies; Arts/cultural programs; Education, association; Education, fund raising; Elementary/secondary education; Early childhood education; Child development, education; Elementary school/education; Secondary school/education; Vocational education; Higher education; Adult education—literacy & basic skills; Libraries/library science; Reading; Education; Natural resource conservation & protection; Environment; Wildlife preservation & protection; Hospitals (general); Dental care; Health care; Substance abuse, services; Mental health/crisis services; Health associations; Cancer; AIDS; Alcoholism; Biomedicine; Health organizations; Medical research; Cancer research; AIDS research; Legal services; Employment; Food services; Nutrition; Housing/shelter, development; Recreation; Human services; Children & youth, services; Child development, services; Family services; Hospices; Aging, centers & services; Women, centers & services; Minorities/immigrants, centers & services; Homeless, human services; Community development; Voluntarism promotion; Federated giving programs; Roman Catholic federated giving programs; Protestant federated giving programs; Religious federated giving programs; Mathematics; Computer science; Government/public administration; Protestant agencies & churches; Roman Catholic agencies & churches; Religion; Minorities; Native Americans; Disabled; Aging; Women; Economically disadvantaged; Homeless; General charitable giving.
Types of support: General/operating support, continuing support, annual campaigns, capital campaigns, building/renovation, equipment, land acquisition, endowment funds, emergency funds, program development, conferences/seminars, seed money, curriculum development, fellowships, scholarship funds, research, matching funds.
Limitations: Giving primarily in the Puget Sound region, especially Seattle, WA. No grants to individuals, or for deficit financing, matching gifts, or scholarships; no loans.
Publications: Program policy statement, application guidelines.
Application information: Application form not required.
Initial approach: Letter
Copies of proposal: 1
Deadline(s): None
Board meeting date(s): As required
Final notification: 8 to 12 weeks
Officers and Trustees:* Ann Pigott Wyckoff,* Pres.; Arline Hefferline, Secy. and Fdn. Mgr.; Theiline P. Scheumann,* Treas.; Mary Ellen Hughes, Charles M. Pigott, Dana Pigott, James C. Pigott, Susan W. Pohl.
Number of staff: 1 full-time professional.
EIN: 916029352
Grants for Aging:
Mount Saint Vincent Foundation, Seattle, WA, $50,000. For general support. 94.

1038
SAFECO Corporate Giving Program
Community Relations
SAFECO Plaza
Seattle 98185 (206) 545-5015
Contact: Jill A. Ryan, Mgr., Community Rels.
Fax: (206) 545-5730

Financial data (yr. ended 12/31/95): Total giving, $6,600,000, including $6,175,000 for grants and $425,000 for employee matching gifts.
Purpose and activities: SAFECO takes a "hand-on approach to our communities because it allows us to affect, in a significant way, the environment in which we conduct business." Grants fall into three basic areas: corporate contributions, involvement grants, and matching gifts. The Home Office Contributions Program gives in Seattle under the guidance of an employee committee made up of senior management. Public health is one area of great interest, including AIDS. For the Branch Contributions Program, employee committees in the branch offices consider requests from local nonprofits. In the Community Involvement Program, employees combine their volunteer time and the corporation's financial resources to undertake charitable projects. The Volunteer Involvement Program (VIP) matches Seattle Area employees with a nonprofit that needs their skills. The 12 Days of Christmas Program is a package of 12 different holiday projects for community groups. The Matching Gift Programs includes Your Gifts Plus which matches employees' cash gifts of $25 or more and Your Time Plus which donates $100 to a nonprofit for which an employee has volunteered 25 hours or more during a 12-month period. SAFECO also participates in the annual United Way Drive each year, raising employee dollars and making direct grants. Each branch has an employee committee to decide grants.
Fields of interest: Museums; Performing arts; Arts/cultural programs; Libraries/library science; Education; Health care; Substance abuse, services; Mental health/crisis services; AIDS; Alcoholism; Health organizations; Medical research; AIDS research; Human services; Aging, centers & services; Federated giving programs; Government/public administration; Aging; Canada.
Types of support: Building/renovation, program development, fellowships, scholarship funds, employee volunteer services, employee matching gifts, matching funds.
Limitations: Giving limited to areas where a significant number of employees live and work; eligible locations are: Richmond, VA; Nashville, TN; Atlanta, GA; Maitland, FL; Dallas, TX; Chicago, IL; Cincinnati, OH; St. Louis, MO; Denver, CO; Portland, OR; Spokane, WA; Los Angeles, Fountain Valley, and San Ramone, CA. No support for national organizations, projects or programs operating outside the U.S. or Canada. No grants to individuals, or for endowment funds, loans and investments, general fundraising events and advertising associated with such events, or unrestricted operating funds for United Way agencies.
Application information: Community Rels. Dept. handles giving.
Initial approach: Brief letter of inquiry (no more than 2 pages) describing organization, proposed program, amount requested, geographic area and people to be served, how project will be evaluated, and 501(c)(3)
Deadline(s): None
Board meeting date(s): All requests are evaluated either in SAFECO's Home Office or in the branch office closest to the requesting organizations
Final notification: 6 weeks
Corporate Contributions Committee: Roger H. Eigsti, Chair. and C.E.O.; Bob Dickey, Sr. V.P. and C.F.O.; Dan McLean, Pres. and C.E.O., Safeco Insurance Companies; Richard "Duke" Campbell II, V.P., Personnel; Gordon Hamilton, V.P., Public Rels.; Jill A. Ryan, Asst. V.P., Public Rels.; Robert C. Alexander, Seattle Branch V.P.

1039
Sherwood Trust
P.O. Box 1855
Walla Walla 99362 (509) 337-6316
Contact: Leona Clarno, Secy.-Treas.
Application address: Route 1, Box 48, Waitsburg, WA 99361; Tel.: (509) 337-6316

Established in 1991 in WA.
Donor(s): Donald Sherwood.
Financial data (yr. ended 12/31/94): Assets, $13,703,661 (M); gifts received, $13,208,597; expenditures, $311,641; qualifying distributions, $295,068, including $291,807 for 3 grants (high: $280,000; low: $2,500).
Fields of interest: Higher education; Human services; Aging; Christian agencies & churches.
Types of support: General/operating support.
Limitations: Giving primarily in Walla Walla, WA. No grants to individuals.
Application information: Application form not required.
Deadline(s): None
Officers: Bert R. Edwards, Pres.; W.B. Harris, V.P.; Leona M. Clarno, Secy.-Treas.
Director: R.R. Reid.
EIN: 916337526
Grants for Aging:
Walla Walla Senior Citizens Center, Walla Walla, WA, $2,500. 94.

1040
Skamania Mason's Trust
104 Crews Rd.
Stevenson 98648

Financial data (yr. ended 12/31/92): Assets, $52,652 (M); expenditures, $6,232; qualifying distributions, $6,232, including $6,193 for 10 grants to individuals (high: $1,144; low: $50).
Purpose and activities: Support for payments for prescription medication for needy senior citizens in Skamania County, WA.
Fields of interest: Aging, centers & services; Aging; Economically disadvantaged.
Types of support: Grants to individuals.
Limitations: Giving limited to residents of Skamania County, WA.
Application information: Grants are made through physician referrals. Application form not required.
Deadline(s): None

Officers and Trustees:* Irvin W. Sterns,* Pres.; Marion Crews,* Secy.-Treas.; Ed Callahan, George F. Christensen.
EIN: 911533656

1041
The Greater Tacoma Community Foundation

P.O. Box 1995
Tacoma 98401-1995 (206) 383-5622
Contact: Margy McGroarty, Pres.

Incorporated in 1977 in WA.
Foundation type: Community
Financial data (yr. ended 06/30/95): Assets, $22,676,798 (M); gifts received, $3,540,270; expenditures, $2,157,181, including $1,240,089 for 469 grants (high: $20,000; low: $100; average: $100-$7,500) and $25,000 for 2 loans.
Fields of interest: Museums; Performing arts; Theater; Historic preservation/historical societies; Arts/cultural programs; Child development, education; Higher education; Adult/continuing education; Libraries/library science; Education; Natural resource conservation & protection; Environment; Hospitals (general); Health care; Substance abuse, services; Mental health/crisis services; AIDS; Health organizations; AIDS research; Food services; Housing/shelter, development; Recreation; Youth development, services; Human services; Children & youth, services; Child development, services; Family services; Hospices; Aging, centers & services; Homeless, human services; Community development; Voluntarism promotion; Government/public administration; Leadership development; Disabled; Aging; Economically disadvantaged; Homeless.
Types of support: General/operating support, continuing support, capital campaigns, building/renovation, equipment, emergency funds, program development, seed money, technical assistance, consulting services, program-related investments/loans, employee matching gifts, grants to individuals, matching funds.
Limitations: Giving limited to Pierce County, WA. No support for religious, political, or lobbying activities. No grants for annual campaigns, scholarships, fellowships, or publications, unless specified by donor.
Publications: Annual report, informational brochure (including application guidelines), newsletter, application guidelines.
Application information: Application form required.
Initial approach: Letter, due 1 month prior to deadlines
Copies of proposal: 2
Deadline(s): Mar. 15, July 15, and Nov. 15
Board meeting date(s): 5 times yearly
Final notification: Within 3 months
Officers and Directors:* Mary W. Green,* Chair.; Kathryn Van Wagenen,* Vice-Chair.; Margy McGroarty, Pres.; Ray E. Corpuz, Jr.,* Secy.; William T. Weyerhaeuser,* Treas.; Francie Carr, Compt.; Barbara P. Bingham, Susan Foster, Bill Gill, Steven Hill, Bill Moss, Lyle Quasim, Patricia D. Smith, Janet Stanley, Gregory M. Tanbara, S. Alan Weaver, Donald R. Williams.
Staff: Lynne Rumball, Prog. Officer.
Number of staff: 3 full-time professional; 1 part-time professional; 1 part-time support.
EIN: 911007459

1042
The Wells Charitable Trust

129 West Main St.
Walla Walla 99362 (509) 527-0477
Contact: Larry Siegel, Trustee

Established in 1992 in WA.
Financial data (yr. ended 12/31/95): Assets, $636,616 (M); expenditures, $55,916; qualifying distributions, $48,645, including $46,813 for 22 grants (high: $20,000; low: $400).
Fields of interest: Orchestra (symphony); Elementary/secondary education; Higher education; Family planning; YM/YWCAs & YM/YWHAs; Aging, centers & services; Federated giving programs.
Limitations: Giving limited to the Walla Walla, WA, area.
Application information:
Initial approach: Letter
Deadline(s): None
Trustee: Larry Siegel.
EIN: 916349205

1043
Greater Wenatchee Community Foundation

Seven North Wenatchee Ave., Suite 201
P.O. Box 3332
Wenatchee 98807-3332 (509) 663-7716
Contact: G. Raymond Taylor, C.E.O. and Pres.
FAX: (509) 664-9569

Incorporated in 1986 in WA.
Foundation type: Community
Financial data (yr. ended 06/30/95): Assets, $4,323,891 (M); gifts received, $361,904; expenditures, $340,852, including $215,526 for 41 grants (high: $40,000; low: $85; average: $1,000-$5,000), $14,650 for 15 grants to individuals (high: $5,100; low: $250; average: $400-$1,000) and $16,000 for 2 loans.
Purpose and activities: Primary areas of interest include the arts, education, and the disadvantaged, with emphasis on child welfare and the elderly.
Fields of interest: Media/communications; Visual arts; Museums; Performing arts; Theater; Music; Humanities; History & archaeology; Historic preservation/historical societies; Arts/cultural programs; Early childhood education; Child development, education; Elementary school/education; Higher education; Adult/continuing education; Adult education—literacy & basic skills; Libraries/library science; Reading; Education; Natural resource conservation & protection; Environment; Animal welfare; Wildlife preservation & protection; Hospitals (general); Family planning; Medical care, rehabilitation; Health care; Substance abuse, services; Mental health/crisis services; AIDS; Alcoholism; AIDS research; Food services; Housing/shelter, development; Safety/disasters; Recreation; Human services; Children & youth, services; Youth, services; Child development, services; Family services; Hospices; Aging, centers & services; Women, centers & services; Minorities/immigrants, centers & services; Homeless, human services; Community development; Voluntarism promotion; Federated giving programs; Economics; Minorities; Disabled; Aging; Women; Economically disadvantaged; Homeless.
Types of support: Capital campaigns, building/renovation, equipment, land acquisition, program development, seed money, research, technical assistance, matching funds.
Limitations: Giving limited to north central WA, especially Chelan, Douglas, Grant, and Okanogan counties. No support for religious sectarian purposes. Generally no grants to individuals, or for continuing support, annual campaigns, general operating budgets, or conferences; no loans.
Publications: Annual report, application guidelines, informational brochure, occasional report, grants list.
Application information: Contact foundation for application guidelines or use the PNGF Common Form. Application form not required.
Initial approach: Telephone or letter
Copies of proposal: 4
Deadline(s): Jan. 5, May 5, and Sept. 5
Board meeting date(s): Quarterly
Final notification: 2 months
Officers and Trustees:* John R. Applegate, M.D.,* Chair.; Gerald L. Copp,* Vice-Chair.; G. Raymond Taylor,* C.E.O. and Pres.; Jane Hensel,* Secy.-Treas.; Lloyd L. Berry, Benjamin Flores, Gerald E. Gibbons, M.D., Douglas B. Harper, Gregory A. Lair, Terrence M. McCawley, Leon McKinney, John C. Merritt, Irma Oliver, Leo A. Sax, Barbara Tilly, Mary Ann Warren, Robert L. White, Wilfred R. Woods.
Number of staff: 1 full-time professional; 1 part-time support.
EIN: 911349486

WEST VIRGINIA

1044
Bernard McDonough Foundation, Inc.

1000 Grand Central Mall
P.O. Box 1825
Parkersburg 26102 (304) 485-4494
Contact: James T. Wakley, Pres.

Incorporated in 1961 in WV.
Donor(s): Bernard P. McDonough.‡
Financial data (yr. ended 12/31/94): Assets, $24,210,548 (M); expenditures, $1,557,000; qualifying distributions, $1,395,997, including $1,267,323 for 114 grants (high: $250,000; low: $25; average: $1,000-$15,000).
Purpose and activities: Priority given to programs with no other source of funding. Support for higher and other education, including building funds; civic and public affairs, community funds, and leadership development programs; the humanities and cultural programs; and health and social service agencies, including rehabilitation programs for

the handicapped and drug abuse, hospital building funds, and the elderly.
Fields of interest: Humanities; Arts/cultural programs; Education, fund raising; Higher education; Education; Hospitals (general); Medical care, rehabilitation; Health care; Substance abuse, services; Health organizations; Youth development, services; Human services; Aging, centers & services; Federated giving programs; Government/public administration; Leadership development; Public affairs; Disabled; Aging; Economically disadvantaged.
Types of support: General/operating support, continuing support, annual campaigns, capital campaigns, building/renovation, equipment, emergency funds, program development.
Limitations: Giving primarily in WV. No support for religious organizations, or national health or welfare campaigns. No grants to individuals, or for personnel, operating expenses, or publications.
Application information: Application form not required.
Initial approach: Letter
Copies of proposal: 1
Deadline(s): Submit proposal preferably in Oct.; no deadline
Board meeting date(s): Dec.
Final notification: 1 to 2 weeks
Officers and Directors:* James T. Wakley,* Pres.; Mary Riccobene, V.P.; Katrina Valentine, Secy.; Carl L. Broughton, Robert E. Evans, Mark C. Kury, F.C. McCusker, T.J. Wilson.
Number of staff: 1 part-time professional.
EIN: 556023693
Grants for Aging:
New Orleans Council on Aging, New Orleans, LA, $30,000. For unrestricted support. 94.

1045
Bernice Pickens Parsons Foundation Trust
c/o Bank One, West Virginia, Charleston, N.A.
P.O. Box 1113
Charleston 25324
Contact: Tod Kaufman, Trustee
Application address: 1206 Virginia St. East, Charleston, WV 25301

Financial data (yr. ended 06/30/95): Assets, $403,908 (M); expenditures, $21,654; qualifying distributions, $18,655, including $15,990 for 21 grants (high: $2,500; low: $100).
Fields of interest: Aging, centers & services; Disabled; Aging.
Limitations: Giving limited to WV.
Application information:
Initial approach: Letter
Deadline(s): None
Trustees: William E. Casto, Judy Fisher, Karen Glazier, Tod Kaufman, James Kessell, William Rossman, Bank One, West Virginia, Charleston, N.A.
EIN: 556026999

WISCONSIN

1046
Joseph & Alice Beller Acherman Memorial Fund Trust
c/o Bank One Wisconsin Trust Co., N.A.
P.O. Box 1308
Milwaukee 53201
Contact: Ron Spielman, Trust Officer, Bank One Wisconsin Trust Co., N.A.
Application address: c/o Bank One Wisconsin Trust Co., N.A., 1717 10th St., Monroe, WI 53566; Tel.: (608) 328-4083

Financial data (yr. ended 12/31/94): Assets, $145,528 (M); expenditures, $7,812; qualifying distributions, $5,794, including $4,741 for grants.
Purpose and activities: Support only for senior citizens of Monroe, WI.
Fields of interest: Aging, centers & services; Aging.
Limitations: Giving limited to Monroe, WI. No grants to individuals.
Application information:
Initial approach: Proposal
Deadline(s): None
Trustee: Bank One Wisconsin Trust Co., N.A.
EIN: 396209178

1047
Appleton Papers Corporate Giving Program
825 East Wisconsin Ave.
P.O. Box 359
Appleton 54912 (414) 734-9841
Contact: Dennis N. Hultgren, Dir., Environmental and Public Affairs

Financial data (yr. ended 12/31/92): Total giving, $402,000, including $300,000 for grants, $79,000 for grants to individuals, $11,000 for employee matching gifts and $12,000 for in-kind gifts.
Fields of interest: Media/communications; Visual arts; Performing arts; Higher education; Education; Natural resource conservation & protection; Hospitals (general); Substance abuse, services; Health associations; AIDS; AIDS research; Food services; Human services; Children & youth, services; Youth, services; Hospices; Aging, centers & services; Federated giving programs; Government/public administration; Aging; General charitable giving.
Types of support: General/operating support, continuing support, annual campaigns, capital campaigns, program development, scholarship funds, employee matching gifts, employee-related scholarships, in-kind gifts.
Limitations: Giving primarily in operating locations in OH, PA, and WI.
Application information: Application form not required.
Initial approach: Telephone or letter
Board meeting date(s): Feb. and Dec.
Administrator: Dennis N. Hultgren, Dir., Environmental and Public Affairs.
Number of staff: 1 full-time professional; 1 full-time support.

1048
Brodbeck Foundation, Inc.
1035 East Hwy. 151, Box 656
Platteville 53818
Contact: Robert J. Brodbeck, Secy.

Established in 1987 in WI.
Donor(s): Brodbeck Enterprises, Inc.
Foundation type: Company-sponsored
Financial data (yr. ended 08/31/94): Assets, $54,141 (M); gifts received, $109,655; expenditures, $104,867; qualifying distributions, $104,847, including $103,837 for 99 grants (high: $5,363; low: $16).
Fields of interest: Arts/cultural programs; Education; Health care; Health organizations; Nutrition; Aging, centers & services; Federated giving programs; Aging.
Types of support: General/operating support.
Limitations: Giving primarily in southwestern WI.
Application information:
Initial approach: Letter
Deadline(s): None
Board meeting date(s): Monthly
Officers: William J. Brodbeck, Pres.; Barry J. Brodbeck, V.P. and Treas.; Robert J. Brodbeck, Secy.
EIN: 391605932
Grants for Aging:
Grant County Commission on Aging, Lancaster, WI, $5,363. 94.
Seniors United for Nutrition Program, Dodgeville, WI, $3,575. 94.

1049
Marjorie L. Christiansen Foundation
(Formerly Arthur J. & Cecelia L. Christiansen Foundation)
c/o Bank One Wisconsin Trust Co., N.A.
P.O. Box 1308
Milwaukee 53201-1308

Established in 1960.
Financial data (yr. ended 05/31/94): Assets, $2,654,972 (M); expenditures, $142,964; qualifying distributions, $121,696, including $114,700 for 12 grants (high: $30,000; low: $2,000).
Purpose and activities: Giving primarily in the area of health care and support of programs geared toward the elderly in the Racine, WI, area; priority given to organizations supported by the founder during her lifetime.
Fields of interest: Aging.
Limitations: Giving limited to the Racine, WI, area.
Application information: Application form not required.
Initial approach: Letter
Copies of proposal: 4
Deadline(s): None
Trustees: Roy D. Stewart, Bank One Wisconsin Trust Co., N.A.
EIN: 396037585
Grants for Aging:
Red Bus Corporation, Milwaukee, WI, $10,000. 94.
Saint Monicas Senior Citizens Home, Racine, WI, $15,000. For security system. 94.
Wisconsin Badger Camp, Racine, WI, $2,000. For elderly campers. 94.

1050
Cremer Foundation, Inc.

P.O. Box 1
Madison 53701 (608) 837-5166
Contact: James A. Berkenstadt, Esq., Administrator
Additional tel.: (608) 837-2124

Established in 1965 in WI.
Financial data (yr. ended 12/31/94): Assets, $2,309,253 (M); expenditures, $179,357; qualifying distributions, $161,021, including $161,000 for 21 grants (high: $50,000; low: $500).
Purpose and activities: Giving primarily to social service agencies, especially those aiding troubled youth, the homeless, the handicapped and senior citizens.
Fields of interest: Child development, education; Alcoholism; Biomedicine; Medical research; Human services; Children & youth, services; Youth, services; Child development, services; Family services; Aging, centers & services; Disabled; Aging.
Types of support: General/operating support, seed money, scholarship funds, matching funds.
Limitations: Giving limited to the northeast Dane County, WI, area. Generally, no support for religious-based programs. No grants to individuals, or generally for deficit financing or conferences or seminars.
Publications: Application guidelines.
Application information: Application form not required.
Initial approach: Letter or proposal
Copies of proposal: 1
Deadline(s): 1 month before meeting
Board meeting date(s): Twice a year; usually in Mar. and Aug.
Officers and Directors:* James T. Sykes,* Pres.; Frederick W. Haberman,* V.P.; Helen K. George,* Secy.; Holly L. Cremer,* Treas.; James A. Berkenstadt,* Administrator; H.B. Klotzbach, Robert R. Stroud.
Number of staff: None.
EIN: 396086822

1051
William J. Cronin Foundation

c/o Valley Trust Co., Trust Dept.
P.O. Box 5000
Janesville 53547-5000
Contact: James P. McGuire, Trustee
Application address: P.O. Box 882, Janesville, WI 53547-0882; Tel.: (608) 756-3151

Established in 1979 in WI.
Donor(s): William J. Cronin.‡
Financial data (yr. ended 11/30/93): Assets, $2,057,465 (M); expenditures, $98,722; qualifying distributions, $78,000, including $78,000 for 24 grants (high: $7,800; low: $500).
Fields of interest: Elementary/secondary education; Nursing care; Recreation; Human services; Youth, services; Hospices; Aging, centers & services; Roman Catholic agencies & churches; Religion; Aging.
Limitations: Giving limited to Janesville, WI.
Application information:
Initial approach: Letter
Deadline(s): Nov. 1
Trustees: James P. McGuire, Valley Trust Co.
EIN: 930782568

1052
Patrick and Anna M. Cudahy Fund

P.O. Box 11978
Milwaukee 53211 (847) 866-0760
Contact: Judith Borchers, Exec. Dir.

Incorporated in 1949 in WI.
Donor(s): Michael F. Cudahy.‡
Financial data (yr. ended 12/31/94): Assets, $20,245,356 (M); expenditures, $2,084,465; qualifying distributions, $1,837,994, including $1,837,994 for 171 grants (high: $109,000; low: $400; average: $5,000-$15,000).
Purpose and activities: Primary areas of interest include the arts, education, youth, international relief, and social services. Support for the homeless, family services, and international development programs; support also for national programs concerned with environmental and public interest issues, and cultural and civic affairs programs.
Fields of interest: Arts/cultural programs; Adult/continuing education; Adult education—literacy & basic skills; Reading; Education; Environment; Food services; Housing/shelter, development; Human services; Youth, services; Family services; Homeless, human services; International economic development; International relief; Human rights (international); Rural development; Public policy, research; Government/public administration; Roman Catholic agencies & churches; Asians/Pacific Islanders; African Americans; Latinos; Native Americans; Disabled; Aging; Women; Immigrants/refugees; Economically disadvantaged; Homeless.
Types of support: General/operating support, continuing support, annual campaigns, building/renovation, equipment, program development, seed money, technical assistance, matching funds.
Limitations: Giving limited to WI and Chicago, IL, for local programs and for international (U.S.-based) programs. No grants to individuals, or for endowments; no loans.
Publications: Application guidelines, grants list.
Application information: Application form required.
Initial approach: Letter
Copies of proposal: 1
Deadline(s): Approximately 8 weeks prior to board meetings
Board meeting date(s): Usually in Mar., June, Sept., and Dec.
Final notification: 2 weeks after meetings
Officers and Directors:* Richard D. Cudahy,* Chair.; Janet S. Cudahy,* Pres.; Louise A. McMenamin, Secy.; Judith Borchers, Exec. Dir.; James Bailey, Michaela Cudahy, Richard D. Cudahy, Jr., Dudley J. Godfrey, Jr., Jean Holtz, Philip Lerman, Wesley Scott, Annette Stoddard-Freeman.
Number of staff: 1 part-time professional; 1 part-time support.
EIN: 390991972
Grants for Aging:
Casa Central, Chicago, IL, $15,000. For capital campaign for multi-purpose building. 95.
Elder Care Line, Milwaukee, WI, $10,000. For vehicles. 95.
Housing Opportunities and Maintenance for the Elderly (HOME), Chicago, IL, $10,000. 95.
Little Brothers Friends of the Elderly, Chicago, IL, $10,000. For operating support. 95.
Little Sisters of the Poor, Palatine, IL, $25,000. For apartment project for low-income elderly. Grant shared with Saint Joseph's Home for the Elderly. 95.
Milwaukee Catholic Home, Milwaukee, WI, $10,000. For Intergenerational Day Care Center. 95.
Saint Ann Adult Day Care, Milwaukee, WI, $17,500. For financial assistance to low-income elderly. 95.

1053
The Evjue Foundation, Inc.

1901 Fish Hatchery Rd.
P.O. Box 8060
Madison 53708 (608) 252-6401
Contact: Marianne D. Pollard, Exec. Dir.

Incorporated in 1958 in WI.
Donor(s): William T. Evjue.‡
Financial data (yr. ended 02/28/94): Assets, $6,695,511 (M); gifts received, $1,553,284; expenditures, $1,464,803; qualifying distributions, $1,397,663, including $1,366,252 for 138 grants (high: $300,000; low: $275; average: $1,000-$5,000).
Purpose and activities: Support for education, including higher education; grants also for mental health, youth, and social service agencies, and for cultural programs.
Fields of interest: Journalism & publishing; Arts/cultural programs; Higher education; Education; Animal welfare; Hospitals (general); Family planning; Substance abuse, services; Mental health/crisis services; Alcoholism; Food services; Human services; Children & youth, services; Youth, services; Family services; Aging, centers & services; Aging.
Types of support: Continuing support, annual campaigns, capital campaigns, endowment funds, emergency funds, program development, conferences/seminars, professorships, publication, seed money, internships, scholarship funds.
Limitations: Giving primarily in Dane County, WI. No support for medical or scientific research. No grants to individuals, or for building funds, equipment, land acquisition, renovation projects, or operating expenses; no loans.
Publications: Program policy statement, application guidelines.
Application information: Application form not required.
Initial approach: Letter
Copies of proposal: 1
Deadline(s): Submit proposal preferably in Nov., Dec., or Jan.
Board meeting date(s): Jan., Mar., June, and Sept., and as required
Final notification: 3 months
Officers and Directors:* John H. Lussier,* Pres.; Nancy Brooke Gage,* V.P.; F.H. Gage,* Secy.; F.W. Miller,* Treas.; Marianne D. Pollard,* Exec. Dir.; James D. Lussier, Laura J. Lussier.
Number of staff: 1 part-time support.
EIN: 396073981

1054
Vernon G. Goelzer Trust
c/o Bank One Wisconsin Trust Co., N.A.
Box 1308
Milwaukee 53201

Financial data (yr. ended 05/31/95): Assets, $689,341 (M); expenditures, $33,405; qualifying distributions, $27,241, including $24,773 for grants.
Fields of interest: Higher education; Housing/shelter, aging.
Limitations: Applications not accepted.
Application information: Contributes only to pre-selected organizations.
Trustee: Bank One Wisconsin Trust Co., N.A.
EIN: 396566242

1055
Greater Green Bay Community Foundation
333 Main St., Suite 177
Green Bay 54301 (414) 432-0800
Contact: Cynthia A. Johnson, Exec. Dir.
FAX: (414) 432-5577

Established in 1991 WI.
Foundation type: Community
Financial data (yr. ended 06/30/95): Assets, $8,552,037 (M); gifts received, $4,208,886; expenditures, $1,124,961, including $988,988 for 74 grants (high: $150,000; low: $25), $12,300 for 20 grants to individuals (high: $1,250; low: $200) and $30,000 for 8 in-kind gifts.
Fields of interest: Historic preservation/historical societies; Arts/cultural programs; Education; Environment; Health care; Youth development; Human services; Aging.
Types of support: Program development, conferences/seminars, seed money, scholarship funds.
Limitations: Giving limited to northeast WI.
Publications: Annual report, newsletter, informational brochure, application guidelines.
Application information: Application form not required.
Initial approach: 1-page letter or telephone
Copies of proposal: 1
Deadline(s): None
Board meeting date(s): Mar., June, Oct., and Dec.
Officers and Directors:* Robert C. Gallagher,* Pres.; Jeffrey C. Beinlich,* V.P. and Secy.; Herbert C. Liebmann III,* V.P.; Jane P. Van Lanen,* V.P.; Daniel P. Bittner,* Treas.; Cynthia A. Johnson, Exec. Dir.
Number of staff: 1 full-time professional; 1 full-time support.
EIN: 391699966
Grants for Aging:
American Red Cross, Lakeland Chapter, WI, $500. For vehicle for elderly and handicapped. 94.
Home Respite Care, Oconto Falls, WI, $1,000. For volunteer training. 94.

1056
Huss Foundation
(Formerly Alvin & Miriam Huss Foundation)
c/o First National Bank of Hudson
P.O. Box 187
Hudson 54016-0187

Established in 1983 in WI.
Donor(s): Alvin J. Huss.
Financial data (yr. ended 12/31/93): Assets, $59,289 (M); gifts received, $70,000; expenditures, $43,779; qualifying distributions, $43,762, including $42,487 for 4 grants (high: $26,641; low: $1,150).
Fields of interest: Arts/cultural programs; Higher education; Environment; Hospitals (general); Alcoholism; Human services; Aging, centers & services; Christian agencies & churches; Aging.
Limitations: Applications not accepted. Giving primarily in MN and WI. No grants to individuals.
Application information: Contributes only to pre-selected organizations.
Trustees: Alvin J. Huss, Alvin J. Huss, Jr., Ruth S. Huss.
EIN: 391474563

1057
Johnson Controls Foundation
5757 North Green Bay Ave.
P.O. Box 591
Milwaukee 53201 (414) 228-2296
Contact: Valerie Adisek, Admin. Secy.

Trust established in 1952 in WI.
Donor(s): Johnson Controls, Inc.
Foundation type: Company-sponsored
Financial data (yr. ended 12/31/94): Assets, $19,506,650 (M); gifts received, $3,200,000; expenditures, $3,846,447; qualifying distributions, $3,761,881, including $3,757,375 for 1,184 grants (high: $250,000; low: $13; average: $500-$100,000).
Purpose and activities: Grants for higher education; health and hospitals; community funds; social services, including aid to the handicapped, care of children, and the aged; and civic, arts, and cultural organizations.
Fields of interest: Performing arts; Arts/cultural programs; Higher education; Hospitals (general); Health care; AIDS; Health organizations; AIDS research; Human services; Children & youth, services; Youth, services; Aging, centers & services; Federated giving programs; Government/public administration; Disabled; Aging.
Types of support: General/operating support, continuing support, annual campaigns, capital campaigns, building/renovation, emergency funds, seed money, employee matching gifts, employee-related scholarships, matching funds.
Limitations: No support for religious purposes, public or private preschools, elementary or secondary schools, industrial groups or trade associations supported by industrial groups, foreign-based institutions, or fraternal, veterans', or labor groups. No grants to individuals (except employee-related scholarships), or for fundraising events, courtesy advertising, deficit financing, equipment, land acquisition, special projects, research, publications, conferences, or seminars; no loans.
Publications: Application guidelines.
Application information: Employee-related scholarship awards are paid directly to institutions and not to individuals. Application form not required.
Initial approach: Letter
Copies of proposal: 1
Deadline(s): None
Board meeting date(s): Usually Mar., June, and Nov.
Final notification: Up to 120 days
Advisory Board: Fred Brengel, James H. Keyes, R. Douglas Zeigler, Denise Zutz.
Scholarship Selection Committee: Frederick E. Sperry, Norbert J. Tlachac, Marie Uihlein.
Trustee: Firstar Trust Co.
Number of staff: 1 full-time professional; 3 part-time support.
EIN: 396036639

1058
The Elmer Leach Foundation, Inc.
c/o Firstar Bank Oshkosh, N.A.
P.O. Box 2448
Oshkosh 54903
Contact: Frederick E. Leach, Pres.
Application address: 2737 Harrison St., P.O. Box 2608, Oshkosh, WI 54903

Established in 1965 in WI.
Donor(s): Leach Co.
Financial data (yr. ended 12/31/94): Assets, $2,226,505 (M); gifts received, $790; expenditures, $122,161; qualifying distributions, $113,051, including $113,040 for 24 grants (high: $22,000; low: $100).
Purpose and activities: "To promote mental, moral, and physical improvement to worthy persons to include without limitations, private secondary education, care of sick, aged, or helpless, improvement of living conditions, and provision of recreation for all classes."
Fields of interest: Education; Health associations; Recreation; Human services; Children & youth, services; Aging, centers & services; Federated giving programs; Aging.
Limitations: Giving primarily in Oshkosh, WI.
Application information: Application form not required.
Initial approach: Letter
Deadline(s): Jan. 1 through Nov. 1
Officers: Frederick E. Leach, Pres.; David C. Leach III, Exec. V.P.; Phyllis L. Leach, Secy.; David Fischer, Treas.
EIN: 396093521

1059
Madison Community Foundation
(Formerly United Madison Community Foundation)
615 East Washington Ave.
Madison 53701 (608) 255-0503
Contact: Jane Coleman, Exec. Dir.
Application address: P.O. Box 71, Madison, WI 53701

Established in 1977 in WI; reorganized in 1986.
Foundation type: Community
Financial data (yr. ended 12/31/95): Assets, $38,485,122 (M); gifts received, $5,200,000; expenditures, $3,900,000, including

$3,000,000 for 100 grants (high: $75,000; low: $2,000; average: $2,000-$75,000) and $167,141 for 2 foundation-administered programs.
Purpose and activities: To enhance the quality of life in Dane County, WI, in the areas of arts and culture, economic and community development, education, the environment, the elderly, families, and youth.
Fields of interest: Performing arts; Arts/cultural programs; Education; Environment; Youth, services; Family services; Community development; Aging.
Types of support: Building/renovation, equipment, program development, seed money, technical assistance, matching funds.
Limitations: Giving limited to Dane County, WI. No support for religious purposes. Generally, no grants to individuals, or for annual campaigns, conferences, building or endowment funds, or deficit financing.
Publications: Annual report, application guidelines, informational brochure, newsletter.
Application information: Application form required.
Initial approach: Proposal
Copies of proposal: 5
Deadline(s): Mar. 1 and Sept. 1
Board meeting date(s): 6 times a year
Final notification: May 30 and Nov. 30
Board of Governors: Gary L. Schaefer, Chair.; Terry Haller, Vice-Chair.; Steve Mixtacki, Treas.; Jane T. Coleman, Exec. Dir.; and 12 additional members.
Staff: Amy T. Dally, Prog. Officer; Angela Y. Fussell, Project Assoc.; Juan Jose Lopez, Project Dir.; Joan Klaski, Assoc. Dir.
Number of staff: 5 full-time professional; 2 full-time support.
EIN: 396038248

1060
Marshall & Ilsley Corporate Giving Program

770 North Water St.
Milwaukee 53202 (414) 765-7700
Contact: Harold W. Reiter, V.P.

Fields of interest: Media/communications; Museums; Music; Arts/cultural programs; Secondary school/education; Higher education; Education; Environment; Hospitals (general); Health care; Health organizations; Medical research; Human services; Youth, services; Aging, centers & services; Community development; Federated giving programs; Religious federated giving programs; Economics; Government/public administration; Aging.
Limitations: Giving primarily in the metropolitan Milwaukee, WI, area.
Application information:
Initial approach: Letter
Deadline(s): None
Board meeting date(s): Monthly

1061
Faye McBeath Foundation

1020 North Broadway
Milwaukee 53202 (414) 272-2626
Contact: Sarah M. Dean, Exec. Dir.
FAX: (414) 272-6235

Trust established in 1964 in WI.
Donor(s): Faye McBeath.‡
Financial data (yr. ended 12/31/95): Assets, $14,703,570 (M); expenditures, $1,250,185; qualifying distributions, $1,043,565, including $952,030 for 44 grants (high: $100,000; low: $1,000; average: $20,000-$25,000).
Purpose and activities: To benefit the people of WI by providing homes and care for elderly persons; promoting education in medical science and public health; providing medical, nursing, and hospital care for the sick and disabled; promoting the welfare of children; and promoting research in civics and government directed towards improvement in the efficiency of local government.
Fields of interest: Early childhood education; Elementary school/education; Secondary school/education; Medical school/education; Dental care; Nursing care; Health care; Substance abuse, services; Mental health/crisis services; AIDS; Alcoholism; Biomedicine; Health organizations; Nutrition; Youth development, citizenship; Human services; Children & youth, services; Youth, services; Child development, services; Family services; Hospices; Aging, centers & services; Public policy, research; Government/public administration; Public affairs, citizen participation; Aging.
Types of support: General/operating support, continuing support, program development, seed money, technical assistance, matching funds.
Limitations: Giving limited to WI, with emphasis on the greater Milwaukee area. No grants to individuals, or for annual campaigns, capital projects, endowment funds, scholarships, fellowships, or specific medical or scientific research projects; grants rarely for emergency funds; no loans.
Publications: Annual report, program policy statement, application guidelines.
Application information: Application form required.
Initial approach: 2-page preliminary application
Copies of proposal: 1
Deadline(s): 1 month prior to board meetings
Board meeting date(s): 6 times a year
Final notification: 10 days after meeting
Officers and Trustees:* Thomas J. McCollow,* Chair.; William L. Randall,* Vice-Chair.; Joan Hardy,* Secy.; Sarah M. Dean, Exec. Dir.; Charles A. Krause, Bonnie R. Weigell, Firstar Trust Co.
Number of staff: 1 part-time professional.
EIN: 396074450
Grants for Aging:
YMCA of Metropolitan Milwaukee, Milwaukee, WI, $25,000. For senior housing program. 95.

1062
Milwaukee Foundation

1020 North Broadway
Milwaukee 53202 (414) 272-5805
Contact: Douglas M. Jansson, Exec. Dir.

Established in 1915 in WI by declaration of trust.
Foundation type: Community
Financial data (yr. ended 12/31/94): Assets, $138,428,472 (M); gifts received, $11,858,392; expenditures, $7,192,945, including $5,310,989 for grants (high: $150,000; low: $1,000).
Purpose and activities: Present funds include many discretionary and some funds designated by the donors to benefit specific institutions or for special purposes, including educational institutions, the arts and cultural programs, community development, social services, and health care; support also for conservation and historic preservation.
Fields of interest: Visual arts; Performing arts; Dance; Historic preservation/historical societies; Arts/cultural programs; Early childhood education; Child development, education; Elementary school/education; Secondary school/education; Higher education; Adult/continuing education; Education; Natural resource conservation & protection; Family planning; Health care; Substance abuse, services; Mental health/crisis services; AIDS; Alcoholism; Health organizations; AIDS research; Delinquency prevention/services; Legal services; Employment; Food services; Nutrition; Housing/shelter, development; Recreation; Human services; Children & youth, services; Youth, services; Child development, services; Family services; Aging, centers & services; Women, centers & services; Homeless, human services; Race/intergroup relations; Urban/community development; Community development; Public policy, research; Government/public administration; Minorities; Disabled; Aging; Women; Economically disadvantaged; Homeless.
Types of support: Capital campaigns, building/renovation, equipment, program development, conferences/seminars, seed money, scholarship funds, matching funds.
Limitations: Giving primarily in the greater Milwaukee, WI, area. No support for the general use of churches or for sectarian religious purposes, or for specific medical or scientific projects except from components of the foundation established for such purposes. No grants to individuals (except for established awards), or for operating budgets, continuing support, annual campaigns, endowment funds, or deficit financing.
Publications: Annual report, informational brochure (including application guidelines), grants list, newsletter, program policy statement, application guidelines.
Application information: Capital requests are reviewed at Dec. board meeting. Application form required.
Initial approach: Letter of intent
Copies of proposal: 1
Deadline(s): Submit proposal preferably 10 weeks before board meetings; deadlines Jan. 2, Apr. 1, July 1, and Oct. 1
Board meeting date(s): Mar., June, Sept., Dec., and as needed
Final notification: 2 weeks after board meetings
Officers: Douglas M. Jansson, Pres., Secy., and Exec. Dir.; Wendy Horton, C.F.O.
Directors: Carl A. Weigell, Chair.; Polly H. Van Dyke, Vice-Chair.; William Fitzhugh Fox, John H. Hendee, Jr., Geneva B. Johnson, George Kaiser, Stephen H. Marcus, Charles S. McNeer, Linda T. Mellowes, Jose A. Olivieri.

Trustees: Bank One Wisconsin Trust Co., N.A., First Bank Milwaukee, Firstar Trust Co., Marshall & Ilsley Trust Co.
Staff: James Marks, Assoc. Dir.; Margaret Jane Moore, Sr. Prog. Officer; Sarah Ann Ford, Prog. Officer; Sigfredo Gutierrez, Prog. Officer; Patrice McIntyre, Scholarships Administrator.
Number of staff: 8 full-time professional; 1 part-time professional; 9 full-time support.
EIN: 396036407
Grants for Aging:
Artreach Milwaukee, Milwaukee, WI, $10,000. To develop intergenerational arts project in which older adults share artistic experiences with children. 95.
Family Service of Milwaukee, Milwaukee, WI, $15,000. For training program for Alzheimer's disease caregivers. 95.
S.E.T. Ministry, Milwaukee, WI, $15,000. For continued matching grant for case management demonstration project for elderly and disabled in public housing. 95.

1063
John A. & Evelyn Monahan Memorial Trust

c/o Bank One Wisconsin Trust Co., N.A.
P.O. Box 1308
Milwaukee 53201 (414) 765-2800
Contact: Margaret Paur, Trust Officer, Bank One Wisconsin Trust Co., N.A.

Financial data (yr. ended 04/30/95): Assets, $735,352 (M); expenditures, $32,696; qualifying distributions, $23,299, including $20,880 for 7 grants (high: $4,400; low: $1,780).
Fields of interest: Youth, services; Aging, centers & services; Disabled; Aging.
Limitations: Giving limited to residents of Milwaukee County, WI.
Application information: Application form not required.
Deadline(s): None
Trustee: Bank One Wisconsin Trust Co., N.A.
EIN: 391333780

1064
National Institute of Biogerontology

4610 University Ave.
P.O. Box 55231
Madison 53705
Contact: Dr. Everett L. Smith, Pres.

Established in 1985 in WI.
Financial data (yr. ended 06/30/94): Assets, $6,116 (M); gifts received, $2,520; expenditures, $3,561.
Purpose and activities: Support limited to research on aging and disuse atrophy with emphasis on atrophy and osteoporosis.
Fields of interest: Medical research; Aging, centers & services; Aging.
Types of support: Seed money, curriculum development, research, grants to individuals.
Limitations: Giving primarily in WI.
Application information: No grants paid in fiscal 1994.
Initial approach: Proposal
Deadline(s): None
Officers and Directors:* Everett L. Smith,* Pres.; Robert O. Ray,* V.P.; Patricia Smith,* Secy.-Treas.; Vernon Dodson, William Ershler, William G. Reddan.
Number of staff: None.
EIN: 391484704

1065
NMC Projects, Inc.

P.O. Box 600
Stoughton 53589

Established in 1959 in WI.
Donor(s): Nelson Industries, Inc.
Foundation type: Company-sponsored
Financial data (yr. ended 07/31/93): Assets, $389,642 (M); gifts received, $100,000; expenditures, $103,397; qualifying distributions, $103,397, including $73,592 for 77 grants (high: $10,000; low: $30) and $29,600 for 20 grants to individuals.
Purpose and activities: Support focus is on youth, elderly, education, special community projects, and for health and human services; also awards scholarships at participating high schools for higher and technical education; medical education scholarships handled by the CES Foundation of the State Medical Society of WI. Participating high schools are Arcadia, Bloomer, Mineral Point, Neillsville, Wautoma, Black River, Viroqua, and Stoughton high schools and Riverdale High School in Muscada.
Fields of interest: Historic preservation/historical societies; Arts/cultural programs; Higher education; Education; Natural resource conservation & protection; Wildlife preservation & protection; Hospitals (general); Substance abuse, services; Heart/circulatory disease; Medical research; Heart/circulatory research; Human services; Youth, services; Aging, centers & services; International relief; Federated giving programs; Religion; Aging; Economically disadvantaged; General charitable giving.
Types of support: Continuing support, annual campaigns, capital campaigns, building/renovation, equipment, emergency funds, program development, scholarship funds, employee-related scholarships, scholarships—to individuals, exchange programs.
Limitations: Giving primarily in WI.
Publications: Annual report, 990-PF.
Application information: Decisions on scholarships made by high schools. Application form not required.
Initial approach: Letter with copy of proposal
Deadline(s): Apr. 15 for high school scholarships
Board meeting date(s): Quarterly
Officers: Stephen R. Slinde, Pres. and Treas.; Michael C. Bemis, V.P.; Robert B. Murphy, Secy.
Number of staff: None.
EIN: 396043256

1066
Siebert Lutheran Foundation, Inc.

2600 North Mayfair Rd., Suite 390
Wauwatosa 53226 (414) 257-2656
Contact: Ronald D. Jones, Pres.

Incorporated in 1952 in WI.
Donor(s): A.F. Siebert,‡ Reginald L. Siebert,‡ Milwaukee Electric Tool Corp.
Financial data (yr. ended 12/31/94): Assets, $56,418,205 (M); gifts received, $48,100; expenditures, $3,427,849; qualifying distributions, $2,730,073, including $2,660,116 for 278 grants (high: $250,000; low: $500; average: $2,500-$10,000).
Purpose and activities: Support for Lutheran institutions, including colleges, schools, churches, and Lutheran religious welfare agencies.
Fields of interest: Elementary/secondary education; Early childhood education; Child development, education; Secondary school/education; Higher education; Education; Human services; Child development, services; Aging, centers & services; Protestant federated giving programs; Protestant agencies & churches; Religion; Minorities; Aging.
Types of support: Program development, seed money, consulting services, matching funds.
Limitations: Giving primarily in WI. No grants to individuals, or for endowment funds, scholarships, or fellowships; no loans.
Publications: Program policy statement, application guidelines, informational brochure (including application guidelines).
Application information: Grantees are required to sign Grant Agreement Form. Application form not required.
Initial approach: Letter or telephone
Copies of proposal: 1
Deadline(s): Mar. 15, June 15, Sept. 15, and Dec. 15
Board meeting date(s): Jan., Apr., July, and Oct.
Final notification: 1 week after board meeting
Officers and Directors:* John E. Koenitzer,* Chair.; Frederick H. Groth,* Vice-Chair.; Ronald D. Jones, Pres.; Ned W. Bechtold, Secy.; Armour F. Swanson, Treas.; Richard C. Barkow, Chris M. Bauer, Jack S. Harris, Raymond J. Perry, John C. Zimdars, Jr.
Number of staff: 1 full-time professional; 1 full-time support.
EIN: 396050046

1067
Taylor Family Charitable Irrevocable Trust of 1977

c/o Waukesha State Bank, Trust Dept.
P.O. Box 648
Waukesha 53187

Established in 1977 in WI.
Financial data (yr. ended 12/31/94): Assets, $199,891 (M); expenditures, $12,684; qualifying distributions, $11,459, including $10,313 for grants.
Fields of interest: Aging.
Limitations: Applications not accepted. Giving primarily in Waukesha, WI. No grants to individuals.
Application information: Contributes only to pre-selected organizations.
Trustee: Waukesha State Bank.
Advisory Committee: Velma Geraldson, Don L. Taylor.
EIN: 396297286

1068
James A. Taylor Family Foundation, Inc.

1000 West Donges Bay Rd.
Mequon 53092-5999 (414) 241-4321
Contact: James A. Taylor, Pres.

Established in 1959 in WI.
Donor(s): Taylor Electric Co., James A. Taylor.
Financial data (yr. ended 06/30/92): Assets, $737,744 (M); gifts received, $10,000; expenditures, $45,644; qualifying distributions, $44,305, including $44,175 for 117 grants (high: $10,700; low: $25).
Fields of interest: Visual arts; Museums; Performing arts; Dance; Historic preservation/historical societies; Arts/cultural programs; Elementary/secondary education; Child development, education; Secondary school/education; Higher education; Theological school/education; Adult education—literacy & basic skills; Libraries/library science; Reading; Education; Natural resource conservation & protection; Environment; Animal welfare; Hospitals (general); Family planning; Nursing care; Health care; Substance abuse, services; Mental health/crisis services; Health associations; Cancer; Heart/circulatory disease; Alcoholism; Health organizations; Medical research; Cancer research; Heart/circulatory research; Delinquency prevention/services; Human services; Child development, services; Family services; Aging, centers & services; Federated giving programs; Christian agencies & churches; Religion; Disabled; Aging; Economically disadvantaged; General charitable giving.
Types of support: General/operating support, continuing support, annual campaigns, capital campaigns, building/renovation, emergency funds, seed money, research.
Limitations: Giving primarily in WI.
Application information: Giving to new applicants is very limited. Application form not required.
Deadline(s): None
Officers and Directors:* James A. Taylor,* Pres.; James A. Taylor, Jr.,* V.P.; John W. Taylor,* Secy.-Treas.; Scott A. Nyholm, Jr., Mgr.; Barbara T. Mans.
Number of staff: None.
EIN: 396045247

1069
Unicare Foundation, Inc.

105 West Michigan St.
Milwaukee 53203-2914 (414) 347-4221
Contact: Ronald Retzke, Ph.D., Pres.

Established in 1985 in WI.
Foundation type: Company-sponsored
Financial data (yr. ended 12/31/95): Assets, $303,793 (M); gifts received, $134,675; expenditures, $189,323; qualifying distributions, $189,323, including $127,383 for 16 grants (high: $45,000; low: $2,000).
Purpose and activities: Awards grants for Alzheimer's disease research and services for quality of life in long-term care settings and for care-giver education in communities served by Unicare Health Facilities.
Fields of interest: Health care; Medical research; Aging, centers & services; Aging; General charitable giving.
Types of support: Consulting services, seed money, research, curriculum development, program development, technical assistance, conferences/seminars.
Limitations: Giving primarily in areas served by Unicare Health Facilities. No grants to individuals.
Publications: Annual report (including application guidelines), application guidelines, informational brochure.
Application information: Contact a local Unicare Health Facility for further information. Application form required.
Deadline(s): Quarterly
Officers and Directors:* Guy W. Smith,* C.E.O.; Ronald Retzke, Ph.D.,* Pres.; Nancy A. Wier,* V.P.; Colleen Schroeder,* Treas.; Rob Guilbert, David Gustafson, Ph.D., Margaret Hastings, Ph.D., John Hughes, Tom Kirk, Jeff Minor, Bill Mulligan, Janice Ricchio, Jim Wahner, Lee Wallace.
Staff: Lisa Bittner, Recorder; Scott Miller, Financial Analyst.
Number of staff: None.
EIN: 391549381
Grants for Aging:
Alzheimers Disease and Related Disorders Association, Louisville, KY, $5,000. 94.
Alzheimers Disease and Related Disorders Association, Metropolitan Minneapolis-Saint Paul Chapter, Bloomington, MN, $11,250. 94.
Alzheimers Disease and Related Disorders Association, Tarrant County Chapter, Fort Worth, TX, $2,500. 94.
Alzheimers Treatment and Research Center, Saint Paul, MN, $4,000. 94.
Children of Aging Parents, Levittown, PA, $5,000. 94.
French Foundation for Alzheimer Research, Los Angeles, CA, $22,500. 94.
Wisconsin Alzheimers Information and Training, Milwaukee, WI, $1,900. 94.

1070
United Wisconsin Services Foundation, Inc.

(Formerly Blue Cross and Blue Shield United of Wisconsin Foundation, Inc.)
401 West Michigan St.
Milwaukee 53203 (414) 226-5756
Contact: Tom Luljak, Exec. Dir.

Established in 1984 in WI.
Donor(s): Blue Cross and Blue Shield United of Wisconsin, United Wisconsin Services, Inc.
Foundation type: Company-sponsored
Financial data (yr. ended 12/31/94): Assets, $2,636,760 (M); gifts received, $2,800,000; expenditures, $568,118; qualifying distributions, $539,818, including $539,695 for 147 grants (high: $50,000; low: $100).
Purpose and activities: Giving primarily for education, health services, health clinics, vision, aging and youth.
Fields of interest: Visual arts; Performing arts; Higher education; Education; Health care; Youth, services; Family services; Aging, centers & services; Community development; Voluntarism promotion; Federated giving programs; Aging.
Types of support: Annual campaigns, scholarship funds, research.
Limitations: Giving limited to WI. No grants to individuals.
Application information: Application form required.
Initial approach: Letter
Deadline(s): Varies
Board meeting date(s): Apr. 19, July 14, Oct. 15, and Dec. 7
Officers: Thomas R. Hefty, Chair. and Pres.; Mary Traver, V.P. and Secy.-Treas.; Mark Granoff, V.P.; Jeffrey Nohl, V.P.; Essie M. Whitelaw, V.P.; Tom Luljak, Exec. Dir.
Number of staff: None.
EIN: 391514703
Grants for Aging:
Coalition of Wisconsin Aging Groups, Madison, WI, $18,000. For study on long-term care. 94.

1071
Harriet Brower Warnemuende Charitable Trust

c/o Bank One Wisconsin Trust Co., N.A.
P.O. Box 1308
Milwaukee 53201
Application address: Richard J. Blahnik, Trust Officer, Bank One Wisconsin Trust Co., N.A., P.O. Box 1029, Green Bay, WI 54305; Tel.: (414) 436-2602

Financial data (yr. ended 08/31/93): Assets, $580,016 (M); expenditures, $31,235; qualifying distributions, $26,274.
Purpose and activities: Support to organizations providing services to elderly or sick persons and their immediate families of Brunn County, WI.
Fields of interest: Hospitals (general); Family services; Aging, centers & services; Aging.
Types of support: General/operating support.
Limitations: Giving limited to Brown County, WI.
Publications: Application guidelines.
Application information:
Initial approach: Proposal
Deadline(s): None
Trustee: Bank One Wisconsin Trust Co., N.A.
EIN: 396443109

WYOMING

1072
The Goodstein Foundation

P.O. Box 2773
Casper 82602 (307) 234-0821
Contact: Robert W. Miracle, Pres.

Incorporated in 1952 in CO.
Donor(s): J.M. Goodstein.‡
Financial data (yr. ended 06/30/95): Assets, $4,932,492 (M); expenditures, $332,227; qualifying distributions, $277,845, including $277,845 for 53 grants (high: $130,000; low: $100).
Purpose and activities: Giving primarily to Jewish causes in the metropolitan Denver, CO, area. Giving also for education, health, human

services and civic projects which initiate, additional philanthropic giving, such as matching grants, in Natrona County, WY.
Fields of interest: Higher education; Hospitals (general); Human services; Jewish federated giving programs; Aging.
Types of support: General/operating support, capital campaigns, building/renovation, equipment, matching funds.
Limitations: Giving primarily in the metropolitan Denver, CO, area and Natrona County, WY. No grants to individuals.
Publications: Annual report.
Application information:
Initial approach: Letter
Deadline(s): None
Officers: Robert W. Miracle, Pres.; Lucy M. Goodstein, V.P. and Secy.
EIN: 836003815
Grants for Aging:
Beth Israel at Shalom Park, Aurora, CO, $100,000. 94.
Seniors, Denver, CO, $5,000. 95.
Seniors, Denver, CO, $3,000. 94.

1073
Hazel Patterson Memorial Trust

130 South Main St.
Buffalo 82834 (307) 684-2207
Contact: William D. Omohundro, Trustee

Established in 1989 in WY.
Financial data (yr. ended 09/30/95): Assets, $1,015,520 (M); expenditures, $52,423; qualifying distributions, $46,546, including $45,608 for 16 grants (high: $8,000; low: $400).
Fields of interest: Museums; Education; Hospitals (general); Mental health/crisis services; Human services; Children & youth, services; Aging, centers & services.
Limitations: Giving limited to Buffalo, WY. No grants to individuals.
Application information:
Initial approach: Letter
Deadline(s): None
Trustees: Don Kraen, William D. Omohundro, Sandra Todd.
EIN: 742557301

SECTION II: VOLUNTARY ORGANIZATIONS

VOLUNTARY ORGANIZATIONS

ACADEMIC AND RESEARCH CENTERS

1074
Bowling Green State University Gerontology Program
Bowling Green, OH 43403 (419)372-2326
Contact: Dr. Jennifer Kinney

Purpose and activities: Program of education, training, and service within a public university.
Geographic focus: Active in OH, nationally and internationally.
Technical assistance: Gerontology faculty provides training and service programs of benefit to the aging, to public service providers, and others.
Publications: Informational brochure, course listings and other material.

1075
Brookdale Center on Aging of Hunter College
425 East 25th St.
New York, NY 10010-2590 (212)481-4426
Contact: Rose Doborf, Exec. Dir.

Purpose and activities: Provides professional training for and advice to those providing social services to the elderly.

1076
Case Western Reserve University Senior Scholars Program
103 Guilford House
10900 Euclid Ave.
Cleveland, OH 44106-7116 (216)368-2090
FAX: (216)368-1861
Contact: Kathy Manos, Dir.

Established in 1979.
Purpose and activities: Provides university level programs for those age 50 and older who do not wish to enroll in a full semester program. Classes are comprised of three 11-week semesters. Three topic-specific courses are offered each semester. Program also includes a winter intersession. Courses are non-credit with no exams or papers required. There is a single nominal fee per semester with limited scholarship funds; assigned books are available at a discount. Courses for the Fall, 1996 semester include: Literature Anthropology, Psychology, Political Science, Economics.
Geographic focus: Active in the Cleveland, OH, area.
Publications: Informational brochure. Course lists describing upcoming courses are available.

1077
Duke University Center for the Study of Aging and Human Development
Duke University Medical Center
Box 3003
Durham, NC 27710 (919)660-7500
Additional tel.: (919)660-7502;
FAX: (919)684-8569
Contact: Harvey Jay Cohen, M.D., Dir.

Established in 1955.
Purpose and activities: Serves as a national resource for information and as a training ground for future generations of research investigators, teachers, practitioners, and planners. Stimulates and supports research in the field of aging, disseminates information resulting from studies at the university, and develops interest in the field of aging through lectures, seminars, conferences, and institutes. Basic research includes human and animal physiology, Alzheimer's Disease, family structure and intergenerational relationships, and the demographics and economics of aging populations. The non-degree training program includes advanced research training, apprenticeships, and continuing education. Direct services include clinical services, geriatric consultation, and a family support program which provides a model for community support groups assisting families caring for persons with Alzheimer's Disease at home.
Geographic focus: Active regionally and nationally, with direct service programs for the elderly and their families in the Durham, NC area.
Publications: Informational brochure, newsletter, occasional report. "Center Report" presents brief summaries of the implications and applications of research findings (quarterly newsletter). Additionally publishes technical reports and the proceedings of conferences and seminars. Current publications include: "Mobilizing Networks of Mutual Support: How to Develop Alzheimer Caregivers Support Groups," "Families and Older Persons: Policy, Research, and Practice" and MULTIDIMENSIONAL FUNCTIONAL ASSESSMENT: THE OARS METHODOLOGY, edited by Gerda Fillenbaum (1988 edition). This manual presents a tested, reliable, and valid methodology for the assessment of impaired adults generally, and of the elderly in particular. The Older Americans Resources and Services (OARS) Multidimensional Functional Assessment Questionnaire is designed to provide systematic information on the level of functioning in each of five areas: physical health, mental health, social resources, economic resources, and self-care capacity. Another major segment of the questionnaire is designed for the assessment of need for services. The volume discusses the range of application of the assessment methodology, from the use as a clinical intake instrument of survey work to impact-of-intervention studies. The volume contains reliability and validity data; illustrations of three applications of the methodology; and an interview instruction chapter. Write for publications list.

1078
Florida State University Pepper Institute on Aging and Public Policy
647 Bellamy Bldg.
Tallahassee, FL 32306-3055 (904)644-2831
Contact: Melissa Hardy, Dir.

Established in 1976.
Purpose and activities: Provides gerontological policy research and education for professionals and students and offers technical expertise and service to policymakers and service providers. Fosters educational programs in gerontology through graduate and undergraduate certificate programs and with conferences and workshops, and promotes faculty and graduate student research.
Geographic focus: Active in FL, nationally and internationally.
Technical assistance: Provides consultation and service to state and federal government and the aging services network.
Publications: Informational brochure.

1079
Institute for Retired Professionals, New School for Social Research
66 West 12th St.
New York, NY 10011 (212)229-5682
Contact: Michael Markowitz, Dir.

Established in 1962.
Purpose and activities: The first peer-coordinated adult education program in the U.S., offering an opportunity for many highly trained retired professionals to renew their education at the university level without the usual course procedures. Members are both students and teachers, enabling retirees to be leaders in second careers as educators. Program is comprised of weekly discussion and study groups on selected academic subjects ranging from African-American

authors to workshops in poetry and writing memoirs. Additional social activities and cultural events are included. An annual fixed fee entitles members to participate in all phases of the program and to enroll in one New School Adult Division course each semester. Membership is open to those recently retired from a professional or executive career. Members offer public programs quarterly (which have included Women's Poetry readings, Holocaust memorial, and since 1988, a reading of African-American Poetry).
Geographic focus: Active in the metropolitan New York, NY, area.
Publications: Informational brochure, newsletter. An annual literary magazine, "IRP Voices," edited by retired members, publishes the work of creative writers in the program.

1080
Long Island University Center on Aging

C. W. Post Campus, Roth Hall
Brookville, NY 11548 (516)299-2716
FAX: (516)299-2587
Contact: Ilene Nathanson, D.S.W., Dept. of Health Care and Public Administration, College of Management

Established in 1987.
Purpose and activities: Develops and implements programs related to older people in three areas: (1) public policy and public service; (2) research and evaluation; and (3) education and training. Provides educational programs and training in gerontology, particulary on social work with the elderly.
Geographic focus: Active primarily in the Long Island, NY, area; also active in the metropolitan New York, NY, area.
Funding activities: Support includes technical assistance, training, use of University facilities, managerial assistance and interns.
Technical assistance: Provided to nonprofit agencies, businesses, and governmental agencies.
Publications: Brochure on the Center on Aging and the gerontology programs in the Department of Health Care and Public Administration on the C.W. Post Campus of Long Island University; technical reports; and gerantological social work materials.

1081
Portland State University Institute on Aging

P.O. Box 751
Portland, OR 97207 (503)725-3952
Contact: Elizabeth A. Kutza, Ph.D., Dir.

Established in 1969.
Purpose and activities: A multi-disciplinary research and training unit housed within the university's School of Urban and Public Affairs. Objectives are: to design, carry out, and facilitate research on adult development and aging; to develop and implement training for persons interested in gerontological careers; and to provide community services in the form of short-term training and technical assistance as well as by sponsoring specific service organizations for the aged. Sponsors the Senior Adult Learning Center, an adult education and inter-generational program.
Geographic focus: Active nationally but with regional emphasis; community service programs in the Portland, OR, area.
Technical assistance: Staff regularly provide technical assistance to community organizations as well as short-term training sessions on topics such as pre-retirement planning, widowhood adjustment, and long-term care. Partner with the Oregon Health Sciences University and the VAMC at Portland in the Oregon Geriatric Education Center.
Publications: Informational brochure, newsletter. Publishes "IOA Report," a periodic newsletter describing research and training activities of the Institute, and "GeriTRACS," a newsletter of the Oregon Geriatrics Education Center.

1082
Syracuse University All-University Gerontology Center

426 Eggers Hall
Syracuse, NY 13244-1090 (315)443-2703
FAX: (315)443-1081
Contact: Richard V. Burkhauser, Dir.

Established in 1972.
Purpose and activities: The Center, located in the Maxwell School of Citizenship and Public Affairs, has been a leader in public policy analysis and professional education to benefit the elderly since its inception in 1972. The Center administers an academic concentration in gerontology for both graduate and undergradute students.
Publications: Informational brochure.

1083
University of Florida Center for Gerontological Studies

3355 Turlington Hall
Gainesville, FL 32611 (904)392-2116
FAX: (352)392-8524
Contact: Raymond T. Coward, Ph.D., Dir.

Purpose and activities: Serves as a center for research, training, and service in all areas of gerontology, with an emphasis on the social-behavioral and allied health sciences.
Geographic focus: Active nationally with emphasis on FL.
Publications: Newsletter and occasional papers.

1084
University of Georgia Gerontology Center

100 Candler Hall
Athens, GA 30602 (706)542-3954
FAX: (706)542-4805
Contact: Dr. Leonard W. Poon, Dir.

Purpose and activities: Coordinates graduate and postdoctoral training and research at the University of Georgia in the field of gerontology. The Faculty of Gerontology consists of 47 faculty members from 28 departments, and ten Colleges and Schools. The faculty focuses training and research in four areas: 1) the oldest-old; 2) cognitive aging; 3) applied gerontology; and 4) demography.
Geographic focus: Active in GA and at national and international levels.

1085
University of Maryland Center on Aging

University of Maryland
College Park, MD 20742-2611 (301)405-2543
Contact: Dr. Laura B. Wilson, Dir.

Purpose and activities: Coordinates graduate certificate in aging programs for the university and involved in aging research and community service. Although some programs involve contact with the elderly regarding specific programs or services, the Center is primarily involved with the training of professionals.
Publications: An information packet is available.

1086
University of Nebraska at Omaha, Department of Gerontology

Omaha, NE 68182 (402)554-2272
Contact: Dr. James Thorson

Purpose and activities: An academic department offering undergraduate and graduate training in gerontology and research into aspects of social gerontology, death, and dying.
Geographic focus: Active in the Midwest.

1087
University of North Texas, Department of Applied Gerontology

P.O. Box 13438
Denton, TX 76203-6438 (817)565-2765
FAX: (817)565-4370
Contact: Dr. Richard A. Lusky, Dir.

Purpose and activities: An undergraduate and graduate program of education in administration, long-term care and retirement facility administration of community-based programs for the aged, and direct services to the elderly.

1088
University of Rhode Island Program in Gerontology

608 Chafee Bldg.
Kingston, RI 02881 (401)792-2792

Purpose and activities: An academic program offering both an undergraduate major & minor, and a graduate certificate in gerontology in Master's programs in Human Development, Adult Education, and Nursing.
Geographic focus: Active primarily in RI.
Publications: 1) Health promotion information packets are occasionally distributed when students are in programs with direct contact with the elderly; 2) Academic publications include journal articles, chapters, and books authored by faculty members; 3) Grant-funded project educational materials are available in the areas of geriatric health promotion and the field of aging and developmental disabilities.

1089
University of South Florida — SOC 107

College of Arts & Sciences
Tampa, FL 33620-8100 (813)974-2414
Contact: William E. Haley, Chair.

Purpose and activities: Gerontology is the study of the process of human aging in all its many aspects: physical, psychological, and social. In the Department of Gerontology particular emphasis is placed upon applied gerontology, with the goal of educating students who, in their professional careers in the field of aging, will work to sustain or improve the quality of life of older persons. To this end the Department offers the degree of Bachelor of Arts in Gerontology, Bachelor of Science in Gerontology, and Master of Arts in Gerontology. The Department of Gerontology also hosts the University-wide Ph.D. in aging studies.

1090
University of Southern California — Ethel Percy Andrus Gerontology Center

University Park, Mail Code 0191
Los Angeles, CA 90089-0191 (213)740-6060
FAX: (213)740-8241
Contact: Edward L. Schneider, Dean

Established in 1965.
Purpose and activities: Provides research, education, and service in the field of aging. The Gerontology Research Institute administers research under three program areas: neurogerontology, social and behavioral sciences, and policy and services. In 1991-1992, instructional activities included: advanced study, research training, a bachelor's, master's, and doctoral degree program, management training, internships, and the Gerontology Library.
Geographic focus: Active nationally, with international students and fellows; also offers direct service activities in the Los Angeles, CA, area.
Technical assistance: Service activities include Andrus Volunteers who provide lectures and workshops in the community as well as technical assistance to groups wishing to develop similar programs for older adults. The Andrus Older Adult Center provides caregiver classes and counseling for older adults and those responsible for their care and also provides telephone referral on community resources. The Business Institute on Aging is a corporate support group offering seminars and workshops to corporate executives interested in older worker and older consumer issues.
Publications: Annual report, informational brochure. Issues a Dissemination List covering numerous published project reports in the areas of: case management, employment and retirement, housing, intergenerational studies, long-term care, senior centers, and service delivery systems. The Andrus Volunteer Program has separate publications on working with the aging, with titles including "Caregivers: An Annotated Bibliography" and "Sample Programs for Caregivers." Write for Dissemination List.

1091
University of Utah Gerontology Center

College of Nursing, Rm. 316
Salt Lake City, UT 84112 (801)581-8198
Contact: Dale Lund, Dir.

Purpose and activities: Conducts research, education/training, and service in the field of gerontology. Offers gerontology certificate and Master's Degree. Specific areas of expertise are bereavement, caregiving, and health promotion, and video respite.
Geographic focus: Active regionally, serving basically UT, CO, MT, ND, SD, WY.
Publications: Numerous publications of research done at the university are available.

1092
University of Wisconsin Institute on Aging

Medical Services Ctr.
1300 University Ave.
Madison, WI 53706 (608)262-1818
Contact: Carol Ruff, Interim Dir.

Purpose and activities: The Institute on Aging is a multidisciplinary research and graduate training unit within both the Graduate School and Medical School of the University of Wisconsin at Madison. Its main function is to encourage and coordinate a campus-wide effort to promote innovative multidisciplinary research by faculty and graduate students about aging and the adult life course. It also is a liaison to funding sources and serves as adminstrative center for interdepartmental and intercollegiate projects. Research emphases about aging and adult development are many, including clinical research in behavorial medicine, basic studies of biological aging, historical and sociodemographic research on the life courses of birth cohorts, behavioral research on effective cognitive functioning and optimal aging, and sociobehavioral studies of the life, world, well-being, and residential environments of the older population. While the Institute does not offer its own degrees in gerontology or lifespan development, it coordinates a broad array of courses and degree programs that are taught and offered by Institute-affiliated faculty within nearly all colleges and schools on the Madison campus. Four area groups of affiliated faculty members adminster a non-degree certificate program within the Institute. For graduate and advanced professional students, certificates in "biology of aging," "life-span development," "social gerontology," and "clinical geriatrics," are awarded by the Institute. For returning "Special" students not pursuing a specific graduate degree, and for undergraduate students, a Specialist in Gerontology certificate program.
Geographic focus: Serves the entire University of Wisconsin system.
Technical assistance: Provides faculty with material and administrative resources and computing.

DENOMINATIONAL ORGANIZATIONS

1093
American Jewish Congress

Stephen Wise Congress House
15 East 84th St.
New York, NY 10028 (212)879-4500
FAX: (212)249-3672
Contact: Phil Baum, Exec. Dir.

Purpose and activities: A charitable and educational organization with a total membership of 50,000, including 14 regions nationwide. Objectives include creative survival of the Jewish people. A major part of domestic program is devoted to improving the quality of life of the elderly.
Funding activities: Works collaboratively with other organizations on volunteer programs for the elderly.
Technical assistance: Staff provides printed material, consultation, and loan of personnel to both members and nonmembers in the areas of education, employment, health, housing, research, and volunteer programs.

1094
B'nai B'rith

1640 Rhode Island Ave., N.W.
Washington, DC 20036 (202)857-6581

Purpose and activities: Largest Jewish sponsor of federally subsidized housing in the U.S. Also provides community action programs and advocacy and seeks to improve community affairs and living.
Funding activities: Received HUD funding for senior citizens housing. Works collaboratively with other gerontological and housing organizations.
Technical assistance: Provides printed material and consultation to members and nonmembers in the areas of community development, housing, and volunteer programs.

1095
Church of the Nazarene

6401 The Paseo
Kansas City, MO 64131 (816)333-7000
FAX: (816)361-4983
Contact: Dr. Jack Stone, General Secy., HQ Operations Officer

Purpose and activities: Religious organization with over 1,000,000 members and 11,482 affiliates worldwide. Committed to outreach and specific religious purposes. The General Church has a retirement center for those who have served in overseas missionary work, and it also has pensions and retirement programs for those in career ministries in the church.
Geographic focus: Active worldwide.
Funding activities: Supports conferences and publications. At the local level churches may sponsor nutrition programs, nursing homes, retirement towers or apartments, transportation, and recreational activities.

Technical assistance: Printed materials and consultation in the areas of education and training, housing, and nutrition.
Publications: Publishes "Herald of Holiness" in English, Portuguese & Spanish.

1096
Daughters of Isabella
375 Whitney Ave.
New Haven, CT 06511 (203)865-2570
Additional address: P.O. Box 9585, New Haven, CT 06535

Established in 1897.
Purpose and activities: Catholic women's fraternal organization, founded as an auxiliary of the Knights of Columbus. Objectives are to unite all Catholic women for spiritual benefits, promote higher ideals within the society, and provide charity work for the well-being of society. Membership consists of the International Circle which supervises the entire order, State, and 804 individual circles. In addition to special charitable and apostolic activities worldwide, the society is raising a $1 million endowment for the National Center for Family Studies at Catholic University.
Geographic focus: Active membership primarily in the U.S. and Canada, with charitable and apostolic activities worldwide.
Funding activities: Individual circles, i.e., local chapters, may or may not provide funding on a local basis for programs such as Meals on Wheels. Contact local chapter for further information.
Publications: Informational brochure.

1097
Episcopal Society for Ministry on Aging
(also known as ESMA)
323 Wyandotte St.
Bethlehem, PA 18015-1527 (610)868-5400

Established in 1964.
Purpose and activities: The Episcopal Church's national agency on aging for the development and support of ministries with and for older adults. EMSA is a volunteer organization of bishops, clergy and lay persons. In fulfilling its responsibility, EMSA initiates and implements programs with and through provinces, dioceses, congregations, agencies and units of the Episcopal Church to seek a more positive image of aging and greater justice for the elderly; and to equip bishops, clergy and lay leaders with knowledge and skills to strengthen their ministry on aging. EMSA works to serve the spiritual, psychological and physical needs of older persons and to maximize the use of their unique gifts and talents in continuing contributions to church and society.
Publications: AFFIRMATIVE AGING: A CREATIVE APPROACH TO LONGER LIFE (Morehouse Publishing); OLDER ADULT MINISTRY: A RESOURCE FOR PROGRAM DEVELOPMENT (Presbyterian Publishing House); the videotape, "The (In)Dignity of Aging"; and yearly Age in Action materials. Publication order form available.

1098
Evangelical Good Samaritan Society
4800 West 57th St.
Sioux Falls, SD 57106 (605)362-3100
FAX: (605)362-3356
Contact: Dr. Mark Jerstad, Pres.

Established in 1922.
Purpose and activities: A Christian service organization operating over 240 long-term care facilities in 26 states. Society places special emphasis on the spiritual, emotional, and social needs of the aged.
Funding activities: For member facilities only. The central office provides support to the local facilities for staff development. Member facilities collaborate with other community organizations to develop nutrition, transportation, and outreach services.
Technical assistance: Primarily for member facilities, with assistance to other organizations available on a cost basis. Includes printed material and consultation in the areas of community development, education, health, housing, nutrition, and volunteer programs. A continuing priority is to provide quality educational programs and materials for facilities' staff, with workshops for Directors of Nursing Services, Social Service Directors, and Program/Activity Coordinators. Seminars in resource development, marketing, and bookkeeping are offered.
Publications: Newsletter. "The Good Samaritan," official publication of the Society. Write to be placed on mailing list.

1099
Friends United Meeting
101 Quaker Hill Dr.
Richmond, IN 47374

Purpose and activities: Acts as headquarters for overseas missions. Supports hospitals and community based health care programs and other agencies that benefit the aging.
Geographic focus: Kenya, Uganda, Tanzania, Belize, Jamaica, Cuba, Palestine, USA, Canada, and Mexico.
Limitations: Support for Friends (Quaker) institutions affiliated with Friends United Meeting only.

1100
Jewish Association for Services for the Aged
(also known as JASA)
40 West 68th St.
New York, NY 10023 (212)724-3200
FAX: (212)721-6612
Contact: David J. Stern, Exec. V.P.

Purpose and activities: Assists the elderly to remain in their communities, maximize their independence and avoid unnecessary institutionalization. Services and programs include specialized housing, social services (information and referral, casework, protective services, legal services, guardainship, financial management, mental health, victim's assistance, and crime prevention); group work (life-long education; intergenerational, wellness and educational programs; recreation; volunteer activities and nutrition programs); home delivered meals and home care programs; and grassroots advocacy & training through JPAC (Joint Public Affairs Committee for Older Adults).
Geographic focus: Active in New York City and Nassau and Suffolk counties, NY.
Publications: Public affairs newsletter.

1101
Lutheran Service Society of Western Pennsylvania
440 Lincoln Ave.
Pittsburgh, PA 15202 (412)734-9330
FAX: (412)231-6258
Contact: Robert Sprague, Dir.

Purpose and activities: A regional social service agency for the elderly. Programs and services include: Meals-on-Wheels, Protective Service, Care Management, transportation coordination, senior center services, volunteer programs, outreach and Personal Assistance Service.
Geographic focus: Active in the Pittsburgh, PA, area.
Publications: Informational brochure.

1102
Mennonite Health Services
(also known as MHS)
2160 Lincoln Hwy. East, Box 6
Lancaster, PA 17602-1150 (717)293-7125
FAX: (717)293-7854

Established in 1947.
Purpose and activities: Mennonite Health Services (MHS) is a health and human service organization which provides service to both Mennonite and Brethern in Christ churches in the U.S. and to society at large. MHS was created out of a 1947 call from Mennonite churches to respond to the needs of persons with mental illness. In 1989 MHS expanded to become a larger church-sponsored health and human service organization. Serving in the name of Christ and recognizing the value of all human life, MHS carries out the Biblical injunction to help people toward health and hope by guiding institutions, promoting the potential of Christian community for healing, and fostering new opportunites for service. Governed by a board of directors appointed by its constituent churches, MHS serves a variety of nationally recognized and fully accredited human service institutions, including: psychiatric hospitals, retirement homes, youth services programs, acute care hospitals, and developmental disability services providers. MHS links the Christian philosophy of its constituent churches with member institutions by holding reserved powers for its partner members. These powers include appointment of the member institution's board members and approval of its by-laws, chief executive officer, and mission statement. By giving these powers to MHS, the partner institutions indicate their commitment to the church's mission of integrative healing as well as stringent secular accreditation. Other categories of membership are available that give collaboration between institutions with a similiar orientation. MHS facilitates these links in order to

find solutions to problems which utilize resources well and empower people within its institutions to function as a Christian community. MHS provides for institutional councils for chief executive officers to interact and solve problems. Other activities include staff exchange between institutions to share expertise and joint corporate ventures.
Technical assistance: MHS delivers a variety of corporate services to its member organizations. The MHS medical expense plan provides inexpensive yet comprehensive health insurance coverage for the employees of member institutions. In addition to experiencing cost benefits, participating members have the opportunity to influence the plan's components and overall direction. MHS' personnel recruitment program established by the psychiatric centers of MHS connects qualified Christian psychiatric professionals and professionals-in-training with employment opportunities in the participating centers. The MHS staff are also available for consulation and support when difficulties are encountered by leadership of member institutions.

1103
Presbyterian Health, Education, and Welfare Association
(also known as PHEWA)
100 Witherspoon St.
Louisville, KY 40202-1396 (502)569-5794

Purpose and activities: Brings together the separate PHEWA networks under one united entity. Subsidary networks of PHEWA may offer specific programs or services that benefit the elderly, but main office does not.

1104
The National Benevolent Association of the Christian Church (Disciples of Christ)
11780 Borman Dr., Suite 200
St. Louis, MO 63146-4157 (314)993-9000
Contact: Cindy R. Dougherty, Pres.

Established in 1887.
Purpose and activities: A nationwide organization with facilities and community-based programs for the care of older adults, persons who are physically and mentally handicapped, and children who are abused, neglected, and emotionally disturbed. For older adults, care units include independent living, nursing care, and multi-level care facilities, some specializing in the care of Alzheimer's disease patients. Additionally, community programs include services such as Meals on Wheels, pre-retirement planning clinics, seminars on working with older adults, and education programs on Alzheimer's disease. NBA services are available to both members and nonmembers of the Christian Church (Disciples of Christ).
Geographic focus: Active nationally, with care units and community-based programs in 27 states.
Funding activities: Funding limited to NBA programs.
Publications: Informational brochure. Publishes a facility directory and numerous brochures on the NBA care units. Also, "Family Talk," a semi-annual magazine.

GERONTOLOGICAL ORGANIZATIONS

1105
AARP Andrus Foundation
601 E St., N.W.
Washington, DC 20049 (202)434-6190
Contact: Dr. John Feather, Dir.

Established in 1968.
Purpose and activities: The AARP Andrus Foundation was established in 1968 as a memorial to Dr. Ethel Percy Andrus, founder of AARP. In the Spring of 1996, the Foundation Board adopted the following mission: The AARP Foundation enhances the lives of older persons through research on aging. Future support will be provided for research that produces new knowledge on aging; efforts that make currently available research accessible to the AARP membership, professionals serving the aged and the general public; and, preparation of the next generation of researchers in aging. Under these new initiatives, the AARP Andrus Foundation has awarded three grants to date, one is to establish quality assurance standards in managed care and the other two are for minority fellowships under the auspices of national aging organizations.
Funding activities: The Foundation is undergoing major changes in its funding programs and is currently developing a new strategic plan.
Limitations: No grants to individuals, or for non-expendable equipment or graduate assistants' tuition, fees or stipends.
Application information: Not accepting unsolicited proposals at this time; contact the Foundation for further information.

1106
Administration on Aging
Cohen Bldg.
3300 Independence Ave., S.W.
Washington, DC 20201 (202)619-0556
FAX: (202)619-7586
Contact: Joyce P. Berry, Ph.D., U.S. Commissioner on Aging

Purpose and activities: An agency of the Department of Health and Human Services that develops federal programs and coordinates community services for older persons.
Geographic focus: National.

1107
American Association for International Aging
(also known as AAIA)
1900 L St., N.W.
Suite 510
Washington, DC 20036-8762 (202)833-8893
Contact: Dr. Helen K. Kerschner, Exec. Dir.

Established in 1983.
Purpose and activities: Established to initiate a creative U.S. response to the challenges set forth in the International Plan of Action developed at the United Nations World Assembly on Aging. Provides support for economic development, senior volunteer and limited health-related programs for the elderly in Third World countries. Seeks to educate the American public, corporate and governmental sectors about international aging issues, and to implement in the U.S. those concepts and programs involving older people that have been successful in other nations.
Geographic focus: Active internationally. Grants program limited to Colombia, Ecuador, Ghana, India, Indonesia, Jamaica, Kenya, and Sri Lanka; projects in other Third World countries will be considered on a case-by-case basis.
Funding activities: Funds may be for entire projects or portions thereof. Grants made to small scale humanitarian and development projects designed to reach low-income, aged people in Third World countries. Preference to three types of projects: those which encourage continued activity and self-sufficiency, projects focused on economic development efforts, and projects which involve older women in planning as well as implementation. Areas of particular interest include: entrepreneurial, group and sponsored enterprises and low-tech food production. Grants can range from $500 to $10,000.
Limitations: No grants for labor costs or food, and in most cases, for construction. No multi-year grants.
Application information: Application guidelines available. Proposals must be written in English, with financial requests presented in U.S. currency equivalents. Application form required.
Deadlines: None
Publications: Informational brochure, program policy statement (including application guidelines). Publishes a quarterly newsletter, "AAIA Reports." Has also published AN INTERNATIONAL DIRECTORY OF ORGANIZATIONS IN AGING; A U.S. DIRECTORY AND SOURCE BOOK ON AGING, and a background paper in aging for the House Select Committee on Aging. Also available: "Retired Americans Look at International Development;" "65 Ways to Be Involved in International Development: A Retired American's Guide to Participation in Local, National and International Activities;" "An Organizing Guide for Community-Based Education and International Action;" "Focus Groups: Three Organizing Steps for Education Design and Delivery" "A Primer on International Development;" a compilation of demographic data on international aging; and a report, "Aging and the Global Agenda of Women: Conversations in Nairobi".

1108
American Association of Homes and Services for the Aging
(also known as AAHSA)
901 E St., N.W., Suite 500
Washington, DC 20004-2011 (202)783-2242
FAX: (202)783-2255
Contact: Sheldon L. Goldberg, Pres.

Established in 1961.
Purpose and activities: National association representing more than 5,000 community-based

not-for-profit nursing homes, independent housing, continuing care retirement communities, assisted living facilities, and community service programs for the elderly. Provides leadership in representing and promoting the interests of its constituents through advocacy, education, professional development, research, and services. Enhances members' ability to meet the social, health, environmental, and quality of living needs of individuals and communities they serve. Through direct delivery of services in their facilities, members care for over one million senior adults each year, while also meeting the needs of many more through outreach programs.
Technical assistance: Generally, restricted to members. Provides timely information and assistance in interpreting relevant legislation and regulations. The Professional Development Institute delivers educational programs at the spring conference and annual meeting, as well as seminars on topics of special interest throughout the year. AAHSA sponsors a national accreditation program for continuing care retirement communities and a national certification program for retirement housing professionals. Assistance with finding low-cost financing is offered through the AAHSA Development Corporation. Several insurance programs and a national group purchasing program are also offered to AAHSA members. Collaborative Innovations, Inc., an AAHSA subsidiary provides turnkey development of assisted living facilities.
Publications: Informational and consumer brochures, newsletters. Membership includes subscriptions to "Currents" (monthly), "Washington Report" (biweekly) and the "Directory of Members" (bi-annual). Also available are videos, reference materials and books in subject areas including managed care, continuing care, long-term care, housing, Alzheimer's disease, public and community relations, and management practices. Write for resource catalog.

1109
American Association of Retired Persons

(also known as AARP)
601 E St., N.W.
Washington, DC 20049 (202)434-2277
FAX: (202)434-6408
Contact: Horace Deets, Exec. Dir.

Established in 1958.
Purpose and activities: AARP is a nonprofit, nonpartisan membership organization dedicated to addressing the needs and interests of older Americans through education, advocacy, and community service. With a membership of more than 33 million, AARP is open to anyone age 50 or older, both working and retired. Members are actively involved in community, state, and national affairs, and AARP's 4,000 chapters and 2,500 Retired Teacher Association units throughout the U.S. provide opportunities for volunteer service and fellowship. Its vision is to excel as a dynamic presence in every community, shaping and enriching this experience of aging for each member and for society. Long-term goals include: continuing to provide quality service to members, communities, volunteers and staff; working to achieve universal access to comprehensive, affordable health and long-term care for all; assisting employers to recruit, manage, train, and retain an older work force and to increase work options available to older persons; working to reduce poverty and promoting economic security for individuals of all generations; conducting and supporting research to understand and meet AARP members' needs and those of an aging population; and to maximize the effectiveness of AARP's volunteers, staff, and technological resources.
Technical assistance: AARP provides legislative advocacy by developing policy recommendations on behalf of the diverse group of older Americans it represents and advocates their needs with federal and state legislators. AARP's programs and departments include: consumer affairs, criminal justice services, health advocacy services, housing, interreligious liaison, Legal Counsel for the Elderly, Research Information Center, Senior Community Service Employment Program, Tax-Aide program, Senior Environmental Employment Program, and the Widowed Persons Service. Member benefits include: motoring plan; discounts on auto rentals, lodging, and sightseeing; group health, auto, homeowners, and mobile home insurance programs; mail-order pharmacy service with home delivery; an investment program; and AARP Visa card.
Publications: Members receive bimonthly the nation's most widely circulated magazine, "Modern Maturity," and the "AARP Bulletin," 11 times per year. In addition, more than 175 specialized publications about health, consumer affairs, crime prevention, retirement planning, lifetime learning, and driver re-education are available free of charge to members and the public. Also available are slide-tape and videocassette programs on issues of importance to older people.

1110
American Association of Retired Persons (AARP) Foundation

601 E St., N.W.
Washington, DC 20049 (202)434-2000
Contact: C. Anne Harvey

Purpose and activities: A funding entity of AARP established to promote the economic and social well-being of older persons.
Funding activities: Grants made to tax-exempt organizations and programs identified as serving older persons for the development or maintenance of projects and community-service endeavors. the foundation also receives funds from external sources for the support of AARP programs.
Application information: The foundation is not accepting grant applications at the present time.

1111
American Geriatrics Society, Inc.

770 Lexington Ave., Suite 300
New York, NY 10021 (212)308-1414
FAX: (212)832-8646
Contact: Linda Hiddemen, Exec. V.P.

Purpose and activities: Medical society composed of physicians and other health professionals active in the field of clinical geriatrics. Conducts continuing education programs with hospitals, long-term care facilities, universities, and other medical societies. Encourages greater interest in and integration of geriatrics into medical education, and stimulates faculty development in the field.
Technical assistance: Services for health professionals only. Public information referalls and physician for the lay consumer public.
Publications: Monthly medical journal, "Journal of the American Geriatrics Society," on the newest methods for treating and preventing disease in the aged. The monthly newsletter covers meetings, seminars, and current events in the field of geriatric medicine. Physician Self-Assessment Program, the Geriatrics Review Syllabus. The "American Geriatrics Society's Complete Guide to Aging & Health", by Mark E. Williams, M.D., published by Harmony Books, 1995.

1112
American Society for Geriatric Dentistry

(also known as ASGD)
211 East Chicago Ave., Suite 948
Chicago, IL 60611 (312)440-2660
Contact: Dr. John S. Rutkauskas

Established in 1965.
Purpose and activities: Professional society dedicated to the maintenance and improvement of the oral health of the elderly. Members include dental practitioners, dental school faculty, researchers, auxiliaries, and other health care professionals. Improves the management and treatment of the geriatric dental patient by disseminating knowledge and skills, and promotes access to oral health care for the elderly by helping to overcome obstacles such as fear, physical barriers, and finances. Advocates for the expansion of dental benefits in legislation and social planning, encourages dental schools to provide education and clinical training, and sponsors and contributes to many national symposia.
Geographic focus: Active in the U.S. and Canada, with some foreign activities.
Publications: Informational brochure, newsletter. Subscriptions to "Special Care in Dentistry" (bimonthly) as well as an informational newsletter are included with membership.

1113
American Society on Aging

833 Market St., Suite 511
San Francisco, CA 94103-1824 (415)974-9600
FAX: (415)974-0300

Purpose and activities: Seeks to improve the lives of older Americans by providing training and education for those working with and for the elderly.
Publications: "Generations," a quarterly journal, and "Aging Today," a bimonthly newspaper, are available by subscription.

1114
Children of Aging Parents

(also known as CAPS)
1609 Woodbourne Rd., Suite 302A
Levittown, PA 19057 (215)945-6900
Contact: Thomas Humphrey, Exec. Dir.

Purpose and activities: A national nonprofit, tax-exempt organization dedicated to the needs of the caregivers of the elderly. Provides resource information and referrals while developing nationally a network of support groups.
Publications: Newsletter (available through membership only). Also available: Starting a Self-Help Group for Caregivers manual, Instant Aging Workshop manual, Care Sharing Directory of Geriatric Care Managers and Caregivers Support groups nationwide, and many information sheets to help caregivers and professionals.

1115
Daughters of the Elderly Bridging the Unknown Together

(also known as DEBUT)
Area 10 Agency on Aging
2129 Yost Ave.
Bloomington, IN 47401 (812)876-5319
Contact: Pat Meier

Established in 1981.
Purpose and activities: Support group designed by and for women struggling with the responsibilities, emotions, and decisions involved in the care of aging parents. Focuses on education regarding aging and related issues, support for caregivers in their multiple roles, and respite, time away from the caregiving for self-renewal and other responsibilities. Offers information and support, in a non-judgmental atmosphere, to daughters, daughters-in-law, and granddaughters who are concerned about and caring for aging parents at home, in health care centers, and at a distance. Program includes weekly meetings.
Geographic focus: Active primarily in Bloomington, IN, but has helped to organize other groups in various areas and receives correspondence from throughout the U.S. and Canada.
Publications: Informational brochure. Also DAUGHTERS OF THE ELDERLY: Building Partnerships in Caregiving, edited by Jane Norris, published by I.U. Press, is available in bookstores.

1116
Elder Craftsmen, Inc.

921 Madison Ave.
New York, NY 10021 (212)861-5260
FAX: (212)772-9717
Contact: Janet Langlois, Exec. Dir.

Established in 1955.
Purpose and activities: This organization's mission is to help men and women 55 and over to be creative, productive and independent, and to seek broader recognition by the general public of the skills and capabilities of older people. Programs include: 1) training in various crafts for representatives and or members of agencies serving older adults, mainly senior citizens and nursing homes, 2) community service projects for older crafters in senior programs in the NYC area, sometimes including their frail and homebound elderly members, as well unaffiliated seniors from around the country, to make items for needy families, 3) an Intergenerational program bringing together older crafters with teens and pre-teens and 4) exhibits of crafts produced by older crafters.
Technical assistance: The training studio program offers courses in a variety of different crafts for representatives of agencies serving older adults. Staff offers site visits as well as consultation on topics including equipment use, organizing crafts sales, and managing crafts programs. A reference library and slide collection is available to other agencies planning programs relating to crafts. Staff advises organizations interested in establishing similiar operations.
Publications: Informational brochure, newsletter, annual report. "The Official Sales and Planning Guide for Senior Craft Programs" is a manual on craft sales, record keeping techniques, and scheduling. "Opportunities in Crafts for Older Adults," is a partial listing of nationwide shops and cooperatives.

1117
Elderhostel

P.O. Box 1959
Wakefield, MA 01880-5959 (617)426-7788
URL: http://www.elderhostel.org;
FAX: (617)426-8351
Contact: William Berkeley, Pres.

Purpose and activities: Elderhostel is a non-profit educational organization that provides short term, residential educational programs throughout the world for people aged 55 and older.

1118
Federal Council on Aging

330 Independence Ave., S.W., Suite 4280 HHS-N
Washington, DC 20201 (202)619-2451
Contact: Kevin W. Parks, Exec. Dir.

Purpose and activities: An advisory group authorized by the Older Americans Act of 1965 that is selected by the President and Congress. The fifteen members represent a cross-section of rural and urban older Americans, national organizations with an interest in aging, business, labor and the general public.

1119
Gerontological Society of America

1275 K St., N.W., Suite 350
Washington, DC 20005-4006 (202)842-1275
FAX: (202)842-1150; E-mail: geron@geron.org;
URL: http://www.geron.org
Contact: Carol A. Schutz, Exec. Dir.

Purpose and activities: A multidisciplinary professional organization that promotes the scientific study of aging in the bio-medical and social sciences, and its translation.

1120
Gray Panthers Project Fund

P.O. Box 21477
Washington, DC 20009 (202)466-3132
Contact: Charlotte Flynn, Chair.

Purpose and activities: Intergenerational coalition working to build an America that serves people at every age, with 45,000 members nationally. Coordinates public education efforts seeking to end harmful myths about the elderly. Advocates against budget reductions in Social Security and Medicare. Additionally, efforts in cities across America include nursing home reform, adequate nutrition for the poor, and developing housing alternatives for homeless people of all ages. Mobilizes both young and old, with motto, "Age and Youth in Action." Offers specific programs or services that benefit the aging, with activities depending on programs of local chapters.
Publications: Informational brochure. "Network" (a quarterly news journal), "Maggie Kuhn on Aging" on what people can do to combat agism through their churches. Also, Maggie Kuhn's new book, NO STONE UNTURNED, the story of her life and activism thus far.

1121
Legal Services for the Elderly

(also known as LSE)
130 West 42nd St., 17th Fl.
New York, NY 10036 (212)391-0120
FAX: (212)719-1939
Contact: Jonathan A. Weiss, Dir.

Purpose and activities: Provides quality legal representation to the elderly and assists other legal services attorneys. Current cases are in four main areas: pensions; government benefits and entitlements (including Social Security and medicaid benefits); discrimination and adverse treatment; and health and long term care. Assists through training and lecturing, litigation and support.
Technical assistance: Available to assist legal services attorneys with research and advice in the field.
Publications: Informational brochure. Reports including "A Survey of the Legal Problems of the Elderly," and "How to Handle a Social Security Disability Case" are available. Write for publications list.

1122
National Association for Hispanic Elderly

3225 Wilshire Blvd., Suite 800
Los Angeles, CA 90010 (213)487-1922
FAX: (213)385-3014
Contact: Carmela G. Lacayo, Pres. and C.E.O.

Purpose and activities: Works to ensure that older Hispanic citizens are included in all social service programs for older Americans.

1123
National Association of Area Agencies on Aging

(also known as N4A)
1112 16th St., N.W.
Washington, DC 20036-4823 (202)294-8130
FAX: (202)296-8134
Contact: Janice Fiegener, Exec. Dir.

Established in 1974.
Purpose and activities: Represents the interest of approximately 670 Area Agencies on Aging nationwide which were established to implement local programs under the Older Americans Act. Promotes national policy that would allow elderly Americans to remain independent in their communities and homes for as long as possible, with the primary objectives of providing leadership to Area Agencies and enhancing their central role within the national network on aging. N4A takes an active national advocacy role working with key Congressional and Administration officials and other national organizations on legislative, regulatory, and policy issues.
Technical assistance: Provides training services and materials as well as technical assistance specifically geared to Area Agency operations. Additionally, offers Area Agencies a number of management services to aid in problem solving.
Publications: Informational brochures and a Bi-monthly newsletter. Also publishes general and technical brochures, reports, and training manuals. Additional information brochures available. Write for publications list.

1124
National Association of Retired Federal Employees

1533 New Hampshire Ave., N.W.
Washington, DC 20036-1279 (202)234-0832
FAX: (202)797-9697
Contact: Judy Park, Legislative Dir.

Purpose and activities: A service organization protecting the interests of persons covered by the Civil Service Retirement and Federal Employees Retirement systems. Represents federal retirees spouses and survivors with the Office of Personnel Management, Executive Branch and Congress. Supports legislation beneficial to federal retirees and opposes legislation detrimental to them. Average annual membership: 460,000.
Publications: "Retirement Life," monthly magazine.

1125
National Association of State Units on Aging

(also known as NASUA)
1225 I St., N.W., Suite 725
Washington, DC 20005 (202)898-2578
Fax: (202)898-2583
Contact: Daniel Quirk, Exec. Dir.

Purpose and activities: National, nonprofit, public interest organization dedicated to providing general and specialized information, technical assistance and professional development support to State Units on Aging. The membership of the Association is comprised of the 57 state and territorial government agencies charged with advancing the social and economic agendas of older persons in their respective states.
Technical assistance: Organizational units of NASUA include: communications and development, community services and long term care systems development, program management and administration, and elder rights system development. Member services include regular information and reports on current legislative/regulatory issues and policies affecting state programs; training/technical assistance and publications on a wide range of program/management issues such as Older Americans Act, State Unit program operations, home and community based long term care, older worker issues, elder abuse, state long term care ombudsman programs, information and referal, employee caregiving, state tax policies, health care cost containment, resource allocation, state leadership in minority aging and nutrition programs; convening of an annual membership meeting; orientation and training for State Unit directors and staff; and regular communication with the Congress and the Administration, as well as national aging organizations, other human service networks and organizations representing business, industry and philanthropic interests.

1126
National Caucus and Center on Black Aged

1424 K St., N.W., Suite 500
Washington, DC 20005 (202)637-8400
FAX: (202)347-0895
Contact: Samuel J. Simmons, Pres.

Purpose and activities: NCBA administers advocacy and services concerned with issues and programs affecting the low income elderly with primary attention to the unique needs of the Black elderly. Its advocacy activities relate to monitoring programs for the elderly at various federal agencies and consults with Congress on issues concerned with the low income elderly. NCBA operates direct services concerned with the following: 1) employment programs for persons 55 years of age and over; 2) wellness promotion and disease prevention services; 3) the ownership and management of housing projects for the elderly; and 4) internship and training programs in long term care services.
Geographic focus: Active nationwide.
Publications: Quarterly newsletter. Special reports on various aspects of aging.

1127
National Council on Teacher Retirement

P.O. Box 202243
Austin, TX 78720 (512)335-0055

Purpose and activities: Provides guidance in the development and maintenance of fair and equitable retirement plans for qualified career public employees and promotes levels of benefits for members and beneficiaries to assure them economic security. Encourages plan trustees, directors, and administrators to provide progressive leadership and sound management to ensure that the objectives of the plans are attained.

1128
National Council on the Aging, Inc.

(also known as NCOA)
409 Third St., S.W.
Washington, DC 20024 (202)479-1200
Contact: Dr. Daniel Thursz, Pres.

Established in 1950.
Purpose and activities: NCOA is a center of leadership, innovation, and nationwide expertise in the issues of aging. A membership of more than 7,500 organizations and individuals (professionals and volunteers, service providers, consumer and labor groups, businesses, government agencies, religious groups, and voluntary organizations) who work with and on behalf of older persons. NCOA's programs include: Family Friends, an intergenerational volunteer program that matches mature men and women with children and families at risk; Retirement and Life Planning, seminars delivered in 100+ corporations annually; initiatives in support of caregivers and consumer-directed choices in community-based long-term care; national standards and training for adult day services and for senior centers; Discovery Through the Humanities community discussion series; interfaith program resources for Faith in Action and the National Clergy Leadership Project; older worker training and placement, a program assisting 10,000 low-income participants annually and providing technical assistance to employers and training specialists.
Funding activities: NCOA maintains the Ollie A. Randall Library-12,000 volumes on aging, with primary emphasis on the psychosocial, economic, and health aspects; employment and training; retirement, corporate programs; education; and demographics.
Technical assistance: Provides training, education, technical assistance, and consultation for those working with current and future generations of older persons.
Publications: Subscription to three periodicals is via membership, NCOA NETWORKS, monthly newspaper (9 issues/year); Perspective on Aging, quarterly magazine; and Abstracts in Social Gerontology: Current Literature on Aging, quarterly journal. NCOA PUBLICATIONS - a catalog of books and reports (including the NCOA Public Policy Agenda 1995-1996), brochures, program resources and kits, and videos-is available free upon request.

1129
National Hispanic Council on Aging

2713 Ontario Rd., N.W.
Washington, DC 20009 (202)265-1288
Contact: Marta Sotomayor, Ph.D., Pres. and C.E.O.

Purpose and activities: A private nonprofit organization that works to promote the well-being of older Hispanic individuals.

1130
National Indian Council on Aging, Inc.
(also known as NICOA)
6400 Uptown Blvd., N.E.
City Centre, Suite 510-W
Albuquerque, NM 87110 (505)888-3302
FAX: (505)888-3276
Contact: Dave Baldridge, Exec. Dir.

Purpose and activities: An Advocacy organization representing American Indian and Alaska Native elders nationwide. Seeks the provision of improved comprehensive services to Indian and Alaska Native elderly through information dissemination, testimony before Congress, and participation with provider agencies and advocacy groups. Provides employment training in 12 states under the Senior Community Service Employment Program.
Technical assistance: Information, identification of resources, presentation at conferences and seminars, etc. Consultation available re: health, housing, nutrition, and other issues affecting Indian Program.
Publications: "Elder Voices," quarterly newsletter (subscription). "The NICOA Report: Health and Long-Term Care for Indian Elders" (1996, $10), "Mapping Indian Elders" (1996, $25), "A National Indian Aging Agenda for the Future" (1994). Written testimonies and position statements upon request.

1131
National Senior Citizen Law Center
(also known as NSCLC)
1815 H St., N.W., Suite 700
Washington, DC 20006 (202)887-5280

Purpose and activities: A technical support center for legal services programs and state and area agencies on aging. Provides substantial assistance to legal services corporation attorneys so that they can better serve the elderly poor. Promotes expansion of legal service delivery to the elderly.
Technical assistance: Upon request, will provide basic technical assistance, draft pleadings, write memoranda and briefs, assist with litigation, act as co-counsel, and otherwise participate in cases affecting the elderly. Printed material and consultation on education/training and research also provided.

1132
Northeastern Gerontological Society
Boston University Gerontology Center
53 Bay State Rd.
Boston, MA 02215 (617)353-5045
FAX: (617)353-5047
Contact: Liz Markson, Pres.

Purpose and activities: Provides a forum for practitioners, academics, older adults and others interested in the field of aging. Specific programs and services include committees that establish programs for the elderly, an annual conference, and a mid-life and older women's committee. Also focuses on biomedical aspects of aging, public relations, long-term care, research, social policy, and corporate relations.
Geographic focus: Active in the northeastern states from ME to DE.
Funding activities: Provides awards for research and also scholarships to enable students to attend conference.
Publications: Informational brochure, newsletter.

1133
Older Women's League
(also known as OWL)
666 11th St., N.W.
Suite 700
Washington, DC 20009 (202)783-6686
Contact: Deborah Briceland-Betts

Purpose and activities: Through a network of national chapters, OWL seeks to educate the public about the problems and issues of concern to mid-life and older women.

1134
Operation ABLE
180 North Wabash Ave., Suite 802
Chicago, IL 60601 (312)782-3335
Hotline: (312)782-7700; *FAX:* (312)580-0348
Contact: Shirley Brussell, Exec. Dir.

Purpose and activities: Provides part-time, full-time and temporary job positions, including outplacement, counseling and training work opportunities with special emphasis on the older worker.

1135
Shepherd's Centers of America
6700 Troost, Suite 616
Kansas City, MO 64131 (816)523-1080
Toll Free: (800)547-7073; *FAX:* (816)523-5790; or URL: http://www.qni.com/~shepherd
Contact: Dr. Elbert C. Cole, Exec. Dir.

Purpose and activities: Organizes a community for the most effective use of its resources in meeting the needs of older adults. The Shepherd's Centers focus on a limited service area, work in partnership with other agencies, vest reponsibility in the elderly, create volunteer service opportunities, and involve coalitions of religious congregations for basic support. Currently there are 85 centers in 25 states.
Technical assistance: Assists network centers in promoting growth in programs and services, develops new centers, and provides training and consultation to professionals and volunteers. Offers workshops and consultations in areas including fundraising, community-based support, program planning, and ministry by and for older adults.
Publications: Informational brochure, Internet Home Page with extensive information about the organization; individual centers; and programs, activities, and services.

1136
The Retired Officers Association
(also known as TROA)
201 North Washington St.
Alexandria, VA 22314-2539 (703)549-2311
Additional tel.: (800)245-8762

Purpose and activities: Dedicated to maintaining a strong national defense and to preserving the earned entitlements and benefits of members of the uniformed services and their families, with 428 chapters in the U.S. and abroad. Activities and services include legislative action regarding retired and active uniformed services personnel; retirement information, advice and assistance; dependent educational assistance; and survivor assistance.
Geographic focus: Active internationally.
Publications: "The Retired Officer Magazine" (monthly publication). Booklets include "Help Your Widow," "Reserve Retirement Benefits," "SBP Made Easy," "Planning For Military Retirement," "Marketing Yourself for a Second Career," and "To Your Good Health" (free to members). Write for publications list or go to our web page, http://www.troa.org.

PROFESSIONAL AND SERVICE ORGANIZATIONS

1137
American Association for Adult and Continuing Education
(also known as AAACE)
1200 19th St. N.W., Suite 300
Washington, DC 20036-2422 (202)429-5131
FAX: (202)223-4579
Contact: Dr. Drew Allbritten, Exec. Dir.

Purpose and activities: Promotes the growth of and provides support for the field of adult and continuing education. Maintains a program unit, Aging issues.
Publications: Publications available, write for details.

1138
American Bar Association Commission on Legal Problems of the Elderly
740 15th St., N.W., 8th Fl.
Washington, DC 20005-1009 (202)662-8690
FAX: (202)662-1032;
E-mail: abaelderly@attmail.com
Contact: Nancy Coleman, Staff Dir.

Established in 1978.
Purpose and activities: Established by the ABA to examine the law-related concerns of older persons in the U.S. Goal is to encourage and improve the delivery of legal services to the elderly particularly through involvement of the private bar, and to explore legal issues surrounding long-term care, home care, guardianship, home equity conversion, surrogate decision-making, and Social Security due process. Serves as a resource for state and local bar

associations, state and area agencies on aging, legal sevices programs, law firms, corporate law departments, law schools and others interested in the legal problems of the elderly. The following projects are currently in progress and will result in specific products: 1) state courts involvement in elder abuse cases; 2) mediation of bioethical disputes in nursing homes; 3) legal/liability questions in the use of independent contractors for the provision of home care to the elderly and persons with disabilities; and 4) making juries accessible to the elderly and persons with disabilities.
Technical assistance: Provides information and guidance in emerging areas of law and seeks to generate pro bono, reduced-fee, and community education programs for senior citizens, as well as relevant continuing education programs for attorneys. Acts as a clearinghouse for private bar activities to assist the elderly, and seeks to implement models which afford maximum cooperation among legal services projects, the private bar, and the Older Americans Act network of state and area agencies on aging.
Publications: "Bifocal," quarterly newsletter. "In Your Hands: The Tools for Preserving Personal Autonomy," community & professional education video narrated by the late Helen Hayes with epilogue by her son James MacArthur, that addresses legal aspects of planning for incapacity and emphasizes the autonomy enhancing value of legal planning tools. Over 800,000 copies of 1990 booklet, Health Care Power of Attorney-An Introduction and Sample Form. 1992 video package, "Downsizing in an Aging Workforce: The Law, the Limits and the Lessons," narrated by Harvard University professor Arthur Miller, targets business & industry leaders & senior through mid-level managers and introduces their obligations under the Age Discrimination in Employment Act. "Giving Something Back-Pro Bono for the Elderly," a joint video project of the Commission and AARP Legal Counsel for the Elderly, narrated by Vernon Jordan, emphasizes multiple benefits of pro bono service to older persons by law firms and attorneys. Court-Related needs of the Elderly and Persons with Disabilities: A Blueprint for the Future (91), includes recommendations for improving the judicial system's accessibility for the elderly & persons with disabilities. Guardianship of the Elderly: A Primer for Attorneys (91); Steps to Enhance Guardianship Monitoring (91); & Alternatives to Guardianship-Substantive Training Materials & Module for Professionals Working with the Elderly & Persons with Disabilities (92), are designed to assist professionals to serve best interests of their elderly clients. The Patient Self-Determination Act State Law Guide (91) is designed to help states develop statement of patient's rights to make medical treatment decisions in order to comply with the implementation of federal Act (PL 101-508). Opening the Courthouse Door: An ADA Guide for State Courts (92) explains compliance in the courthouse with public access provisions of Americans with Disabilities Act. Attorney's Guide to home Equity Conversion (92) compares federal and lender-insured mortgages, provides overview of issues to be addressed when considering a sale-leaseback or sale of remainder interest, and includes current information on income tax and government benefit issues. Targetting Disability needs: A Guide for Dispute Resolution Programs on the Americans with Disabilities Act (94) presents an overview ADA/ADR map, answers critical questions about ADA, describes range of disabilities, offers ideas on ways dispute resolution programs can overcome barriers and enhance access, gives practical tips for communicating with persons with disablilities and suggests useful community resources. Ethical Issues in Representing Older Clients (Fordham Law Review, Vol. LXII, No. 5, March 1994) a special issue that contains recommendations of two day conference, articles prepared in connection with the conference, and summaries of the efforts of working groups. Shape your Health Care Future with Health Care Advance Directives: produced jointly by the ABA Commission on Legal Problems of the Elderly, Legal Counsel for the Elderly and the American Medical Association - a revised edition of Health Care Power of Attorney Booklet (95). Recommendations for State Courts Handling Elder Abuse Cases: culminates a two-year project by the State Justice Institute and offers 29 recommendations to enhance the ability of the state courts' to handle cases involving elder abuse (96). Effective Counseling of Older Cleints the Attorney-Client Relationship: informs attorneys of best ways to accomadate older clients and focuses on attorney's ability to communicate clearly and sensitively with this often-neglected client population (95). Legal Issues and Resources: An introduction for Professionals Working with Older Persons or their Families-designed to assist non-legal staff of aging services programs to identify common legal problems and direct clients to appropriate legal assistance. (1996).

1139
American College of Health Care Administrators

325 South Patrick St.
Alexandria, VA 22314 (703)739-7900
FAX: (703)739-7901;
E-mail: achca@achca.usa.com
Contact: Richard L. Thorpe, Exec. Dir.

Established in 1962.
Purpose and activities: The association for professional administrators of long-term health care organizations and facilities, with membership over 6,500 in the U.S., Canada, and other countries. Furthers the profession of providing comprehensive medical, personal, and social services for persons who require various therapeutic, protective, and supervised environments and milieus in a long term care setting. Advances the general welfare through education, research, and the maintenance of standards of professional competence and achievement and a code of ethics. Additionally, advocates for the profession through coordinated action and communication.
Technical assistance: Administers the Professional Certification Program for Nursing Home Administrators and the Assisted Living Administrators Certificate Program.
Publications: Membership includes subscriptions to "The Journal of Long-Term Care Administration" (quarterly) and a newsletter, "The Long-Term Care Administrator" (8 times/year). A series of self-instruction programs, symposium proceedings, and cassette tapes of educational sessions and policy and procedure manuals are also available.

1140
American Dietetic Association

216 West Jackson Blvd., Suite 800
Chicago, IL 60606 (312)899-0040
FAX: (312)899-1979

Purpose and activities: Professional society of dieticians professionals who work in health care, business, and education. Dietitians are the leading resource anywhere there is a need for nutrition research, evaluation and education to promote health, prevent disease, and speed recovery from illness. ADA launched its Nutrition & Health Campaign for Older Americans in 1996.
Publications: A complete catalog of educational materials for professionals and consumers is available from ADA. For the consumer: Pass the Calories Please! A cookbook and problem-solving guide for people who need to eat more or gain weight; The Health Weigh: A Pratical Food Guide. The first half of this weight control booklet includes information diets, healthy weight charts, changing your habits, and ways to evaluate popular diets. The second half includes cooking tips, recipes, and a week of menu ideas. Skim the Fat: A Preatical and Up-to-Date Food Guide is available at bookstores. Building a lower-fat diet is explained with many pratical applications for shopping, label reading, cooking, and eating on the go. Explores the relationship between dietary fat and cancer, hypertension, diabetes, atherosclerosis, perpheral artery disease, and stroke, with an entire chapter dedicated to heart disease. For answers to your food and nutrition questions and for a referral to a registered detitian in your area, call the Consumer Nutrition Hot Line at (800)366-1655 weekdays, 9am-4pm Central.

1141
American Foundation for the Blind

(also known as AFB)
11 Penn Plaza, Suite 300
New York, NY 10001-2018 (212)502-7600
TDD: (212)502-7662
Contact: Carl Augusto, Exec. Dir.

Established in 1921.
Purpose and activities: AFB takes a national leadership role in developing public policy and legislation, public education about blindness and visual impairment, and serving as a leading information source about resources and services related to blindness and visual impairment. AFB's national headquarters is in New York City; Government Relations office in Washington, D.C., its National Braille Literacy Center in Atlanta, Georgia, and offices in San Francisco, Dallas, and Chicago. AFB also conducts, evaluates, and publishes social research on visual impairment and blindness, and records and duplicates approximately 400 Talking Book titles each year under contract with the Library of Congress. AFB convenes the Josephine L. Taylor Leadership Institute, the leading national policy-focused conference for the vision field.
Technical assistance: AFB's Aging Program: AFB's aging and vision loss specialists carry out public education and advocacy to expand the

availability of vision-related rehabilitation for older adults. Current activities include; A campaign, "We Help Those Who Don't See Well, Live Like Those Who Do." providing public service announcements with the message that vision loss does not have to mean the end of one's way of life. A consumer information packet is available on request from AFB's Information Center (800)232-5463. Development of a curriculum and video on aging and vision loss, designed for use in university gerontology programs and in-service training (National Institute on Disability and Rehabilition Research grant H133G30053). The team convenes the National Aging and Vision Network, a leading national resource on vision-related rehabilitation for older adults. The Network's goal is to increase the availability of responsive, high quality services for older adults who are visually impaired, through the health care system, the rehabilitation system, and the aging network. Provides members with regular policy updates and timely legislative alerts, and it serves as a vehicle for information exchange about program innovations; interagency collaboration, and funding strategies that expand access to services.
Publications: AFB News — a semi-annual newsletter; Current Projects and Activities; JLTLI Bullentin, and AFB annual report. AFB Press is the leading publisher of textbooks in the audiences, including professionals, people who are visually impaired and their families, and the general public. Titles in Aging include: Vision and Aging: Crossroads to Service Delivery; Prescriptions for Independence, Out of the Corner of my Eye. AFB Press also publishes the Journal of Visual Impairment & Blindness. The AFB Information Center and Migel Memorial Library serve as a centralized clearinghouse for dissemination of information about blindness and low vision including fact sheets, position papers and bibliographies of vision topics. Visit the AFB gopher and web site on the internet including the Resources on Aging section. URL: http://www.afb.org/afb; For more information about AFB's Aging Program and the National Aging and Vision Network please contact: Albert L. Orr, American Foundation for the Blind, 11 Penn Plaza, Suite 300, New York, NY 10001, Phone: (212)502-7634; FAX: (212)502-7773; E-mail: alorr@afb.org; Lorraine Lidoff, American Foundation for the Blind, 15 Mechanic St., No. 3, Provincetown, MA 02657, Phone and FAX: (508)487-5815; E-mail: lidoff@afb.org; Judy Scott (AFB Southwest) 260 Treadway Plaza, Exchange Park, Dallas, TX 75235, Phone: (214)352-7222; FAX: (214)352-3214; E-mail: afbdallas@atb.org.

1142
American Parkinson's Disease Association
1250 Hylan Blvd., Suite 4B
Staten Island, NY 10305 (800)223-2732

Purpose and activities: Provides support to families and patients coping with Parkinson's Disease. Funds medical research on this neurological disease.

1143
American Red Cross
430 17th St., N.W.
Washington, DC 20006 (202)737-8300

Purpose and activities: A humanitarian service organization which, guided by its Congressional Charter and the principles of the International Red Cross Movement, provides relief to victims of disasters, and helps people prevent, prepare for, and respond to emergencies. The American Red Cross provides its services through a network of 1400 chapters, 1.4 million volunteers, and 32,000 paid staff. Its services to the elderly include transportation nutrition, telephone reassurance and friendly visits to the homebound, personal emergency response systems, meals, social events, and opportunities for volunteer involvement. In addition, the elderly benefit from the Red Cross nursing, health, safety, blood, and disaster services, as well as its volunteer services in hospitals and nursing homes.
Technical assistance: The Red Cross provides training courses, printed material, consultation and referral, and loan of personnel. It can best be accessed through its local chapters which in addition to Red Cross mandated services, offer service menus tailored specifically to their communities.

1144
Cancer Care, Inc.
1180 Ave. of the Americas
New York, NY 10036 (212)302-2400
FAX: (212)719-0263; E-Mail: Cancercare@aol.com
Contact: Diane Blum, A.C.S.W., Exec. Dir.

Established in 1944.
Purpose and activities: A nonprofit organization founded to help people with cancer and their families cope with the impact of cancer. Through professional one-to-one counseling, specialized support groups, educational programs, and telephone and internet contact, Cancer Care provides support, guidance, information and referrals, all free of charge. Cancer Care also offers financial assistance for treatment-related costs on a restricted basis. Sponsors groups, educational, and public information programs to help older adults deal with cancer. Cancer Care, Inc. is separate and apart from any other organization.
Geographic focus: National programs provided from twelve offices in NY, NJ, and CT, through a national toll-free counseling line, and through the internet.
Funding activities: Financial support to cancer patients on a restricted basis to help pay for treatment-related costs.

1145
Concerned Relatives of Nursing Home Patients
P.O. Box 18820
Cleveland Heights, OH 44118 (216)321-0403
Contact: Mary Adelaide Mendelson, Exec. Dir.

Purpose and activities: Support group for those who have had, currently have, or will soon have a family member in a nursing home.

1146
Corporation for National Service
1100 Vermont Ave., N.W.
Washington, DC 20525 (202)606-4851
FAX: (202)565-2794

Purpose and activities: Administers the following locally directed but federally legislated grant programs: Foster Grandparent Program, Retired Senior Volunteer Program (RSVP), and the Senior Companion Program.

1147
Loyal Order of Moose
Supreme Lodge Bldg.
Mooseheart, IL 60539 (708)859-2000
Contact: Frank A. Sarnecki, Dir. General

Purpose and activities: An international family fraternal organization which provides social and philanthropic programs for its 1.8 million members in 4,000 lodges and chapters. Owns and operates a self-contained model retirement community, Moosehaven, in Orange Park, FL, that exists for members in need of this care. The community has a capacity of 550, including a health care facility for 160 individuals, and residence eligibility is restricted to members of the Order continuously for 15 years immediately preceding application.
Geographic focus: Active in the U.S., Canada, Bermuda, and Great Britain.
Publications: Informational brochure. Write to the Public Relations Department for additional information.

1148
National Association for Continence
(also known as NAFC)
P.O. Box 8310
Spartanburg, SC 29305 (864)579-7900
FAX: (864)579-7902

Purpose and activities: Works to educate the general public and health professionals about the prevalence, diagnosis, and treatment of urinary incontinence.
Publications: Publishes a quarterly newsletter. Also have various leaflets about incontinence.

1149
National Association of Life Underwriters
(also known as NALU)
1922 F St., N.W.
Washington, DC 20006-4387 (202)331-6000
Contact: William Regan, Exec. V.P.

Established in 1890.
Purpose and activities: This professional organization is a federation whose members are 1,000 state and local associations. The 140,000 members of the local associations are professionals who sell life and health insurance and other related financial products. Objectives include contributing to national and community well-being through organized programs of public service and political involvement.

Funding activities: Local associations sponsor fundraising campaigns for the Red Cross, United Fund, Heart Association, and Cancer Society. Supports public education efforts on blood donor needs, home and highway safety, human organ transplant donor solicitation, activities for the aging, and Medic-Alert. Emphasis is on local community service programs, with some assistance to national projects such as the Medic-Alert Foundation. Also sponsors the Senior Citizens Health Insurance Counseling (SCHIC) Program.
Technical assistance: Provided through NALU's Community Service Program which prepares and distributes project resource material that affiliated members need to implement community service projects. Printed material and consultation, available to both members and nonmembers, exists in the areas of health, support and protective services, and volunteer programs.

1150
National Governors' Association

444 North Capitol St., Suite 267
Washington, DC 20001-1572 (202)624-5300
FAX: (202)624-5825
Contact: Raymond C. Scheppach, Exec. Dir.

Established in 1908.
Purpose and activities: A national organization of the governors of the 50 states and the five territories. Assists the nation's governors to influence collectively the development and implementation of national policy and to apply creative leadership to state problems.
Technical assistance: Serves as a vehicle for sharing the knowledge of innovative programs among the states and provides technical assistance and consultant services to governors on management and policy issues.
Publications: Informational brochure, newsletter. Numerous health policy studies include: "Strategies for Improving State Perinatal Programs," a seven-part series, and "State Long-Term Care Reform: Development of Community Care Systems in Six States." Write for publication list.

1151
National Institute on Aging

Public Information Office
Bldg. 31, Rm. 5C27, 31 Center Dr., MSC 2292
Bethesda, MD 20892-2292 (301)496-1752

Purpose and activities: As part of the National Institutes of Health, the National Institute on Aging is the federal government's principal agency for conducting and supporting biomedical research, social and behavioral research related to the aging process, and the diseases and special problems of older individuals.

1152
National Society to Prevent Blindness

(also known as NSPB)
500 East Remington Rd.
Schaumberg, IL 60173 (800)331-2020

Purpose and activities: National Society to Prevent Blindness (dba Prevent Blindness America) is a national voluntary health organization dedicated to eliminating preventable causes of vision loss and blindness through comprehensive programs of public and professional education and information, community services, and research.

1153
National Women's Health Network

514 10th St., N.W., Suite 400
Washington, DC 20004 (202)347-1140
FAX: (202)347-1168

Purpose and activities: To ensure that women have access to quality, affordable health care. Also serves as an information clearinghouse on women's health issues.

1154
Self-Help for Hard of Hearing People, Inc.

(also known as SHHH)
7910 Woodmont Ave., Suite 1200
Bethesda, MD 20812

Purpose and activities: An international nonprofit volunteer educational organization for hard of hearing people, their relatives and friends. SHHH is devoted to the interests of those who cannot hear well but who are committed to participating in the heaing world.

1155
The American Speech - Language - Hearing Association

(also known as ASHA)
10801 Rockville Pike
Rockville, MD 20852 (301)897-5700
Contact: Dr. Frederick T. Spahr, Exec. Dir.

Purpose and activities: A scientific organization of 83,994 professional members in the field of human communication. Conducts national projects in the field of aging. Encourages basic scientific study of the processes of individual human communication, with special reference to speech, hearing, and language. Promotes investigation of disorders of human communication, fosters improvement of clinical procedures with such disorders, and stimulates exchange of information among persons and organizations thus engaged, disseminating such information.

Funding activities: Support for conferences, staff development, publications, and research and demonstration projects.
Technical assistance: Provided by staff to members and nonmembers through printed material and consultation in the areas of education, training and health.

1156
U.S. Senate Special Committee on Aging

SD-G31
Washington, DC 20510 (202)224-5364
FAX: (202)224-8660
Contact: Senator William S. Cohen, Chair.

Purpose and activities: Provides Congressional oversight of all programs providing services for older Americans. Not a legislative committee but acts as a resource to other Senate committees, members, and the nation. Conducts hearings and provides written information on pertinent current issues.
Publications: Offers numerous publications on issues affecting the aging, including employment, retirement, housing and health care.

1157
United Seniors Health Cooperative

1331 H St., N.W., Suite 500
Washington, DC 20005-4706 (202)393-6222
FAX: (202)783-0588

Purpose and activities: United Seniors Health Cooperative (USHC) is a nonprofit independent consumer organization. For the past decade it has been at the vanguard of helping older adults achieve health, independence, and financial security.
Publications: Eldergames; Home Care for Older People: A Consumer's Guide; Long-Term Care: A Dollar and Sense Guide; Long-Term Care Insurance: A Professional's Guide to Selecting Policies; Managing your Health Care Finances; United Seniors Health Report Newsletter. Forthcoming publications include: The Dictionary of Eldercare Terminology and the Elder Care Primer Series.

1158
The National Academy on Aging

1275 K St. N.W., Suite 350
Washington, DC 20005 (202)408-3375
FAX: (202)842-1150
Contact: Robert B. Friedland, Ph.D., Director

Established in 1994.
Purpose and activities: The National Academy on Aging was originally established in October 1994 through a cooperative agreement between the Gerontological Society of America and the United States Administration on Aging. By serving as a national forum for policy analysis and debate, the Academy seeks to encourage innovative and

responsible thinking on critical aging policy issues. Such issues include health care, long-term care, and income security in an intergenerational context. The Academy explores a number of areas, including the needs of older persons and their families, the appropriate balance between risk and security in preparing for those needs, and how public and private institutions might respond to the aging of our society, the balance between community, state, and federal authority, and the implications for public policy and programs; the values underlying our views about aging and the responsibility of individuals, families, employers, and government; and changes in the delivery of health and long-term care and the implications for financing of appropriate care. The Academy is governed by a steering committee, and assisted by panels of expert advisors. In addition to The Department of Health and Human Services, funding is provided by donations and grants from private foundations.

APPENDIX

STATE GOVERNMENT AGENCIES

While the vast majority of funds for aging projects comes from Federal sources, state and local agencies are intimately involved with the grants process. For reasons of cost efficiency, convenience, and political expediency, local agencies often administer programs rather than increasing the federal administrative network. This arrangement highlights the political mood of "cooperative Federalism." By such an arrangement, each level of government functions to maximize the allocation of resources and the monitoring of operations and results.

In this section, state agencies are listed that offer assistance for projects and programs related to the aged. The grants seeker should contact the appropriate state agency for the most recent data on the status of listed or planned programs, as well as be aware of the state's priorities for the aged, such as housing, health, transportation, etc.

ALABAMA

State of Alabama, Commission on Aging

Ms. Martha Murph Beck, Exec. Dir.
RSA Plaza
770 Washington Ave., Suite 470
Montgomery, AL 36130 (334)242-5743

ALASKA

State of Alaska, Alaska Commission on Aging

P.O. Box C
Juneau, AK 99811 (907)465-3250

AMERICAN SAMOA

American Samoa, Territorial Administration on Aging

John E. Suisala, Dir.
Pago Pago, AS 96799 (684)633-1251

ARIZONA

State of Arizona, Aging and Adult Administration

1789 West Jefferson, 2SW, 950A
Phoenix, AZ 85007 (602)542-4446

ARKANSAS

State of Arkansas, Department of Human Services, Division of Aging and Adult Services

P.O. Box 1437, Slot 1412
Little Rock, AR 72203-1437 (501)682-2441

CALIFORNIA

ADULT DAY HEALTH CARE BRANCH

State of California, Department of Aging

1600 K St.
Sacramento, CA 95814 (916)445-4600

MULTIPURPOSE SENIOR SERVICES PROGRAM

State of California, Department of Aging

1600 K St.
Sacramento, CA 95814 (916)322-7200

PREVENTIVE HEALTH CARE FOR THE AGING PROGRAMS

State of California, Department of Health and Welfare Agency

P.O. Box 942732
Sacramento, CA 94234-7320 (916)324-2281

COLORADO

State of Colorado, Department of Social Services, Aging and Adult Services

110 16th St., 2nd Fl.
Denver, CO 80203-1714 (303)620-4147

CONNECTICUT

ELDERLY SERVICES DIVISION

State of Connecticut, Department of Social Services

Christine M. Lewis, Dept. of Social Services
25 Sigourney St.
Hartford, CT 06106 (860)424-5274

DELAWARE

Delaware Health and Social Services, Division of Services for Aging and Adults with Physical Disabilities

1901 North Dupont Hwy.
Administration Bldg. Annex
New Castle, DE 19720 (302)577-4791

DISTRICT OF COLUMBIA

District of Columbia, Office on Aging

One Judiciary Sq.
441 4th St., N.W.
Suite 900
Washington, DC 20001 (202)724-5622

FLORIDA

ADULT PROTECTIVE SERVICES

State of Florida, Department of Health and Rehabilitative Services (HRS)

1317 Winewood Blvd.
Bldg. 5, Rm. 200
Tallahassee, FL 32399-0700

State of Florida, Department of Elder Affairs

4040 Esplanade Way
Suite 215
Tallahassee, FL 32399-7000

GEORGIA

State of Georgia, Department of Human Resources, Division of Aging Services

Two Peachtree St., N.W.
Suite 18-403
Atlanta, GA 30303-3176 (404)657-5258

Other State agencies providing direct services to the elderly

Georgia Department of Human Resources
Public Health Division
Two Peachtree St., N.W., 7th Fl.
Atlanta, GA 30303-3176 (404)657-2700

Rehabilitative Services Division
Two Peachtree St., N.W., 23rd Fl.
Atlanta, GA 30303-3176 (404)657-3000

Family and Children Services
Two Peachtree St., N.W., 16th Fl.
Atlanta, GA 30303-3176 (404)657-5180

Mental Health, Mental Retardation, & Substance Abuse
Two Peachtree St., N.W., 4th Fl.
Atlanta, GA 30303-3176 (404)657-2260

GUAM

Government of Guam, Department of Public Health and Social Services, Division of Senior Services

P.O. Box 2816
Agana, GU 96910

IDAHO

State of Idaho, Commission on Aging

State House, Rm. 108
Boise, ID 83720 (208)334-3033

ILLINOIS

State of Illinois, Department on Aging

421 East Capitol Ave., No. 100
Springfield, IL 62701-1789 (217)785-3356

Other agencies in Illinois that provide services to seniors

Attorney General's Office
Protection from Consumer Fraud
Chicago (800)243-5377
Springfield: (800)252-2518

County Supervisor of Assessments
Homestead Exemption
Contact county tax assessor's office or county supervisor of assessment

Department of Commerce & Community Affairs (DCCA)
Energy and Weatherization Assistance and Tourism
(800)252-8643

Department of Insurance (Complaints and information about insurance companies)
320 West Washington
Springfield, IL 62767
Senior Health Insurance Program (SHIP):
(800)548-9043
Chicago (312)814-2420
Springfield: (217)782-4515

Department of Public Aid
Food Stamps, medical assistance, financial assistance, SSI
(217)782-3458
(800)252-4343 Toll-free within IL

Regulates nursing homes, operates a nursing home complaint hotline
(217)785-0321
(800)252-4343 Toll-free in IL only

Department of Rehabilitation Services
Client Assistance Program (CAP)
100 North 1st St., 1st Fl. West
Springfield, IL 62702-5197 (800)641-3929
Toll-free in IL only

(800)275-3677

Department of Revenue
Circuit Breaker Tax Relief and Pharmaceutical Assistance Program
(800)624-2459
TDD: (800)544-5304

Local Social Security Offices
Medicare and Social Security benefit information
(800)772-1213

Secretary of State's Office
Photo I.D.'s, Driving Courses, and Veteran's Services
(800)252-2904

INDIANA

BUREAU OF AGING AND IN-HOME SERVICES

State of Indiana, Family and Social Services Administration, Division of Disability, Aging and Rehabilitative Services

402 West Washington St.
P.O. Box 7083
Indianapolis, IN 46207-7083 (317)232-7020

IOWA

State of Iowa, Department of Elder Affairs

914 Grand Ave., Suite 236
Des Moines, IA 50319 (515)281-5187

KANSAS

State of Kansas, Department on Aging

Docking State Office Bldg.
915 S.W. Harrison, No. 150-S
Topeka, KS 66612 (913)296-4986

KENTUCKY

Cabinet for Families and Children, Department for Social Services/Division of Aging Services

275 East Main St.
Frankfort, KY 40621 (502)564-6930

LOUISIANA

State of Louisiana, Governor's Office of Elderly Affairs

P.O. Box 80374
Baton Rouge, LA 70898-0374 (504)925-1700

Names of other state agencies that provide direct services to the elderly are:

Department of Health and Hospitals
Office of Mental Health
P.O. Box 4049, Bin 12
Baton Rouge, LA 70821-4049

Department of Social Services
Office of Community Services
P.O. Box 3318
Baton Rouge, LA 70821

MAINE

The Bureau of Elder and Adult Services

Department of Human Services
State House
Station No. 11
Augusta, ME 04333-0011 (207)624-5335

MARYLAND

State of Maryland, Office on Aging

State Office Building, Room 1007
301 West Preston Street
Baltimore, MD 21201 (410)767-1100

MASSACHUSETTS

The Executive Office of Elder Affairs

One Ashburton Place
Boston, MA 02108 (617)727-7750

MICHIGAN

State of Michigan, Office of Services to the Aging

P.O. Box 30026
Lansing, MI 48909 (517)373-8230

MINNESOTA

Minnesota Board on Aging

Human Services Bldg.
444 Lafayette Rd.
St. Paul, MN 55155-3843 (612)296-2770

MISSISSIPPI

AGING PROGRAMS FOR ELDER CITIZENS

State of Mississippi, Department of Human Services, Division of Aging and Adult Services

750 North State St.
Jackson, MS 39202 (601)359-4929

MISSOURI

State of Missouri, Division on Aging

615 Howerton Court
P.O. Box 1337
Jefferson City, MO 65102 (314)751-3082

MONTANA

State of Montana, Office on Aging, Senior and Long Term Care Division, Department of Public Health and Human Services

P.O. Box 4210
Helena, MT 59604 (406)444-4077

NEBRASKA

State of Nebraska, Department on Aging

P.O. Box 95044
301 Centennial Mall South
Lincoln, NE 68509-5044 (402)471-2306

There are several departments that provide direct service to the elderly as a part of a more general program (in terms of age) such as:

Department of Health & Human Services (HHS)
P.O. Box 95007
Lincoln, NE 68509-5007

Department of HHS Finance & Support
P.O. Box 95026
Lincoln, NE 68509-5206

Department of HHS Regulation & Licensure
P.O. Box 94728
Lincoln, NE 68509-4728

NEVADA

State of Nevada, Division for Aging Services

340 North 11th St., Suite 203
Las Vegas, NV 89101 (702)486-3545

NEW HAMPSHIRE

State of New Hampshire, Department of Health and Human Services, Division of Elderly and Adult Services

115 Pleasant St., Annex No. 1
Concord, NH 03301-3843 (603)271-4394

NEW JERSEY

CONGREGATE SERVICES PROGRAM

New Jersey Department of Health and Senior Services

CN 807
Trenton, NJ 08625-0807 (609)292-1876

FEDERAL AID TO COUNTY OFFICES ON AGING

New Jersey Department of Health and Senior Services, Division of Senior Affairs

CN 807
Trenton, NJ 08625-0807 (609)292-6193

LEGAL SERVICE DEVELOPMENT FOR THE ELDERLY

New Jersey Department of Health and Senior Services, Division of Senior Affairs Elder Rights Unit

CN 807
Trenton, NJ 08625

NUTRITION (CONGREGATE AND HOME DELIVERED MEALS)

New Jersey Department of Health and Senior Services, Division of Senior Affairs

CN 807
Trenton, NJ 08625 (609)292-6192

OMBUDSMAN FOR THE INSTITUTIONALIZED ELDERLY

New Jersey Department of Health and Senior Services

Office of the Ombudsman for the Institutionalized Elderly
101 South Broad St.
CN 807
Trenton, NJ 08625-0807 (609)292-8016

SENIOR COMMUNITY SERVICES EMPLOYMENT

New Jersey Department of Health and Senior Services, Division of Senior Affairs

CN 807
Trenton, NJ 08625-0807 (609)292-6193

STATE AID TO COUNTY OFFICES ON AGING

New Jersey Department of Health and Senior Services

CN 807
Trenton, NJ 08625-0807 (609)292-6193

TECHNICAL ASSISTANCE TO PROGRAMS ON AGING

New Jersey Department of Health and Senior Services, Division of Senior Affairs

CN 807
Trenton, NJ 08625 (609)292-6193

NEW MEXICO

New Mexico State Agency on Aging

228 East Palace Ave., Ground Fl.
Santa Fe, NM 87501 (505)827-7640

NEW YORK

New York State Office for the Aging

Two Empire State Plaza
Albany, NY 12223-1251 (800)342-9871

NORTH CAROLINA

State of North Carolina, Department of Human Resources, Division of Aging

693 Palmer Dr.
Caller Box 29531
Raleigh, NC 27626-0531

NORTH DAKOTA

State of North Dakota, Department of Human Services, Aging Services Division

600 South 2nd St., Suite 1C
Bismarck, ND 58504-5729 (701)328-8910

OHIO

State of Ohio, Department of Aging

50 West Broad St., 9th Fl.
Columbus, OH 43266-0501 (614)466-5500

OKLAHOMA

State of Oklahoma, Department of Human Services, Aging Services Division

312 N.E. 28th St.
Oklahoma City, OK 73105

OREGON

State of Oregon, Department of Human Resources, Senior Services Division

500 Summer St., N.E.
Salem, OR 97310 (503)945-5811

PENNSYLVANIA

Pennsylvania Department of Aging

400 Market St.
Harrisburg, PA 17101 (717)783-1549

PUERTO RICO

Governor's Office of Elderly Affairs

P.O. Box 50063
Old San Juan Station
San Juan, PR 00902 (787)721-6121

RHODE ISLAND

State of Rhode Island, Department of Elderly Affairs

160 Pine St.
Providence, RI 02903-3708 (401)277-2858

SOUTH CAROLINA

State of South Carolina, Governor's Office, Division on Aging

202 Arbor Lake Dr., Suite 301
Columbia, SC 29223 (803)737-7500

SOUTH DAKOTA

State of South Dakota, Department of Social Services, Office of Adult Services and Aging

Kneip Bldg.
700 Governors Dr.
Pierre, SD 57501 (605)773-3656

TENNESSEE

Tennessee Commission on Aging

500 Deaderick St., 9th Fl.
Nashville, TN 37243-0860 (615)741-2056

Area Offices on Aging

Dir.
First Tennessee Development District
207 North Boone St.
Johnson City, TN 37601

Dir.
East Tennessee HRA
408 North Cedar Bluff Rd., Suite 150
Knoxville, TN 37923

Dir.
Southeast Tennessee Development District
25 Cherokee Blvd.
P.O. Box 4757
Chattanooga, TN 37405

Dir.
Upper Cumberland Development District
1225 Burgess Falls Rd.
Cookeville, TN 38501

Dir.
Greater Nashville Region Council
700 Stahlman Bldg., Box 233
211 Union St.
Nashville, TN 37201

Dir.
South Central Development District
P.O. Box 1346
815 South Main
Columbia, TN 38401

Dir.
Northwest Tennessee Development District
P.O. Box 963
Martin, TN 38237

Dir.
Southwest Tennessee Developmental District
27 Conrad Dr., Suite 150
Jackson, TN 38301

Dir.
Delta Area
125 Mid-America Mall
Penthouse
Memphis, TN 38103-2084

TEXAS

Texas Department on Aging

P.O. Box 12786
Austin, TX 78711 (512)424-6840

TRUST TERRITORY OF THE PACIFIC ISLANDS

Trust Territory of the Pacific Islands, Division of Aging

Office of Grants Management
Government of the Trust Territory of the Pacific Islands
Saipan, CM 96950

Northern Mariana Islands, Department of Community and Cultural Affairs, Office on Aging

Civic Center - Susupe
Saipan, CM 96960

UTAH

State of Utah, Division of Aging and Adult Services

120 North 200 West
Salt Lake City, UT 84103 (801)538-3910

VERMONT

State of Vermont, Department of Aging and Disabilities

103 South Main St.
Waterbury, VT 05671-2301 (802)241-2400

VIRGIN ISLANDS

DIVISION OF SENIOR CITIZENS AFFAIRS

Government of the Virgin Islands of the United States, Department of Human Services

No. 19 Estate Diamond, Frederiksted
St. Croix, VI 00840 (809)692-5950

VIRGINIA

THE AGING NETWORK

Virginia Department for the Aging

700 East Franklin St., 10th Fl.
Richmond, VA 23219-2327 (804)225-2271

WASHINGTON

WASHINGTON STATE SENIOR CITIZENS SERVICES ACT

State of Washington, Department of Social and Health Services, Aging and Adult Services Administration

P.O. Box 45600
Olympia, WA 98504-5600 (800)422-3263

State of Washington, Department of Social and Health Services, Aging and Adult Services Administration

P.O. Box 45600
Olympia, WA 98504-5600 (206)493-2549

WEST VIRGINIA

West Virginia Office of Aging, Commission on Aging

1900 Kanawha Blvd., East
Holly Grove Bldg. 10
Charleston, WV 25305-0160 (304)558-3317

WISCONSIN

State of Wisconsin, Bureau on Aging

Department of Health and Family Services
Division of Supportive Living
One West Wilson St.
P.O. Box 7851
Madison, WI 53707-7851 (608)266-2536

WYOMING

Wyoming Division on Aging

Deborah Fleming, Administrator
Hathaway Bldg., Suite 139
Cheyenne, WY 82002-0480 (307)777-7986

INDEX

INDEX